Diseases
of Cage and Aviary
Birds

Margaret L. Petrak, V.M.D., Editor

Staff Member Angell Memorial Animal Hospital
Boston, Massachusetts

315 Illustrations—12 in Color

LEA & FEBIGER · PHILADELPHIA

1969

SBN 8121-0187-1

All Rights Reserved

Copyright © 1969 Lea & Febiger

Library of Congress Catalog Card Number 68:18856

PRINTED IN THE UNITED STATES OF AMERICA

Preface

In early 1963, Mr. Theodore Phillips, then on the editorial staff at Lea and Febiger, asked me to edit a book on diseases of cage birds. The interest in the subject shown by veterinarians throughout the United States and his own knowledge of veterinary literature had convinced him of the need for such a book. My developing concern in both medical and surgical treatment of cage birds and my frustration at the unavailability of pertinent literature influenced my decision to acquiesce. A table of contents was formulated, the project was approved, and work was begun. Mr. Phillips sought constructive criticism from veterinarians, ornithologists, nutritionists, and zoologists, and selected the majority of the American contributors.

We received some early criticism for presuming to write a book on a field of medicine still in its infancy. However, in the five years since the book's conception all criticism has disappeared, to be replaced by encouragement and, gratifyingly, by impatience for publication of the work.

The book is directed primarily toward the clinician and the student. To the clinician as a reference book, to the student as a text, and to both with the hope of stimulating interest in the care of cage birds. Others who will find this text to be of use in their professions include research workers, zoologists, and aviculturists.

Because the treatment of cage birds has not generally been taught in veterinary schools it was decided to make the book as broadly informative as possible. Hence the non-clinical chapters dealing with identification and general information on the more common species of cage birds, their behavior, care and management, and nutrition were included. Information on anatomy, physiology, and genetics provided in texts on poultry is not completely applicable to cage birds. Therefore chapters have been included on these subjects as well. In particular, the Chapter on the Anatomy of the Budgerigar by Howard Evans represents a totally original contribution.

Being a compilation of the work of many people, the book necessarily varies in style and in some instances is repetitive. An effort was made to allow each author's individuality to be evident. Since this is a first endeavor, the reader will find deficiencies, but it is hoped that these will stimulate further research in the field and subsequent publications.

I wish to express my gratitude to all of the contributors for their willingness to take time from their busy lives to help make this a volume of merit; to Bill Dilger for his help and encouragement, especially in the initial stages of development; Leslie Arnall for his help in the selection of British authors and for his generous contribution of a chapter at the eleventh hour; David Blackmore for graciously responding to my numerous questions and requests; Ted Phillips for his early assistance and continuing inspiration; Ken Bussy for his editorial capabilities and vision; Emily Anderson for her fine editorial assistance; Jean Husted for her remarkable researching, questioning, and editing abilities; and Helen Hickey for her secretarial work and for aiding me in maintaining enthusiasm over five long years.

Boston, Massachusetts   Margaret L. Petrak

Contributors

IRVING E. ALTMAN, D.V.M.
Brooklyn, New York

ROBERT B. ALTMAN, D.V.M.
Codirector, A & A Veterinary Hospital,
and Long Island Pet Hospital
Brooklyn, New York

LESLIE ARNALL, B.V.Sc., M.R.C.V.S.
"Mayfields," 83 Lacey Green
Wilmslow, Cheshire, England

PAUL ARNSTEIN, D.V.M., M.P.H.
U.S. Department of Health, Education, and Welfare,
Public Health Service, Communicable Disease Center, at the
George William Hooper Foundation
University of California, San Francisco Medical Center
San Francisco, California

DAVID K. BLACKMORE, B.Sc., Ph.D., F.R.C.V.S.
Laboratory Animals Centre,
Medical Research Council Laboratories
Carshalton, England

PAUL A. BUCKLEY, Ph.D.
Assistant Professor of Biology,
Department of Biology
Hofstra University
Hempstead, Long Island, New York

JOHN P. CAVILL, M.R.C.V.S.
The Veterinary Investigation Officer
Woodthorne, Wolverhampton
Staffordshire, England

WILLIAM C. DILGER, Ph.D.
Associate Professor of Ethology and
Assistant Director of Research,
Laboratory of Ornithology
Cornell University
Ithaca, New York

HOWARD E. EVANS, Ph.D.
Professor of Veterinary Anatomy,
New York State Veterinary College
Cornell University
Ithaca, New York

DONALD S. FARNER, Ph.D.
Professor of Zoophysiology and
Chairman, Department of Zoology
University of Washington
Seattle, Washington

R. N. T-W-FIENNES, M.A., M.R.C.V.S.
Head of Department of Pathology,
Nuffield Institute of Comparative Medicine
Regent's Park, London, England

CHARLES P. GANDAL, D.V.M.
Veterinarian, The New York Zoological Society
New York, New York

CHARLEY E. GILMORE, D.V.M.
Pathologist, Angell Memorial Animal Hospital
Instructor in Pathology, Harvard Medical School
Research Associate in Pathology,
Massachusetts Institute of Technology
Boston, Massachusetts

DR. JENS HASHOLT
Small Animal Clinic,
Royal Veterinary College
Copenhagen, Denmark

CARLTON M. HERMAN, Sc.D.
Chief, Section of Wildlife Disease and Parasite Studies
Patuxent Wildlife Research Center
Laurel, Maryland

I. F. KEYMER, M.R.C.V.S., Ph.D.
Department of Pathology,
The Zoological Society of London
Regent's Park
London, England

JOHN LYNN LEONARD, D.V.M.
Instructor, Small Animal Surgery and Medicine,
School of Veterinary Medicine
Auburn University
Auburn, Alabama

KARL F. MEYER, M.D., D.V.M.
Director Emeritus, Hooper Foundation
Professor Emeritus of Experimental Pathology,
University of California
San Francisco Medical Center
San Francisco, California

LAWRENCE MINSKY, D.V.M.
San Gabriel, California

MARGARET L. PETRAK, V.M.D.
Staff Member,
Angell Memorial Animal Hospital
Boston, Massachusetts

ERWIN SMALL, D.V.M., M.S.
Professor, Veterinary Clinical Medicine
College of Veterinary Medicine, University of Illinois
Urbana, Illinois

ROBERT M. STONE, D.V.M.
Detroit, Michigan

DR. T. GEOFFREY TAYLOR
Department of Physiology and Biochemistry
The University
Reading, England

C. IVAR TOLLEFSON, Ph.D.
The R. T. French Company
Rochester, New York

MRS. KATHARINE TOTTENHAM
Bideford Zoo
Devon, England

Contents

Part I–Non-Clinical Aspects

Part II–Clinical Considerations

PART I

NON-CLINICAL ASPECTS

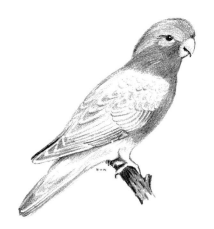

1

Common Types of Cage Birds

William C. Dilger

Approximately 8600 different species of birds exist in the world today, all placed in the Class Aves. Many hundreds of these species are kept by bird fanciers, some more or less commonly and others rarely. The species discussed in this Chapter are those that are most often encountered, and they are representative of the larger groups, other species of which are also quite popular.

CLASSIFICATION

The Class Aves is subdivided into about 27 Orders, 160 Families, and some 1800 Genera. All Order names end in "formes," and all Family names end in "idae." The names of Orders, Families, and Genera are always capitalized; in addition, genus and species names are always italicized.* One or more subpopulations, called subspecies, have been recognized in some species, resulting in a third word in the full scientific name. For example, *Turdus migratorius achrusterus* (the southern robin).

Other subdivisions are sometimes recognized, such as Subclasses, Superorders, Suborders, Tribes, and Subfamilies. These categories represent attempts at expressing relationships even more exactly, but such subdivisions need not concern us here.

*For example, the canary is in the Order Passeriformes (perching birds), Family Fringillidae (including certain finches, sparrows, buntings, cardinals, and serins), and the Genus *Serinus* (serins), the full name being *Serinus canarius.*

REPRESENTATIVE CAGE BIRDS
Order: Psittaciformes

Family: Psittacidae (including parrots, cockatoos, parakeets, macaws, lorikeets, and similar birds)

BUDGERIGAR (MELOPSITTACUS UNDULATUS)

This bird, a native of the drier portions of Australia, is easily the most popular parakeet* kept as a pet. Budgerigars, which are also called budgies, parakeets, shell parakeets, and undulating grass parakeets, are slender, long-tailed birds about 7½ inches long. The wild type is green with barrings of darker color on the back and wings, and finer barrings on the crown, nape, and cheeks. The forehead is clear yellow, as is the "bib." The central tail feathers are blue, the others being patterned in yellow, green, and black. At the lower margin of the bib are a few round black spots. A bluish streak extends backward from near the corner of the mouth. Male and female birds look alike, except that the bare thick skin adjoining the forehead at the base of the upper mandible (known as the cere) is blue in males and brownish or pinkish in females. The feet of males are bluish grey, whereas those of females are pink-hued. Immature birds are difficult to sex, as the cere is always pinkish brown. However, the nostrils of immature females tend to be rimmed with white. Immature birds have the forehead finely barred, which should be remembered when one is purchasing a bird.

---

*The term "parakeet" generally applies to a long-tailed, slender bird belonging to the Family Psittacidae, occurring in Central and South America, Africa, Asia, Australia, and many islands of these areas. One species, *Conuropsis carolinensis*, or Carolina parakeet, once lived in the southern United States but is now extinct.

During the process of domestication of these birds, a number of color varieties have become established—white, yellow, blue, and various shades of green.

Budgerigars are extremely easy to breed, but not as solitary pairs. They are highly social in their breeding in the wild, and at least three pairs must be present within sight and sound of each other in order for breeding to occur. Since this species is domesticated, they do not need large breeding cages. Standard breeding cages and nest boxes are available commercially.

Budgerigars are not particularly messy, although, like most other seed-eaters, they do scatter seed hulls around. Their droppings are small and dry.

Some budgerigars, particularly if acquired young, can learn to talk quite well, and a few develop astounding vocabularies. In training a young bird to talk it is best to keep it out of hearing distance of other birds of its kind and to patiently repeat over and over the word that is being taught. It is best to speak more slowly than normal, because the birds have a tendency to speed up words when they repeat them. As soon as one word is learned, teaching can begin on another. Contrary to popular opinion, there is no proved sex difference in ability of the birds to mimic. They can also be taught to perform various tricks, and will become extremely tame with careful handling.

LOVEBIRDS (AGAPORNIS SPP.)

These birds deserve to be more popular as cage birds than they are. The genus includes nine different forms, but one form, *Agapornis swinderniana* (Swindern's lovebird), is not known in captivity. Four kinds are usually available from animal suppliers in the United States. These are the peach-faced lovebird (*A. roseicollis*), black-masked lovebird (*A. personata*), blue-masked lovebird (mutant from *A. personata*), and

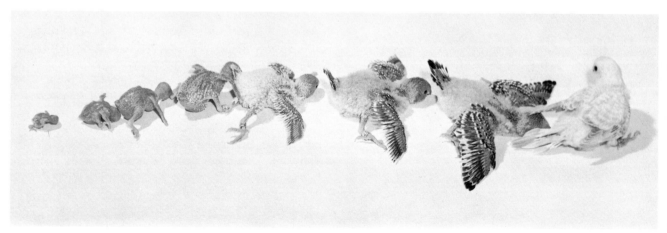

Fig. 1-1. *Budgerigar young at the age of 5 hours, 3 days, 6 days, 9 days, 12 days, 14 days, 16 days, and 21 days.* (*Photograph by George L. Wetzel. Courtesy of R. T. French Co.*)

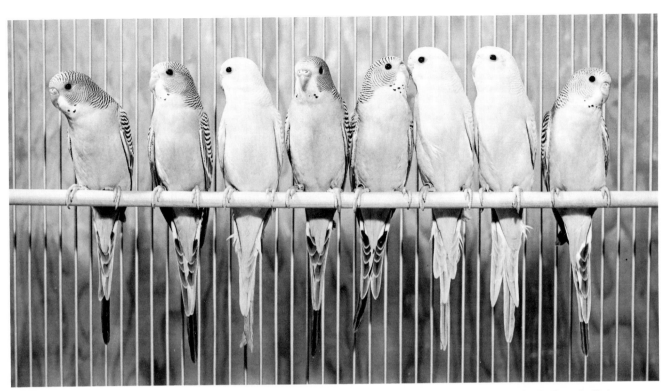

Fig. 1-2. *Budgerigars at the age of 9 weeks. (Photograph by George L. Wetzel. Courtesy of R. T. French Co.)*

Fischer's lovebird (*A. fischeri*). Occasionally the Nyassaland lovebird (*A. lilianae*) and the black-cheeked lovebird (*A. nigrigenis*) are available, especially in California. The red-faced lovebird (*A. pullaria*), the Madagascar, or grey-headed, lovebird (*A. cana*), and the Abyssinian lovebird (*A. taranta*) are practically unknown as cage birds in North America, because of the U.S. Public Health Service restrictions on the importation of parrots. The species that are available here are those for which breeding stocks happened to be available before the restrictions went into effect.

The peach-faced, black-masked, and Fischer's lovebirds are all small, short-tailed parrots, ranging from 6 to 7 inches long, and mainly green in color. The peach-faced lovebird is light green with a whitish bill, red forehead, peach-colored cheeks and throat, and a blue rump. The black-masked and Fischer's lovebirds have red bills and a broad area of naked white skin around the eyes. The black-masked lovebird has a black head bordered behind by a yellow collar, which extends below as a rather broad yellow band separating the contrasting colors of head and chest. Fischer's lovebird has the fore parts of the head red and has less yellow on the breast and neck. The crown and back part of the head are a bronzy green color. There is no sex difference in the appearance of birds of these three species, and there is no reliable way to determine their sex except by surgery or by observa-

tion of their behavior. Some bird fanciers believe that if the pelvic bones almost touch (pelvic bone test) the bird is probably a male, whereas if they are more than an eighth of an inch apart it is probably a female. Basing determination of sex on behavior is tricky, because these birds have a propensity for forming homosexual pairs.

Immature peach-faced lovebirds have a dark-brown "saddle" on the bill and lack the red forehead characteristic of the adult bird. Otherwise they are paler editions of the adults. Immature black-masked and Fischer's lovebirds are merely paler replicas of the parents. The blue-masked lovebird, established as a mutant of the black-masked form, differs from it primarily in the deletion of all yellow color; blue appears where the black-masked is green, and an off-white replaces yellow. The bill is pink instead of red.

All forms breed freely in captivity and are managed in the same way as budgerigars, except that it is not necessary to have several pairs for breeding to take place. Nest boxes should be more spacious and have larger entrance holes than the boxes used for budgerigars, but except for this requirement lovebirds are completely satisfied with almost any box. All should be provided with sheets of paper or large leaves, from which they cut strips of nesting material. The peach-faced lovebird females carry these strips, several at a time, tucked in the feathers of their rumps. The black-masked and Fischer's lovebirds carry them one at a time in their bills; these two species also need a supply of short, slender twigs for their nests. The twigs should be green, because moisture is essential to the hatching of the thick-shelled eggs.

The three to eight white eggs are laid one every other day. The incubation period is about 23 days. The newly hatched young are covered with a rather dense coat of reddish down. The young leave the nest at about five weeks of age and are weaned approximately two weeks later. When they are raised by hand they become incredibly tame but rarely, if ever, learn to talk. Lovebirds can learn to perform tricks and to talk, but their voices are harsh and objectionable at close range.

Like budgerigars, they are not messy birds, except for the scattering of seed hulls. Their droppings are dry and odorless.

Their vicious habits preclude caging them with birds of other species.

All lovebirds are native to Africa or Madagascar. *A. personata* and *A. fischeri* are found in the lightly wooded plains southeast of Lake Victoria. *A. roseicollis* is found in Angola.

COCKATIEL (NYMPHICUS HOLLANDICUS)

This native of the dry interior of Australia is probably the most popular psittacine in captivity, except for the ubiquitous budgerigar.

It is a slender bird about 12 inches long. The tail is long and tapering. The head has a long, pointed crest. Most of the body is a soft grey, and the wings have a conspicuous white patch beginning at the wrist and extending back through the secondaries. The face in adult males is bright yellow, and this color extends upward onto the crest. The cheeks have a circular patch of orange, and the under portions of the tail are dark grey. Adult females have only a slight tinge of yellow on the face, and the circular patch is a much duller orange. The under side of the tail has irregular bars of a yellowish color. Immature birds resemble adult females. Males require nearly two years to reach their brightest plumage, but begin to be distinguishable at about six months. Before this time, there is no reliable method of sexing them except surgically. Many aviculturists think that immature male birds have slightly yellower faces than do the females. Others try to sex cockatiels and other parrots by the "pelvic bone test," mentioned earlier in the discussion of lovebirds. This entails determining the distance between the tips of the pelvic bones, which are farther apart in females. This is extremely difficult to do reliably, and may even be dangerous in the larger parrots.

Cockatiels are among the easiest of all birds to breed in captivity. A large breeding cage should be provided, the larger the better. A nest box should be hung high, either inside the cage or outside with an opening cut in the wires of the cage to correspond with the entrance to the box. The box should be about 9 inches wide by 9 inches deep by 15 inches high. The entrance hole should be located high up on one side, and just wide enough to allow the birds passage. The back should be hinged to permit cleaning and inspection of the box. The bottom should be covered to a depth of two or three inches with coarse sawdust, wood chips, peat, or similar material. A ladder of hardware cloth or other material should be stapled inside the box from the entrance hole to the bottom of the box.

Once a pair has shown interest in the nest box it is best to inspect the box *daily* or leave it completely alone. A tame pair of birds become accustomed to daily attention, but if inspection is sporadic the birds are disturbed and may desert the box and its contents. This rule applies in the case of other birds as well. It is always better to curb one's curiosity and leave the birds alone.

These birds are extremely peaceable and can be kept with small finches and other non-aggressive birds. This is not true of most other parrots.

Cockatiels make excellent pets. They are not excessively messy, since their droppings are rather small and dry, a condition typical of desert birds which must conserve water. They become quite tame and affectionate, and can be taught to mimic and do tricks. One of their less-endearing qualities is their tendency to whistle loudly when the spirit moves them.

If cockatiels are kept for breeding it is best to avoid handling them or attempting to train them, for they become more interested in the attentions of their owner than in their mate.

AFRICAN GREY PARROT (PSITTACUS ERITHACUS)

This species has a wide distribution in the forested areas of Africa and is one of the most commonly kept of the larger parrots. Its popularity stems from the fact that it is probably the best talker of all the parrots.

It is a rather heavily built, short-tailed bird, about 14 to 15 inches long. There is no sexual dimorphism, the birds of both sexes being mainly grey with a red tail. A bare area around the eye is whitish; the bill is black. Immature birds have dark eyes, which gradually turn a pale straw color as they mature. It is best to buy a young bird, as adult birds, caught wild, never really become tame. African grey parrots have been bred in captivity, but their breeding is best attempted by specialists with much experience.

Like all other large parrots, they should be kept in a roomy cage, allowing them freedom of movement and at least short flights. They are fond of chewing on pieces of tree branches, and these should be provided and renewed frequently. Only non-toxic branches must be used, such as maple, elm, birch, or any of the fruit woods.

Young birds raised with gentle attention become extremely tame and make wonderful pets. They can be taught to talk by the same methods employed with budgerigars. Like most other large parrots, they may be very long-lived. Extreme claims are hard to prove, but a life span of 50 or more years is not an unreasonable expectation.

YELLOW-HEADED AMAZON
(AMAZONA OCHROCEPHALA)

The yellow-headed amazon is found in the tropical forests of Central and South America. It is a large bird, about 15 inches long. Its coloration varies, but it is primarily green with varying amounts of yellow on the head. The amount of yellow, indeed its coloration in general, depends on the subspecies; in some birds the entire head is yellow, whereas in others the amount of yellow is less. There are touches of red in the wrist area, and some blue in the wings. The tail has a bold pattern of black, green, and red. The sexes are alike in appearance.

Birds of this species are known by a number of different common names, depending on the subspecies they belong to—for example, Levaillant's amazon, Mexican double yellow head, yellow-naped amazon, Panama amazon, and yellow-fronted amazon. Yellow-headed amazons make fine pets and generally develop into good talkers if they are obtained young. These birds do not breed readily in captivity.

MACAWS (ANDORHYNCHUS AND ARA)

These very large, long-tailed parrots are often kept as pets, their fairly high cost probably being the chief deterrent to their greater popularity. Several species, all native to the forests of tropical America, are commonly available. The largest is the hyacinthine macaw (*Andorhynchus hyacinthinus*). It is a deep hyacinth blue all over and has a massive black bill. There is some bright yellow naked skin around the eyes and at the base of the lower mandible.

The genus *Ara* contains several species commonly seen in captivity. Among the more common of these are the blue and gold macaw (*A. ararauna*) and the scarlet macaw (*A. macao*). Both species are approximately 3 feet long, the blue and gold having a slightly

longer tail. The tail accounts for about half of the length. The blue and gold macaw is a rich blue color on the nape and back, and the dorsal wing and tail feathers. The crown is green, a black chin strap is present, and the remainder of the under side is yellow, except on the tail, which is blue tinged with yellow. The face has naked white skin, with three rows of tiny black feathers below the eye and similar lines between the eyes and the nostrils. The massive bill is black, the eyes are grey, and the feet are black.

The scarlet macaw is scarlet on the body and deeper scarlet on the head. Bright yellow and blue are splashed on the wings, and the rump is pale blue. The tail is red and blue. The upper mandible is a white horn color, and the lower mandible is black; the large bare cheek patches are white. The young of both species are similar to the parents in color but have duller plumage. Male and female birds are colored alike, with the male bird slightly larger.

Another species, the military macaw (*Ara militaris*), is generally dull olive-green in color, with a red forehead and with red in the wings and tail.

Macaws generally are hardy and have a long life span. All are exceptionally intelligent and, despite their large size and formidable bill, make docile and charming pets. Their natural sounds are harsh and loud, but their speaking voices are pleasant and soft. They require a great deal of attention and care if they are to remain desirable pets. Like some other parrots, they scream if they are frustrated or unhappy. They are commonly kept in cages much too small for them, and chaining them to a perch is an inhumane practice. They are seen at their best at liberty or in a large aviary. All can become ridiculously tame with careful handling, but great care should be taken when handling newly acquired birds, because of the very large and powerful bill. Even tame birds should be carefully watched as they, like other birds of the parrot family, have a propensity for chewing up almost everything in sight in order to keep the upper mandible from becoming too long. For this reason their perches should be of very hard wood. Wood scraps may be used to satisfy the need of the birds for something to chew on.

These birds are seldom bred except by specialists. Those interested in breeding them should consult some specialized source, such as *Parrots and Related Birds*, by Henry Bates and Robert Busenbark (T. F. H. Publications, Inc., Jersey City, N.J.), which contains information on aviary construction and nesting material.

Macaws are good mimics and some individuals might even be described as gifted. The technique for teaching them is the same as that described for budgerigars.

There is no sexual dimorphism in any of the macaws, and there is no reliable way to ascertain the sex of a bird except surgically. The slight differences in proportion that may exist are only suggestive rather than certain criteria.

The macaws are not particularly messy birds, but their large size and chewing behavior make them more troublesome in this respect than the smaller parrots.

Order: Passeriformes (perching birds)

Family: Fringillidae (certain finches, sparrows, buntings, serins, and related birds)

CANARY (SERINUS CANARIUS)

This species is the second most popular cage bird, the budgerigar being number one. Canaries are most often kept for their beautiful song, but many specialists value them also for some of the many colors and shapes developed during the process of their domestication. In the wild they occur widely over Europe and adjacent islands. The wild type is greenish yellow above and yellow below, with darker streaking. The sexes are alike in appearance. Most canaries are from 5 to $5\frac{1}{2}$ inches long.

They breed readily in captivity, as do all domesticated species. A roomy cage equipped with a nest bowl should be provided. Nesting material consists of yarn, grass, and the like. Cages, nest bowls, and nesting material are available commercially. The clutch comprises three to five bluish-green eggs spotted with reddish brown.

Canaries become good pets but never become as desirous of human company as do the various parrots and insectivorous birds.

Family: Estrildidae (estrildine finches)

ZEBRA FINCH (POEPHILA CASTANOTIS)

The zebra finch is a very popular cage bird and is representative of a large group of related birds, all requiring similar care. Some of its commonly seen relatives are the various mannikins, cutthroat finch, various waxbills, Java sparrow, Bengalese finch, and cordon bleu.

The zebra finch occurs in the drier parts of Australia and, like most of its relatives, is highly social. This species has become domesticated in captivity, and several color varieties have been established. One of these is white; the others are mainly diluted versions of the wild type, occurring in various shades of grey, tan, cream, or buff. The wild type, or "grey,"

zebra finch is a handsome bird, only $4\frac{1}{2}$ inches long. Adult males have red bills, greyish crowns, brownish backs, white bellies, and chestnut flanks spotted with white. The tail is black with large white spots. There is a vertical white stripe below the eye, which is bordered with black. The cheeks are chestnut. The breast is finely barred black and white. Adult females lack the chestnut flanks and cheeks, as well as the barred breasts. Juvenile birds resemble adult females, but their bills are black.

Zebra finches breed freely in captivity. Most prefer to nest in a finch-type nest box, which is simply a small wooden box with the front extending only about two-thirds of the way to the top. Nesting material such as long, dry blades of grass, burlap ravelings, bits of yarn, and weed stems should be provided. The male builds the nest, which is a hollow sphere with an entrance on one side. The eggs are white, and hatch in about 12 days. The young fledge when they are between two and three weeks old.

Zebra finches are small, beautiful birds, which are not messy or noisy.

BENGALESE FINCH (LONCHURA DOMESTICA)

The Bengalese finch, or society finch, has been domesticated for so long that its origins are lost in antiquity. Its wild ancestor is consequently a subject of argument. However, the most recent investigations seem to indicate that it is a domesticated form of the sharp-tailed finch (*Lonchura striata*), which occurs in tropical Asia.

These birds are only about $4\frac{1}{2}$ inches long. The sexes are alike, but the color and pattern show extreme variation. Most of the birds are white more or less blotched with black, tan, or brown. They breed freely, and are often used as foster parents for some of the finches that are difficult to rear in captivity. The principles governing their care and breeding are the same as those for the zebra finch.

JAVA SPARROW (PADDA ORYZIVORA)

The Java sparrow, which is native to tropical southern Asia and Java, is larger than the zebra and Bengalese finches, being about 5 to $5\frac{1}{2}$ inches long. These birds are mostly grey, with black heads and pink-tinged bellies. The bill is red, the cheeks are white, and the tail is black.

They are not easy to breed, but a domesticated all-white variety is said to breed fairly freely. They can be cared for in the same way as zebra finches.

Java sparrows are not noisy, and they make good pets. They always appear to be in good condition, for their plumage is naturally smooth and silky.

Family: Timaliidae (babblers)

PEKIN ROBIN (LEIOTHRIX LUTEA)

This so-called robin is not a member of the thrush family, but is one of the large family of babblers. It is a small bird, about 6 inches long. In the wild it occurs in Asia from the Himalayan mountains to southern China. The sexes are alike. The bill is red toward the tip, but black at the base. The upper parts of the bird are olivaceous. The tip of the tail is blackish; the flight feathers are washed with rusty orange and finely edged with yellow. There is a limited yellow bar across the secondary feathers near the secondary coverts. A light area occurs in front of and over the eyes. The throat and breast are deep yellow, the color becoming still deeper toward the rear of the body. The rest of the under parts are pale olivaceous, becoming nearly white under the tail.

Pekin robins breed more readily in captivity than do most other insectivorous birds. They should be kept in a roomy, planted aviary. The small, cup-shaped nest is built concealed in a bush. Breeding birds require large quantities of live insects to feed their young.

These birds make delightful, affectionate pets for those who have the time to cater to their needs, and the song of the male is delightfully melodious. This species is probably the most commonly kept of the small insectivorous birds.

Family: Sturnidae (starlings, mynahs, and related birds)

TALKING MYNAH (OR MYNA) (GRACULA RELIGIOSA)

This species is probably the best talking-bird available. Unlike parrots, whose mimicry approximates human speech, the voice of the mynah comes close to duplicating human tonal qualities. The mynah is a member of the starling family; individual birds vary greatly in size, depending on the subspecies they belong to. In the wild this species occurs in the forested tropical areas of India, Ceylon, Burma, Malay Peninsula, and the East Indian islands. All forms, contrary to some opinion, are equally good at learning to talk.

They are large black birds, 12 to 18 inches long. The bill and feet are yellow, as are the bare wattles around the face and nape. There is a white patch on each wing. The sexes look alike. Young birds have stubby tails and, if young enough, will still gape for food.

For the best results in teaching mynahs to talk, they should be obtained when young. The same techniques are used as in teaching the psittacine birds.

Mynahs are heavy feeders and rather messy, with loose droppings. The cage must be cleaned daily, but the handsome appearance and great powers of mimicry of the bird more than offset the extra care that is required.

Breeding of mynahs in captivity has rarely occurred, but success has been achieved in large aviaries affording maximal privacy. They need a large nest box, as they are hole nesters.

These birds make wonderful pets, and soon become very tame.

Order: Piciformes

Family: Ramphastidae (toucans, toucanettes, and aracaris)

There are about 5 genera and nearly 40 species of birds in the family Ramphastidae, the 3 genera that are discussed below being those most commonly kept in captivity. All are brightly colored and boldly patterned, with huge but surprisingly light-weight bills. All are active birds, with rather jerky, precise movements. They get along with other largish soft-billed birds, but when birds are newly introduced the group should be watched very carefully for signs of friction. The various species in this family can be housed in mixed flocks, but again caution should be exercised in case any individuals have a penchant for bullying or for being bullied. Birds which are added to existing groups should be watched with special care. Several birds introduced to new quarters at the same time seldom give any trouble. Unless a bird is already quite tame and steady, it will do better in a large aviary than in a smaller cage, because of its awkward and damaging flights when frightened.

The sexes are alike in all the species discussed below. Immature birds tend to be smaller, especially the bills, and they are duller in color than the adults.

It seems to be generally agreed that, with patience and gentleness, toucans and toucanettes can be tamed even when they are caught as adults. The aracaris apparently only become really tame when they are hand-raised.

All these birds can be fed a ration of mynah pellets as a basic diet, augmented by a variety of fruits (apple, peach, banana, pear, and the like), along with some raw meat. It is better to provide more than the necessary amount of food in order to ensure their eating enough. If several are kept together, it is wise to watch them carefully in order to determine if any dominant individual is keeping the others from eating. If this happens, food should be provided at several spots at the same time.

The breeding of these birds is something to be attempted only by specialists. All are hole-nesters in the wild, and lay white eggs.

All of them make lively, amusing pets, but they should not be kept by anyone not willing to devote much time to them. They are extremely messy birds that require daily cleaning of their cages and immediate environment. Even though all are native to the tropical forests of the Americas, they are reasonably hardy if they are kept from drafts and the temperature does not go below about 40°F.

TOUCANS (RAMPHASTOS)

The Toco toucan (*Ramphastos toco*) and the sulfur-breasted toucan (*R. sulfuratus*) are perhaps the commonest toucans in captivity. Both are around 16 inches long, including the bill. The Toco toucan is black, with a white bib shaded yellow on the breast, a white rump, and the under tail coverts red. The huge bill is bright orange with darker markings. The naked skin around the eyes is blue. The sulfur-breasted toucan is mostly black with a white rump, and a yellow face and throat. The bill and the naked skin around the eyes are bright green. There is also some orange in the bill, and it has a maroon tip.

TOUCANETTES (AULACORHYNCHUS)

The emerald toucanette (*Aulacorhynchus prasinus*) is the commonest toucanette seen in captivity. It is much smaller than the toucans. Its bill is blackish, with a broad yellow swath covering much of the upper mandible. The edges of the bill are jagged. The bare skin around the eyes is greyish green. The remainder of the bird is a pastel green, darker above. There is some red in the under tail coverts.

ARACARIS (PTEROGLOSSUS)

The collared aracari (*Pteroglossus torquatus*) is the commonest aracari seen in captivity, and it also is smaller than the toucans. The bill is even more jagged than that of the toucanettes, and is blackish with the upper portion of the upper mandible and the entire base of the bill yellowish. The edges of the bill are greyish. The bare area around the eyes is bluish in front, shading to red behind the eyes. The upper parts, head, throat, and chest are black. The under parts are basically yellow smudged with red, particularly around a blackish spot on the breast. A broad black band separates the yellow area of the breast from that of the abdomen.

Suggested Reading

BATES, H., and BUSENBARK, R.: *Parrots and Related Birds.* Jersey City, T. F. H. Publications, Inc., 1959. 373 pp.

BATES, H., and BUSENBARK, R.: *Finches and Soft-billed Birds.* Jersey City, T. F. H. Publications, Inc., 1963. 703 pp.

BOOSEY, E. J.: *Foreign Bird Keeping. A Complete Guide to Breeding and Management.* London, Iliffe Books Ltd., 1962. 384 pp.

CLEAR, VAL: *Common Cagebirds in America.* Chicago. Ill., Audubon Publ. Co., 1966. 142 pp.

NAETHER, C.: *Soft-billed Birds.* Fond du Lac, Wis., All-Pets Books, Inc., 1955. 64 pp.

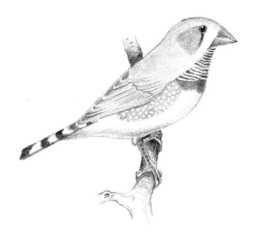

2

Caging
and
Environment

William C. Dilger

Keeping a bird healthy in captivity requires serious consideration of its accommodations and immediate environment. It is not at all difficult to provide a proper situation for most birds, but their requirements must be thoroughly understood from the first. More captive animals are cruelly kept out of mistaken kindness than for any other reason. The principal source of difficulty is the adoption of an anthropomorphic viewpoint when considering the needs of the bird or other animal. A moment's reflection should suffice to prompt the realization that all animals differ in their requirements, and that not many of these requirements are the same as man's.

Both the physical and psychological needs of an animal must be met if it is to be kept healthy and comfortable. It is, fortunately, not ordinarily necessary to duplicate its normal habitat in order to accomplish this. When the needs of an animal are not precisely known, the normal wild habitat should be recreated as closely as possible, in an effort to include all of the features absolutely necessary for its well-being. On the other hand, birds which have been bred in captivity for many generations, such as canaries and budgerigars, are quite simple to care for. The requirements of most other birds fall somewhere between these two extremes.

The available avicultural and ornithological literature provides much useful information for anyone who is dealing with a species not ordinarily kept in captivity or for the novice who is dealing with birds whose needs are well understood.

UNIQUE ENVIRONMENTAL REQUIREMENTS

Each species of bird, or of any other animal for that matter, lives in a unique world of its own. This world is potentially made up of all the impressions the animal is capable of receiving through its sense organs. In birds these impressions are chiefly received through the organs of seeing and hearing—much as man's are. Other senses play a comparatively minor role in building up a picture of the world, but this participation varies from species to species. However, it is a characteristic of the behavior of animals that they respond to only a comparatively narrow range of stimuli among those which are potentially available. The stimuli to which they do respond are those to which response has evolved in order to ensure that the species behaves properly with respect to all the needs it has for maintaining itself in a normally healthy state and for reproducing its kind. Stimuli that are "irrelevant" are ignored as if they did not exist. This "stimulus filtration" is the subject of intensive investigation; it is now known that some of it occurs peripherally in the sense organs themselves, and some of it occurs in the central nervous system.

In a way, this sensory selectivity makes the task of providing an animal's requirements much simpler and is the reason that we do not ordinarily have to duplicate in great detail all the features of its normal habitat. It is necessary only that we recognize the comparatively few environmental features on which the animal depends for a normal existence. For instance, the requirements of African lovebirds, such as the popular peach-faced lovebird and black-masked lovebird, include simply an adequate diet, fresh water, ample room, a nest box, a firm horizontal perch of proper diameter, nest material, and a mate. This is obviously a much smaller number of items than are found in their native habitat. With provision of these few features the birds keep in perfect health and breed freely—the ultimate criteria for the proper maintenance of any species.

Cage Requirements

SIZE

Most birds are accustomed to flying and should be housed so that they can fly easily from one perch to another. Birds should be provided with all the room possible, thus, the minimal space in which they can be successfully maintained becomes the important consideration. This of course varies with the species being kept. When considering the minimal space requirements

possible, it is important to keep in mind that the *proportions* of a cage are more critical than is the absolute *volume* enclosed. Volumes being equal, a cage with greater length in relation to its height and width is better than one of more nearly equal dimensions. The greater length allows more room for flying and for other exercise.

A cage should be wide enough to allow the bird to spread its wings fully and have ample room to spare. It should also be wide enough to allow the bird to retreat a secure distance from a disturbance from any direction. Tame birds with a large wing span can be comfortable in a narrower cage than can a rather nervous bird with a smaller wing span. Generally less room is required for domesticated or aviary-raised birds than for their wild counterparts. Everyone is familiar with the size of cages in which domesticated canaries and budgerigars are customarily kept. These cages are ordinarily large enough if they are properly arranged inside; they would be much too small for undomesticated canaries or budgerigars.

It is difficult to give minimal measurements for cage sizes, but, as a rule of thumb, enclosures for the various small finches should be at least 24 inches long, 12 inches wide, and 12 inches high. Larger finches should have a cage approximately 4 feet long, with the other dimensions increased in proportion. Birds the size of grosbeaks should not be kept in anything smaller than this. Larger birds naturally need proportionately larger cages.

PERCHES

Perches should be placed at the same height and as far apart as possible. They should not, however, be placed so near the end of the cage that the bird will rub its tail against the cage when it is turning around on the perch. Such contact quickly results in an unsightly, frayed tail. These perches should be placed rather high in the cage. If other perches are placed lower, care should be taken to arrange them so that they, or a bird sitting on them, cannot be defecated on by a bird sitting on one of the higher perches.

Perches are usually fashioned from wooden dowels. These are easy to scrub, but have serious disadvantages. Besides being too smooth for secure footing, they are all of the same diameter and curvature, which forces the bird always to bend its toes in the same way and frequently leads to foot trouble. Perches made from natural twigs or branches cut from non-toxic trees and shrubs, such as fruit trees, or elm, ash, maple, willow, and nut trees, are much better. Such material provides a much more natural perch, gives the bird perches of a variety of diameters to grip, and is rough enough to provide secure footing. Such perches are more difficult to clean, but they can easily be replaced instead. The sand-coated perches commercially available are of dubious utility. They may even cause foot trouble in tender-footed species, or aggravate already sore feet. Since parrots of the various species are fond of chewing on everything they can reach, their perches should be of the hardest wood available in order to minimize the replacement problem. This is also true for some cardueline finches, such as crossbills.

BAR SPACING

Cages should be fashioned with bar spacing appropriate to the species being kept. The smaller waxbills can escape between bars spaced only ½ inch apart. Birds always look larger than they really are, because of their feathers. Bar spacing should not be decreased more than necessary, however, to ensure that one's view of the bird is not unnecessarily restricted. Painting the bars with flat black paint surprisingly increases the visibility into the cage. Only a non-toxic paint should be used.

TYPES OF CAGES

There are two main types of cages. One made entirely of wire is perhaps the most familiar type. It has the advantage of providing visibility of the occupant from all directions; it has the disadvantage of denying the bird a feeling of security, as there is no escape from disturbance from any direction. Also, it is difficult to protect the bird from dangerous drafts. This, however, is the type of cage most commonly available commercially, and such cages are often very decorative. Cage decorations, however, are usually difficult to clean adequately and are therefore best avoided. Many cages are hopelessly proportioned, some even being built as narrow, vertical cylinders. Any poorly proportioned or unnecessarily ornamented cage should be scrupulously avoided. If an all-wire cage is used, it should be placed so it is completely out of drafts at all times, and should also be placed so that the occupant is free from disturbance on at least one side.

The other major type of cage is the box cage. This is an opaque box constructed of thin wood or metal, with the front fitted with bars or screening (Fig. 2-1). Such a cage eliminates the danger of drafts, provides security for the bird, and is simple to construct. The inside is customarily painted some light color; the outside can be finished in any manner desirable, but the use of non-toxic paints is extremely important. Local paint suppliers can give the necessary advice for this, the paints used for painting baby toys and furniture being safe for this purpose.

Modified box cages are often constructed (Figs. 2-2, 2-3). In these cages the top and one or more additional

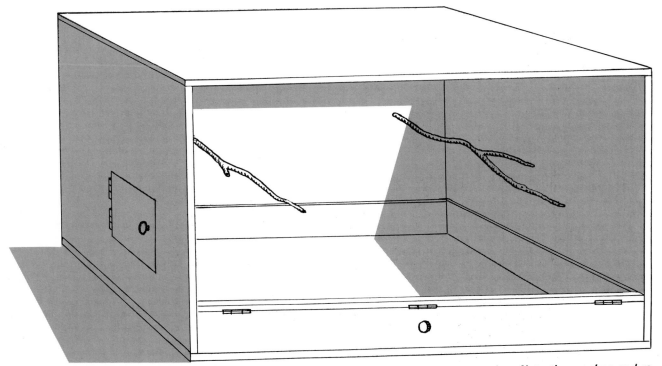

Fig. 2-1. Box Cage: *Only the front is open and may be fitted with either bars or screening. Note the perches and removable metal tray.*

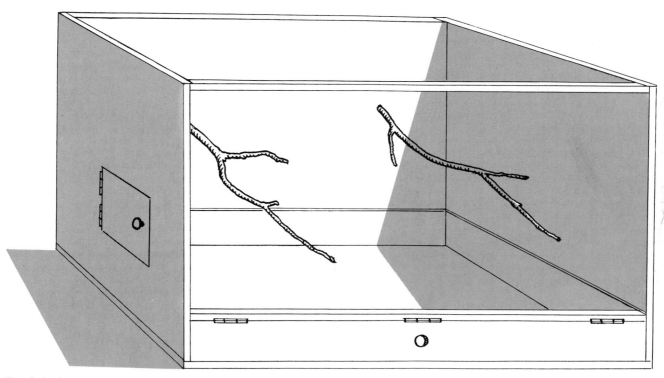

Fig. 2-2. Semi-box Cage: *Both the top and front are open and may be fitted with either glass or screening.*

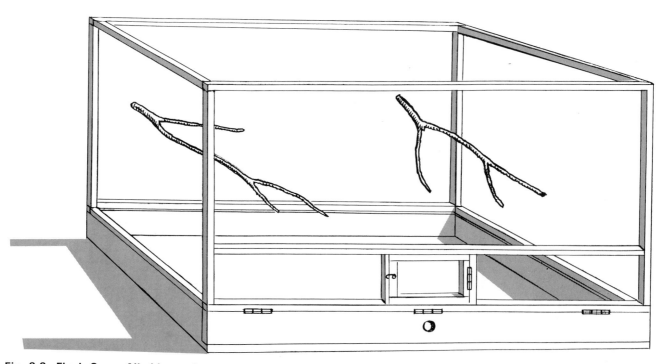

Fig. 2-3. Finch Cage: *All sides and top are open and may be screened or have a glass front.*

sides may be screened, in addition to the front. At least two adjacent sides, however, should always be made of solid material. Such cages are usually referred to as "semi-box cages."

FACILITIES FOR CLEANING

No matter what type of cage is used, it should have a bottom that is easy to remove and clean without danger of the bird escaping during the procedure. Ordinarily a sliding metal tray is used. This tray can be painted for easy maintenance, and it should be touched up whenever bare patches appear. The tray should be deep enough to contain accumulated seed husks and bird droppings without danger of their being unduly scattered about the room as a result of the bird's movements. This is less of a problem with box cages than with all-wire cages.

FACILITIES FOR FEEDING

Food and water containers should be made so that they are easy to clean thoroughly. They should have no narrow, hard-to-reach corners and crevices in which dirt can accumulate. They should be sturdy and, of course, should be made of non-toxic materials. Their placement is important. They should be so situated that the bird has easy access to them but cannot defecate into them. They should be easy to remove and to replace. Some bird fanciers favor small, self-feeding hoppers for seeds (Fig. 2-4). These have the advantage of holding a large amount of food, thus minimizing the danger of the supply running out. One need only glance at the open portion of the hopper to see if any food remains. However, one must look carefully, because seed husks can give the superficial impression of food remaining when, in fact, there is none. Hoppers also keep the food supply cleaner by minimizing the danger of its being contaminated by droppings.

OTHER REQUIREMENTS

Sharp projections in a cage, such as nail points, broken wires, wood splinters, and the like, can be dangerous and these should be looked for and removed or the cage be repaired as necessary.

Ordinarily, the bottom of the cage is covered with a layer or two of paper on which a little grit is sprinkled. For most birds this type of substrate is suitable, but in a few cases it is deleterious. For instance, some birds such as pittas spend much or all of their time on the floor of the cage and their feet become sore very easily if they are not on something softer, such

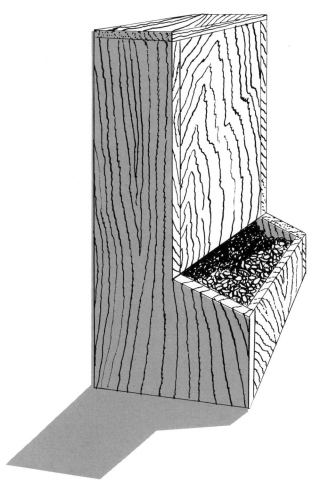

Fig. 2-4. *Food hopper. Such a hopper can easily be made at home; it is suitable for any dry food, such as seeds or pellets.*

as an inch or so of dampened peat moss. Most birds seem to benefit if a piece of growing sod is placed in the cage from time to time. Fruit-, nectar-, and meat-eating species must have their cages cleaned very frequently, often daily, in order to maintain sanitary conditions. This is true of toucans, honey-eaters, hanging parakeets, lories, mynahs, fruit-suckers, and all similar species.

Routine of Care

It is a good policy to do feeding, watering, and cleaning at the same time each day. Birds quickly become accustomed to such routine, and may become disturbed if these operations are performed at unpredictable times. They also are suspicious of anything different, such as use of strange containers for food or water. The consequences of this are probably not serious, but it can cause a sharp drop in consumption of food or water for a short period. One should always remember to move slowly and deliberately around birds and not make sudden loud sounds as birds are very easily frightened by unaccustomed movement or sound.

Freedom from Cage

Pet birds derive some healthful exercise from being allowed to fly at liberty in the home, and they are often seen at their best in this way. However, birds enjoying such liberty have an almost uncanny ability to get themselves injured or killed. They get caught in closing doors, fall into pots of boiling liquid or open toilets, get caught by cats, get stepped or sat on, eat poisonous house plants, are sucked up in vacuum cleaners, or simply escape through an open door or window. If a bird is allowed freedom from its cage it should be constantly watched in order to avoid any serious consequences to the bird or damage to the house and its furnishings. Such vigilance is particularly necessary with parrots, because of their propensity for chewing on almost anything within their reach.

Aviaries

Many people would like to construct an aviary in which to keep larger numbers of birds or for breeding of birds needing roomier accommodations. Such an aviary consists of a flight space and a shelter. Plans for building single or multiple units for various purposes are readily available, but some general considerations may properly be discussed here. Such an aviary can be from but a few feet long and wide up to almost any dimension desired. It should be remembered that the cost of construction becomes relatively less as the size of the enclosed area increases.

FLIGHT SPACE

The frame for the flight space can be made of wood or of metal such as angle irons or pipes. If destructive birds such as parrots, crossbills, or woodpeckers are to be kept, it is easier to construct the frame of metal than it is to devise inexpensive ways to protect the wood.

The considerations governing the proportions of cages apply to aviaries as well; a longish, narrow flight space is preferable to one more nearly cubical, especially if the size is comparatively small. Eight feet or more is a good height for an aviary. Birds, when frightened by someone entering the flight space, feel more secure if they can fly above the source of the disturb-

ance. Also, because of this propensity of birds for flying upward when disturbed, the door into the flight space should be only about 4 feet high. This helps to prevent birds from escaping past the person who is entering or leaving. However, it is best in this connection to construct a "bird lock," consisting of a small entrance chamber, with its own outside door. In this way, a person can enter the lock, close the outside door, and then open the door leading into the flight space. This is good insurance against possible escape of any bird.

FLOOR

The floor of the aviary can be of earth, concrete, or wood. Each has its advantages and disadvantages. Earthen floors tend to become contaminated and may become a source of disease, especially if many birds are kept. This is not so serious a feature if only one or two pairs occupy the space. Earthen floors have the advantage that they can easily be planted with various shrubs, vines, and herbaceous plants. Concrete floors are hard on birds' feet, but they can be spread with a litter of some sort, such as peat, ground corn cobs, or shredded sugar cane. This can easily be removed and replaced as the need demands. Wooden floors are difficult to maintain, especially if dampness is a problem. They also tend to harbor dirt in the cracks and are difficult to clean. Neither wood nor concrete floors can be planted, but plants can be placed in large tubs and this gives the advantage of mobility if one wants to shift the plantings about. Either wood or concrete is better protection against vermin attempting to burrow in from outside. If a wood or earth floor is used, the wire mesh of the sides of the flight space should extend $1\frac{1}{2}$ to 2 feet down into the ground and then be turned outward at a right angle. This prevents rats, weasels, and other burrowing pests from gaining entrance.

SHELTER

The sheltered portion of the aviary should be part of an existing building or a separate shed built at one end of the flight space. The juncture of the shelter and flight space should be tight and sturdy, to prevent vermin from entering or birds from escaping. The interior of the shelter should be provided with perches placed as high as possible, and there should be small openings through its wall into the flight space through which the birds can enter to roost or to escape inclement weather. Most birds dislike flying downward, especially when preparing to roost, so the perches inside the shelter should be placed higher than the nearer outside ones, with the access holes on a line between them. Some birds are reluctant to use a shelter and must be coaxed or gently driven in before they are shut in at night. It is a good plan to roof over 4 or 5 feet of the flight space immediately adjacent to the shelter, thus providing protection from rain and snow. A portion of the upper sides of the flight space below the roofed portion can also be profitably sheltered with some transparent material, such as fiber glass panels or clear plastic sheeting stretched over wooden frames.

Unless the shelter is roomy and dependably heated, birds that are susceptible to cold must be kept indoors during the winter. Thermostatically controlled electric heat is the best, but gas or oil heaters are satisfactory if they are controlled thermostatically and properly vented to the outside. If a shelter is to be heated, for the sake of economy it should also be insulated.

An aviary should be placed so that it is protected from the prevailing winds and still receive several hours of sunlight each day.

Mice are nearly impossible to keep out of an aviary. Juvenile mice can easily pass through ½-inch netting or bar spacing. Even pregnant house mice can squeeze through a 1 by ½-inch opening. These rodents do not attack the birds, but they eat much of their food and foul the remainder. They also disturb the birds by running about the aviary and perches during the night. This, done night after night, can actually cause the death of birds both from the physiological stresses imposed on them and from the accumulated effects of multiple small injuries, particularly to the brain, caused by the birds blindly flying into objects in the dark.

TEMPERATURE AND HUMIDITY

Birds, being warm-blooded animals, are relatively independent of environmental temperatures and humidity. Extremes, of course, are to be avoided. In general birds do better at the cooler and drier ends of their preferred temperature and humidity ranges. It is surprising how tolerant even many tropical birds are to cold, short of actual freezing temperatures, if they are adequately sheltered at night and kept free from drafts.

Suggested Reading

SODERBERG, P. M.: *Foreign Birds for Cage and Aviary.* London, Cassell and Co. Ltd., 1956. Book I, *Care and Management*, 88 pp.

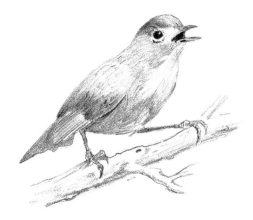

3

Behavioral Aspects

William C. Dilger

If a bird is not physically and psychologically healthy there is usually something wrong with the way it is being kept. It is necessary to develop some knowledge of the behavioral characteristics of one's captive birds and be constantly sensitive to them in order to manage their environment properly. Some of the necessary considerations were treated in Chapter 2, on Caging and Environment.

As stated there, it is a mistake to consider a bird's needs from an anthropomorphic viewpoint. The same applies to bird behavior. Birds do get hungry, thirsty, cold, hot, afraid, aggressive, and the like, but they do not have the higher feelings of humans, such as altruism and love, nor do they feel hate. Birds can become frustrated, however, and unresolved frustrations are responsible for many of the difficulties encountered in keeping them.

CAUSES OF ABNORMAL BEHAVIOR

FRUSTRATION

Birds may, for instance, become frustrated in their attempts to escape from their cages. This occurs when the cage is not suitable for the occupant. The most frequent faults are small size, poor proportions, or unsuitable arrangement of perches and other items inside the cage.

Frustrated escape behavior provides one of the most difficult problems for both the aviculturist and the bird. Birds in small cages soon learn they cannot escape, and they even come to feel a measure of security. Their escape behavior is usually soon reduced to rather agitated hopping from perch to perch, or to short flights from perch to perch without colliding with the bars or wire netting.

Birds in large bare aviaries tend to remain rather wild and commonly fly headlong into the netting when they are frightened. It is important to provide escape routes by having the flight space high enough (8 feet or more) and to provide shelter from disturbance, as by opaque baffles hanging from the roof in front of some of the perches. Planted aviaries are much better than bare, and birds in them soon become much steadier when subject to disturbance.

The larger parrots are commonly kept in cages too small for them, and initially spend much time in attempts to escape. These escape movements in time become stereotyped and, in the end, become so ritualized that it is often difficult to recognize them for what they are. Some birds make figure-of-eight-on-its-side movements with the head, others perform a stilted form of bowing, and still others repeatedly and rhythmically bow or tip the head from side to side. Such parrots often become so psychologically disturbed that they will not fly even when they are finally given the opportunity.

ABSENCE OF SENSORY STIMULI

Another frequent problem with parrots, particularly birds of the larger species such as amazons or macaws, stems from the failure to give them a stimulus-rich environment. Species of animals that are particularly intelligent (for example, large parrots, crows, ravens, jays, monkeys, apes, men) require an environment rich in stimuli appealing to their dominant senses. Such animals just have to see, hear, and handle a great variety of objects in order to maintain mental health. The larger parrots are denied these experiences more frequently than not. The result is a seriously disturbed animal very refractory to efforts designed to improve the situation. The commonest result is self-mutilation, probably stemming from an effort to find something of interest to do. The commonest type of self-mutilation is feather plucking. Some birds render themselves practically nude. Less commonly, the bird may chew its toes, causing the loss of one or more toes or even of an entire foot. All of this can be avoided by providing a large enough cage containing an ample number of objects for the bird to explore. These objects should be renewed frequently, in order to provide novelty.

Feather loss and other physical damage may, of course, result also from disease and injury. These subjects are treated in other chapters.

CHANGES FROM NATIVE EATING HABITS

The food of most seed-eating birds occurs in relative concentration in the wild, and such birds eat at definite periods during the day, the remainder of the time being taken up with other necessary activities. Conditions in captivity usually approximate this situation, and no special problems are ordinarily encountered.

Birds that normally eat other foods, particularly animals, usually have to hunt assiduously for their meals and spend much of their waking hours foraging, performing their other necessary activities as best they can. Such species in captivity are usually provided with their food *ad libitum*, so that they have a propensity for over-eating. The result is obesity, particularly in those kept in cages, the problem usually not being as serious in birds kept in large aviaries. These birds may become so fat they cannot fly, and the obesity may also result in gastrointestinal trouble or cardiovascular malfunction. The obvious solution is to limit the amount of food provided for them.

There also seems to be a psychological necessity for such birds to hunt and capture live food, regardless of how nutritionally perfect the substitute diet may be. Insectivorous birds should frequently be given opportunity to catch their own live food. Mealworms, flies, maggots, crickets, and cockroaches are commonly utilized for this purpose. Such birds in smaller cages or unplanted aviaries need this opportunity more than do birds in planted aviaries, where usually enough natural food can be found to supplement their normal diet.

Most insectivorous birds offered for sale have been caught in the wild and are not accustomed to the various artificial diets designed to nutritionally approximate the one naturally consumed. It is often difficult to get such birds to eat these mixtures. For this purpose aviculturists employ a technique they term "meating off," a process which entails liberally sprinkling a dish of the proprietary mixture with live food. The birds are attracted to this, and while eating they usually, probably by accident, ingest some of the mixture. The amount of live food can be gradually reduced each day, until the birds are feeding freely on the proprietary mixture.

The same technique can be used to make rather drastic changes in the diets of other birds as well, if any such change becomes necessary. It may, for instance, sometimes be desirable to medicate seed-eating birds by mixing the medication in a damp mash of some sort. Such birds can first be led to eat the mash by sprinkling it with seeds which, like the insects, are gradually reduced until the mash is taken freely. Even such inveterate seed-eaters as budgerigars can be induced to eat a mash by use of this technique.

It is important to provide food at appropriate heights, depending on where the birds are primarily adapted to feed. Ground-foraging birds should be fed on the ground. Those which normally forage in trees or bushes should have their food placed accordingly.

ISOLATION

Highly social species such as budgerigars and the colonial lovebirds should not be isolated from their own kind while still being able to hear and see each other. Birds so isolated will frequently gradually decline in general health and may eventually die. The actual physiological changes that take place are not known. It is perfectly all right to keep such birds as individual pets away from their own kind so long as they do not have the frustration of being able to see or hear the other birds without being able to achieve physical contact.

INTERINDIVIDUAL AND INTERSPECIES RELATIONSHIPS

One must be alert to guard against individuals or species which tend to bully others. If the aggression is immediate and obvious, it is easy to identify and re-move the offenders. On the other hand, the behavior of some individuals is much more insidious. They may monopolize the food and water containers, for instance, and keep other birds away from them. Such habits should be carefully watched for, especially among newly acquired birds. Several dishes of food and water may be provided, or, once it is identified, the offending bird can be removed.

Some birds seem to get along with others for long periods and then suddenly turn on their companions. Many parrots have a propensity for doing this, as do many other species which may be territorial during their reproductive cycles. Most parrots and highly territorial species are best kept apart from others.

PRESERVATION OF PSYCHIC AND PHYSICAL HEALTH

As emphasized in Chapter 2, it is not often necessary to exactly duplicate a bird's wild habitat, but one must be aware of the items essential in its life and provide them in an acceptable manner. One must keep in mind that, if certain conditions are not provided, a bird can become frustrated, frightened, or unduly aggressive. In such event a bird can easily become psychotic and even suffer a decline in physical health. A thorough knowledge of the bird's wild environment, combined with a sincere desire to make the bird comfortable, should enable an owner to keep any species in good condition.

Suggested Reading

HARWOOD, P. M. A.: Bird psychology and aviculture. Avic. Mag. *64:*9–17, 1958.

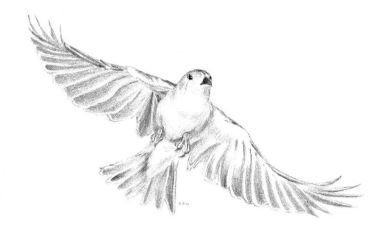

4

Genetics

Paul A. Buckley

Of all major groups of animals, birds are probably the best known taxonomically and evolutionarily, but, paradoxically, they are the least known genetically. This is unfortunate, since ideal evaluation of taxonomic inferences is facilitated by knowledge of the genetic system involved. There has, however, been a great surge of research in avian genetics, attacks being made from two widely separated fronts.

Studies on the inheritance of avian morphological characters—now at the stage that study of genetics in *Drosophila* was in the first 20 years of this century—have been done by poultrymen and by aviculturists, usually from a practical, applied viewpoint. Fowl breeders studied chickens (*Gallus gallus*), turkeys (*Meleagris gallopavo*), domestic, or Pekin, ducks (*Anas platyrhynchos domesticus*), pheasants (*Phasianus* spp.), and pigeons (*Columba livia*), and more recently have studied the Eurasian migratory quail (*Coturnix* spp.). Aviculturists have worked with pigeons and with canaries (*Serinus canarius*), budgerigars (*Melopsittacus undulatus*), and other commonly kept cage birds. It is largely from these writings that the material in this Chapter has been drawn.

THE AVIAN GENETIC SYSTEM

CYTOLOGY

The genetic system of birds—the cytological configuration of the chromosomes that determines the passage of hereditary material from generation to generation—was not accurately unravelled by microscopists until 1963. That year, for the first time, unequivocal cytological proof was offered for the existence of fe-

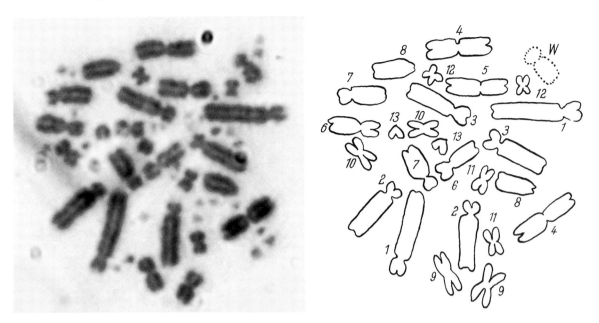

Fig. 4-1. *Photograph and drawing of female chromosome complement (budgerigar kidney 4). X3650. Note distinctive morphology of W(Y) chromosome. (Rothfels, K., Aspden, M., and Mollison, M.: Chromosoma* **14**: *463, 1963.)*

male heterogamety in birds, with demonstration of an X(Z) and a Y(W) chromosome in female budgerigars and two X(Z) chromosomes in males.[46] Prior to this time, it had been demonstrated genetically on the basis of progeny test results that females were either XO(ZO) or XY(ZW), but owing to the confusing array of avian chromosomes, it had not been possible to decide finally if females did indeed possess a Y(W). Since most animals have XY rather than XO systems, possession of the XY(ZW) seemed more likely.

Shortly after the Y(W) chromosome had been found in budgerigars, Ohno *et al.,*[39] using the same reliable, replicable techniques, found that female pigeons and canaries also have an XY(ZW) system. It is almost certain that all birds will be found to have the same configuration, since genetic systems are usually evolutionarily conservative.

In the first attempt to use comparative cytology as a tool in avian taxonomy after identification of the Y(W) in the three kinds of birds mentioned above, Beçak *et al.*[1a] compared the karyotypes* of birds from diverse orders with those of several families of snakes. They found the closest similarity to those of the colubrid snakes (racers and allies). However, these data are only fragmentary and, although they indicate from still another line of evidence the phyletic affinity of birds and snakes, they must be evaluated with circumspection.

Karyotype: the complete description of the numbers and types of chromosomes in the nucleus in male and female somatic cells in an organism.

SEX-LINKAGE AND SEX-INFLUENCED INHERITANCE

A distinction between "sex-linkage" and "sex-influenced inheritance," often confused by non-geneticists, is important. "Sex-linkage" refers to the location of genes on either the X or the Y chromosome. In all the well-studied *Drosophila* species only about 40 different genes (almost all related with fertility or fecundity) have been located on the Y, in contrast to several scores or more on the X. Any evidence of genes located on the Y(W) chromosome in birds would be of immense interest. Such a gene *might* be indicated by the presence of a character expressed *only in females* and *in all females in the line.*

"Sex-influenced inheritance" refers to the expression of genes which are located on either autosomes or sex chromosomes (and hence in all cells of every animal), but whose *expression* is influenced by the genetic sex of the animal. All mammals have genes for ovaries and testes in all cells, yet only in the aberrant and exceedingly rare true hermaphrodite are both organ systems present simultaneously. Their expression is sex-influenced.

Sex-linkage is relatively common in birds. A point to be stressed is that there is no intrinsic relationship between a sexual character and the chromosomal location of the gene affecting it, many genes affecting sexual characters being located on autosomes.

The first suggestion that a gene might be sex-linked

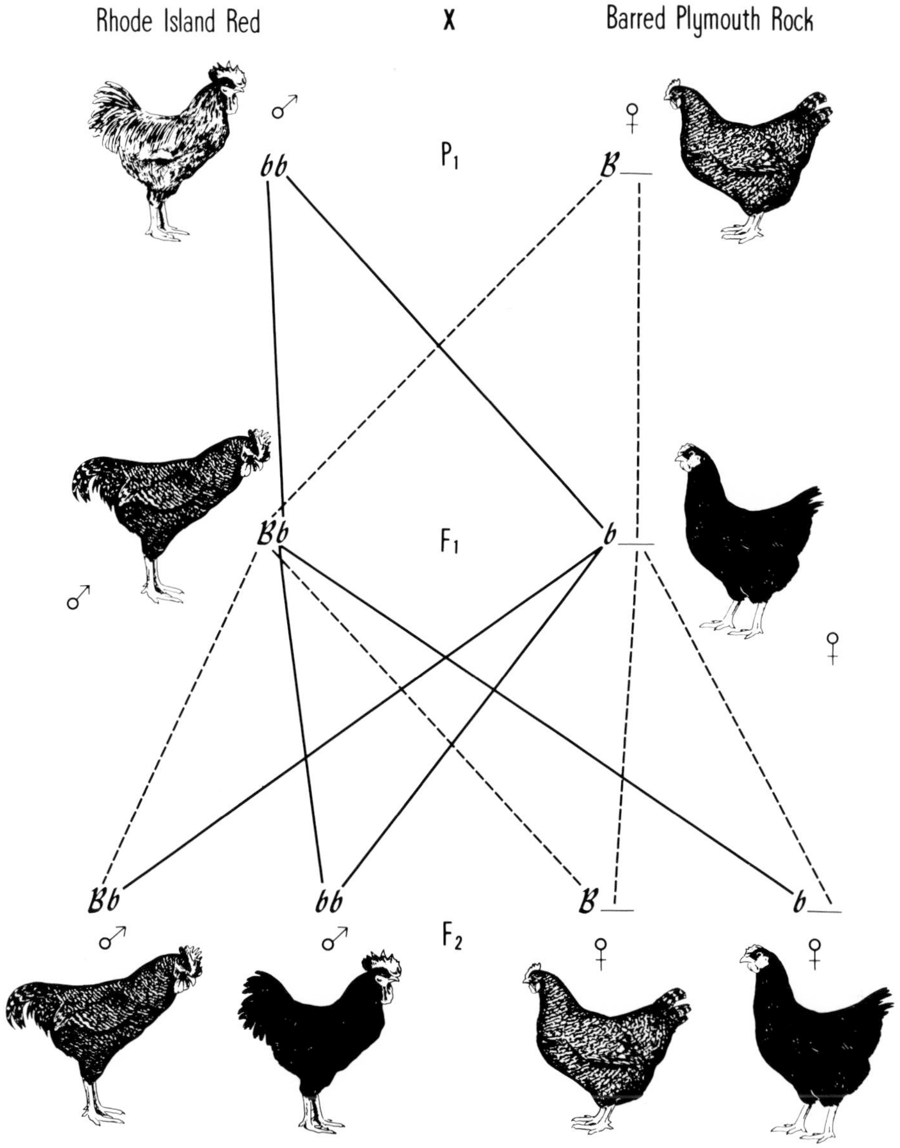

Rhode Island Red   **X**   Barred Plymouth Rock

Fig. 4-2. *Sex-linked transmission of barring in the cross of Rhode Island red ♂ × barred Plymouth Rock ♀. (Hutt, Frederick B.: Animal Genetics. Copyright © 1964. The Ronald Press Company, New York.)*

would be the appearance of phenotypes* in numbers deviating from the expected 3 to 1 ratio for completely dominant autosomal genes in the F_2. This is often the result of differential mortality in the sexes if the gene is lethal when homozygous.† If a gene is sex-linked and recessive in birds, it will be expressed in males only when it occurs in double dose—one received from

Phenotype: the observable characters of an animal, that is, the discernible results of the interactions between the genotype and the environment of the animal.

†*Homozygous:* of a diploid, sexually reproducing organism, possessing identical alleles at a given locus on both members of a pair of homologous chromosomes.

each parent; however, females will always express every gene on their single X chromosome since there isn't a second X to mask any of its genes. If the gene is lethal, all females will be born dead, or no females will even appear as offspring. Such findings immediately implicate a sex-linked recessive. Dominance in sex-linkage is not so easily separated from autosomal dominance, unless one uses reciprocal cross tests. In such tests a male of Type A is mated with a female of Type B, and a male of Type B with a female of Type A. With easily observable characters, identical results from the two crosses suggest autosomal inheritance; different results indicate probable sex-linkage.

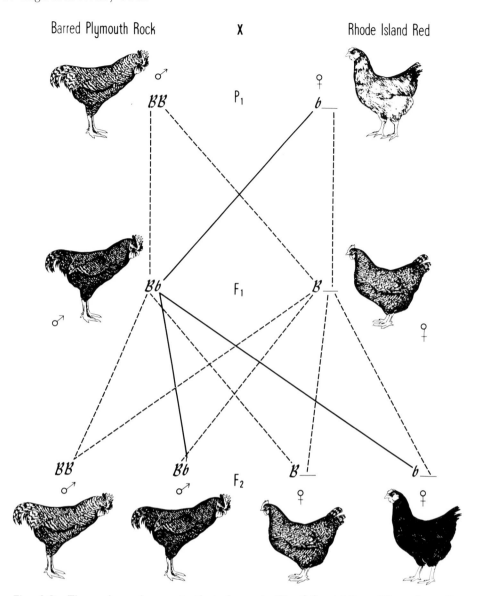

Fig. 4-3. *The reciprocal cross to that shown in Fig. 4-2, yielding different results in the F₁ and F₂ generations. (Hutt, Frederick B.: Animal Genetics. Copyright © 1964. The Ronald Press Company, New York.)*

It should be pointed out that most but not all mutant genes are recessive. There is good reason for this, since a mutation usually disrupts a delicate balance of genes that have evolved to work together as a unit. In nature, strong selection will be apparent for additional genes, called modifiers, to change an undesirable but not lethal gene from an original dominance to a later recessiveness. This suppresses deleterious effects but at the same time preserves variation in the population and any effects of hybrid vigor, or heterosis, that heterozygous* individuals (heterozygotes) might

show. The same mechanism can operate in reverse on an initially recessive mutation that is more advantageous than its wild-type, dominant, allele†: in time, the originally recessive allele will have become dominant to the concomitantly recessive wild-type allele. This is not an invariable rule, nor is the commonest allele always dominant. The most frequent allele of those determining human blood groups is recessive, and persons homozygous for that allele (blood group Type O) constitute the greatest number of the population.

Many other factors affect intergenic and intragenic

Heterozygous: of a diploid, sexually reproducing organism, possessing different alleles at a given locus on both members of a pair of homologous chromosomes.

†*Allele:* one of the possible variants of a particular gene, only one of which can occupy a given locus at a given time. A gene may have one or many alleles.

relationships, and the interested reader should consult one of the general works included among the references at the end of the Chapter.[9,10,11,22,25,37]

EXTRACHROMOSOMAL INHERITANCE

It is possible for 'genes' to be passed on from a female organism to its young and yet never be located on chromosomes. These factors can be located in cytoplasm of the egg. Mitochondria, Golgi bodies, and, in plants, various plastids, among others, are inherited in this way. In addition, extraneous bodies such as bacteria and viruses are transmitted from mother to offspring not only in the cytoplasm of the egg but in the yolk, in milk in mammals, and in crop milk in pigeons and doves. Although not related to the genome* of the animal in the conventional sense, the genomes of such bacteria and viruses are nevertheless expressed through their hosts, and their presence or absence can have marked effects on production, fecundity, survival, and resistance to epidemic diseases, or have influence in other economically important ways.

Maternal inheritance, as it is also called, gives results similar to the findings associated with sex-linkage when reciprocal tests are performed. Since it at present seems to be uncommon in most animals, with the few exceptions listed above, maternal inheritance should be considered only after exhaustive tests have ruled out normal sex-linkage. (For details see Hutt.[25]) Nevertheless, several cases from the fowl have been reported in issues of *Poultry Science*. As examples, in one case extrachromosomal control of the rate of egg production was involved, and in another the amount of estrogen present in certain double-yolked eggs. It is probable that as techniques for study are refined the list of cases of maternal inheritance will be extended to include both other birds and other characters.

LINKAGE AND MAPPING

Although a number of genes have been identified in several species of birds, none has been assigned to any specific chromosome, with the obvious exception of the X-linked genes. When two or more genes are known to be linked—that is, located on the same chromosome and therefore more likely to be inherited together—a beginning linkage map can be constructed by using methods shown in any genetics textbook. As more and more genes are found to behave as if linked, they will be organized into separate linkage groups, each representing a different autosome. If the cytology of the organism is well known, and minor peculiarities of the structure of the individual chromosomes are

*Genome: a single set of chromosomes, implying the genetic potential therein.

detailed, correlations can be made between visible chromosomal damage or duplication, and the effects of known genes. In this way, once one gene of a linkage group can be cytologically identified with a certain chromosome, the remainder of the linkage group can be assigned linear positions on the same chromosome. This has been done with many *Drosophila* and other dipteran species whose giant salivary gland chromosomes facilitate pictorial mapping. But even in vertebrates as well studied as the house (or laboratory) mouse (*Mus musculus*), only 18 of the 19 possible autosomal linkage groups had been recognized, and, prior to 1964, none had been assigned to an individual autosome.[25] In the fowl, virtually the only bird in which any autosomal linkage groups have been found, at least five are known.[22] With the study of avian karyotypes still in its infancy, it may be some time before any avian genes can be assigned to autosomes. In the meantime, while awaiting the cytologists' progress, we can gather as much information as possible about bird genes and their mode of action.

It is a handy rule of thumb to remember that in sexually dimorphic birds the young of both sexes tend to resemble the female parent, and in sexually monomorphic forms the young tend to have no plumage different from their parents. Early, rapid, and accurate determination of sex by external methods is important in young domestic birds, and laparotomy is often inadvisable or inconclusive. For these reasons, fowl and pigeon breeders have developed "auto-sexing" breeds, or lines having sex-linked genes controlling down feather patterns that on inspection reveal the sex of the chick. (An example of this type in the rock dove is illustrated in Figure 4-4.) Unfortunately, this technique has not yet been extended to many other birds, but careful breeding programs with elaborate screening and mapping procedures should make possible the recognition and fixation of genes of this nature in other breeds and species of birds.

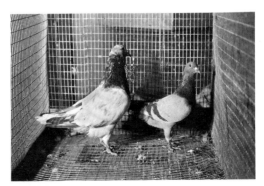

Fig. 4-4. *Rock dove, showing an auto-sexing breed.*

PIGMENTATION

PIGMENTS AND STRUCTURAL COLORS

Birds are rich in colors and color patterns, relying largely on visual as well as vocal communication. A great many variations of normal plumage, many with a genetic basis, have arisen in birds; others are transitory responses to local environmental variables. In any event, before plumage variation in birds is discussed, a brief description of avian pigments and the physical phenomena responsible for the coloration of birds is essential. For greater detail, including chemical structure of the compounds and tests for their presence, see Fox and Vevers,[10] from which this discussion is largely adapted.

The most common bird pigments are the *melanins*. *Eumelanin* is blackish, *phaeomelanin* is brownish, and the more recently named *erythromelanin*[17] is chestnut-red. Birds synthesize melanins, which are deposited as granules in the skin and feathers. The melanins, depending on the amount present, give all shades from light grey and yellow to jet black.

The next most common pigments are the red, orange, and yellow *carotenoids,* giving all shades from pale red, yellow, and orange to the intense colors of South American tanagers (Thraupidae). Many of the numerous avian carotenoids are restricted to certain genera or families. As a class these compounds can be divided into the hydrocarbon *carotenes,* giving red-orange hues, and the oxygen-containing carotene derivatives: *xanthophylls* (yellow and orange) and *carotenoid acids* (red). Carotenoids are deposited in diffuse, non-granular form and, for the most part, cannot be synthesized by birds. They are ingested in plant and some animal foods and are deposited, often unaltered chemically, in feathers and soft parts.

These basic pigments alone, or in conjunction with the physical phenomena discussed in the following paragraphs, can act to produce a startling array of colors, textures, and patterns.

The phenomenon of light scattering, with innumerable small particles scattering incident light in various ways, is responsible for blue of the sky, snow whiteness, blue of bird feathers, and the whiteness of albinism. When the scattered light is blue, it is said to be produced by Tyndall scattering; when white, by "ordinary" scattering. If the particles causing the scattering are smaller in diameter than a wavelength of red or yellow light—about 0.6 micron—they will scatter far more light at the blue/violet end of the spectrum. Since the size of air-borne particles is in this range, the scattered light makes the sky appear blue. In ordinary scattering, the particles are small enough to scat-

ter light, but too large to scatter it differentially; hence all incident light is reflected equally, giving whiteness.

Minute, air-filled cavities within the keratin of the barbs are the Tyndall-scattering agents in birds' feathers. If these cavities are filled with a suitable liquid, the blue color gives way to a dull brown, returning again to blue when the liquid has evaporated. All whiteness in birds is caused by feather barbules—in this case colorless from lack of pigments—which reflect light diffusely from their surfaces. Whiteness of snow is the result of action of the same principle. If a white feather is immersed in a liquid with the same refractive index as keratin, it becomes translucent, the whiteness returning when the feather is removed from the liquid.

However, the colors usually produced by each type of scattering can be modified. If Tyndall scattering occurs in the presence of a yellow carotenoid pigment, the combination will give a green color that is further accentuated by the sensitivity of the human eye to green. Most green color in birds is produced in this way. Olive-green is usually produced by yellow pigments overlying melanin, with no scattering effects, and some of the African touracos (Musophagidae) have one of the few green pigments known in birds, turacoverdin, a porphyrin. Blue or violet in birds is due to Tyndall scattering or interference (see below), with the sole exception of a blue-violet carotenoid in the fruit pigeon, *Ptilinopus.* Purple, not a true spectral color, is usually the result of Tyndall scattering on melanins or carotenoids, but true purple pigments may exist. Ordinary scattering may not produce whiteness if the material responsible for the scattering absorbs certain wavelengths differentially as a result of its own physical nature, but in birds this condition probably rarely exists.

The metallic, scintillating colors seen in hummingbirds (Trochilidae), sunbirds (Nectariniidae), and in peacock (*Pavo*) tails and mallard (*Anas platyrhynchos*) heads are due to *interference phenomena.* The following quotation from Fox and Vevers[10] explains them best:

"The interference of light is responsible for the colours of a soap bubble and of a film of oil on water. White light is reflected from both outer and inner surfaces of the bubble or film, that reflected from the inner surface travelling further. If the distance between the surfaces is such that the optical retardation is an odd number of half wavelengths, part of the spectrum is reduced or cancelled out and we see the sum of the remainder. Since the distance between the surfaces varies in different parts of the film, and in the soap bubble changes with time, there results a play of colours. The colours also vary with the angle from which the object is viewed, since a change of angle alters the path difference between the interfering rays of light."

In bird's feathers interference takes place in the barbules, which are flattened and widened along part of their length and then twisted 90 degrees so that their flat surfaces face the viewer. The two layers causing the interference are the top and bottom of the pigment crystals—usually melanin. In some birds lacking pigment crystals there is occasional iridescence, probably caused by interference between keratin layers of the feather. The exact shade of the iridescent color is, naturally, a function of the underlying pigment.

ABNORMALITIES OF PIGMENTATION

Albinism, used here in its limited sense, is the abnormal total loss of all pigments (in both plumage and body tissue), resulting in an all-white animal with pink eyes and light bill, legs, and feet. In animals with multiple pigment systems, an albino is lacking the alleles for all normally found pigments. The condition can be produced by genes at several different loci, but I know of no case of albinism in birds that is not recessive to normal, or wild-type, coloration. It may be autosomal or sex-linked, both types occurring with about the same frequency. A given population may contain genes for albinism at several different loci, and perplexing ratios might be obtained if two genetically different albinos were bred. All-white plumage associated with dark eyes, or otherwise normal plumage with patches of white, should not be called partial or incomplete albinism, but rather *leucism.*

Abnormal loss of pigmentation is known as either *leucism* or *albinism.* Albinism was considered above. *Complete leucism* is the loss of all pigments (melanic and carotenoid) in the plumage but not in the soft parts. *Partial leucism,* often incorrectly called partial

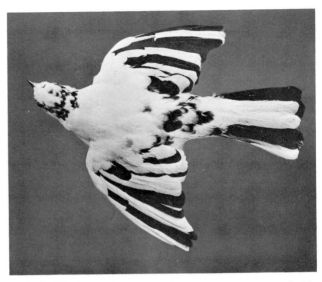

Fig. 4-6. *European blackbird* (Turdus merula)—*remarkably symmetrical, yet "patchy" leucism.* (*Sage, B. L.: Brit. Birds* 55:*201, 1962.*)

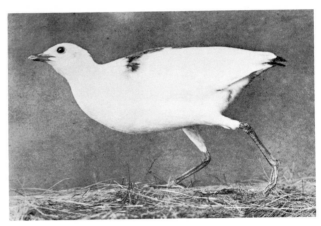

Fig. 4-7. *Corn crake* (Crex crex)—*almost fully leucistic.* (*Sage, B. L.: Brit. Birds* 55:*201, 1962.*)

albinism, is a localized, often symmetrical loss of all pigments in the plumage. *Melanic leucism* is the loss of all melanins but not of carotenoids, when each is normally found in different parts of the plumage. An all-white redpoll (*Acanthis flammea*) with a normal red cap would be a melanic leucino. *Carotenoid leucism* is the loss of all carotenoids but not of melanins, when each is normally found in different parts of the plumage. An otherwise normal redpoll with a white cap would be a carotenoid leucino. Leucism, unlike albinism, is often dominant to normal, or wild-type, coloration, and, since genes at different loci are involved, it is possible for an animal to be leucistic in one part of the plumage and melanistic in another. Such cases are not infrequently observed.[47]

The loss of one pigment (such as a melanin or a

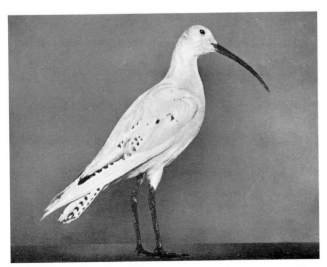

Fig. 4-5. *Eurasian curlew* (Numenius arquata)—*almost fully leucistic.* (*Sage, B. L.: Brit. Birds* 55:*201, 1962.*)

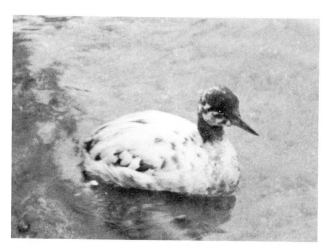

Fig. 4-8. *Red-necked grebe (Podiceps grisgena)—partial leucism of body and wings apparently also associated with dark feathers in the cheeks, normally white all year round. (Sage, B. L.: Brit. Birds 55:202, 1962.)*

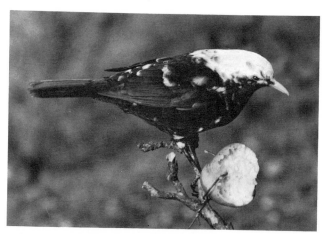

Fig. 4-10. *European blackbird (Turdus merula)—partial leucism, but restricted to the head area. Nine months after this picture was taken white feathers had become so extensive that only the underparts remained largely black, instead of the whole bird. (Sage, B. L.: Brit. Birds 55:201, 1962. Photo by C. W. Teager.)*

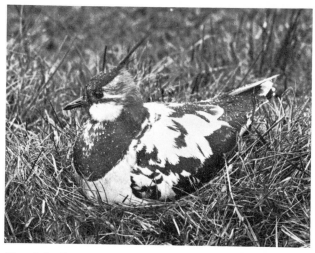

Fig. 4-9. *Eurasian lapwing (Vanellus vanellus)—partial leucism on the wings and back (blotches). (Sage, B. L.: Brit. Birds 55:201, 1962. Photo by Walter E. Higham.)*

carotenoid) in an organism which normally has more than one such pigment located in separate areas, or one overlying another, results in the condition known as *schizochroism*. Since the two more common melanins are each controlled by separate genes, it is possible for birds to lack one or the other in cells that normally have both. This results in melanic-melanic schizochroism, usually called just *melanic schizochroism,* of two forms[15]: *grey variants,** which have lost phaeomelanins, and *fawn variants,* which lack eumelanins. In cardueline finches the grey condition is inherited as an autosomal recessive, the fawn condition as a sex-linked

Grey variants: not to be confused with species normally colored grey, for which other mechanisms are responsible, usually just reduction in the amounts of eumelanin.

recessive. Harrison[17] has recorded more complicated cases of birds which still retained their erythromelanin but exhibited leucism or melanic schizochroism in other areas of their plumage.

In *melano-carotenoid schizochroism,* either melanin or the carotenoid normally found in the same cell is lost, completely unmasking the pigment remaining. In budgerigars loss of melanin yields yellow in normally green birds, and loss of the carotenoid yellow pigment yields blue. (White birds are recessive for loss of both pigments, but having dark eyes are properly considered completely leucistic.) Terms for all the various permutations of pigment schizochroism are so far lacking, most of them being exceedingly rare or unknown.

When melanins replace the carotenoids normally present in some or all parts of the plumage, or are deposited in abnormally increased amounts in areas where the melanins are normally present, the condition is called *melanism.*

Carotenism, an abnormality of carotenoid pigmentation, according to Harrison[16] may result from one of four causes, which may overlap: (*a*) changes in normal distribution of carotenoid pigments; (*b*) increase in amount of pigment, that is, an increase in intensity of color; (*c*) change in the color of the pigment; or (*d*) replacement of melanin by a carotenoid in an area that is normally melanic.

Erythrism is the abnormal replacement of all or almost all eumelanin (and possibly phaeomelanin) by erythromelanin, giving chestnut-red feathers or plumage. Erythrism and partial leucism have been found

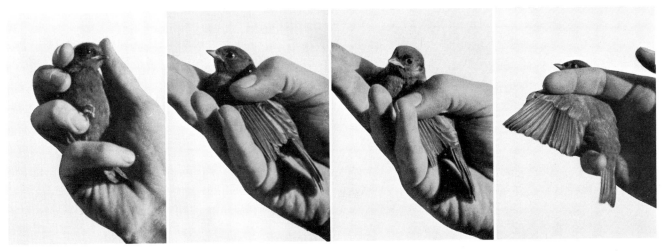

Fig. 4-11. *Great tit* (Parus major)—*melanism in one of eight young similarly colored, out of nine, whose mother was normal and father not seen. Entire bird blackish, even where normally white and yellow. (Sage, B. L.: Brit. Birds 55:201, 1962. Photos by Eric Hosking.)*

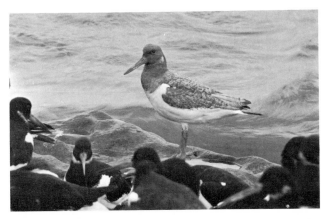

Fig. 4-12. *Eurasian oystercatcher* (Haemotopus ostralegus)—*probably dilution of the entire plumage, although possibly schizochroism with the loss of one melanin over the entire body. (Sage, B. L.: Brit. Birds 55:201, 1962. Photo by Eric Hosking.)*

simultaneously in the so-called "Cory's" least bittern (*Ixobrychus exilis*), a now probably extinct local color phase of this North American heron.[60] Erythrism is not uncommon in other herons (Ardeidae), hawks (Accipitridae), owls (Tytonidae and Strigidae), and nightjars (Caprimulgidae), but is relatively rare in most commonly kept cage birds. Little is known of the inheritance of erythrism, but some evidence suggests that its expression may vary.

Cyanism, an abnormal amount of blue color, can result from melano-carotenoid schizochroism. *Xanthism,* abnormal amounts of yellow-orange, can result from either melano-carotenoid schizochroism or carotenism; depending on its etiology, it may show qualitative differences.

Dilution is an abnormality that is genetically distinct from any of those discussed previously. It denotes an over-all reduction in quantity of all pigments present in the animal, producing a faded appearance but with the original patterns and colors retained. Dilution in zebra finches (*Poephila castanotis*) is incompletely dominant, but whether this is true also in other birds is unknown. It is important, if confusing, to keep in mind that grey and fawn variants—themselves the result of an abnormality, melanic schizochroism—can be further subject to dilution, as result of the action of a dilution gene at another locus.

The foregoing discussion emphasizes that genes at a number of different loci are responsible for these aberrations, and that, although it is unlikely, it is possible for an individual bird to be homozygous for a few or even for several of them.

Often associated with many of the above conditions are other manifestations of physical abnormality, whether the direct result of the same allele (pleiotropism), or of genes linked to those directly controlling color. Partial deafness and blindness, bill and foot deformities, and even lethality and sublethality are often noted in association with plumage changes.[47] Concomitant behavioral changes, other than increased predation of albinos and leucinos, have rarely been investigated, but Keeler[26] found albino doves (*Streptopelia* sp.) had food preferences differing markedly from those of normal birds. Even the casual breeder could easily contribute meaningful data of this sort.

Leucism or melanism can occur normally in the development of individuals of certain strains of domestic birds, disappearing with age. In addition, diet, increased humidity, localized trauma, and other non-genetic factors may cause the appearance of deviant

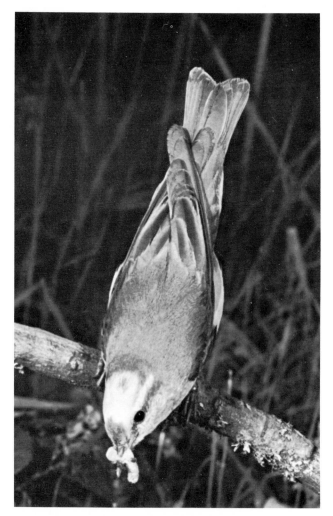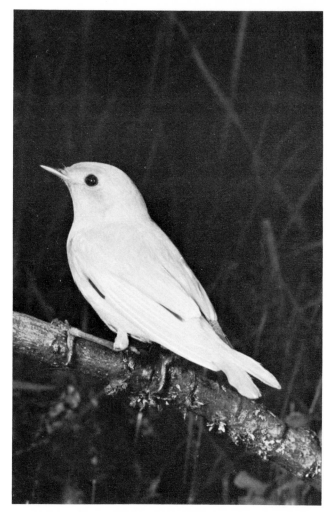

Fig. 4-13. *European wood warblers (Phylloscopus sibilatrix)—xanthism, partial in both sexes (left, male; right, female), but almost complete in the female. Both sexes are normally dull olive drab above and dingy white below. The male shown here is normal except for a straw-colored cap, but the female has a primrose head and back, darker yellow shoulders and upper-tail coverts and white underparts. Her bill and legs are abnormally colored, but not her eyes. The bill, eyes, and legs of the male are unaffected. (Sage, B. L.: Brit. Birds 55:201, 1962. Photos by Eric Hosking.)*

plumages. However, its genotype* will affect the degree to which an animal responds to environmental pressures, and this aspect of the problem should be investigated.

The genetics of plumage characters in wild birds, especially of passerine birds, has been little studied. For the most part data have come from study of a single hybrid or occasionally populations of hybrids, and usually plumage characters are inherited in additive or polygenic† fashion. In a series of papers concerning the rejoining of eastern and western North American populations separated by Pleistocene glaciation, Sibley, Short, and West[50-55,63] have found polygenic inheritance of these characters to be the rule, with hybrids and backcrosses exhibiting the full range of recombinant types from one parental extreme to the other. Yellow wagtail races (*Motacilla flava*) in Eurasia usually inherit head color independently of body color.[38] On the other hand, in the softbill *Zosterops* of South Africa there seems to be some simple dominance in the inheritance of breast color, although the matter is not clear cut.[56] These are only a few examples. Very little work has been done in this area, and the apparently overwhelmingly higher incidence of polygenic versus simple Mendelian inheritance of plumage patterns may be diminished as more data are made available. For a full treatment of the evolu-

Genotype: the actual genetic constitution of an animal, including both Mendelian and non-Mendelian factors.

†*Polygenic inheritance:* the inheritance of a characteristic when controlled jointly by two or more genes (= multifactorial inheritance, quantitative inheritance).

tionary implications of plumage variation, especially the occurrence of other than sexual polymorphisms in nature, see Mayr[37] and Ford.[9]

It should be mentioned that the mature feather is a dead structure, sealed off from the body and receiving no nourishment from it. Therefore, it has been assumed that the fully formed feather can undergo no further change in color, with the obvious exceptions of changes from foxing (fading) due to sunlight, and wear of the tips. However, controversy has arisen over the validity of this assumption, and although some circumstantial evidence has been adduced in support of the opposite view, the occurrence of a change with time in the color or pattern in one mature feather has yet to be documented. Any one believing he has such an example should submit photographic and feather evidence to one of the ornithological or avicultural journals.

BODY ABNORMALITIES

STRUCTURAL AND PHYSIOLOGICAL ABNORMALITIES

Anatomical abnormalities can be either hereditary or ontogenetic (that is, result from abnormal individual development). Since data on each type are meager, and non-existent for most non-game birds commonly kept in captivity, information is necessarily drawn from the scattered literature on pigeons and doves, and domestic fowls.

Too little is known about most reported defects for them to be classified with certainty as hereditary or ontogenetic, especially in the wild, since parentage and even the nesting area of the parent birds are usually unknown. In poultry, however, defects are usually developmental, with obviously heavy selection pressure against hereditary conditions. The bill and feet are most often affected in the birds that survive; because these

are the organs of food procurement, unfavorable alleles are undoubtedly subject to direct, intense selection. An animal unable to eat is also unable to find a mate, breed, and pass on its genes. It is likely that the relative incidence of hereditary defects is lower in wild birds than in domestic birds, for man can often bypass abnormalities that are disadvantageous under wild conditions, and heterozygotes may have economically desirable characteristics.

Several foot disorders are recurrent in domestic birds. In the fowl, splitfoot is an autosomal recessive trait, lethal when homozygous. The foot is cloven and toes are missing. Other mutations cause the absence of varying numbers of toes, and a mutation in turkeys produces a bizarre combination of nakedness and polydactyly. This is the loss of all feathers and scales (embryonically derived from the same type of cell), and presence of an increased number of toes. It is an autosomal recessive, but is different from two others that are often paired—one a sex-linked recessive called naked, and the other an autosomal recessive called scaleless. Sex-linkage and recessiveness characterize wingless, a poultry disorder, and paroxysm, a behavioral condition in fowl marked by tetany and inability to stand or walk normally. In ducks a semilethal autosomal recessive causes head tremors; micromelia (reduced forelimbs) in Japanese quail is another autosomal recessive, lethal when homozygous. So-called silky plumage in doves is an autosomal dominant, and a related condition in fowl—the famous frizzling—is incompletely dominant. These and many more fowl and dove mutations are recorded in the *Journal of Heredity*, Volumes 47 to 54 (1956 to 1963), and by Hutt.[22] Table 4-1 lists known mutations in domestic pigeons, giving a good picture of their distribution, and indicating whether they are dominant or recessive, autosomal or sex-linked. Similar information could be assembled for chickens, ducks, and turkeys.

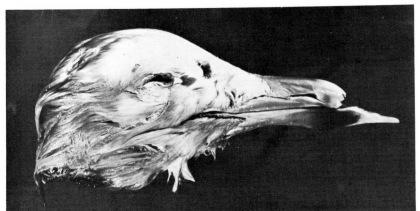 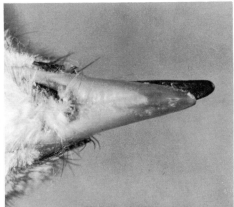

Fig. 4-14. *Bill deformities. (Sage, B. L.: Brit. Birds* 55:*201, 1962.)*

Table 4-1. Genetic Characters*

Phenotype	Factor Symbols	Relation to Normal Blue Pigeon	Found Commonly In	Sex-Linked?
Color:				
Black (solid)	S	Dom.	Many breeds	No
Black blue-tail or black check (T-pattern)	C^T	Dom.	Many breeds	No
Blue checker	C	Dom.	Many breeds	No
Blue barless	c	Rec.	Strassers, swallows, ice pigeons, larks	No
Red (ash)	B^A	Dom.	Many breeds	Yes
Red (solid)	e	Rec.	Many breeds	No
Brown (chocolate)	b	Rec. (Allele of B^A)	Silver kings, etc.	Yes
Silver (true)	d	Rec.	Tumblers, giant homers, etc.	Yes
Yellow	$d\begin{Bmatrix}B^A\\e\end{Bmatrix}$	(Combination)	Carneaux, etc.	Yes
Dun	d, S	(Combination)	Carneaux, etc.	Yes
Khaki and Drab	d, b	(Combination)	Oriental frills	Yes
Grizzle	G	Dom.	Dragoons, etc.	No
Smoky	sy	Rec.	Carriers, barbs, magpies, archangels, etc.	No
Opal ("mosaic")	o	Rec.	Racing homers (rare)	No
Dominant Opal	Od	Dom.	Strassers	No
Almond	St	Dom. (Allele of St^F)	S. F. Tumblers, etc.	Yes
Faded	St^F	Dom. (Allele of St)	Auto-sexing types	Yes
Milky	my	Rec.	Fantails, Lahore	No
Pale	d^P	Rec. (Allele of d)	Light bronze archangels	Yes
Indigo	In	Dom.	Carneaux	No
Pearl eye	tr	Rec.	Tumblers, etc.	No
Albino	al	Rec.	(Rare)	No
Pink-eyed-dilute	pd	Rec.	(Rare)	No
Gazzi	z	Rec.	Many breeds	No
Reduced	r	Rec.	(Rare)	Yes
Structure:				
Crest (any kind)	cr	Rec.	Nuns, etc.	No
Hood	cr and ?	Rec.	Jacobins	No
Frill	....	Rec. (But not simple)	Oriental frills, owls, etc.	Possibly in part
Silky (Lace)	L	Dom.	Fantails	No
Porcupine	p	Rec.	(Rare)	No
Feathered legs (Grouse)	gr	Rec. or partial dom.	Oriental frills, etc.	No
Feathered legs (Slipper)	....	Partial dom.	Pigmy pouters	No
Extra tail feathers	....	Partial dom.	Fantails, etc.	No
Oil Gland (absence)	n	Rec.	Fantails, maltese, etc.	No
Web-foot	w	Rec.	(Rare)	No
Polydactyly	py	Rec.	Kings (rare)	No
Outer toe repeat	t	Rec.	Homers (rare)	No
Scraggly	sc	Rec.	(Rare)	No
Achondroplasia	ac	Rec.	(Rare)	No
Microphthalmia	mi	Rec.	Giant homers (rare)	No
Functional:				
Ataxia	at	Rec.	(Rare)	No
Clumsy	cl	Rec.	(Rare)	No

*From Levi, W. M.: The Pigeon. Sumter, S.C., Levi Publishing Co., Inc., 1957.

In wild birds occasional instances of foot or bill deformities are known, one of the more frequent being a split upper or lower mandible, resulting in malocclusion and overgrowth. Death by starvation or puncture of the throat by the upper mandible usually ensues. Most of the birds that die as the result of such deformities are probably never seen. Bill abnormalities in British waterfowl (Anatidae) have been recorded,[18] the data being obtained from unhatched young at a wildfowl preserve. One of the most common defects found by Harrison and Kear[18] is called short upper beak, occurring by itself or with acrania or meningocele. This beak defect is thought to be identical to a similar condition in fowl, in which it is often associated with micromelia and other skeletal anomalies.[28] It is inducible with insulin in 4–5 day embryos[29]; if insulin is given to 3–4 day embryos, hereditary polydactyly is affected.[30] These data indicate the possibility of both a genetic and an environmental basis for apparently identical abnormalities.

ABNORMALITY OF SIZE AND SEX

Gigantism and dwarfism in birds may occur more often than has been reported. The hereditary basis of each, if similar to that of human stature, would depend on a number of genes. On the other hand, extreme variation in size in some or even all cases may be due to one gene controlling synthesis of pituitary growth hormone, size of the pituitary itself, or the production of an individual enzyme that is necessary for synthesis of the growth hormone. Dwarfism is a sex-linked recessive in fowl, first reported by Hutt.[24] A few cases are known from the wild, involving dwarf ring-necked pheasants (*Phasianus colchicus*)[1] and black-headed gulls (*Larus ridibundus*).[1,21] A giant least sandpiper (*Erolia minutilla*) reportedly was collected on Long Island, N.Y., some years ago by Dr. W. T. Helmuth, but no further data are available.[49] Any cases of gigantism or dwarfism in cage birds should be reported in detail, and such birds should be bred whenever possible.

Mosaicism—the appearance of gonads or patches of plumage normally associated with the opposite sex—is uncommon in birds.[58,64] Not more than a dozen gynanders, as animals with bilateral hermaphroditism, the extreme condition, are called, have been reported. Cardueline finches (bullfinches [*Pyrrhula pyrrhula*], chaffinches [*Fringilla coelebs*]), estrildids (Gouldian finch [*Poephila gouldiae*]), and some woodpeckers and game birds have shown the condition. It usually appears as a left ovary and a right testis in the same bird; the reverse of this has been reported but apparently was

never documented anatomically. Body size and skeletal peculiarities, two criteria of sexual difference in many birds, conform to gonad placement in gynanders. When sex-linked differences in plumage exist they too will reflect externally the placement of the gonads, with one side showing the characteristic male plumage, and the other the female.[64]

At least eight different and not mutually exclusive mechanisms have been proposed to explain the production of gynanders and mosaics.[13,64] None of these mechanisms have been thoroughly investigated cytologically or embryologically, but probably all are known to have occurred at one time or another. They are: (1) loss of one sex chromosome in embryogenesis, (2) double fertilization of an egg with two male pronuclei, (3) non-disjunction of sex chromosomes, (4) triploidy, (5) "bipaternity," with non-degenerate merocytes acting as mosaic grafts, (6) polyspermy with one ovum, (7) development of supernumerary sperm into patches of engrafted tissue, and (8) a mechanism analogous to that which is responsible for the production of a "freemartin" in cattle.

Hereditary hermaphroditism in birds is known only in pigeons, where in one race 80 per cent of the males had a left ovotestis, with complete oviduct and ovocytes, and a right testis with accessory structures.[42] In addition, in certain smaller breeds of domestic fowl there is a dominant gene, often associated with some modifiers, that suppresses male plumage in cocks.[22] Accidental anomalous development might result in a condition resembling true genetic hermaphroditism, and in some breeds of fowl old hens have been reported to undergo sex reversal and begin crowing. However, true sex reversal that cannot be explained by hermaphroditism is apparently still unknown in birds.[59] For a fuller treatment of the subject, see Witschi[64] and Taber.[58]

A variety of systems control secondary sexual characters in birds. Hormonal control (found in fowl and "lower" orders of birds) is evolutionarily more primitive, sexual morphology being the result of a precise but all-too-easily-shifted balance between the medullary (male) and the cortical (female) elements of the gonads, a balance which is often disturbed during development of the individual. In the more advanced and more stable condition (found in the "higher" perching birds such as sparrows [Fringillidae]) sex determination depends only on presence of the sex chromosomes, and cannot be appreciably overridden by hormonal imbalance. Both extremes and conditions intermediate between them have been found in unrelated families of birds, but the distribution of mechanisms determining secondary sexual characters in birds is largely unstudied.[64]

GENETICS AND DISEASE

Little information is available on the relationship between genotype and disease susceptibility in domestic birds other than the fowl, and none at all is available for wild birds. There is, however, literature available[23,40] which deals exclusively with this topic, but mostly in mammals, not birds. Since the late 1950's *Poultry Science* has with increasing frequency included papers on the genetic aspects of disease resistance and control. Most of what follows has been drawn from the three publications referred to; Warren's review paper[62] is also a useful reference.

Any character or trait that can be successfully selected for or against has a genetic basis. The converse of this statement, that inability to successfully select for a character or trait implies no genetic basis, is incorrect. Selection for a gene acts only on the character or trait for which the gene is most directly responsible. For this reason, unless the selective pressure is exerted on the one phenotype that is effected by the gene in question, there will be no change in the condition to be selected for. Once the proper phenotypic "lever" is found, the selection for or against the trait can then proceed apace.

On the basis of the above criteria, a genetic background has been shown to exist for susceptibilities and resistances to a broad spectrum of diseases. Most such traits are not inherited in simple Mendelian fashion, and probably all will eventually be shown to be polygenically determined, even if the actual number of loci cannot be identified. In the domestic fowl, strains susceptible or resistant to heat prostration, slipped tendon (perosis), blue comb (monocytosis), coccidiosis, bacterial white dysentery (pullorum disease), and fowl typhoid, or showing abnormal riboflavin requirements and thiamine metabolism, to name a few characteristics, are already known. Some neurological dysfunctions have a genetic basis. Congenital loco is a simple autosomal recessive, lethal when homozygous. Achondroplasia is incompletely dominant, and the individuals heterozygous for the condition are called creepers because of their peculiar stance and gait.

Differences in susceptibility and resistance depend on many factors other than the direct expression of the genes controlling them. Female fowl, for example, are more likely to develop lymphomatosis than are males, and fowl leukosis is most lethal at the time of hatching. Hutt[23] pointed out one interesting behavioral correlate: males in breeding condition normally fight much more than females, and hence are more liable to scratches and infection resulting from them. Other such differences are correlated with species and genus distinctions. In other words, the expression of a given gene can vary with the different genetic, temporal, and physical environments in which it is placed.

To give an idea of the wide range of characters and conditions in chickens known to be subject to genetic control, the following list was extracted from the index to Volumes 32 to 41 (1952 to 1961) of *Poultry Science:*

ability to taste $FeCl_2$	molt speed and timing
abnormal sex ratios	prenatal death
body and egg size	semen yield
cholesterol levels	shell characters
drug sensitivities	social aggressiveness
early and late breeding	sterility
energy and protein	tumor susceptibility
requirements of chicks	vitamin deficiencies and
growth rates	other metabolic disorders
hereditary French molt	weights of certain glands

This list is by no means exhaustive, and it could be extended from chickens to ducks and turkeys. There the extension would stop, because almost no information is available on small cage birds.

GENETICS AND BEHAVIOR

The field of behavioral genetics is relatively new, with an upsurge of interest and research occurring only since the late 1950's. The only text on the subject is Fuller and Thompson's *Behavior Genetics*,[11] but another book, *Genetics and the Social Behavior of the Dog*,[48] has also appeared. Most of the work has been done with domestic mammals. The index of Fuller and Thompson's book lacks an entry for "birds," although there are three page references for "fowl" and one for "ducks." Work in the Laboratory of Ornithology at Cornell has focused on the inheritance of species-typical behavior in *Agapornis* parrots (the African lovebirds). Most of this work is so far unpublished, but we can make some generalizations from analyses which were made by Dilger, Ficken, Angstadt, and Buckley.

Several *Agapornis* species cut strips of paper which they carry to their nest boxes, where they construct elaborate nests. (See Dilger,[5,7] for a review of the genus and its behavior.) Behavior of hybrids between male *A. roseicollis* and female *A. personata fischeri* has been studied.[2a,2b] *A. roseicollis* carries several strips at a time, tucked in the feathers of the lower back and rump; *fischeri* carries them one at a time in the bill. Both either fly up to the nest box, or walk up the cage sides, depending on motivation. At six months of age, by which time the cutting and tucking habits of birds of the parent species have generally become fixed for life, F_1 hybrids try to tuck the strips in their rumps, as *A. roseicollis* do, but they have lost, probably as a result of the genetic "upset" of hybridization, one of the acts in the tucking sequence that ensures the strip's staying in the feathers. As a result, strips usually fall out as soon as the bird's head is brought forward. Since natural selection would act heavily against any bird whose genotype would not permit normal nest construction, with the consequent death of the young by smothering, we see one example of how interspecific hybrids can be selected against by means other than sterility.

Although in the case of these hybrids it is reasonably certain that the loss of the act in question has a genetic basis, since it occurs in all of them, regardless of the species rearing them, nothing is known of its actual inheritance. We have not been able to obtain offspring from the reciprocal cross (male *fischeri* and female *roseicollis*) to settle the question of sex-linkage or maternal inheritance. In addition, we have been unable to obtain fertile F_2 eggs, which complicates—or rather limits—genetic analysis.

Little work has been done on behavioral changes in birds associated (linked?) with mutations affecting plumage or other aspects of external morphology. As mentioned earlier Keeler[26] found different food preferences in albino doves, but this could very likely have been due to visual difficulties resulting from lack of pigmentation in the albinos' eyes. An albino mutation reported in *Coturnix* quails[32] offers a chance for a similar study early in the history of the strain. Any changes in sexual behavior should also be looked for. Crawford and Smyth[4] investigated social and sexual behavior changes in barred and in white (autosomal recessive) Fayoumi fowl. They found homozygous white hens socially dominant to barred when all were reared together, but, when they were reared separately and put together as adults, the barred hens dominated the white. To the investigators, sexual behavior appeared the same in both the barred and the white type individuals. I suspect that quantitative study of the individual acts that make up sexual behavior would reveal strain differences. An interesting sidelight that emerged from these same studies was the observation that socially dominant females laid more eggs than did their subordinates, a difference that may be of considerable evolutionary significance if it holds true for wild populations of fowl. Crawford and Smyth's study[4] is another in the growing list reporting modification in the phenotypic expression of genotypes by experiential influences, discussed in a later section. Profitable work of this same nature could easily be done with zebra finches, budgerigars, and other common cage birds, whose normal behavior has already been worked out by ethologists.

For more complete reviews of the genetics of behavior in birds and other animals, consult references 2, 11, 43, and 48.

HYBRIDS AND HETEROSIS

When two animals that are homozygous for a single gene locus, one possessing two dominant and the other, two recessive alleles, are crossed, all F_1 individuals are heterozygous for that locus, having received one dominant and one recessive from the respective parents. Whether at one locus, along one chromosome, or in an entire genome, heterozygosity sometimes gives abnormal phenotypes. Where dominance is incomplete, if the character is not "all-or-nothing," the F_1 heterozygote should be intermediate between the two parental types. When the heterozygote is not intermediate but surpasses both parental values for the trait, the animal expresses hybrid vigor, or heterosis, for that trait. The biochemical and genetic mechanisms producing heterosis have been widely debated, the arguments having been presented by Mayr.[37] The phenomenon itself is of considerable practical interest to breeders. Most of the corn grown in the United States today is hybrid corn, showing heterosis for size, color, and other commercially desirable characteristics. Animal breeders, especially poultrymen and cattlemen, have developed special breeds by crossing two lines and then maintaining the heterotic F_1s as a new breed. Often these are four-way crosses by which effort is made to combine in one breed the best qualities of four. However, unlike the situation in plants, in which the heterotic F_1 can be perpetuated indefinitely by vegetative propagation, hybrid vigor is often quickly lost in animals after the first generation hybrid. The original cross must be repeated over and over to replenish the F_1 stock. Some true-breeding cattle strains are obviously not heterozygous at desirable loci, but rather they have inherited from each parent desirable traits that are inherited differently from one another. A true heterozygote will never breed true, the traits always segregating out in the F_2, unless both homozygous conditions are incompatible with life.

There is little evidence of heterosis in non-commercial birds. We are currently looking for heterosis in body size in our *Agapornis* hybrids; we already have evidence that hybrids cut longer strips of nest paper than does either parent,[2a] but more data are desirable. This is one of the few cases of behavioral heterosis known in vertebrates, and is probably the first in birds. In other behavioral characters, such as frequency and duration of courtship displays, and in external morphology, the hybrids are intermediate; they are, however, duskier about the head than either parent.

Generally, if the expression of a behavioral character shows continuous variation in F_1s, F_2s, and backcrosses, the character is probably inherited polygenically. However, Scott and Fuller[48] demonstrated almost continuous variation in behavioral characteristics in dog "hybrids," even though they were able to show that only one or two genes controlled the system. This possibility should be borne in mind in future genetic studies, especially in studies of behavioral characteristics.

Two or more genes probably participate in influencing the inheritance of most traits. Since in the normal course of time particular alleles achieve distinct frequencies in discrete natural populations, some can become fixed in a population at the expense of others that are lost and that arise again in the particular population only through mutation. When genes controlling a bird's plumage pattern are represented by one series of alleles in one population and by another series in another population, it is interesting to observe the product when they are recombined in a mixed mating.

Lorenz et al.[36] described the phenotypes of hybrid turkeys, from male *Meleagris ocellata* × female *M. gallopavo*. Although reporting only briefly and not giving much detail, the authors did show that the hybrids were essentially intermediate between the parent species on all but one point. The voice was described (no audio-spectrograms were presented) as close to or identical with that of the male parent. If these hybrids are easy to obtain, further studies should be made of the inheritance of voice and plumage color in these obviously closely related birds.

In the lovebirds, what we call the "white eye-ringed forms" (*A. personata personata, p. fischeri, p. lilianae,* and *p. nigrigenis*) are races of the same species occurring in different parts of central East Africa. The courtship behavior in the different races varies only quantitatively. Birds of the different races are fully interfertile, and they are otherwise dissimilar only in obvious but evolutionarily minor plumage patterns. Two races (*fischeri* and *lilianae*) lack the dusky heads of the other two (*personata* and *nigrigenis*). Young produced by mating of non-dusky *fischeri* and non-dusky *roseicollis* are invariably dusky about the head, and young *lilianae* are normally quite dusky-headed, losing this coloration in adult plumage. In the *personata* group, and probably in *roseicollis* as well, all members carry some part of the complex of genes that is responsible for dusky-headedness; when such a bird mates with another carrying either another part or more of the same part of the gene complex, the trait is expressed in the offspring.

This sort of "plumage atavism" has been used to throw light on the phylogeny of several groups of birds, on the assumption that primitive or early evolutionary characters of a polygenic nature will often be shown by hybrids. J. M. Harrison and J. G. Harrison[19,20,20a] have noted the remarkable resemblance of a great num-

ber of *Anas* (*sensu lato*) duck hybrids to Baikal teal (*A. formosa*), and have deduced the *formosa* pattern to be, if not ancestral, at least primitive among contemporary *Anas* ducks. Characters appearing in hybrids have also aided workers in reaching a conclusion regarding the probable ancestral plumage of several forms of bullfinch, although the evidence is not as extensive and convincing as it is in the ducks.[19] Because of the potential taxonomic value of such findings, all bird hybrids should be reported in detail in the literature, especially if they are not listed in Gray's *Bird Hybrids*.[14]

If parts of genotypes for ancestral plumages can be reassembled in some hybrids, such birds can also show abnormalities of pigmentation. It is not uncommon to find patches of white feathering (partial leucism) or extreme melanic pigmentation in hybrids for the same reason that causes atavism: disruption of gene complexes, permitting covert recessives and old combinations to express themselves. In our *Agapornis*, excessive hepatic adiposity, a strong tendency to partial or complete defeathering, and sterility or reduced viability are other undesirable effects of hybridization.[2a]

In nature, when separated populations that have not achieved specific status again come in contact, the initially sharp zone of recombinant (hybrid) types will in time blend imperceptibly on either side into the two parental forms, and the actual contact zone may no longer be discernible. Occurring concomitantly with this blending process will be a re-adaptation of reconstituted gene complexes, and a return again to a more steady, undisrupted state.

GENOTYPE-ENVIRONMENT INTERACTIONS

This discussion will consider interactions between the genotype and the animal's experience or environment which may modify the expression of the genotype. In introduction, it should be stated that the following four assumptions, adapted from Dobzhansky,[8] are agreed on by most evolutionary biologists:

(1) almost every trait or character is the product of the interaction of a gene and the environment in which it is expressed;

(2) almost every trait or character is determined in the final analysis by many genes;

(3) probably all genes determine or affect many characters or traits (pleiotropy);

(4) certain genes, called modifiers, change or control the expression of other genes. (Modifiers and other regulatory genes are discussed in more detail, with examples, by Stent[57] and Kettlewell.[27])

Although the complexity of these statements may disturb one's acceptance of the seeming simplicity of the genetic control of various traits or characters mentioned earlier, they present a more realistic picture of actual genetic action and interaction. But the genotype of an individual or even of a population may be so thoroughly coadapted to act in integrated fashion that a great deal of the variability that should follow from the above four assumptions is damped out. This allows "simple Mendelian inheritance," especially in populations that are almost genetically uniform and where all individuals are raised under similar, controlled conditions. Considerations inherent in such a theoretical situation should not disturb the picture of mechanisms probably operating most of the time in the wild.

PLUMAGE COLOR AND ENVIRONMENT

Many cases of effect of diet on plumage are known to aviculturists; only a few will be mentioned. In the course of studies on a flock of newly captured wild redpolls,[6] several were placed in small cages for close observation. They soon lost their red colors, a not uncommon occurrence in cage birds, but since the diet of the birds contained carotenoids it was a surprising one. After one phase of the studies was over, the birds were liberated in large flight cages. In a short time they had regained their color, although they were on the same diet as before. Their color paled again when they were returned to the small cages. Dilger believed that the activity of extended flights in the larger areas allowed return of the normal color. Indeed, this phenomenon has been reported in red crossbills (*Loxia curvirostra*) and other carduelines, and is probably the correct interpretation.

Several other authors[3,41,61] have referred to the deplorable color of flamingos (Phoenicopteridae) in captivity, where they do not have a supply of carotenoids from the planktonic algae that are the mainstay of their natural diet. If they are given "synthetic" sources of carotenoids in brine shrimp and shredded carrots, their natural color returns and remains as long as this type of food is available. The birds possess the genetic mechanism for producing their natural pigmentation, but this system is ineffective when the carotenoids are unavailable. Here the interaction of the environment with the genome is not as subtle as it is in some other cases.

Excessive melanin deposition (not genetic melanism) is easily caused by oily diets.[47] A combination of oily foods and lack of exercise caused temporary melanism in spotted doves (*Streptopelia chinensis*).[12] An oily-food melanism was reported in the weaver finch *Quelea*

quelea, but Lofts[35] was able to reverse it by temporary exposure to ultraviolet radiation during molting. Sage[47] and Rollin[44] treated the subject in greater detail.

DISEASE CONDITIONS AND ENVIRONMENT

Nakedness—a recessive, sex-linked, sublethal condition in fowl—can be completely overcome by raising the chicks at 100°F. instead of the normal 90°. The birds then feather normally, but at a later date. White leghorns are well known for their ability to survive better than other breeds under heat-wave conditions, and selection for "survivability" trait produced most significant results when more frequent drinking in heat was used as the selection "marker." An autosomal dominant causing partly naked fowls can be overcome if the chicks are fed wet mash, instead of the more usual dry mash, on which only normal birds can live. A condition in turkeys called pendulous crop was by chance found to be dependent on the relative humidity of the region where the birds grow up. Hutt[23] discusses these and similar conditions, mostly in fowl. Literature on other than domestic birds is non-existent. Probably the unusual circumstances required for alleviating the conditions caused by these deleterious genes would never arise in the wild, and then selection would rapidly remove the affected animals and lower the frequency of the responsible alleles.

EXPERIENCE AND ENDOCRINE PHYSIOLOGY

The types of hormones secreted by the endocrine glands in different animals vary only little between species and some phylogenetic inferences can be drawn from comparison of the same hormone derived from distantly and closely related animals. The chemistry of these compounds is genetically determined, but the extent of their actions can be remarkably affected by the experiences of the animal. Lehrman[33] studied prolactin, the anterior pituitary hormone that causes lactation in mammals and the secretion of crop milk in pigeons. In ring-necked doves (*Streptopelia risoria*) he found that adult doves without previous experience raising young would not, when injected with prolactin, feed or even approach the squabs. Once they had successfully raised a brood, however, they responded to prolactin injections by caring for young and immediately secreting crop milk. Somehow, the prolactin effected secretion only in birds with the proper experiences. How this happens is unknown, but a similar phenomenon is known in other animals. Rosenblatt and Aronson[45] discovered that the response to androgens by male domestic cats (*Felis catus*) was contingent on prior sexual experience. This interrelationship of endocrine function and experience is being investigated by a number of workers.

EXPERIENCE AND GENETICALLY CONTROLLED BEHAVIOR

In recent years a number of behavior patterns that were long thought to be non-learned have been found to be inherited but still subject to refinement and modification by experiences the animals undergo. This interaction has de-emphasized the old distinction between "innate" and "learned" behavior and has provided a fruitful approach to animal behavior problems that a few years ago were not even known to exist.

The predisposition of most birds to mate only with their own species was long thought to be genetically determined. Indeed it probably is in part, but experience can alter the situation appreciably. If young *Agapornis* parrots are given to a foster species shortly after they have hatched, they will probably become imprinted on the foster species and will be more likely to form mixed pairs and produce hybrid young. In this way we have obtained all our hybrids. The process is facilitated by the proclivity of *Agapornis* to pair with fellow nestlings. Many animal breeders have discovered the same trick and routinely produce unusual mixed matings in this way.

In at least two species it is not as easy to override inherited qualities that keep species apart. Lanyon[31] studied eastern and western meadowlarks (*Sturnella magna* and *S. neglecta*) in an area of sympatry* in Wisconsin. The "primary songs" of the two species sound quite different to the human ear, but one male eastern there had a "bivalent" repertory, singing both eastern and western meadowlark songs. His eastern songs were normal, but his western songs were about halfway between the average frequencies for the two species. Another male eastern, hand-raised and exposed to mostly male westerns when young, also developed a bivalent song repertory. His eastern songs were in the expected frequency range, but his western songs were never as low as a typical male western's. These cases demonstrate the hand-in-glove interaction between learning (ability to sing either meadowlark's song) and genotype (restriction of whatever song learned to certain frequency ranges). Additional cases of learning-

---

Sympatry: in the natural environment, the existence of individuals of one population within the cruising range of any other populations at breeding or pair-formation time. When the sympatric populations are of different species, the geographic potential exists for their interbreeding, but as a result of biological factors such interbreeding fails to occur. *Ant.:* allopatry.

genotype interactions involving vocalizations are known in other species, and the phenomenon is probably not extremely unusual.

Three concluding examples will be taken from our *Agapornis* studies, in part from Dilger[7] and the remainder from unpublished material.[2a,2b] As mentioned earlier, F_1 hybrids between male *A. roseicollis* and female *A. personata fischeri* do not show one of the elements of successful rump-tucking of paper strips. When four to six months old they start out trying to rump-tuck, but they never quite make it. In their attempts to get the strips rearward, they will run backward, as if that would get their head closer to their rump. They tuck in many inappropriate places like the throat and axillary feathers, which are normal tucking locations in the more primitive members of the genus. But, some (not all), left to their own devices and examined after three years had elapsed, showed remarkably changed behavior. They no longer made many abortive rump-tucks; most of their energies were channeled into carrying the strips to the box one at a time in their bills—just like the other parental species (*fischeri*). Although we do know there is some "learning" that successful rump-tucking is impossible, it may be that all hybrids carry *fischeri* genes for bill-carrying, these genes expressing themselves later, but only in the development of some individuals.

Other experiments we have done with *A. roseicollis* have shown another genotype-experience interaction. In one experiment the rump feathers were shaved off and allowed to regrow. Birds that had never been through a nesting cycle before being shaved never became normal in their tucking behavior even when they were allowed to complete several nesting cycles after the feathers had regrown. Birds that had been through five or six nesting cycles before being shaved were of course just as "frustrated" for the period of their featherless condition as the inexperienced birds were, but resumed normal tucking as soon as their feathers were fully regrown, showing little if any lingering effects of the experimental procedure. Birds of intermediate numbers of nesting cycles and degrees of tucking experience showed intermediate effects of their rump-shaving, on the continuum from the condition of no prior cycles completed, to about six or more cycles completed. (However, later, when seven full-sister hybrids of varying ages and experience were rump-shaved, no consistent response was observed.[2b]) It is also noteworthy that young birds of *roseicollis* seem to have a critical period, some time before the age of six months, during which they must have paper to "practice on," or they will never be able to cut normal strips, no matter how long they live or how much they practice afterward. This is another example of the effect of experience on the development of a behavior pattern that is certainly inherited.

Lastly, in their precopulatory behavior, *A. roseicollis* and *A. fischeri* and their hybrids use a display called Switch-sidling.[5] In normal *roseicollis* pairs, about 32 per cent of the precopulatory displays of the males are Switch-sidlings; in *fischeri* the figure is 51 per cent. Male hybrids of the two species paired with female hybrids Switch-sidle about 40 per cent of the time. But when backcrosses were attempted between the male hybrids and female *roseicollis*, the figure quickly fell from 40 to 33 per cent; in the mating of male hybrids with female *fischeri*, it rose to 50 per cent.[7] Obviously, the frequency of this particular display, although it has a genetic basis, is still remarkably dependent on response frequency feedback from the female involved, the result being an admixture of gen-

otype and experience, fortunately resolvable in this case.

ACKNOWLEDGMENTS

Helpful comments and criticism were received from Allan Brush, Francine G. Buckley, Kendall W. Corbin, William C. Dilger, Paul J. Homsher, Ari van Tienhoven, and Bruce Wallace, and I wish to express my thanks to them. Robert B. Angstadt deserves special gratitude for having read the chapter at several stages and having made material improvement on each occasion. The research staff and technical librarian of the R. T. French Company loaned numerous journals and books that proved invaluable. The National Science Foundation grants G-14205, G-5518, and GB-253, which supported the research on *Agapornis* reported here, are gratefully acknowledged.

References

1. ASH, J. S.: Another dwarf pheasant. Bull. Br. Orn. Club *86:*95–96, 1966.

1a. BEÇAK, W., BEÇAK, M. L., NAZARETH, H. R. S., and OHNO, S.: Close karyological kinship between the reptilian suborder Serpentes and the class Aves. Chromosoma *15:*606–617, 1964.

2. BLISS, E. L., ed.: *Roots of Behavior.* New York, Hoeber Medical Books (Harper & Bros.), 1962. 339 pp.

2a. BUCKLEY, P. A.: Disruption of species-typical behavior patterns in F_1 hybrid *Agapornis* parrots. Zeitschr. f. Tierpsych. (In press.)

2b. BUCKLEY, P. A.: A study of the variation in nest material preparation by F_1 hybrid *Agapornis* parrots. Ph.D. thesis, Cornell University, Ithaca, N.Y., 1966. 102 pp.

3. CONWAY, W. G.: A new ration for flamingos. Avic. Mag *65:*108–112, 1959.

4. CRAWFORD, R. D., and SMYTH, J. R., Jr.: Social and sexual behavior as related to plumage pattern in the Fayoumi fowl. Poultry Sci. *43:*1193–1199, 1964.

5. DILGER, W. C.: The comparative ethology of the African parrot genus *Agapornis*. Z. f. Tierpsych. *17:*649–685, 1960.

6. DILGER, W. C.: Agonistic and social behavior of captive Redpolls. Wilson Bull. *72:*114–132, 1960.

7. DILGER, W. C.: Behavior and Genetics. In *Roots of Behavior,* E. L. Bliss, ed. New York, Hoeber Medical Books (Harper & Bros.), 1962. Pp. 35–47.

8. DOBZHANSKY, Th.: Adaptation in Man and Animals A synthesis. In *Genetic Perspectives in Disease Resistance and Susceptibility,* R. H. Osborne, ed. Ann. N.Y. Acad. Sci. *91:*595–818, 1961. Pp. 634–636.

9. FORD, E. B.: *Ecological Genetics.* New York, J. Wiley, 1964. 335 pp.

10. FOX, H. M., and VEVERS, G.: *The Nature of Animal Colours.* London, Sidgwick and Jackson Limited, 1960. 246 pp.

11. FULLER, J. W., and THOMPSON, W. R.: *Behavior Genetics.* New York, Wiley & Sons, 1960. 396 pp.

12. GOODWIN, D.: Temporary melanism in a Spotted Dove. Bull. Br. Orn. Club *77:*3–5, 1957.

13. GOWEN, J. W.: Genetic and Cytologic Foundations for Sex. In *Sex and Internal Secretions,* 3rd ed., W. C. Young, ed. Baltimore, Williams & Wilkins Co., 1961. Vol. 1, pp. 3–75.

14. GRAY, A. P.: *Bird Hybrids; A Checklist with Bibliography.* Commonwealth Agric. Bur., England. 1958. 390 pp.

15. HARRISON, C. J. O.: Grey and fawn variant plumages. Bird Study *10:*219–233, 1963.

16. HARRISON, C. J. O.: Non-melanic, carotenistic and allied variant plumages in birds. Bull. Br. Orn. Club *83:*90–96, 1963.

17. HARRISON, C. J. O.: The chestnut-red melanin in schizochroic plumages. Ibis *107:*106–108, 1965.

18. HARRISON, J. G., and KEAR, J.: Some congenital abnormalities in the beaks and skulls of wildfowl. Vet. Rec. *74:*632–633. 1962.

19. HARRISON, J. M.: On the populations of the Bullfinch, *Pyrrhula pyrrhula* Brisson in Western Europe, and the possible significance of certain aberrant characters in that species. Bull. Br. Orn. Club *78:*9–14, 23–28, 1958.

20. HARRISON, J. M., and HARRISON, J. G.: Albinism and melanism in birds (as illustrated by the Mallard) and their possible significance. Bull. Br. Orn. Club *82:*101–109, 1962.

20a. HARRISON, J. M., and HARRISON, J. G.: A Gadwall with a white neck ring and a review of plumage variants in wildfowl. Bull. Br. Orn. Club *83:*101–108, 1963.

21. HAZELWOOD, A., and HARRISON, J. M.: A note on *Larus "capistratus"* Temminck. Bull. Br. Orn. Club *73:* 98–100, 1953.

22. HUTT, F. B.: *Genetics of the Fowl.* New York, McGraw-Hill, 1949. 590 pp.

23. HUTT, F. B.: *Genetic Resistance to Disease in Domestic Animals.* Ithaca, N.Y., Comstock Publishing Associates, 1958. 198 pp.

24. HUTT, F. B.: Sex-linked dwarfism in the fowl. J. Hered. *50:*209–221, 1959.

25. HUTT, F. B.: *Animal Genetics.* New York, Ronald Press Co., 1964. 546 pp.

26. KEELER, C. E.: Albinism and diet choice in the ring neck dove. J. Hered. *54:*289–291, 1963.

27. KETTLEWELL, H. B. D.: Insect survival and selection for pattern. Science *148:*1290–1296, 1965.

28. LANDAUER, W.: A semi-lethal mutation in fowl affecting length of the upper beak and of the long bones. Genetics *26:*426–439, 1941.

29. LANDAUER, W.: Insulin-induced abnormalities of beak, extremities and eyes in chickens. J. Exp. Zool. *105:* 145–172, 1947.

30. LANDAUER, W.: The phenotypic modification of hereditary polydactylism of fowl by selection and by insulin. Genetics *33:*133–157, 1948.

31. LANYON, W. E.: The comparative biology of the meadowlarks (*Sturnella*) in Wisconsin. Publ. Nuttall Orn. Club *1:*1–67, 1957.

32. LAUBER, J. K.: Sex-linked albinism in the Japanese Quail. Science *146:*948–950, 1964.

33. LEHRMAN, D. S.: The physiological basis of parental feeding behavior in the Ring Dove (*Streptopelia risoria*). Behaviour *7:*241–286, 1955.

34. LEVI, W. M.: *The Pigeon.* 2nd ed., revised. Sumter, S.C., Levi Publ. Co., 1957. 667 pp. (See esp. Genetics, pp. 298–345.)

35. LOFTS, B.: Melanism in captive weaver-finches (*Quelea quelea*). Nature *191:*993–994, 1964.

36. LORENZ, F. W., ASMUNDSON, V. S., and WILSON, N. E.: Turkey hybrids (*Meleagris ocellata* x *Meleagris gallopavo*). J. Hered. *47:*143–146, 1956.

37. MAYR, E.: *Animal Species and Evolution.* Cambridge, Mass., Belknap Press of Harvard University Press, 1963. 797 pp.

38. MILNE, B.: Variation in a population of Yellow Wagtails. Brit. Birds *52:*281–295, 1959.

39. OHNO, S., STENIUS, C., CHRISTIAN, L. C., BEÇAK, W., and BEÇAK, M. L.: Chromosomal uniformity in the avian subclass *Carinatae.* Chromosoma *15:*280–288, 1964.

40. OSBORNE, R. H., ed.: *Genetic Perspectives in Disease Resistance and Susceptibility.* Ann. N.Y. Acad. Sci. *91:*595–818, 1961.

41. POULSEN, H.: Colour feeding of flamingos. Avic. Mag. *66:*48–51, 1960.

42. RIDDLE, O., HOLLANDER, W., and SCHOOLEY, J.: A race of hermaphrodite-producing pigeons. Anat. Rec. *92:*401–423, 1945.

43. ROE, A., and SIMPSON, G. G., eds.: *Behavior and Evolution.* New Haven, Yale University Press, 1958. 557 pp.

44. ROLLIN, N.: Non-hereditary and hereditary abnormal plumage. Bird Research *2:*1–44, 1964.

45. ROSENBLATT, J. S., and ARONSON, L. R.: The influence of experience on the behavioural effects of androgen in prepuberally castrated male cats. Anim. Behav. *6:*171–182, 1958.

46. ROTHFELS, K., ASPDEN, M., and MOLLISON, M.: The W-chromosome of the budgerigar, *Melopsittacus undulatus.* Chromosoma *14:*459–467, 1963.

47. SAGE, B. L.: Albinism and melanism in birds. Brit. Birds *55:*201–225, 1962.

48. SCOTT, J. P., and FULLER, J. L.: *Genetics and the Social Behavior of the Dog.* Chicago, University of Chicago Press, 1965. 468 pp.

49. SEDWITZ, W.: Personal communication.

50. SHORT, L. L., Jr.: Hybridization in the wood warblers *Vermivora pinus* and *V. chrysoptera.* Proc. XIII Int. Orn. Cong., Vol. I, pp. 147–160, 1963.

51. SHORT, L. L., Jr.: Hybridization in the flickers (*Colaptes*) of North America. Bull. Amer. Mus. Nat. Hist. *129:*307–428, 1965.

52. SIBLEY, C. G.: Species formation in the red-eyed towhees of Mexico. Univ. Calif. Publ. Zool. *50:*109–194, 1950.

53. SIBLEY, C. G., and SHORT, L. L., Jr.: Hybridization in the buntings (*Passerina*) of the Great Plains. Auk *76:*443–463, 1959.

54. SIBLEY, C. G., and SHORT, L. L., Jr.: Hybridization in the orioles of the Great Plains. Condor *66:*130–150, 1964.

55. SIBLEY, C. G., and WEST, D. A.: Hybridization in the

red-eyed towhees of Mexico: The eastern plateau populations. Condor *60:*85–104, 1958.

56. SKEAD, C. J., and RANGER, G. A.: A contribution to the biology of the Cape Province White-eyes (*Zosterops*). Ibis *100:*319–333, 1958.

57. STENT, G. S.: The operon: on its third anniversary. Science *144:*816–820, 1964.

58. TABER, E.: Intersexuality in Birds. In *Intersexuality in Vertebrates Including Man,* C. N. Armstrong and A. J. Marshall, eds. New York, Academic Press, 1964. Pp. 285–310.

59. VAN TIENHOVEN, A.: Reproduction in the Domestic Fowl: Physiology of the Female. In *Reproduction in Domestic Animals.* H. H. Cole and P. T. Cupps, eds. New York, Academic Press, 1959. Pp. 305–342.

60. VAN TYNE, J., and BERGER, A.: *Fundamentals of Ornithology.* New York, J. Wiley & Sons, 1959. 624 pp.

61. WACKERNAGEL, H.: Some results with colour feeding of carotenoids in birds at the Basel Zoological Garden. Avic. Mag. *65:*20–21, 1959.

62. WARREN, D. C.: A half century of advances in the genetics and breeding improvement of poultry. Poultry Sci. *37:*3–20, 1958.

63. WEST, D. A.: Hybridization in Grosbeaks (*Pheucticus*) of the Great Plains. Auk *79:*399–424, 1962.

64. WITSCHI, E.: Sex and Secondary Sexual Characters. In *Biology and Comparative Physiology of Birds,* A. J. Marshall, ed. Academic Press, 1961. Vol. 2, pp. 115–168.

Additional References

BERTHOLD, P.: On adherent colors of the plumage. Bull. Br. Orn. Club *87:*89–90, 1967.

BERTHOLD, P.: Uber Haftfarben bei Vögeln: Rostfarbung durch Eisenoxid beim Bartgeier (*Gypaetus barbatus*) und bei anderen Arten. Zool. Jahrb. *93:*507–595, 1967.

DUNMORE, R.: Plumage polymorphism in a feral population of the rock pigeon. Amer. Midl. Nat. *79:*1–7, 1968.

FORD, E. B.: *Genetic Polymorphism.* London, Faber and Faber, 1965. 101 pp.

HARRISON, J. M.: Three Wigeon and Pintail hybrid siblings: a study in "intersexuality." Bull. Br. Orn. Club *87:* 25–33, 1967.

LANCASTER, F. M.: The inheritance of plumage color in the common [= Mallard] duck (*Anas platyrhynchos*). Bibliographica genetica *29:*317–404, 1963.

LEVI, W. M.: *Encyclopedia of Pigeon Breeds.* Jersey City, T. F. H. Publications, Inc., 1965. 790 pp.

NORRIS, R. A.: A preliminary study of avian blood groups, with special reference to Passeriformes. Bull. Tall Timbers Rsch. Sta. *4:*1–71, 1963.

SHARPE, R. S., and JOHNSGARD, P. A.: Inheritance of behavioral characters in F$_2$ Mallard x Pintail (*Anas platyrhynchos* L. x *Anas acuta* L.) hybrids. Behaviour *27:*259–272, 1966.

THORNYCROFT, H. B.: Chromosomal polymorphism in the White-throated Sparrow, *Zonotrichia albicollis*. Science *154:*1571–1572, 1966.

THOMSON, A. L., ed.: A New Dictionary of Birds. New York, McGraw-Hill Book Co., 1964. 928 pp.

VOITKEVICH, A. A.: *The Feathers and Plumages of Birds.* London, Sidgwick and Jackson, 1966. 365 pp.

VÖLKER, O.: Die gelben Mutanten des Rotbauchwürgers (*Laniarius atrococcineus*) und der Gouldamadine (*Chloebia gouldiae*) in biochemischer Sicht. J. f. Orn. *105:*186–189, 1964.

NOTE: This chapter was written in late 1964.

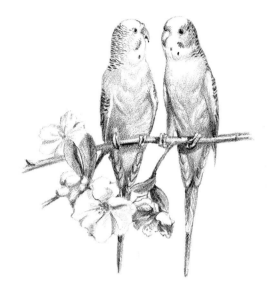

5

Anatomy
of the
Budgerigar

Howard E. Evans

INTRODUCTION

Birds may be characterized anatomically as feathered vertebrates primarily specialized for flight as a means of locomotion. They are more primitive phylogenetically than mammals, and have close affinities with their progenitors, the reptiles. Several of the organ systems of birds are quite different, structurally and functionally, from their counterparts in mammals. The considerable structural diversity found within the Class Aves similarly makes it difficult to generalize among groups, each species having distinctive features. This Chapter is limited to consideration of the specific morphology of the budgerigar, *Melopsittacus undulatus.* The drawings, by Marion Newson, Medical Illustrator in the Department of Anatomy, New York State Veterinary College, were based on 20 budgerigars prepared by various techniques for dissection and illustration.

The generally recognized earliest fossil bird, *Archaeopteryx,* was in most respects reptilian, and it was fortunate that feather impressions were present to indicate the significance of this fossil found in 1861. This specimen, and two similar ones found several years apart in the lithographic limestone of Bavaria, possessed toothed jaws, three clawed digits on each wing, and a long tail of articulating vertebrae which bore feathers along its length.

A fuller appreciation of the behavioral, physiological, and pathological attributes of birds requires examination of their specialized organ systems. Table 5-1, listing by systems some of the principal anatomical features of the bird and mammal, highlights some of the major differences between the two Classes.

Table 5-1. Major Anatomical Differences between Birds and Mammals

Bird	Mammal
INTEGUMENT	
horny beak	no beak
cere	no cere
feathers	hair
sweat glands absent	sweat glands present
uropygial gland present	uropygial gland absent
SKELETON	
light, pneumatic bones	heavy, marrow-filled bones
kinetic skull	akinetic skull
single occipital condyle	double occipital condyles
no cranial sutures	distinct cranial sutures
jaw articulation between quadrate and articular	jaw articulation between dentary and temporal
vertebral regions variously fused	vertebral regions distinct
sternum large and keeled	sternum small and segmental
forelimb with three digits	forelimb usually with more than three digits
fusions of limb bones result in a carpometacarpus, tibiotarsus, and tarsometatarsus	separate carpus and metacarpus, tibia, tarsus, and metatarsus
pelvic symphysis usually absent	pelvic symphysis always present
"wishbone" (clavicles and interclavicle) usually present	"wishbone" never present
coracoid bone large	coracoid bone absent (incorporated into scapula)
phalangeal formula of digits 1 to 4 of pelvic limb is 2-3-4-5	phalangeal formula of digits 1 to 5 is 2-3-3-3-3
ankle joint is intratarsal	functional ankle joint is intertarsal
sacral vertebrae without expanded articular surfaces	sacral vertebrae with expanded articular surfaces
pubis directed caudally	pubis directed cranially
MUSCLES	
pectoral musculature most massive of all	pectoral musculature not largest muscle mass
limb tendons often ossified	limb tendons not ossified
epaxial musculature reduced and of little function	large mass of epaxial musculature of great function in locomotion
DIGESTIVE SYSTEM	
teeth lacking	teeth present
crop usually present	crop absent
stomach in two parts: (a) glandular, (b) grinding	stomach usually single, without grinding portion
colic cecae usually paired or absent	cecum usually single or absent
cloaca always present	cloaca usually absent
UROGENITAL SYSTEM	
elongate kidney with three or more lobes	kidney in one unit, although it may be lobulated
bladder absent	bladder present
penis absent in most	penis always present
all egg laying	only monotremes lay eggs
functional ovary and oviduct only on left side	functional ovary and oviduct on each side
mammary glands absent	mammary glands present
testes internal	testes usually external
female heterogametic	male heterogametic
embryo derives nutrition from yolk	embryo derives nutrition by placental transfer

Table 5-1 (Continued)

Bird	Mammal
RESPIRATORY SYSTEM	
epiglottis absent	epiglottis present
vocal cords absent	vocal cords usually present
thyroid cartilage absent	thyroid cartilage present
tracheal rings complete	tracheal "rings" open dorsally
syrinx present	syrinx absent
small compact lung	large vacuolated lung
slightly expansible lung	greatly expansible lung
anastomosing parabronchi	dead-end alveoli
air sacs present	air sacs lacking
rudimentary diaphragm	strong diaphragm
CIRCULATORY SYSTEM	
aorta derived from right 4th arch	aorta derived from left 4th arch
right and left precavae present	only right precava present
nucleated erythrocytes	non-nucleated erythrocytes
few if any lymph nodes	many lymph nodes
two portal systems (renal and hepatic)	only hepatic portal system
NERVOUS SYSTEM	
cerebral cortex thin	cerebral cortex thick
corpus callosum lacking	corpus callosum present
smooth cerebrum	cerebral gyri and sulci present
optic lobes large	optic lobes small
corpus striatum large	corpus striatum relatively small
small olfactory lobes	large olfactory lobes
EAR	
lack external pinna	have large external pinna
single auditory ossicle: columella	three auditory ossicles: malleus, incus, and stapes
short cochlea	long, coiled cochlea
tympanic membrane convex	tympanic membrane concave
EYE	
bony sclerotic ossicles	no sclerotic ring
ciliary body in contact with lens and by contraction forces it to become round	contraction of ciliary body relaxes fibers which suspend lens, allowing it to become round
pecten present in vitreous chamber	lack pecten
large Harder's glands present	Harder's glands small or absent
nasal glands prominent	nasal glands indistinct

Bibliographic Sources

The literature on avian anatomy appears in diverse journals, proceedings, and transactions. There is no serial publication devoted primarily to the anatomy of birds, although much work is currently being done, and many problems remain.

The most complete classified reference source on birds, including their anatomy, is the four-part Chicago Field Museum publication, *A Bibliography of Birds*,[145] by Ruben M. Strong. This cross-referenced work was published between 1939 and 1959, but all the literature cited appeared before 1940.

In the early part of the 19th century the study of ornithic anatomy was being vigorously pursued in Germany and France. Similar studies soon appeared in England in the Proceedings and Transactions of the Zoological Society of London. The incentive for many of the early studies of comparative anatomy was the need to substantiate or disprove the various taxonomic proposals being advanced.

A publication which is unique in many respects, and which transmits the flavor of the anatomical work and thought of the times, is *A Dictionary of Birds,* by A. Newton,[117] assisted by H. Gadow, published in London from 1893 to 1896. This volume contains concise summaries of many anatomical features and many specific references to morphological works on birds. The 124-page introduction with an index reviews the history of ornithotomy (dissection of birds) as it relates to the various schemes which have been used in the classification of birds. Such features as the presence or absence of the ambiens muscle, aftershaft, cecae, oil gland, or the branching of the carotid arteries have figured prominently in studies performed in the past. This publication is outstanding for its many citations of early anatomical writings and its illustrations of specific morphological features.

Much general information on bird anatomy can be found in standard zoological and veterinary texts, such as Grassé *Traité de Zoologie,*[58] Owen *On the Anatomy of Vertebrates,*[122] Stresemann "Aves," in Kükenthal and Krumbach *Handbuch der Zoologie,*[144] and Ellenberger and Baum *Handbuch der vergleichenden Anatomie der Haustiere.*[38]

Several more recent publications have added greatly to the available anatomical reference material on a variety of birds. Examples include Romanoff *The Avian Embryo,*[132] an anatomicophysiological compendium which includes many references to adult structures and an extensive bibliography, and a two-volume work by twenty contributing authors, *Biology and Comparative Physiology of Birds,* edited by A. J. Marshall.[97] This is the most complete modern treatment of bird structure and function. Each volume has an author and subject index. Darling and Darling's *Bird,*[33] a most readable book by two professional illustrators, contains an entire section of 105 pages devoted to anatomy and physiology and presented in a manner which is both clear and stimulating. The second edition of Sturkie's *Avian Physiology*[146] provides an expanded coverage, with subject additions to the 1954 edition. George and Berger's *Avian Myology*[54] summarizes much current information on the histology, biochemistry, and anatomy of the muscular system of birds.

A series of detailed monographs on the anatomy of the chicken, turkey, duck, coturnix quail, and pigeon are currently in press or preparation by Lucas and Stettenheim, under the sponsorship of the U.S. Department of Agriculture. A chapter on the anatomy of the fowl by Lucas and Stettenheim[90] is included in *Dis-eases of Poultry,* edited by Biester and Schwarte. Other sources of information on anatomy of domestic birds include Kaupp,[78] Chamberlain,[24] Bradley and Grahame,[18] McLeod *et al.,*[93] and Ede.[35]

Anatomical Nomenclature

The description of anatomical structures requires the use of a specialized vocabulary. Vertebrate structures are numerous, and in many instances common names are not available or are so vague as to be meaningless. Early writings in anatomy were almost entirely in Latin, and as a consequence Latin names were applied to most structures and constitute an international glossary. For convenience vernacular terms are often substituted, and in this Chapter "anglicized" terms are used.

Although anatomical terminology has been rather uniform, differences in terms have arisen between different fields of interest and in different countries. The third edition of the *Nomina Anatomica* (1966), prepared by the International Anatomical Nomenclature Committee and approved by the International Congress of Anatomists, includes over 5600 standard terms for man. It is available from the Excerpta Medica Foundation.

A Committee on International Veterinary Anatomical Nomenclature appointed by the World Association of Veterinary Anatomists has recently completed a *Nomina Anatomica Veterinaria for Domestic Animals.* A subcommittee on Avian Nomenclature is currently preparing a list of gross anatomical terms for birds.

It is accepted procedure in anatomical nomenclature to apply the same name to the same structure in different animals even though its appearance may be radically different, so long as there is no question of the homology or similarity in developmental history of the structure. If a structure encountered in a lower animal has no mammalian counterpart, a new term must be coined.

There is still considerable confusion of anatomical terms for avian structures because of uncertain homologies or the lack of corresponding structures in mammals. The present status of muscle terminology poses some serious problems, and most authors find it expedient to list synonymous terms credited to the authors who have figured in the original investigations. Because no standard list was available Fisher[45] chose to use the nomenclature of Howard[63] for bones, of Howell[64,65] for muscles of the shoulder, arm, hip, and thigh, of Shufeldt[138] for muscles of the forearm and hand, and of Hudson[66] for muscles of the shank and foot.

The principles which formed the basis for the establishment of the present international list of anatomical terms (P.N.A.) are:

"(1) As few changes as possible should be made in anatomical nomenclature and well-established and familiar terms should not be altered merely on pedantic or etymological grounds.

"(2) Each structure should be designated by one term only, with a very limited number of exceptions in the form of official alternatives, and each term should be as short and simple as possible and have some informative or descriptive value.

"(3) No attempt should be made to name every minute structure or feature ever discovered and described.

"(4) In general, differentiating adjectives should be arranged as opposites, e.g., major and minor, superficialis and profundus, etc.

"(5) Every term should be in Latin and this form should be used at all international meetings and in all scientific publications with an international circulation, although for national or local meetings and journals, teaching purposes and so on, the terms could be translated into the vernacular equivalents."[71]

Although less than 20 per cent of the terms in the present list are changes from the older B.N.A. nomenclature, several basic differences are apparent. Eponyms were discarded because they are often incorrect by honoring the wrong person, and they vary from country to country. All diphthongs have been eliminated (*e.g., oesophagus* became *esophagus, caecum* became *cecum*), and all hyphens between vowels in the middle of words were omitted (*e.g., infra-orbitalis* became *infraorbitalis*).

General Terms

The longitudinal axis of the body is the vertebral column, with the head at the cranial end and the tail at the caudal end. Structures of the head proper are referred to as anterior or rostral and posterior or caudal in position.

Dorsal refers to the top of the head, and the back of the neck, trunk, and tail. Ventral relates to the under side of the neck, sternum, abdomen, and tail.

The terms proximal and distal are used in reference to the longitudinal axis of the body, thus the distal end of the femur articulates with the proximal end of the tibiotarsus. When using directional terms it is assumed that the bird is in the normal standing position.

The median or sagittal plane passes longitudinally through the body and divides it into right and left halves. A transverse plane is perpendicular to the long axis and divides the body into cranial and caudal

portions or a limb into proximal and distal parts. The frontal plane passes longitudinally through the body and divides it into dorsal and ventral halves.

Tools and Techniques

The structure of a bird can be easily studied with a minimum of equipment and preparation, although many sophisticated techniques are available for special purposes. Most techniques (injection, clearing, reconstruction, etc.) enable one to visualize structures that are too small or too hidden to observe without their use. Some structures can best be seen in a fresh specimen, whereas others are more prominent after preservation.

EUTHANASIA

The standard procedures of an anesthetic overdose with inhaled ether or chloroform or the injection of pentobarbital are suitable for birds. If such agents are not available, illuminating gas for small birds and electric shock for large birds are efficient methods if used with caution. It is not necessary to desanguinate the bird before embalming or injection. Because of the efficient nature of the bird's respiratory system agents administered by inhalation take effect rapidly.

FRESH SPECIMENS

Although freshly killed specimens are preferred for purposes of embalming or preservation, it is also possible to utilize birds that have died of natural causes. One should, if possible, become familiar with the appearance of fresh viscera before proceeding with the study of preserved specimens. The color and consistency of unpreserved organs, blood vessels, and nerves, as well as the ease with which such structures are manipulated and displaced, facilitate their recognition. A helpful procedure at times is the dissection of a fresh specimen while it is held under fluid (saline or water). It may be necessary to change the fluid several times because of leakage of blood, but the visibility of small vessels and nerves is improved and desiccation with consequent distortion of the structures is prevented. When the body cavity is opened under fluid the organs tend to spread apart, facilitating observation and subsequent preservation. An opened specimen pinned to a board and floated upside down in a pan of formalin will harden with the organs extended, and can then be mounted in a museum jar.

The freezing of freshly killed or recently dead birds for subsequent dissection is a practical procedure for many purposes, but it has its limitations. Such a specimen when thawed will be similar in condition to the recently killed animal except that the blood will be clotted and it will not be possible to inject the vessels. The frozen specimen can be cut with a band saw in various planes and placed in preservative to thaw. This procedure will produce excellent permanent specimens for the study of deep organs or of internal topography. Advantages offered by the frozen specimen are the options, after dissection, of preservation of soft parts, skinning and mounting of a study skin, or the preparation of a skeleton.

PRESERVATION

Although many chemicals or combinations of chemicals have been used for preserving animal tissues, the chemical of choice for preserving specimens for purposes of dissection is 5% to 10% formalin. If formalin is not available one can substitute 70% ethyl alcohol, 50% isopropyl alcohol, rum, or bourbon. Small birds such as the budgerigar or canary can be preserved by opening the body cavity and immersing the entire specimen in formalin, by injecting the formalin into the body cavity, or most efficiently by embalming via an artery. The purpose of injecting formalin into an artery is to ensure immediate preservation in all parts of the body rather than relying on diffusion of the preservative fluid through the tissues. Tracheal injection is often sufficient for adequate preservation since the extensive network of air spaces and sacs is in close relation to the viscera. The brain, protected by a tight-fitting skull, will not be sufficiently preserved unless an arterial injection is made or the cranial cavity is opened.

For the injection of the arterial system it is most convenient to reflect the skin of the throat to expose the common carotid arteries as they emerge from the mid-ventral neck muscles (Fig. 5-1). Care must be taken not to rupture the large, thin-walled jugular veins which are located superficially at either side of the neck. Either carotid artery may be injected, and this is best accomplished by using a 26-gauge, $\frac{1}{4}$-inch cutting-tip needle under a dissecting microscope. The needle tip is used for entry into the vessel and is directed toward the heart. Since the 26-gauge needle fills the lumen of the budgerigar's carotid artery so completely, it is not necessary to tie a ligature around this small vessel. For ease of injection the anesthetized bird can be positioned over the back of the hand so that the neck passes over the index finger and the head can be depressed into the palm of the hand by the thumb. This allows the carotid artery to be tensed for insertion of the needle and permits a straight line approach toward the heart. It may be advisable, for

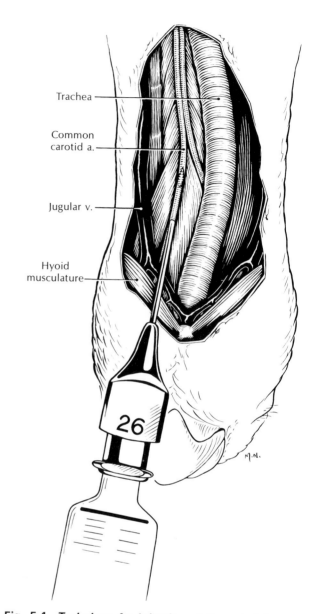

Trachea

Common carotid a.

Jugular v.

Hyoid musculature

Fig. 5-1. *Technique for injection of the arterial system.*

better visibility, to free the artery from its associated muscles by means of a pointed forceps.

A most satisfactory injection instrument is a disposable 2.5 or 3 ml. rubber-plungered syringe. A glass-plungered syringe is satisfactory for injection of formalin but not of latex, which tends to stick in such a syringe. The small plastic disposable syringes are so light and maneuverable that they are ideally suited for small birds. One consideration is the injection medium being used. Liquid rubber (latex) is thicker than embalming fluid, and even after being filtered through cheesecloth it is difficult to aspirate through a 26-gauge needle. This problem can be obviated by removing the needle when filling the syringe or by removing the plunger and filling the syringe with a dropper. Liquid latex is miscible with water prior to the polymerization or setting. Ammonium hydroxide inhibits setting, whereas acetic acid promotes it. While using latex for injection it is advisable to constantly rinse the needle tip and flush the emptied syringe in cold water.

By observing the filling of the contralateral common carotid artery and surrounding cervical vessels one can see the effects of the injection. The amount of material injected will vary with the size of the bird and the patency of the vessels. Only experience with the back-pressure and turgidity of the specimen will indicate when an adequate injection has been made. A budgerigar will require about 1.5 ml. of latex, whereas a large parrot may require 30 ml.

If visualization of the smallest blood vessels is important, it may be advisable to use a suspension of mercuric oxide or India ink, neither of which hardens in the vessels. Various plastics have been used for injection purposes and may be colored as desired. Since they are usually not water-miscible it is necessary to flush the vessels with a solvent such as acetone to prevent clotting and assure a complete injection. Acetate and polystyrene solutions form rigid casts which are ideally suited for subsequent corrosion with acids or alkalis, maceration in water, or preparation with beetle larvae. Other rigid or semi-rigid injection materials include Wood's metal, wax, silicone rubber, and glue. For a discussion of injection techniques and materials see Edwards and Edwards[36] or Tompsett.[152]

The respiratory passageways, lungs, and air sacs can best be studied after injection of latex or Vinylite into the trachea of an unembalmed bird. A ligature should be tied on the trachea after removal of the injection cannula, to prevent backflow. Since the volume of the air sacs is considerable, the latex will harden slowly, and several days should elapse before dissection or corrosion is attempted. During this time the specimen can be kept in a cooler or immersed in alcohol or formalin.

PREPARATION OF STUDY SKINS

The preservation of the skin with its plumage and appendages is of prime importance to museums and research institutions concerned with birds. Although a "mounted" bird implies a stuffed specimen in a life-like position, the great majority of research specimens are prepared as cotton-filled "study skins" in a manner that is standard all over the world. A study skin is prepared by opening the bird along the mid-ventral line to expose the body, severing the pelvic limb at the knee, the tail at the pygostyle, and the wing at the shoulder. The body is removed by turning the skin inside out. This exposes the skull, which allows the

eyelids to be freed from the orbits for removal of the eyes. The posterior portion of the skull is removed with the neck, allowing for removal of the brain and tongue. The attached but everted humerus and femur are scraped to remove the muscles, dusted with borax and naphthalene (or a similar drying and insect-repelling substance), and wrapped with cotton to replace the muscle mass. Various techniques are employed to keep the feathers clean, remove dirt and grease, and preserve the external contours. The skin is stuffed with cotton to approximate natural size, strengthened within the neck by a wire, and stitched along the line of the incision. It is then dried in an extended position with the limbs directed caudally, the wings close to the body, and the beak closed. The eyes appear white since the cotton stuffing can be seen through the open eyelids. If at a later date a mounted specimen in life-like pose is desired, the study skin can be relaxed in a humid chamber and remounted with the addition of some internal wires and glass eyes. A well-illustrated account of methods of skinning and mounting birds appears in Anderson.[5] Museum preparation methods and taxidermy procedures are best described by Rowley.[133] A newer method,[102] still in an experimental stage, eliminates the need for skinning and removal of the body. It involves posing the body by freezing the joints with liquid nitrogen and freeze-drying the entire animal. One advantage of the latter technique is the availability of the skeleton and viscera for study later if desired.

SKELETAL PREPARATION

There are several ways of preparing the skeleton of a bird for study, but the most satisfactory method involves the use of dermestid beetles. Bird bones are delicate and require more gentle treatment than do mammal bones of comparable size. With a properly managed dermestid beetle box (Fig. 5-2) one can process several bird skeletons per week. Dermestid beetles (*Dermestes* and *Attagenus* species), otherwise known as leather, museum, or carpet beetles, will not eat moist flesh but thrive on dry animal products. Since the adult beetles can fly they quickly find suitable sites to lay their eggs, and one can utilize this characteristic by placing a dried carcass on a barn rafter or in an attic to start a colony. Once secured, the beetles will go through their life cycle in a container, so long as they are kept dry and are supplied with dried carcasses. The growing larvae are the most active eaters and are largely responsible for the skeletonizing activity. Care must be taken to prevent escapees from becoming serious house pests in rugs and leather or serious laboratory pests in dried skins, feathers, or dried organs.

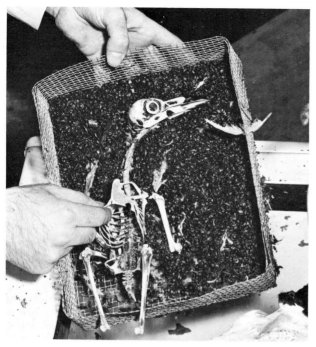

Fig. 5-2. *Skeleton of crow being removed from a dermestid beetle box.*

To prepare a fresh bird for the beetles it should be skinned, eviscerated, and dried in a fly-free environment. Use of a heat lamp and fan speeds the process. With large birds it is advisable to remove the brain from the skull, pierce the eyeball to release the fluid (without injuring the sclerotic ring), and remove the breast and leg muscles. The bird may be posed in a natural position prior to drying by pinning it to a perch and using Styrofoam or cardboard to hold it in place. It is much easier to position the skeleton while it is fresh than it is to moisten and reset all of the joints after the skeleton is removed from the beetle culture. The longer a specimen remains in the culture the more disarticulated it will become, since the beetles attack the ligaments after the flesh is gone. The proper time for removal depends on the larval population, and only by frequent inspection can one determine when the specimen should be turned or removed. On removal from the beetle box the skeleton should be placed in a metal pan under a heat lamp, to drive all larvae out of the interstices of the bones. Failure to do this before immersion of the skeleton in a degreaser (solvent or carbon tetrachloride) or a bleach (hydrogen peroxide) will result in unsightly dead larvae trapped within the bones. Almost all museums and other institutions requiring skeletal preparations of small vertebrates practice dermestid beetle husbandry, and they are usually quite willing to provide one with a starter culture.

Other methods of skeletal preparation include maceration in water, soaking in alkali or ammonia, simmering in detergent, and pressure cooking. For a discussion of these methods, see *How To Make Skeletons,* Turtox Service Leaflet number 9,* or Ward's Service Bulletin number 1.†

The best method of preparing bodies of small birds, especially those of nestlings, is by clearing in 2% potassium hydroxide until translucent, staining the bones with Alizarine red S and clearing in glycerin.[42] This method, combined with vascular or respiratory-tract injections, allows for the visualization of organs in situ. Such preparations, known as clearings, are the most illuminating anatomical preparations because under the dissecting microscope organs, bones, blood vessels, and nerves can be seen and manipulated.

EXTERNAL TOPOGRAPHY AND BODY FORM

EXTERNAL TOPOGRAPHY

The major regions of the body are the head, neck, trunk, and tail. Various body regions have characteristic feathers or markings, and are known by standardized terms since they are indispensable for descriptive purposes. Most ornithological manuals and bird guides illustrate or describe how topographical information is used (see, for example, Friedmann *The Birds of North and Middle America*[49]).

Descriptions and illustrations of regional surface areas based on underlying structures (topographic anatomy) are provided by Komarék[81] and also by Lucas and Stettenheim.[91] Since these regions often have no visible boundaries, the interpretations of various authors and the nomenclature they use will vary. In the living bird, surface reference points so necessary for surgical or experimental procedures may be established by palpation or radiography of the underlying bony structures.

BODY FORM

The head of the budgerigar is nearly spherical and is completely feathered except for a small patch beneath the chin. The eyelid forms a ring around the protruding eye and bears bristle-like lashes. Behind and below the level of the eye is the circular opening of the external auditory meatus, which is covered by feathers and thus hidden from view.

The bill, or beak, is short, broad, hooked, and sharp-pointed. It is hinged at the fronto-nasal suture, and in

*Obtainable from General Biol. Supply House, 8200 S. Hoyne Avenue, Chicago, Ill. 60620.

†Obtainable from Ward's Natural Science Establishment, Inc., P.O. Box 1712. Rochester, N.Y. 14603.

profile it forms a quarter of the circumference of the head. The lower jaw is not visible, due to feathering. It is horseshoe-shaped, fits within the upper jaws, is loosely articulated, and is capable of being opened widely.

The nostrils lie at the base of the bill, enclosed in the soft protruding cere. The color of the cere in the normal adult bird is blue in the male and pink or brown in the female.

The body is short and broad with a straight back line and a deep breast. In the normal perching position the longitudinal axis of the body is held at a 45-degree angle to the ground. Since the sternum is large and extends caudally almost to the pubis, there is very little ventral abdominal wall.

The tail, or uropygium, is the shortened, swollen, and movable terminal portion of the longitudinal axis. It bears the long, pointed tail feathers and oil (uropygial) gland dorsally and the cloacal opening ventrally. Its internal support consists of articulated caudal vertebrae and the blade-like pygostyle. Several overlapping muscle fascicles associated with the tail originate on the pelvis or basal caudal vertebrae and insert on the pygostyle.

The wings are long and the tips of the primary feathers are held over the rump. In the normal perching position (see Fig. 5-6) the humerus, radius, and ulna are held parallel to the line of the back. The distal portion of the wing skeleton (carpometacarpus and digits) is held at a 45-degree angle to the forearm (radius-ulna). The large flight feathers which originate on the distal portion of the wing are directed caudo-dorsally and cross the line of the back at a 45-degree angle.

The legs, when the bird is perching, are held in a flexed position, with the femur and tarsometatarsus parallel to the ground. The flexion angle of the hip joint is approximately 45 degrees, knee joint 75 degrees, and tarsometatarsal joint 45 degrees. This crouched position is in contrast to the more erect posture of many other birds. To grasp the perch the budgerigar uses the second and third toes around the front, to oppose the first and fourth toes around the back of the perch. The third toe is the longest, and each of the four digits bears a sharp claw.

STRUCTURES OF BODY

Integument

The skin or integument of birds consists, as in mammals, of an outer thin epidermis and an underlying thicker dermis. In brooding birds the dermis may thicken and vascularize to form an incubation patch. Subcutaneous fat is common in rather specific loca-

tions beneath the dermis in each species. Over most parts of the body the skin is thin, loosely attached, dry, and quite inelastic. Delicate dermal muscles originate and insert on feather follicles and provide a mechanism for puckering the skin and ruffling the feathers. These smooth muscles crisscrossing in a network act synergistically on neighboring feathers. In several locations there are also dermo-osseus muscles which originate on bones and insert on the skin. Since such muscles have a fixed origin they are capable of pulling the skin or body part toward the site of their origin with considerable force, thus erecting a crest or raising the hackles.

The epidermis gives rise to many structures which we commonly speak of as integumental derivatives. Such structures include feathers, glands, scales, beak, cere, claws, spurs, wattles, combs, and ear lobes. Sengel[137] and Rawles[130] investigated the mutual influences between the epidermis and dermis in the organization of feather tracts and gradients of morphological characteristics.

Beak

The beak, or bill, is a keratinized covering of the jaws common to turtles and birds. It grows constantly in the budgerigar and is worn down accordingly by feeding, grooming, climbing, and purposeful rubbing on parts of the cage or a cuttlefish bone. The size and shape of the beak vary greatly in birds and are correlated with feeding habits. The cutting edges, or tomia, may be serrate, ridged, or smooth. Probably no other organ of the bird exhibits such diverse structural modifications as does the horny beak.

In parrots the upper beak is massive and curved, whereas the lower is small and horseshoe-shaped. The upper beak of the budgerigar is sharp-tipped and closes over the lower beak, hiding most of the latter from view. At the base of the upper beak is the soft, tumescent cere through which the nostrils open. Both the upper and lower beak act as extensions of the jaws. The tips of each are composed of thicker horn, which often remains (Fig. 5-8 B) even after skeletal preparation by dermestid beetles has eliminated other nonmineralized tissues.

Feathers

The characteristic feature of birds shared by no other vertebrate is the presence of feathers. These epidermal structures are similar in derivation to reptilian and mammalian scales. In some species of birds the appearance of feathers on the legs between the scales or on the edge of a scale indicates the similarity of these two types of keratinized epidermis. Rawles[130] performed some interesting experiments which shed new light on the relationship between scales and feathers. The method involved exchanging tissue separated from prospective feathered and scaled regions at various developmental stages. The observations suggested that the prospective skin of the foot, unlike that of other body regions, is capable of giving rise to either or both feathers and scales.

Feathers function as efficient insulators to maintain the high body temperature (105–109°F.) of birds. They also serve in courtship and aggressive displays, nest building activities, and most importantly for flight. Structurally they are complex, light in weight, and of high tensile strength. A fully formed feather is not capable of further growth. It may be modified as a consequence of wear or use or of mechanical manipulation by the bird.

Chandler,[25] in his detailed study of the structure of feathers, reviewed the history of feather studies and discussed the general morphology of feathers. The focus of this work was on the significance of feather structure in the taxonomic classification of birds. Although many Orders of birds were considered, the parrots were not included.

For purposes of orientation, when speaking of a feather or any of its structures, the terms "dorsal" and "ventral" are used relative to the feather itself regardless of the position of the bird. The dorsal surface is the external or exposed surface of the feather, directed away from the body of the bird.

TYPES OF FEATHERS

Three main types of feathers are distinguished: (1) the contour feather, or penna; (2) the plumule, or down feather; and (3) the filoplume, or tufted bristle.

CONTOUR FEATHERS. Contour feathers are so named because they sheathe the body, wings, and tail, and are thus responsible for the external appearance of the adult bird. They are fairly constant in number for each region.

The axis of the feather is the shaft. The bare portion of the shaft, closest to the body, is the calamus, or quill, which is a hollow cylinder filled with cellular pith. At the base of the calamus is an opening, the inferior umbilicus, through which a mesodermal papilla extends during development of the feather. At the upper end the calamus merges with the rachis, as the shaft of the expanded portion of the feather, the vane or vexillum, is known. A small opening, known as the superior umbilicus, or umbilical pit, is present on the under side of the feather at the junction of the calamus and rachis, and in some feathers a small secondary axis, or aftershaft, arises at this spot.

A shallow furrow extends from the superior umbilicus distally along the ventral surface of the shaft. From each side of the shaft, at a 45-degree angle, extend the closely arranged barbs. At the base of a contour feather the lowermost barbs appear fluffy or plumulaceous, but higher up the barbs appear to form a continuous sheet, or vane. Close inspection shows that barbules arise on each side of the barbs, and by a system of hooks and notches the barbules of adjacent barbs interlock. In life, a disruption of this interlocking arrangement, with "splitting" of the vane, can be repaired by pulling the vane through the beak in a direction parallel to the barbs. This function is performed by the bird when "preening." In the ostrich there is little development of the barbule hooks, and thus the contour feathers appear as fluffy plumes.

PLUMULES. The plumule, or down feather, lacks a shaft beyond the calamus or has a very short shaft. It consists of slender barbs and filamentous barbules which do not interlock. These feathers form the covering of a nestling and underlie the contour feathers of the adult. They may be distributed over the whole body, in both the apteria and pterylae, be confined to either, or be absent entirely.

FILOPLUMES. The filoplumes are hairlike, degenerate feathers consisting of a slender shaft or several shafts terminating in a tiny tuft of barbs. They are always associated with contour feather follicles. Further modifications of a feather may result in a shaft lacking barbs so that the feather appears as a bristle. Such bristles are commonly present on the head and neck; more rarely, as in the budgerigar, the eyelashes on the lids are of this type.

WING FEATHERS

The wing skeleton and its associated muscles, blood vessels, and nerves are covered by a thin skin, clothed with feathers. Connecting the shoulder with the wrist across the flexor surface of the elbow is a web of skin called the prepatagium. Tensing this membrane is the function of the tensor patagii longus and brevis muscles. A similar skin web, the postpatagium, stretches between the body and the elbow. On the trailing edge of the wing are the large flight feathers, or remiges, whose quills are firmly anchored in deep follicles which overlie the forearm and digits. Those attached to the hand or pinion (carpometacarpus and digits) are the primaries, and those overlying the ulna are the secondaries (Fig. 5-3). Feathers that lie over the elbow or humerus are called tertiaries, those above the shoulder are the scapulars, and those between the shoulders are the interscapulars.

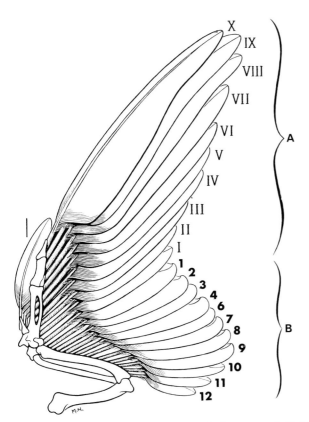

Fig. 5-3. *Ventral view of the wing skeleton, and flight feathers. Note absence of fifth secondary. A, Primaries, or pinion feathers. B, Secondaries, or cubital feathers.*

The numbering of the remiges begins at the carpus and proceeds distally for the primaries and proximally for the secondaries. Depending on the species, there may be from 9 to 16 primaries and 6 to 40 secondaries. The budgerigar has 10 primaries, numbered I to X, and 11 secondaries, numbered 1 to 12, with the 5th missing. This condition of a missing 5th secondary feather is characteristic of several families of long-winged birds, and is known as a diastataxic, or aquincubital, condition. When the 5th secondary is present the condition is called eutaxic, or quincubital. In the budgerigar the space between the 4th and 6th secondaries differs little from that between other adjacent secondaries. Some authors believe a loss of the 5th feather has occurred whereas other believe a shifting of feather rows has taken place. Steiner[142] discussed the ontogeny of the condition, and Miller[105] has tabulated the distribution of eutaxic and diastataxic birds by Family.

On both upper and lower surfaces of the wing there are overlapping contour feathers, or coverts, which complete the flight surface. The caudo-dorsal coverts in particular are linked with their adjacent remiges by interlacing smooth muscle bundles and delicate connective tissue strands which are visible as soon as the skin is removed. Such an arrangement ensures the synergistic action of neighboring feathers.

Attached to the rudimentary 2nd digit (1st digit, or thumb, according to some authors) of the budgerigar are four contour feathers (alulars) constituting the alula, or ala spuria (spurious wing). In most birds there are three or four feathers in the alula, but there may be as many as six or as few as two.

TAIL FEATHERS

Attached to the swollen uropygium are the tail feathers, or rectrices, which are bilaterally paired. Although there may be 4 to 10 pairs of rectrices in birds, the usual number is 6 pairs, as in the budgerigar (see Fig. 5-4 A). The tail is capable of considerable move-

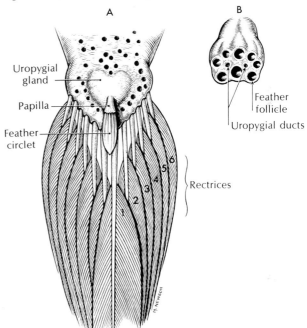

Fig. 5-4. *A. Dorsal view of the uropygium, partially plucked. B. Enlarged view of uropygial papilla, showing uropygial ducts and follicles of feather circlet.*

ment, owing to the freely articulating caudal vertebrae and their associated muscles. It is used as a rudder in flight, as an air brake when landing, and for balance when climbing. Elevation of the tail tends to raise the cloaca and aids in defecation as well as in copulation. The 12 rectrices are strongly attached to the pygostyle and are interconnected basally by fibrous tissue and dermal muscles. Above and below the rectrices are tail coverts, filling out the contour.

PIGMENTATION OF FEATHERS

The color of the plumage may be due to pigments or to structural colors caused by cell or oil layers which diffract light and result in iridescent hues. Pigments include carotenoids or lipochromes which are fat-soluble and usually produce red, orange, and yellow; melanins which are rather insoluble and produce black, gray, and brown; and a rare green pigment, turacoverdin, in the Musophagidae. For a discussion of pigments and structural colors see Mason[18] and Fox.[47] The color pattern of feathers can be altered by hormone treatment. According to Chandler,[25] the delicate blue-green color of the budgerigar results from a blue refraction color in the barbs, coupled with a greenish-yellow pigment in the barbules. Portmann[125] noted that the uniform dark gray wavy pattern of the whole head in the young budgerigar changes at maturity, as the immature feathers are shed, into the vivid black markings of the face and clear yellow of the forehead.

Rawles[131] has described and illustrated the development of a feather and the succession of feather types. This description of feather development is based on her studies. Each feather papilla produces a succession of plumage types (down, juvenile, adult) via an interaction of the dermal papilla and the epidermis. The feather germ of a down feather first appears on the surface of the skin as a slight papilla which elongates to form an epidermal cylinder enclosing a dermal pulp richly supplied with blood vessels. The epidermal cylinder sinks into the skin to form a follicle with a basal collar surrounding the dermal papilla. There are three layers forming the walls of the epidermal cylinder: an outer protective sheath, a middle layer which forms the barbs, and an inner layer which surrounds the pulp. When the outer sheath ruptures and falls off, the barbs are released and when dry they have a fluffy appearance.

From deep within the feather follicle formed originally by the down feather, a contour feather will be produced by a thickening of the epidermal cells surrounding and covering the dermal papilla. The collar of cells thus formed elongates as an epidermal cylinder filled with the growing mesodermal core. The dorsal wall of the growing cyclinder elongates faster than the remaining portion of the collar and forms the rachis, or shaft. On both sides of the growing shaft, barb-ridges form; as shaft growth proceeds additional barb-ridges are added from the collar until the definitive length of the feather is reached. The feather tip therefore has the oldest, or first-formed, barbs. The fluffy basal portions of a contour feather are the last portions to be formed. Prior to rupture of the outer protective sheath the closely packed structure which emerges from the feather follicle is known as a pin feather. It has a turgid pulpy core filled with blood vessels and pigment granules.

Lafeber[83] found that down feathers begin to cover the skin of a nestling budgerigar on about the 12th day, and pin feathers are $\frac{1}{4}$ to $\frac{1}{2}$ inch long on the head, wings, and tail at 17 days. The plumage is complete at about one month of age.

The juvenile feathers which replace the down are of the contour type. They are softer, have fewer barbs, and are more fluffy at the base than are the adult definitive feathers. Usually there are several changes of juvenile feathers before the adult contour and color pattern is attained. A feather papilla located within a feather follicle produces succeeding generations of feathers throughout life. Feathers are shed or molted either at regular intervals or continuously at a predetermined rate or at a certain stage of the follicle. Watson[162] found that during natural juvenile feather replacement in many birds the loss of the old feather is brought about by the growth of the new feather. This is in contradiction to the theory that, except for the first molt of the natal down, the natural molt is a two-part process entailing passive loss of old feathers and subsequent growth of new feathers.

ARRANGEMENT OF FEATHERS, OR PTERYLOSIS

Feathers develop in rows or tracts, called pterylae, or "feather forests," by Nitzsch, their arrangement, known as pterylosis, being characteristic for each species. Study of the number and arrangement of feathers is known as pterylography. Sites of these tracts can be easily observed on a nestling or plucked bird. The intervening spaces, known as apteria, may have down feathers indiscriminately distributed over them.

Nitzsch envisioned the study of these characteristic areas of feather attachment as a major tool in elucidating the phylogeny of birds. *Pterylography*[120] was prepared in 1840 from Nitzsch's manuscript and notes by H. Burmeister, who added a discussion on the development of the feather. In this work the pterylosis of the parrot family is characterized as follows: "Contour-feathers with a large and distinct after-shaft, very sparsely distributed, probably present in smaller comparative number than in any other Birds; and hence there are down-feathers not unfrequently between them, especially on the head and neck, and also on the spaces, and sometimes imperfect powder-down tracts on the pelvis. Oil-gland, when present, with a circlet of feathers on the long, thin, cylindrical tip. There are from *twenty* to *twenty-four* remiges in the wing, but always *four* feathers on the thumb and *twelve* tail-feathers. The form of the tracts varies; they are sometimes remarkably broad, sometimes narrow."

NAMES AND LOCATION OF FEATHER TRACTS

The main feather tracts, or pterylae, are known by several designations and are subdivided in various ways by different authors. A generally acceptable terminology would include capital, spinal, ventral, caudal, brachial, alar, femoral, and crural tracts.

The capital tracts, on the head, include malar, submalar, and inter-ramal regions. The body has spinal tracts, which include dorsal and pelvic areas; the ventral tracts are made up of sternal, pectoral, abdominal, and cloacal feather rows.

The dorsal spinal tract of the budgerigar begins at the occiput four or five feathers wide, passes between the shoulders four feathers wide, and divides into two tracts which separate over the back. These two dorsal tracts coalesce over the ilium and bear small feathers, evenly spaced. On the mid-dorsal rump there are a few large contour feathers in the pelvic spinal tract.

The ventral tract begins on the throat about 4 feathers wide but soon enlarges to 12 feathers in width as it approaches the axilla and passes onto the patagium on each side. The feathering is sparse over the crop, and the midline of the breast is bare except for a few down feathers. The breast is thickly feathered laterally by sternal and pectoral feather rows which continue over the abdomen to the cloaca.

On the tail the caudal tracts include the rectrices and coverts as well as the feather circlet on the papilla of the uropygial gland (see below).

The wing feathers are arranged as brachial tracts of the arm (humeral, subhumeral, and posthumeral) and alar tracts of the forearm, carpometacarpus, and digits (remiges and coverts).

The leg bears a femoral tract on the thigh and a crural tract between the knee and the ankle.

Uropygial Gland

Skin glands are rare in birds and the only conspicuous gland is the uropygial gland (Figs. 5-4, 5-5), known also as the oil, or preen gland. This is a compound alveolar structure, divided into two distinct lobes or paired, and located above the levator muscles of the pygostyle. In the budgerigar the central lumen of each gland is large (Fig. 5-5 C) and filled with secretory material. The duct of each gland opens on the truncate uropygial papilla, which is surmounted by a circlet of feathers (Fig. 5-4). The literature concerning the uropygial gland has been reviewed by Elder.[37] Its function is not certain, but it produces fatty acids, fat, and wax, which act as a waterproofing material when spread on the feathers by means of the bill when the bird is preening. In waterfowl the secretion is essential for feather maintenance and body insulation. It has been suggested that the uropygial gland functions as a source of vitamin D. Contact of the bill with the gland papilla induces a flow of the secretion. The specialized

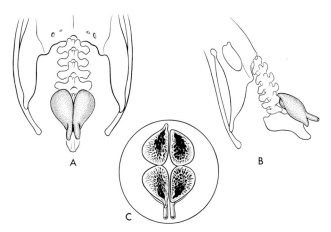

Fig. 5-5. *Uropygial glands and tail skeleton. A. Dorsal view. B. Lateral view. C. Glands sectioned and dorsal portions reflected showing their structure.*

tuft of eight feathers encircling the end of the uropygial papilla in the budgerigar acts as a wick for receiving the secretion. The tail is usually flexed laterally each time the bird reaches over the gland when preening. Not all species of birds have a uropygial gland, and in those that do the tuft of feathers on the papilla is often lacking. The uropygial gland is absent in ostriches, pigeons, and many parrots, as well as in other species.

Skeleton

The bony framework of the body (Fig. 5-6) serves for muscle attachment, protects and supports the viscera, and functions in mineral metabolism. The skeletons of all birds are similar, since the primary modifications for flight are basic. A characteristic feature of bird bones is their lightness due, in large part, to air spaces which are in direct communication with respiratory passageways. These pneumatic bones make possible an increase in bone size for greater muscle or feather attachment without a corresponding increase in weight. As a rule the more efficient large flying birds (albatross) have many pneumatized bones, whereas flightless birds have few. The budgerigar, despite its small size, has many pneumatized vertebrae and ribs, as well as pneumatic spaces in the humerus, coracoid, sternum, ilium, ischium, and pubis (see Fig. 5-22).

The histological structure of the compact bone of birds is similar to that in mammals. In the cortex of a long bone there are outer and inner circumferential lamellae enclosing the spongy bone and marrow spaces in addition to pneumatic channels. Changes in the structure of the bones accompany egg-laying and molting. Occasionally, the mineral drain may prevent the bird from perching or discourage walking. Meister[101]

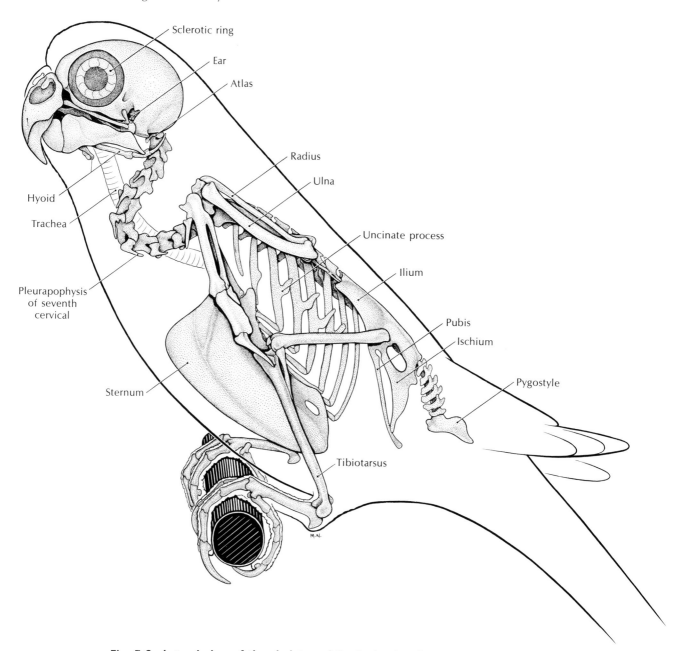

Fig. 5-6. *Lateral view of the skeleton of the budgerigar in normal perching position.*

illustrated some of the histological changes in the long bones of birds during molting, and Bloom *et al.*[13] investigated medullary bone changes during egg formation in the chicken.

The Skull

Although developmentally the bird skull has more individual bones than has the skull of a mammal, great fusions have taken place in the adult bird, reducing the number of components and thus adding strength and rigidity to the brain case. The development of the

chondrocranium and bony skull in birds was reviewed by de Beer,[34] who pointed out the affinities of birds with reptiles in general and with crocodiles in particular. In this work he makes reference to the duck, chicken, pigeon, kiwi, ostrich, kestrel, and sparrow, and presents illustrations of several species. Jollie[72] made a developmental study of the chicken skull and discussed the homologies of skull bones in the reptile, bird, and mammal. An examination of a cleared and stained embryo or recently hatched bird often shows many of the skull sutures which later fusions eliminate in the adult.

KINETICS

The skull of most birds, and that of the parrots in particular, is kinetic rather than fused and rigid as in mammals. This implies that the maxillo-palatal complex is articulated and capable of being moved by muscles in respect to the cranium proper. Observation of a feeding or preening bird discloses that the upper beak or jaw can be raised or lowered to quickly increase the gape or effectively grasp an object. This can also be demonstrated on a fresh skull or on a dried one that has been soaked overnight to soften the articulations.

The pivotal point for the movement of the upper jaw (premaxilla plus nasal) is at the fronto-nasal suture on the dorsal surface of the skull. This movement is brought about by articulating bones that may be seen on the ventral surface of the skull (Fig. 5-7). They consist of the zygomatic arch laterally and the palatine and pterygoid bones medially, meeting the premaxilla anteriorly and the quadrate bone caudally on each

side. The quadrate bone rocks forward or backward with the zygomatic arch and palatal complex. When the zygomatic arch is forced anteriorly it exerts force on the ventro-lateral margins of the premaxilla, thus raising the upper jaw. A similar action is transmitted from the quadrate to the pterygoid to the palatine, which forces the posterior ventral margin of the upper jaw forward and upward. Thus the lateral zygomatic arch and the more medially located pterygoid and palatine bones form a bridge on each side between the upper jaw and the quadrate. The pterygoid and palatine bones slide along the median sphenoidal ridge, which provides stability and an axis of movement. The lower jaw of the budgerigar is rather loosely articulated to the quadrate bone, which allows considerable freedom of forward and backward movement. However, a strong ligament connects the skull to the lower jaw medial to the quadrate bone. Although it is usually true that the lower jaw is raised when the upper jaw is depressed, and vice versa, each jaw is capable of independent movement. The ability to shell seeds re-

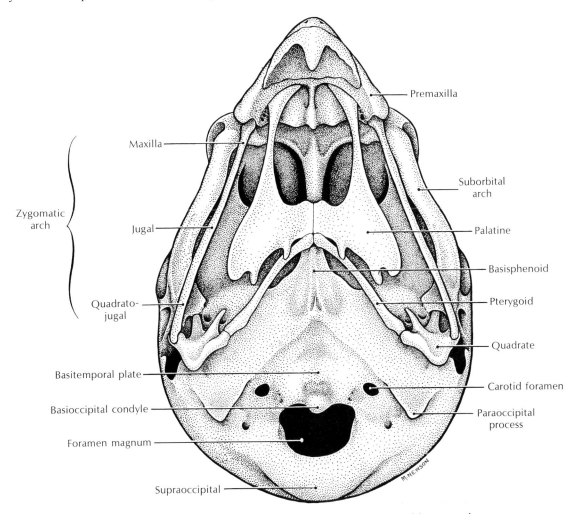

Fig. 5-7. *Ventral view of skull, with mandible and hyoid removed.*

quires this freedom of movement, along with the coordination of the tongue. The horny beak, or rhamphotheca, is vital for seed shelling, since complete removal of the horny beak would leave the jaws incongruent and incapable of such action. The architecture and mechanics of the bird skull have been described by Engels,[41] Beecher,[10,11] Bock,[15] and Spring.[141]

Although many of the individual bones in the skull of the budgerigar have lost their identity because of early fusion, it is still possible to indicate on a drawing where the component parts are located. In lateral view (Fig. 5-8 B) the premaxilla can be seen to form the upper jaw, which in life is completely covered by the horny beak. The premaxillae are paired in the embryo, and each has a frontal, a palatine, and a maxillary process. In the adult they fuse with each other and the nasal bones to form the nasal apertures and house the nasal turbinates. The premaxilla-nasal complex is hinged at the fronto-nasal suture and functions as a pincer.

The orbit is formed primarily by the frontal dorsally and the suborbital arch ventrally. A distinct lacrimal (prefrontal) bone which is so prominent in many birds is not seen in the budgerigar. The interorbital septum between the eyes is formed largely by the perpendicular plate of the ethmoid. At the posterior border of the septum are the olfactory foramen above and the optic foramen below. The frontal bone is the largest bone of the skull and forms the anterior portion of the brain case (Fig. 5-8 A).

The zygomatic arch (Fig. 5-8 B) is a slender, movable rod on each side, between the premaxilla and the quadrate bone. It is actually composed of three elements: the maxilla anteriorly, the jugal in the middle, and the quadratojugal posteriorly. The zygomatic arch functions as a lever to raise the upper jaw.

The quadrate bones function for suspension of the lower jaws and act as pivotal points for upper jaw kinetics. They are roughly X-shaped, articulating with the temporal bone dorsally, the pterygoid anteromedially, the quadratojugal laterally, and the articular bone of the lower jaw ventrally. The quadrate bone is not present as such in the mammal, since it has become the incus of the middle ear. The articular bone is likewise not present in the mammal, since it becomes the malleus of the middle ear. Thus the two bones (quadrate and articular), which in the bird form the jaw joint, in the mammal form a joint between two ossicles of the middle ear—the incus and malleus. The only ear ossicle present in the bird is the slender columella, or stapes, which can be seen in the cavity of the middle ear.

The brain case is formed by the frontals anteriorly, the parietals and occipital posteriorly, the temporals

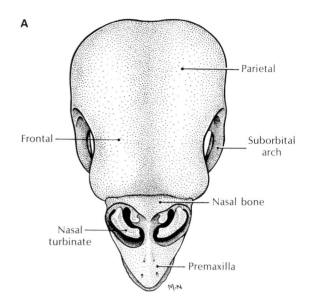

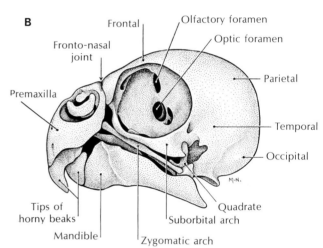

Fig. 5-8. *Dorsal (A) and lateral (B) views of skull, with sclerotic ring and hyoid removed.*

laterally, and the basisphenoid plus basitemporal plate ventrally. In the region of the inner ear the temporal bone is very trabecular internally between an inner and an outer table of bone. The semicircular canals (see Fig. 5-31) can easily be isolated by removing the outer table of the temporal bone to expose the delicate trabeculae. This condition is in contrast to the very dense petrous temporal bone of the mammalian inner ear.

The foramen magnum, through which the spinal cord enters the skull, is formed by the supraoccipital above, the exoccipitals on each side, and the basioccipital below. All components fuse as in the mammal to form an occipital ring. The basioccipital bears a single median condyle for articulation of the skull with the atlas.

The lower jaw of birds is analogous to the mandible

of mammals but not entirely homologous. Although in mammals the dentary bones form the entire lower jaw, in birds six or seven bones join to form it. They are the dentary, splenial, angular, supra-angular, articular, prearticular, and possibly a coronoid. These elements are so firmly fused in the budgerigar that in the adult they appear as one bone.

EYE BONES

The scleral ossicles, which form the sclerotic ring of each eye (see Fig. 5-6), a characteristic feature of some fishes and of all turtles, lizards, and birds, consist in birds of 11 to 15 overlapping plates embedded in the sclera and surrounding the pupil. There are 12 ossicles in each eye of the budgerigar. For a detailed discussion of the sclerotic ring in birds, see Lemmrich[87] and Curtis and Miller.[32]

Hyoid Apparatus

The skeletal support for the tongue and the muscles that move it constitute the bulk of the floor of the pharynx. This portion of the old brachial skeleton (gill arches) is variously modified in birds. Long hyoid horns (cornua) indicate great protrusibility of the tongue, whereas modifications in shape due to muscle attachments usually indicate mobility of the tongue or dexterity of tongue movements.

According to Mivart[109] birds of the Order Psittaciformes are distinguished from birds of every other Order by the shape of the hyoid bones (Figs. 5-9, 5-10). Other workers who have illustrated the hyoids of various parrots include Giebel[55] and Mudge.[115] Mudge reviewed Mivart's findings and added much on lingual musculature.

The characteristics which, taken together, seem to be distinctive of parrots are:

(1) Posterior enlargement of the basihyal.
(2) Growth dorsoanteriorly of a process on each side of the basihyal which Mivart called a parahyal process. In several Australian–South Pacific genera (*Melopsittacus, Eos, Vini, Lorius,* and *Nestor*) the parahyal processes fuse mid-dorsally, forming a parahyal arch.
(3) Presence of an entoglossal in the form of a single broad bone with a large central foramen or, more commonly, paired entoglossals united at the anterior ends by cartilage.

In the budgerigar the basihyal bone is narrow anteriorly and widens to form lateral wings posteriorly (Figs. 5-9, 5-10 A). It is fused inseparably with the urohyal, which tapers to a blunt point (Fig. 5-9). The fusion is such that the basihyal and urohyal appear

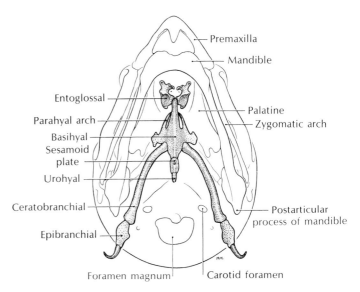

Fig. 5-9. *The hyoid apparatus in relation to the skull, ventral view.*

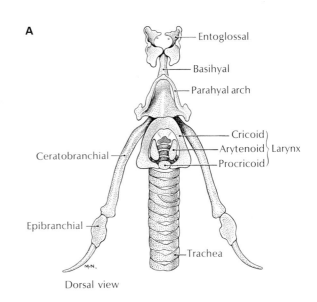

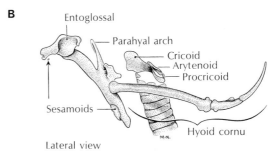

Fig. 5-10. *The bones and calcified cartilages of the hyoid apparatus, larynx, and trachea. A. Dorsal view. B. Lateral view.*

and function as one bone (Fig. 5-10 B). Close inspection of cleared and stained specimens indicates a former suture at the level of the articular facets for the hyoid cornua.

The anterior end of the basihyal bears articular facets for the very movable entoglossal bones and is compressed so that its ventral lip projects beyond the dorsal lip. At the widened region of the basihyal the lateral expansions form a dorsally concave shield or plate from which the parahyal arch takes origin. The parahyal arch extends upward and forward slightly above the body of the basihyal.

The basihyal has a large marrow cavity and a dorsal longitudinal ridge. In lateral view the ventral surface is concave and bears large facets for the articulation of the hyoid horns.

The urohyal functions as a ventrocaudal extension of the basihyal. On its ventral surface there is a close-fitting sesamoid plate, which serves for the attachment of several hyoid muscles (Figs. 5-9, 5-10 B).

The entoglossum consists of paired entoglossal bones. Each is expanded anteriorly and posteriorly, leaving a space between them. The anterior ends of the entoglossals are bifurcate (Fig. 5-10 B), and the inner prongs have a cartilaginous knob. Two or three small sesamoid bones may be embedded in the dense fibrous tissue surrounding the ventral tips of the entoglossum. In most other parrots the two entoglossals are united by a bony isthmus.

Each hyoid horn (cornu) consists of a stout cerato-branchial twice as long as the basihyal, and a short, compressed epibranchial with a long cartilaginous tapered tip. The hyoid horns are not long or greatly curved, which is in keeping with the limited protrusion of the tongue.

Vertebral Column

There is considerable fusion or elongation of the vertebral column in birds as a result of modifications for feeding and locomotion. The movements of the head and neck in birds require freely articulating cervical vertebrae. Although flexibility is of prime importance, strength of the neck must be maintained because of the forceful use of the head in feeding, nest building, and in some instances in climbing. The forces acting upon the rib-cage in respiration and flight require considerable rigidity and result in fusions of the thoracic vertebrae which act as the mid-dorsal fixed attachment. In response to the mechanical problems posed by the impact of landing, bipedal balance, and climbing, there is a fusion of all lumbar and sacral vertebrae to the ilium of the pelvic girdle on either side.

The number of vertebrae in each of the vertebral regions of the bird is usually constant for each species but varies greatly between species. In the budgerigar the numbers generally present are: Cervical 12, Thoracic 8, Lumbar Sacral 8, Caudal 8. Because of the lumbo-sacral fusions in the adult it is difficult to determine the exact number of vertebrae present in this combined region. The only freely moving vertebrae are the cervical and caudal vertebrae.

A typical vertebra has a saddle-shaped body or centrum, a dorsal neural arch (forming the vertebral canal) topped by a spinous process known as a neural spine; it has a mid-ventral spine or keel known as a hypapophysis, lateral transverse processes, and paired cranial and caudal articulating processes called pre- and postzygapophyses.

CERVICAL REGION

The atlas, or 1st cervical vertebra, is a small ring-like bone with a large mid-ventral spur which projects caudally beneath the body of the axis. The atlas forms a ball-and-socket joint with the single basioccipital condyle of the skull, permitting great movement of the head. The axis, or 2nd cervical vertebra, has a process, the odontoid process or dens, projecting cranially from its centrum, and a caudally located ventral hypapophysis. It is at least twice the size of the atlas. Both the atlas and axis lack transverse processes, pleurapophyses, and the transverse foramina that are characteristic of other cervical vertebrae.

The pleurapophyses are conspicuous, caudally directed paired spines which represent fused ribs but function for attachment of cervical muscles. By virtue of the embryonic fusion between each two-headed rib and the transverse process of the corresponding vertebra, a transverse foramen is formed. The successive transverse foramina which pierce the bases of the pleurapophyses form the vertebral canal for the passage of the vertebral artery. The 5th cervical vertebra has the longest pleurapophyses, and a keel-like hypapophysis which extends the full length of the vertebral body. At the caudal end the hypapophysis becomes bulbous and fits into a median notch on the succeeding vertebra. The 6th, 7th, and 8th cervical vertebrae are similar to the 5th. The 9th, 10th, 11th, and 12th cervical vertebrae have anteriorly located keel-like hypapophyses and increasingly broad caudo-ventral articulations in place of the bulbous articulations of the preceding vertebrae. Except for the 12th cervical, they bear pleurapophyses which decrease in size caudally. The last, or 12th, cervical vertebra varies in morphology. In some specimens only a transverse foramen and pleurapophysis remain, whereas in others an articulated rib is present. This cervical rib (about 4 mm. long) is about half as long as the first thoracic rib.

THORACIC REGION

The eight vertebrae making up the thoracic region are characterized by the presence of ribs. The articulations for each rib are seen as lateral facets on the centrum. The capitulum of the rib rests on the centrum, and the tuberculum joins the transverse process (Fig. 5-11). Thoracic vertebrae 1 to 4 have keel-like hypapophyses which serve for the origin of ventral cervical muscles. As the bird ages various fusions of thoracic vertebrae result in a more rigid spine. A spine consisting of fused thoracic vertebrae is sometimes spoken of as an os dorsale, or notarium. There is a movable joint between the 6th and 7th thoracic vertebrae. The 7th and 8th thoracic vertebrae are fused to the lumbar vertebrae, as well as to the overlapping ilia.

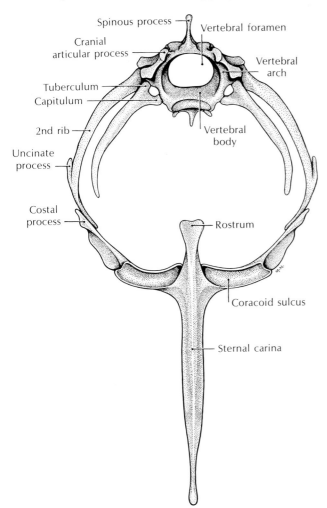

Fig. 5-11. *Cranial aspect of the thoracic inlet, and first thoracic vertebra.*

LUMBAR AND SACRAL REGIONS

The early fusion of lumbar and sacral vertebrae results in a rigid anchorage for the pelvis and pelvic limb. The last few thoracic vertebrae and the first few caudal vertebrae fuse with the combined lumbo-sacral region to form a synsacrum. A developmental study will have to be made to determine the primary number of lumbar and sacral vertebrae, since fusions have eliminated all evidence of intervertebral articulations. There appears to be five lumbar nerves and three sacral nerves. On the ventral surfaces of the vertebrae remnants of transverse processes can be seen. In life the kidney occupies this area, and the transverse processes serve to anchor it firmly in place. Frequently there is a pair of elongate free ribs attached to the first lumbar vertebra.

CAUDAL REGION

The tail or uropygium in all modern birds is relatively short. There are six free caudal or coccygeal vertebrae, plus a terminal keel-shaped pygostyle. Each caudal vertebra has a large neural spine and well-developed transverse processes. The pygostyle, or os uropygii, represents an embryonic fusion of several caudal vertebrae. It serves to support the tail feathers and uropygial gland.

Thorax

The rib cage and sternum of the bird form an expansible cylinder which encloses most of the viscera and acts as a bellows for respiration.

RIBS

The numbering of the ribs in birds presents difficulties not encountered in mammals. Because of the great fusions occurring in regions of the spine and the intermediate characteristics of some vertebrae, there is often uncertainty concerning the numbering of the vertebral elements. In the past ribs have been designated as cervical, cervico-dorsal, thoracic, or lumbar, according to criteria used by the investigator.

Cervical ribs in the budgerigar appear either as fused spines (pleurapophyses) or on the 12th cervical vertebra as articulated short ribs embedded in the ventro-lateral muscles of the neck.

Thoracic ribs articulate with the vertebrae by means of diarthrodial joints and typically join the sternum. The first two of the eight thoracic ribs in the budgerigar are atypical in not articulating with the sternum. They are, however, joined by ligaments to the sternum and function as integral parts of the thoracic cage. (These ribs have been called cervico-dorsal ribs by some authors.)

Lumbar ribs, when present, are very slender and parallel the last thoracic ribs but do not join the sternum. Dorsally the lumbar ribs are fused to the overlying ilium, as is the last thoracic rib (see Fig. 5-14).

A typical rib is bicipital, having a double attachment to the vertebral column by means of a capitulum and a tuberculum. The capitulum, or head of the rib, articulates with the centrum of the vertebra and continues as a cylindrical neck to join the flattened shaft of the rib. At the point where the neck of the rib joins the shaft there is a dorsal articular process, or tuberculum, which meets the transverse process of the vertebra.

The shafts of the 3rd to the 8th thoracic rib are composed of a dorsal, or vertebral, portion and a ventral, or sternal, portion. Although there are two distinct parts to the rib it is not at once apparent, since the acute-angle joint between them lies close to the sternum. From this joint the sternal portion passes cranially to articulate in a facet along the lateral border of the sternum. The hinge joint between the two parts of the rib allows it to be folded or extended, thus raising or lowering the sternum. By this mechanism the size of the thorax can be changed for inspiration and expiration in the manner of a bellows.

Midway on the vertebral portion of the shaft of ribs 2 to 6 there is a flat spur, or uncinate process, which projects from the caudal border of the rib and overlaps the rib behind. This arrangement strengthens the rib cage, provides more attachment for muscles, and assures synchrony of movement of the ribs in respiration.

The ribs have air passageways within them at vertebral and sternal extremities (see Fig. 5-22). Supplying the vertebral ends of ribs 1 to 6 are direct connections from the parabronchi along the medio-dorsal border of the lung. Sternal ribs 3 through 6 receive air connections from the sternum and ventral border of the anterior thoracic air sac.

STERNUM

The sternum, or breastbone, although characteristic for each species, is a variable structure in birds. It may be either elongate or broad, and may have a large keel or a small keel. Lateral processes may be separate and distinct, or they may be fused with the sternal plate. Such fusion is often associated with aging.

Since the sternum is the origin for the flight muscles, it is modified accordingly. In the flightless birds (os-

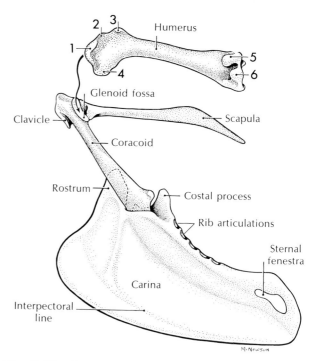

Fig. 5-12. *Bones of pectoral girdle with sternum and disarticulated humerus on which the following landmarks are indicated: 1, head; 2, lesser tuberosity; 3, deltoid crest; 4, greater tuberosity; 5, dorsal condyle; 6, ventral condyle.*

trich) a keel or carina is lacking, whereas in strong fliers (hummingbird) the keel is deeper than the sternum is broad.

The sternum of the budgerigar (Fig. 5-12) is twice as long as it is broad. A large keel, deepest cranially, runs the length of the sternum. Close to the cranial end of the keel there is a perpendicular ridge that indicates the internal air passageway from the sternal diverticulum. A large central pneumatic foramen receives the connecting airway from the sternal diverticulum of the interclavicular air sac. The air passageways of the carina are interconnected with those of the sternal plate (see Fig. 5-22).

Prominent oval apertures, sternal fenestrae, near the caudo-lateral margins of the sternal plate represent the remnants of notches between the anterior and posterior xiphisternal processes.

On the lateral margins of the sternal plate are five facets for receiving the sternal ribs. Each has a pneumatic foramen connecting the sternal diverticulum with the air spaces of the rib.

Cranial to the rib facets on each side there is a dorsally projecting process known as the costal or antero-lateral process. The second thoracic rib is bound to this process by a ligament. The base of the anterior surface of each costal process helps form the coracoid facet.

The coracoid facets of the sternum are the largest articular areas on the skeleton. They face cranially, run transversely, and are separated by a median rostrum. Since the coracoid bones are large and stabilize the pectoral girdle, their articular facets are correspondingly well developed. The rostrum of the sternum is also referred to as the sternal spine, or manubrium. It receives a ligament from each clavicle.

Pectoral Girdle

The pectoral girdle of birds consists of a blade-like scapula parallel to the vertebral column, a stout coracoid bone extending from the sternum, and usually well-developed clavicles fused mid-ventrally by an interclavicle to form a furcula—the wishbone, or the "merry thought" of older works.

The scapula and coracoid together form the glenoid fossa for the reception of the head of the humerus (see Fig. 5-12). Medially the scapula, coracoid, and clavicle form the foramen triosseum for the passage of the tendon of the supracoracoideus muscle. This muscle, which raises the wing, originates on the sternum and attaches to the dorsal surface of the proximal end of the humerus.

The clavicles are reduced to short spurs in the budgerigar, as is common in many parrots (see Fig. 5-13). The base of the reduced clavicle is expanded and bridges the supracoracoid sulcus on the medial surface of the coracoid.

The coracoid bone, characteristic of birds, functions as an extension of the sternum in the form of a "bowsprit" for muscle attachment and a pivotal point for the wing. At its ventral end the coracoid is expanded transversely to articulate with the sternum. Near the dorsal extremity on the medial side there is a foramen through which air from the interclavicular air sac enters the bone.

The scapula, or shoulder blade, is as long as the coracoid but very compressed in contrast. It parallels the vertebral column and lies above the dorsal arches of ribs 1 through 5.

Wing

The wing of birds is characterized by a reduction and fusion of the distal elements (Fig. 5-13).

HUMERUS

The stout humerus is as long as the scapula, and has an ovoid articular head which fits into the shallow glenoid fossa formed by the scapula and coracoid. On the medial surface of the greater tuberosity be-

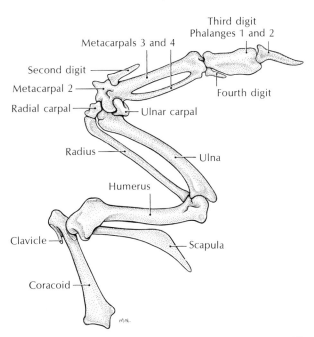

Fig. 5-13. *Left pectoral girdle and wing skeleton. The wing is elevated to show the ventral surface.*

neath the head, the large pneumatic foramen can be seen in the subtrochanteric fossa. Air enters the humerus through this foramen after passing through the axillary diverticulum of the interclavicular air sac.

When the wing is folded, the humerus lies parallel to the scapula. At the proximal end of the humerus the greater tuberosity lies ventral to the head, and the lesser tuberosity (for the supracoracoideus muscle) is dorsal to the head of the humerus. The distal continuation of the lesser tuberosity is the deltoid crest, for the insertion of the pectoralis muscle. On the lateral surface of the humerus, between the head and the greater tuberosity, there is a deep groove for a coraco-humeral ligament.

The distal end of the humerus bears a trochlea in the form of a slightly elongate dorsal condyle (ectepicondyle) for articulation with the radius plus ulna, and a more rounded ventral condyle (entepicondyle) for articulation with the ulna alone.

RADIUS AND ULNA

The radius and ulna are equal in length and slightly longer than the humerus. The radius is straight and more slender than the ulna. It has a shallow fossa proximally for articulation with the humerus, and an oval condyle distally where it joins the radial carpal bone. The ulna is a stout, slightly curved bone with two articular fossae proximally and two articular condyles distally, one of the condyles pivoting on the ulnar carpal and the other on the carpometacarpus.

The olecranon process of the ulna is short and receives the triceps tendon. In the normal folded wing the radius is dorsal to the ulna.

CARPUS

The wrist, or carpus, is greatly reduced and consists of only two free elements, the radial carpal on the outer aspect and the ulnar carpal on the inner, or flexor, surface of the joint.

DIGITS

In the mammalian forelimb the phylogenetic loss of digit I is followed by the loss of digit V. The pattern appears to be similar in the bird wing. Developmental studies by Montagna[111] and Holmgren[62] indicate that the digits remaining are II, III, and IV. (Some authors, including George and Berger,[54] do not consider the evidence presented so far as conclusive, and they prefer to number the digits I, II, and III. The latter system thus justifies retaining the term *pollicis*, for thumb, where appropriate, in naming other structures.)

In the budgerigar three digits remain and are associated with the second, third, and fourth metacarpals. The second metacarpal is the shortest and appears as a tubercle, the extensor process, on the radial side of the carpometacarpus. Articulating with it is the single phalanx of digit II, a triangular element which bears the four feathers of the alula. The third and fourth metacarpals are elongate and fused with each other at their proximal and distal ends. Six of the primary wing feathers attach on the dorsal surface of the third and fourth metacarpals. Metacarpal III is the largest and bears a digit with two phalanges. Phalanx 1 is flat, twice as long as broad, and wider distally than proximally; phalanx 2 is triangular, and forms the tip of the wing skeleton. The third digit, being the longest, is responsible for anchoring 4 of the 10 primary feathers of the wing. Metacarpal IV is slender, and the single phalanx of the fourth digit is closely applied to the proximal inner margin of the first phalanx of the third digit.

Pelvic Girdle

Since the sternum of birds is large and functions to support the viscera, there is little development of the abdominal wall and pubis. In the ostrich-like birds a pelvic symphysis remains, but in others the two halves of the "girdle" are widely separated ventrally. The loss of strength resulting from the lack of a pelvic symphysis is compensated for by the strong fusion of the ilia along their dorsal borders with the synsacrum,

the dorsal plate formed by fusion of a few thoracic, all lumbar, all sacral, and a few caudal vertebrae.

Each of the hip bones composing the pelvic girdle consists of an ilium, ischium, and pubis, meeting at the acetabulum, where the head of the femur articulates.

The dorsal surface of the ilium cranial to the acetabulum is slightly concave, whereas that of the caudal portion is rather flat and level with the synsacrum. The ventral surface of the ilium (Fig. 5-14) can be divided into three regions. An anterior region, traversed by the 6th, 7th, and 8th thoracic ribs, forms an area for anchorage of the cranial lobe of the kidney. A middle region is more deeply recessed on each side of the lumbar vertebrae; in life it houses the middle lobe of the kidney and is traversed by the femoral nerve and artery. The caudo-ventral region of the ilium is the widest and the most deeply recessed of the three regions; it houses the large median caudal lobe of the kidney and is traversed by the ischiatic nerve and artery. The line of sacro-iliac fusion can be seen running longitudinally through the middle of each recess.

The ischium is only half the size of the ilium. The ischiatic foramen through which the sciatic nerve passes is a remnant of the ischiatic notch between the ilium and ischium.

The pubis is reduced to a long splintlike bone along the ventral border of the ischium. It projects caudally and medially as a prominent landmark of the ventral body wall. Between the ischium and pubis are the obturator notch and the ischio-pubic incisure.

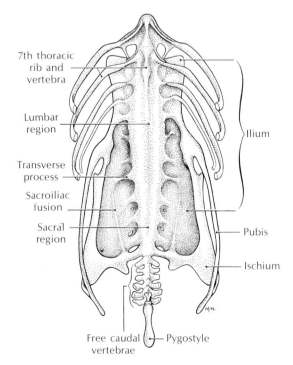

Fig. 5-14. *Synsacrum and pelvis, ventral view.*

Pelvic Limb

The pelvic limb of the bird (Fig. 5-15) consists of the thigh, enclosing the femur, the crus, or leg, containing the fibula and tibiotarsus, and the foot, which includes the tarsometatarsus and digits. A distinct tarsus, as is found in mammals, is lacking in birds. Developmentally the proximal tarsal bones fuse with the tibia and the distal tarsal elements fuse with the metatarsals.

FEMUR

The femur in all birds is shorter than the tibiotarsus. It has a small head, which fits deeply into the perforated acetabulum. The greater trochanter of the femur is prominent, and is located lateral to the head of the femur. The distal end of the femur forms a trochlea cranially and two condyles caudally. On the cranial surface of the knee joint between the medial and lateral ridges of the trochlea rests the patella.

PATELLA

The patella is a sesamoid bone in the tendon of insertion of the femorotibialis plus iliotibialis muscles. The distal part of the tendon of insertion, called the patella ligament, is very firm and keeps the patella at a fixed distance from the tibiotarsus. In some aquatic birds the patella ligament ossifies, fuses with the patella, and acts as a proximal extension of the cnemial crest, providing for greater leverage.

TIBIOTARSUS

The tibiotarsus is the largest bone of the limb. Its proximal end is expanded for articulation with the femur, and it bears a small lateral flange and a cnemial crest on its cranial surface. Many birds have a medial and a lateral cnemial crest. The anterior tibial and long digital extensor muscles take origin from the expanded proximal end of the tibiotarsus and the cnemial crest.

FIBULA

The fibula articulates with the lateral condyle of the femur but is not well developed in birds. It is very reduced in the budgerigar, being only one-third the length of the tibiotarsus. A ligament extends from the tip of the fibula to the lower third of the tibiotarsus. The distal portion of the fibula is attached along part of its length to a ridge on the tibiotarsus.

FOOT, OR PES

The foot of a bird may be well adapted for performing a particular function associated with its habitat or feeding behavior. Several studies have been made in this regard. (See the review of adaptive radiation in birds by Storer.[143]) The foot includes the tar-

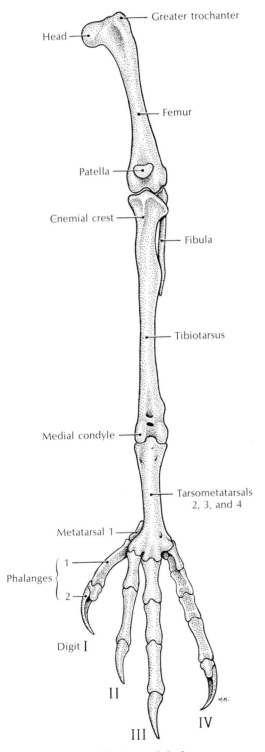

Fig. 5-15. *Left pelvic limb, cranial view.*

Greater trochanter

Head

Femur

Patella

Cnemial crest

Fibula

Tibiotarsus

Medial condyle

Tarsometatarsals 2, 3, and 4

Metatarsal 1

Phalanges { 1 2

Digit I

II

III

IV

sometatarsus, first metatarsal, phalanges of the digits, and the claws.

The 2nd, 3rd, and 4th metatarsal bones are fused with each other and with the tarsus to form a stout tarsometatarsus. The distal extremities of the three fused metatarsals each still have double condylar facets for articulation with the digits.

No bird has more than four toes. The more terrestrial the species, the more rudimentary is the 1st digit, or hallux. The ostrich has the most reduced foot of all birds, with only two digits remaining of the ancestral five. Some birds have three toes, but the great majority of birds have four.

When four toes are present it is rare, as in swifts, to have all of the toes directed forward. Most commonly, as in passerines, toes II, III, and IV are directed forward and toe I is directed backward. In the parrot family, which includes the budgerigar, and several other families, toes II and III are directed forward while toes I and IV are directed backward. (The situation differs in trogons, where III and IV are directed forward, I and II backward.)

Digit I has two phalanges and articulates with a small metatarsal bone attached to the medial side of the tarsometatarsus. Digit II has three phalanges, III has four phalanges, and IV has five phalanges. The third digit is the longest, and the terminal phalanx of each digit is covered by a sharp claw.

Musculature

The muscles comprise the greatest bulk of the body and by their contraction produce movement and heat. All animals owe their very existence to muscles, since they function in parturition or egg laying, circulation, respiration, swallowing, peristalsis and defecation, eye movements, and a host of other activities, in addition to locomotion.

On the basis of their histological structure, muscles may be classified into three types: smooth (non-striated, white, involuntary), cardiac, and striated (skeletal, red, voluntary). Muscles may also be classified on the basis of their embryonic origin and their innervation as somatic or visceral. Somatic muscles are always striated, and are innervated by somatic motor nerves. They include the axial and appendicular muscles, more generally known as skeletal or voluntary muscles. These are the muscles of locomotion and constitute the "flesh." Visceral muscles may be striated or smooth, and are innervated by visceral motor nerves. They include the striated branchial muscles of the face, jaws, pharynx, and larynx, the smooth muscles of the digestive, reproductive, and excretory systems, and the muscle of the heart (cardiac muscle).

The fixed or proximal attachment of a muscle is called the origin, and the other end is the insertion. In the limbs of birds the origin and belly of a muscle are often close to the body, whereas the insertion is via a long tendon acting at a distal point.

Muscles may be named according to their shape, origin, action, or position. No one system of naming muscles is completely satisfactory, and as a result avian myology is overburdened with synonymous terms and homologies of doubtful authenticity. A standardized list is much desired, since about 190 muscles are involved (approximately 10 skin, 35 head, 22 neck, 25 body, 8 tail, 45 wing, and 40 in the pelvic limb).

Reference sources on avian myology include the following: Fürbringer,[50] Shufeldt,[138] Gadow and Selenka,[52] Kaupp,[78] Hudson,[66] Howell,[65] Fisher,[45] Swinebroad,[147] Hudson and Lanzillotti,[67] and Goodman and Fisher.[57]

George and Berger,[54] in their monograph on avian myology, have presented an over-all summary of current information on bird muscles.

Regional Synopsis of the Muscles

MUSCLES OF THE SKIN

Dermal and dermo-osseus muscles have commonly been considered as distinct muscle entities and are usually discussed as a functional group because of their common relationship to the skin and common action upon the feathers. Included in this category are five dermal muscles originating and inserting in the skin and seven dermo-osseus muscles originating on bone and inserting in the skin. Shufeldt[138] and others have dealt with these striated dermal muscles as if they were not related to the skeletal musculature. George and Berger[54] have pointed out that these muscles are simply specialized slips of well-known muscles and they suggest the following relationships:

(1) The dermo-temporalis, dermo-dorsalis, platysma myoides, and dermo-cleido-dorsalis are parts of the cucullaris muscle complex.
(2) The dermo-tensor patagii (see Fig. 5-17) is similarly the propagial part of the cucullaris.
(3) The dermo-iliacus is the dorsocutaneous portion of the latissimus dorsi.
(4) The dermo-ulnaris is the serratus metapatagialis.
(5) The dermo-humeralis and dermo-pectoralis are slips of the pectoral muscle.
(6) The cleidotrachealis is a portion of the sternohyoid-sternotrachealis complex.

These authors doubt the actual existence, as independent muscles, of Shufeldt's dermofrontalis, circumconcha, and dermospinalis muscles.

MUSCLES OF THE HEAD

EYE. Six extraocular muscles move the eyeball (2 oblique and 4 rectus muscles), two muscles operate the nictitating membrane (quadratus and pyramidalis), and three muscles serve the eyelids (orbicularis, levator of upper lid, and depressor of lower lid).

EAR. A small fusiform muscle originates on the ventro-lateral surface of the occipital bone behind the auditory meatus and sends a delicate tendon through a foramen into the tympanic cavity, where it attaches to the extrastapedial cartilage of the columella. Although this muscle has been called the tensor tympani by some authors (a function which it may well perform) it appears to be homologous with the mammalian stapedius (see Fig. 5-30). The dermo-temporalis muscle above the ear appears to be capable of functioning as a constrictor of the auditory meatus, since its contraction would pull the skin forward as an auricular flap.

JAW. Much has been written about the jaw muscles of birds from both a functional and a taxonomic standpoint by Beecher,[10] Fisher and Goodman,[46] and Bock.[14] George and Berger[54] note the present state of confusion regarding the nomenclature of the jaw muscles of birds and suggest the need for a monograph on the subject. The muscles associated with the jaws are: the depressor mandibulae (or digastricus), which arises from the occipital region, inserts on the medial articular process of the mandible and opens the jaws; the adductor mandibulae, a complex rather than a single muscle arising from the temporal fossa, zygomatic bar, and postorbital region and inserting on the mandible to close the jaws; the pterygoideus muscles, pseudotemporal muscles, protractor quadratus, and protractor pterygoideus muscles.

MUSCLES OF THE TONGUE AND INTERMANDIBULAR REGION

The muscles which are associated with the hyoid apparatus are generally considered tongue muscles although they are not all intrinsic components of the tongue. Engels[40] described the tongue muscles in passerine birds, and Mudge[115] illustrated and described the myology of the tongue of several parrots.

The budgerigar has an elaborate muscular suspension of the hyoid apparatus, as do other parrots. There are sesamoid bones in the tendons of insertion of the muscles attaching to the ventral extremity of the entoglossum and a sesamoid plate applied to the urohyal which receives the posterior portion of the mylohyoideus and the posterior part of the serpihyoideus. In all there are approximately 15 hyoid muscles, some single but most paired. The budgerigar tongue muscles and their

functional relationships have not been studied. Closely associated with the muscles of the hyoid apparatus are those of the larynx. These include the cricoarytenoideus (dilator laryngis) and constrictor glottidis (constrictor laryngis). The cleidotrachealis (ypsilotrachealis) is a muscle which originates on the clavicle and passes up the neck to insert on the trachea, skin of the neck, or cricoid cartilage in several different species.

MUSCLES OF THE SYRINX

At the bifurcation of the trachea into bronchi various modifications of the cartilaginous tracheal and bronchial rings and semirings form a vocal apparatus called the syrinx. The muscles which operate this apparatus have a similar pattern in related birds and have been used for a long time in the classification of passerine birds. The naming of the syringeal muscles is in need of clarification, although many studies have been made of their morphology in different groups.[4,50,103,106,107]

There may be from zero to nine pairs of intrinsic syringeal muscles in birds. Maynard[100] discussed the increasing complexity of the syrinx, starting with the voiceless vultures. He noted that "the parrots, in spite of their unrivaled ability to mimic human speech, possess comparatively simple vocal organs." Miskimen[106] concluded from a study of passerine birds that "there is a direct correlation between the degree of development of the syrinx, with respect to muscles and attachments, and the quality (variety of notes) of the song."

In the budgerigar the syrinx consists of an expansion of the trachea followed by paired free semirings, each of which connects with a bronchus via membranous connections (Fig. 5-16). There are two paired muscles intimately associated with the syrinx, and a third pair of muscles which courses over them.

The most superficial muscles in the region of the syrinx appear to be a continuation of the lateral tracheal muscles. These slender and delicate muscles originate on the larynx and are closely applied to the lateral walls of the trachea as they pass caudally. Cranial to the syrinx the muscles from the two sides may join ventrally in some specimens, or the right lateral tracheal muscle may be augmented by a fan of fibers originating on the ventral surface of the trachea. From this point caudally the tracheal muscles diverge, become slender tendons, and pass over the surface of the bronchotracheal muscles. The tendons of insertion of the lateral tracheal muscles blend with the oblique septum (diaphragm) on the ventral surface of the lung at the point of entrance of the pulmonary arteries and bronchi. This muscle, by contraction, can shorten the tracheo-bronchial junction and thus relax the syringeal membranes. The name of this muscle is in question. It appears to be homologous with the

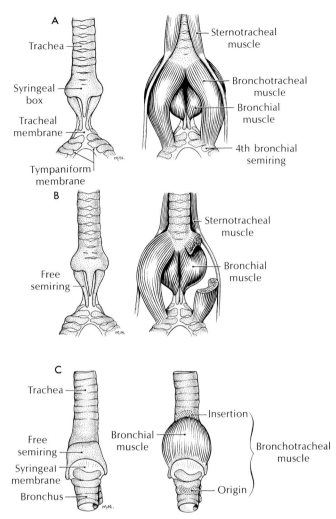

Fig. 5-16. *Ventral (A), dorsal (B), and lateral (C) views of cartilages (left) and muscles (right) of the syrinx.*

sternotracheal muscle, although it has lost its attachment to the sternum.

The bronchotracheal muscles (Fig. 5-16) are stout and arch laterally over the syrinx. Beneath these muscles are the shorter bronchial muscles which originate on the syringeal box of the trachea and insert on the free semirings.

MUSCLES OF NECK

The long neck of birds, with many more cervical vertebrae than are present in mammals, functions as a flexible connector of the head and body by virtue of saddle-shaped articulations of the vertebrae and the numerous overlapping fascicles of cervical muscles.

According to George and Berger,[54] the superficial skin muscles of the neck represent the cucullaris complex. There is an outer, circular layer, which functions as a constrictor colli, and a deeper, longitudinal layer,

which forms the specialized dermal muscles of the head and neck. The latter muscles include the dermo-temporalis and the dermo-tensor patagii, both of which are present in the budgerigar (see Fig. 5-17).

There are about 14 other groups of cervical muscles, most of which are similar in arrangement to those found in mammals. Some of these serially overlapping fascicles, such as the spinalis and iliocostalis, are continuations of the epaxial muscles of the vertebral column. The ventral muscles of the neck are the longus colli fascicles which arise from the hypapophyses of both thoracic and cervical vertebrae. They pass up the neck, inserting on the transverse processes of almost all of the cervical vertebrae.

MUSCLES OF TRUNK

Because of the fusion occurring between many of the vertebrae of the trunk and the consequent loss of flexibility, the musculature of the trunk of birds is very greatly reduced. Muscles seen on the thoracic vertebrae represent epaxial muscles of the transversospinalis, longissimus, and iliocostalis systems. The muscle bundles which make up each of these three systems are given names according to their origins, insertions, and the number of vertebrae spanned. A prominent group of the most medial system (transversospinalis) is the spinalis thoracis musculature, which consists of overlapping fascicles originating from the synsacrum and neural spines and inserting on more cranial vertebrae. Another well-defined group of muscle bundles of the lateral system (iliocostalis) is called the sacrolumbalis. They originate on the ilium or on the transverse processes of thoracic vertebrae and pass forward to insert on transverse processes or ribs of the more cranial vertebrae. The spinalis musculature continues into the neck as the spinalis cervicis.

MUSCLES OF TAIL

The terminal axial muscles originate on the sacrum and caudal vertebrae and insert on more distal caudal vertebrae or on the pygostyle. There is a superficial and a deep dorsal series (levators), a lateral series (abductors), and a ventral series (depressors). All function to control the rectrices and move the tail.

THORACIC MUSCLES

Between adjacent ribs are external and internal intercostal muscles which act to pull the ribs together. Since the most cranial ribs are fixed by the scalene and serratus anterior muscles, the net effect of a contraction of the intercostal muscles is to pull the ribs forward, thus enlarging the thoracic cavity and aiding inspiration. The external intercostal muscles are better developed than are the internal muscles.

From the caudal edge of each uncinate process a band of muscle fibers passes ventro-caudally to the rib behind. These muscles, which strengthen the rib cage, were called the appendico-costales by Shufeldt[138] and Kaupp.[78]

The levatores costarum are a series of muscle slips derived from the dorsal ends of the external intercostal muscles which extend from the transverse process of a vertebra to the dorsal end of a more caudally placed rib. Contraction of these slips pulls the ribs forward and aids inspiration.

ABDOMINAL MUSCLES

The abdominal wall is small in birds, owing to the large sternum. However, the four characteristic abdominal muscles of the mammal are present—an external and internal abdominal oblique, a transversus abdominis, and a rectus abdominis. The abdominal muscles help support the viscera, and by contraction aid in defecation and respiration. They attach to the rib cage, sternum, and pubis. Kadono, Okada, and Ono,[74] utilizing electromyographic techniques, found that the abdominal muscles of the chicken are the principal muscles of expiration, although they are assisted by the 5th and 6th external intercostal muscles.

MUSCLES OF THE WING

The modifications for flight combined with the divergent ancestry of birds result in a muscular pattern of the wing which is very different from the forelimb pattern of other animals. Although in most instances the names used are the same as those for mammals, the homologies are often in doubt. There are about 15 extrinsic and 30 intrinsic muscles of the wing.

BREAST MUSCLES

The most important flight muscles are the two large breast muscles which elevate and depress the humerus. These muscles with opposite actions both originate on the sternum and constitute the largest muscle mass of the body. The pectoralis is the large superficial muscle responsible for the downstroke of the wing, whereas the supracoracoideus, which is considerably smaller, is responsible for the upstroke.

The pectoralis muscle (Figs. 5-17, 5-21) has also been called the superficial pectoral or pectoralis major. It originates primarily on the sternal carina along the entire lower half of the keel. Fiber bundles also orig-

inate from the sternoclavicular ligament, the fascial covering of the supracoracoideus, and the caudal portion of the rib cage. The pectoralis muscle inserts via a short tendon on the ventral surface of the deltoid crest of the humerus.

A characteristic feature of the pectoral muscle of the budgerigar is the ease with which the muscle bundles can be teased apart or dissociated with a weak hydroxide solution. George and Berger[54] have studied the types of fiber found in the pectoralis muscle of birds and propose six groups based on the presence, size, and distribution of white, red, and intermediate types of fibers.

The supracoracoideus, also called the deep pectoral or pectoralis minor, is hidden beneath the pectoralis muscle. It originates on each side of the sternum along the angle formed by the carina and the sternal plate. A few short fiber bundles originate on the base of the coracoid. The insertion of the supracoracoideus is by means of a tendon which passes through the foramen triosseum to attach on the dorsal surface of the humerus distal to the humeral crest. This muscle acts to abduct and elevate the wing.

Although the clavicles of the budgerigar are very reduced, the sternoclavicular ligament is well developed. The thoracic inlet begins at the V formed by the sternoclavicular ligaments.

SHOULDER MUSCLES

The latissimus dorsi is the most superficial muscle of the back and has two distinct parts. An anterior portion originates from the supraspinous ligament and spinous processes of two or three thoracic vertebrae; the posterior portion comes from the median ridge of the synsacrum by means of an aponeurosis common to both the rhomboideus and the sartorius muscle. The tendons of insertion attach to the medial surface of the proximal end of the humerus. The anterior portion has a wide, delicate, fleshy attachment to the humerus immediately distal to the insertion of the supracoracoideus. The posterior portion attaches by a long, narrow, but strong tendon below the attachment of the anterior portion. Both portions pass between the two heads of the triceps to insert.

A narrow latissimus dorsi metapatagialis originates above the posterior portion of the latissimus dorsi, passes distally over its surface, and inserts into the skin along the caudal margin of the humeral feather tract. The muscles function to elevate or adduct the arm and flex the shoulder.

The rhomboideus superficialis is a thin sheet of muscle lying beneath the latissimus dorsi. It is frequently called the trapezius muscle. The muscle origi-

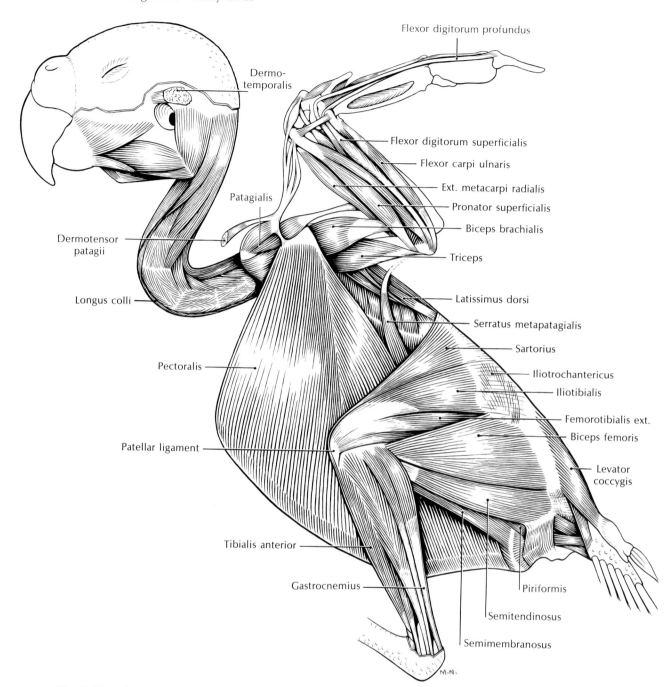

Fig. 5-17. *Superficial muscles of the body, lateral view, with wing elevated, showing ventral aspect.*

nates from the neural spines of the cervical and thoracic vertebrae and inserts along the vertebral border of the scapula. Beneath the superficial rhomboid muscle is the rhomboideus profundus, with a similar but more extensive origin and insertion. Both muscles draw the scapula upward.

Of the many wing muscles, only a few will be considered, to illustrate the functional arrangement of extensors and flexors. A muscle spanning two joints may act as a flexor of one joint and an extensor of the other.

On the dorsal surface of the base of the wing, covering the shoulder joint, two large muscles are visible. They are the patagialis longus et brevis and the triceps brachii in pre- to post-axial sequence. Beneath the origin of the large patagialis muscle are the short coracobrachialis anterior and the deltoideus. Caudal to these muscles the strong tendon of the supracoracoideus muscle can be seen as it emerges from the foramen triosseum and inserts on the dorsal aspect of the humerus.

SPECIFIC WING MUSCLES ON BASIS OF FUNCTION

EXTENSION OF THE SHOULDER JOINT. *Coracobrachialis Anterior (Coracohumeralis).* Origin: On the cranial surface of the coracoid bone at the point where the vestigial clavicle fuses with the head of the coracoid. The muscle caps the cranial surface of the shoulder joint and lies between the pectoralis and the deltoideus in dorsal view.

Insertion: On the dorsal surface of the proximal end of the humerus below the humeral crest and next to the insertion of the pectoralis. In addition to extending the shoulder, it elevates the wing.

Deltoideus (Scapulohumeralis, Deltoideus Minor, D. Brevis, D. Internus, D. Externus, Supraspinatus, Coracobrachialis Internus, Coracobrachialis Anterior). Origin: On the head of the coracoid and clavicle by a short tendon adjacent to and behind the tendon of origin of the patagialis muscle. Only one deltoid muscle is present, but its position would indicate that it is the deltoideus minor of George and Berger.[54]

Insertion: On the humerus cranial to the humeral crest adjacent to but above the insertion of the coracobrachialis anterior.

Patagialis. Although primarily a flexor of the elbow, this muscle, aided by the dermotensor patagii, also acts to extend the shoulder joint.

FLEXION OF THE SHOULDER JOINT. *Dorsalis Scapulae.* Origin: By fleshy fibers from the entire caudolateral surface of the scapula and a part of the lateral rib cage. This is the most massive muscle of the shoulder. The dorsal outline of the muscle is seen as a white raphe and corresponds with the dorsal border of the scapula. The dorsalis scapulae muscle can be seen superficially between the cranial and caudal portions of the latissimus dorsi muscle.

Insertion: By a short, strong tendon to the medial surface of the humerus between the pneumatic foramen and the greater tuberosity. The insertion of this tendon pierces the tendon of origin of the humerotriceps muscle.

Proscapulohumeralis (Scapulohumeralis Anterior, Supraspinatus, Subscapularis Pars Externa). Origin: By fleshy fibers from the cranial third of the scapula ahead of the dorsalis scapulae.

Insertion: By a strong, short tendon to the base of the internal tuberosity of the head of the humerus.

A muscle originating on the entire length of the sternoclavicular ligament passes medial to the coracoid and attaches to the internal tuberosity of the humerus in common with the tendon of the proscapulohumeralis.

Coracobrachialis Posterior (Pectoralis Tertius). Origin: By a close attachment to the base and dorso-lateral surface of the coracoid. Some fibers originate on the sternum.

Insertion: The muscle passes upward and attaches by a strong tendon to the internal tuberosity of the head of the humerus.

Scapulotriceps (Triceps Scapularis, Long Head of Triceps, Anconaeus Scapularis, Anconaeus Longus). Origin: This superficial portion of the triceps brachii muscle originates on a scapulo-coraco-humeral anchor in the form of a stout tripartite tendon between the three bones. The muscle passes along the caudal surface of the humerus and sends a tendon over the lateral surface of the elbow joint.

Insertion: By a strong attachment on the lateral surface of the proximal end of the ulna. It acts as a flexor of the shoulder joint and as an extensor of the elbow joint.

EXTENSION OF THE ELBOW JOINT. *Humerotriceps (Triceps Humeralis, Anconaeus Humeralis).* Origin: On the caudal surface of the humerus over the proximal two-thirds of the bone. This muscle is entirely separate from the scapulotriceps, although the two are in contact with each other over most of their length.

Insertion: On the tip of the olecranon, where it can exert maximum force for extension.

Serratus Metapatagialis. Origin: On the lateral surface of the rib cage above the pectoralis.

Insertion: This narrow and weak muscle has an insertion into the margin of the humeral feather tract. It passes over the extensor surface of the elbow joint, and therefore can act as an extensor of the wing.

FLEXION OF THE ELBOW JOINT. *Patagialis Longus et Brevis.* Origin: This combined muscle arises from a single tendon on the cranial surface of the dorsal end of the clavicle. The muscle soon widens to cover the shoulder joint and head of the humerus. It is more extensive in the budgerigar than in several other birds. The form of the tendons of insertion is variable. There are usually three or four narrow tendons or one narrow and another wide tendon on the cranial border representing the patagialis longus portion and a single, more proximally located tendon of the brevis portion. In some specimens, a strong band from the mid-portion of the patagialis muscle bridges the flexor angle of the forearm and blends with the fascial covering of the extensor metacarpi radialis.

Insertion: The most anterior tendons form the margin of the propatagium and insert on the extensor process of the second metacarpal bone and the distal extremity of the radius (Fig. 5-17). The tendon of the more caudal portion of the muscle inserts on the dorsal surface of the elbow joint by blending with the origin of the extensor metacarpi radialis, and on the distal end of the humerus. In addition to flexing the forearm it tenses the propatagial membrane and extends the shoulder. The longus tendon extends the carpometacarpus.

The dermotensor patagii from the skin of the neck joins the tendon of insertion of the patagialis longus et brevis.

Biceps Brachii. Origin: This prime flexor of the forearm arises as a broad, dense tendon from the head of the coracoid, passes beneath the insertion of the pectoralis, and passes along the ventro-lateral surface of the humerus. It is composed of a single fusiform belly along side of the humerotriceps. At the distal third of the muscle an indication of two bellies can be seen, each of which gives rise to a slender tendon.

Insertion: The tendon of the slightly larger and more ventral belly attaches to the proximal end of the radius; the other tendon attaches to the proximal end of the ulna. Both insertions are close together between the radius and ulna.

EXTENSION OF THE CARPUS. *Extensor Metacarpi Radialis.* Origin: By a strong tendon from the cranial surface of the distal end of the humerus above the lateral epicondyle. This large muscle on the cranial border of the forearm has several tendinous insertions on its surface from the patagialis muscles.

Insertion: On the extensor process of the carpometacarpus by a strong tendon. (This process represents fused metacarpal II.)

A delicate, long tendon from the extensor ossis metacarpi II passes through the carpal canal with the tendon of the extensor metacarpi radialis and joins it prior to insertion.

FLEXION OF THE CARPUS. *Flexor Carpi Ulnaris.* Origin: By a short, stout tendon from the distal end of the medial epicondyle of the humerus, distal to the origin of the flexor digitorum superficialis. This long muscle lies along the caudal border of the forearm.

Insertion: On the proximal surface of the ulnar carpal bone by a strong tendon.

Flexor Metacarpi Radialis (Extensor Metacarpi Ulnaris, Extensor Carpi Ulnaris). Origin: This nomenclaturally controversial muscle originates from the lateral epicondyle of the humerus and the proximal end of the ulna. It runs along the dorsal surface of the ulna, becomes tendinous at the carpal joint, and extends as a narrow tendon around the cranial surface of the ulnar condyle to insert on the carpometacarpus. George and Berger[54] review the status of this muscle, which functions as a flexor although it appears to belong to the extensor group by innervation.

EXTENSION OF THE DIGITS. *Extensor Digitorum Communis.* Origin: On the lateral epicondyle of the humerus, deep to the origin of the flexor metacarpi radialis. The belly of this muscle lies on the dorsal surface of the forearm, between the flexor metacarpi radialis and the extensor metacarpi radialis.

Insertion: The tendon passes through a groove on the ulnar condyle and bifurcates on the proximal end of the carpometacarpus. The short branch inserts on the second digit (first digit or pollex of some authors), and the long tendon continues across the carpometacarpus to the third or longest digit. This digital extensor muscle can also act as an extensor of the carpus.

FLEXION OF THE DIGIT. *Flexor Digitorum Superficialis.* Origin: By a tendon from the medial epicondyle of the humerus distal to the origin of the pronator profundus. The shiny tendon of origin is almost as wide as the muscle and it continues along the surface of the muscle to the distal end of the forearm where it inserts on the ulnar carpal bone and the proximal primary feathers. The main muscle mass passes around the anterior surface of the ulnar carpal bone to enter the carpometacarpus, where it parallels the extensor tendon to the distal phalanx of the third digit.

MUSCLES OF THE PELVIC LIMB

In birds the ilium extends for a considerable distance cranial and caudal to the acetabulum, and thus serves a prime function for attachment of limb muscles. The stresses of walking and landing are transferred from the elongated ilium to the fused synsacrum.

The femur is held close to the body, and the articulation of the head of the femur in the acetabulum (hip or coxal joint) is such that its movement is rather limited to an antero-posterior plane.

The articulation of the tibiotarsus with the femur (knee or stifle joint) allows flexion and extension of the joint with some degree of rotation. There are medial, lateral, and cruciate ligaments, as well as two menisci, a patella, and occasionally other sesamoid bones at the knee joint. The femur rotates laterally as its distal end glides over the tibial articular surface, so that in walking the body is brought over the supporting leg by a rotation at the knee, producing a waddle.

The proximal tarsal bones are fused with the tibia and the distal tarsals are fused with the metatarsus, resulting in an intratarsal joint the movement of which is limited to flexion and extension.

Hudson[66] studied the pelvic muscles in many species of birds. Howell[65] summarized the muscle groups of the hip and thigh in regard to their nerve supply and showed their homology with muscles of the reptile and mammal. As with the wing muscles, the muscles of the pelvic limb are each known by several different names. The discussions of the following muscles exemplify some of the functional relationships in the pelvic limb of the budgerigar.

The flexors of the knee also extend the hip, whereas the extensors of the knee flex the hip.

The muscles seen superficially (see Fig. 5-17) on the lateral surface of the thigh, in cranial to caudal sequence, are the sartorius, iliotibialis, femorotibialis, biceps femoris, semitendinosus, and semimembranosus.

SPECIFIC MUSCLES OF PELVIC LIMB ON BASIS OF FUNCTION

EXTENSION OF THE KNEE. *Sartorius.* Origin: From an aponeurosis attached to the median dorsal ridge of the synsacrum and the anterior iliac crest. This most cranial muscle of the thigh passes medially as it approaches the knee.

Insertion: On the medial surface of the fascia of the knee joint.

Iliotibialis Lateralis. Origin: By an aponeurosis continuous with the origin of the sartorius which extends over the iliac crest to the median ridge of the synsacrum. Beneath the translucent aponeurosis of this muscle the iliotrochantericus posterior can be seen. The wide origin of the muscle narrows as it passes distally. About two-thirds of the length down the thigh, the muscle forms an aponeurosis which blends with the covering of the femorotibialis muscle below.

Insertion: In common with the femorotibialis via the patella ligament to the tibia. The iliotibialis muscle is divided by some workers into an anterior part (sartorius), a medial part (tensor fasciae), and a posterior part (gluteus posterior).

Femorotibialis Externus. Origin: On the greater trochanter of the femur. The proximal portion of this muscle is hidden dorsally by the iliotibialis.

Insertion: By the strong patella tendon, of which it is the principal component, to the cranial surface of the proximal end of the tibia. This muscle is therefore the most powerful extensor of the knee.

FLEXION OF THE KNEE. *Biceps Femoris.* Origin: On the dorsal surface of the ischium and by a broad aponeurosis along the iliac crest. This large laterocaudal thigh muscle tapers as it approaches the back of the knee to insert.

Insertion: The strong tendon of insertion passes through a sling or loop (along with nerves and blood vessels) and attaches to the caudal surface of the proximal portion of the fibula. The sling is formed by a ligament which extends from the lateral condyle of the femur to the head of the tibia. By means of this sling the weight of the body is partially transferred, when the leg is bent, to the distal end of the femur. The biceps muscle, in addition to flexing the knee, rotates the leg outward, abducts the limb, and extends the hip.

Semitendinosus. Origin: By fleshy fibers from the ischium caudal to the origin of the biceps femoris. This caudo-lateral muscle of the thigh crosses superficial to the piriformis as it passes distally toward the popliteal space. A short accessory semitendinosus is present in the budgerigar as a continuation of the parent muscle.

Insertion: The flat tendon of insertion joins that of the semimembranosus and fuses with the sheath of the gastrocnemius muscle. A weak attachment to the femur is seen passing between the pars media and pars externa of the gastrocnemius.

Semimembranosus (Flexor Cruris Medialis, Ischioflexorius). Origin: From the lowermost portion of the ischium. This medial caudal muscle of the thigh is partially visible in lateral view. It has a shorter belly than the semitendinosus, to which it is closely applied.

Insertion: A flat tendon in common with that of the semitendinosus, fusing with the sheath of the gastrocnemius.

EXTENSION OF THE TARSOMETATARSUS. *Gastrocnemius.* Origin: There are three heads and three bellies to the gastrocnemius muscle in the budgerigar.

The pars interna, the largest of the three parts, arises from the medial condyle of the femur, the medial surface of the cnemial crest, and along two-thirds of the length of the tibialis anterior muscle.

The pars externa originates on the lateral side of the ligamentous sling extending from the lateral condyle of the femur to the head of the tibia, halfway between the passage of the biceps tendon and attachment of the sling to the condyle. The belly of the external portion is short and spindle-shaped.

The pars media is the smallest of the heads of the gastrocnemius. It arises from the back of the knee between the pars externa and pars interna.

Insertion: The flat tendon of the pars externa passes along the caudal surface of the crus. Midway down the crus the tendon of the pars media joins it. On the distal third of the crus the tendon of the pars interna also joins the combined tendon and this broad, single tendon of insertion passes over the extensor surface of the tibial cartilage to insert on the caudal surface of the tarsometatarsus. In so doing the gastrocnemius tendon confines the digital flexor tendons on the plantar surface of the tarsometatarsus.

FLEXION OF THE TARSOMETATARSUS. *Tibialis Anterior.* Origin: By two heads. The superficial, or tibial, head arises from the cnemial crest and proximal cranial flange of the tibia. The smaller deep, or femoral, head originates on the lateral femoral condyle. The bellies of the two muscles are quite separate from one another, as are their tendons of insertion, although the tendon of the deep head is very slender. Both tendons are held close to the tibiotarsus by a transverse ligament, located near the distal end of the tibiotarsus.

Insertion: On the cranial surface of the proximal third of the tarsometatarsus.

EXTENSION OF THE DIGITS. *Extensor Digitorum Longus.* Origin: By a wide fleshy attachment on the cranial surface of the tibia medial to the cnemial crest. This muscle, for its full length, lies beneath the tibialis anterior on the cranial surface of the tibiotarsus.

Insertion: The long tendon passes under a bony bridge on the cranial surface of the distal end of the tibiotarsus. The tendon becomes superficial on the cranial surface of the tarsometatarsus and divides into extensor tendons for each of the digits.

FLEXION OF THE DIGITS. *Flexor Digitorum Superficialis.* Origin: From the intercondyloid area of the femur and the caudal surface of the proximal end of the tibia. The muscle passes distally on the tibiotarsus over the flexor digitorum longus, through the tibial cartilage and hypotarsal canal.

Insertion: On the basal phalanges of the toes, where a sheath is formed for the passage of the long digital flexor.

Flexor Digitorum Longus. Origin: By two heads from the fibula and tibiotarsus. This is the deepest muscle of the caudal surface of the crus. The tendon passes through a fibrous canal deep to the tibial cartilage.

Insertion: The tendon of insertion trifurcates and passes to the distal phalanges of digits II, III, and IV.

Digestive System

The components of the digestive apparatus are concerned with the prehension and ingestion of food, its transmission through the alimentary canal, and the process of absorption and elimination. The canal (Fig. 5-18) consists of the mouth, pharynx, esophagus, crop, proventriculus, gizzard, small intestine, cecum, large intestine, and cloaca. Accessory organs include the beak, tongue, salivary glands, pancreas, and liver. Many glands are embedded in the wall of the canal throughout its length.

Joos[73] studied the gross and histological development of the intestinal tract in the budgerigar (*Melopsit-*

tacus undulatus). She found that the establishment of form takes place in three stages. From the 1st to the 5th day the primitive intestinal loop and the duodenum form, from the 6th to the 13th day the group-specific pattern is laid down, and from the 13th day to hatching on the 18th day the tract grows in length and volume. Calhoun[22] described and illustrated the microscopic anatomy of the digestive tract of the chicken.

In birds the alimentary canal consists histologically of an outer tunica serosa, a tunica muscularis composed of an outer longitudinal and an inner circular smooth muscle layer, a tela submucosa of loose fibro-elastic tissue, and a tunica mucosa with folds or villi. The latter consists of longitudinal smooth muscle fibers and tubulo-alveolar glands which open individually onto the stratified squamous epithelium. Isolated lymphatic nodules are also present in the mucosa.

GENERAL TOPOGRAPHY

The mouth is bounded by the horny beaks which grow constantly and must be worn by normal use in order to maintain their shape for optimal function. The blunt tongue on the floor of the mouth is very mobile, but only slightly protrusible. The shelling of seeds requires manipulation between the tongue and beak in such a manner that the husk is cracked, removed, and ejected while the kernel is retained and swallowed. Palatal pads on the roof of the mouth appear to aid in these functions. The hyoid apparatus provides support for the tongue and an attachment for the larynx. Behind the glottis the pharynx narrows to form the esophagus, which passes down the neck, at first dorsal to the trachea, and then to the right. Shortly after reaching the right side of the trachea the esophagus widens to form a large crop, cranial to the thoracic inlet. The crop extends to the left side of the base of the neck, but on the midline it narrows to re-form an esophageal tube, which passes between the coracoid bones to the right of the syrinx and dorsal to the heart.

At the level of the base of the heart and the first ribs the esophagus is continuous with the glandular stomach, or proventriculus. The proventriculus inclines to the left dorsal to the heart and extends to the level of the 6th thoracic vertebra in contact with the left body wall. Here in the thoraco-abdominal cavity it joins the large muscular stomach (ventriculus), or gizzard, which occupies an area bounded cranially by the 5th rib and caudally by the ischium. On a radiograph the gizzard appears more caudally located than one might expect.

The duodenum begins at the cranio-dorsal border of the gizzard, passes ventrally along the surface of the gizzard, and extends caudally to the level of the inter-

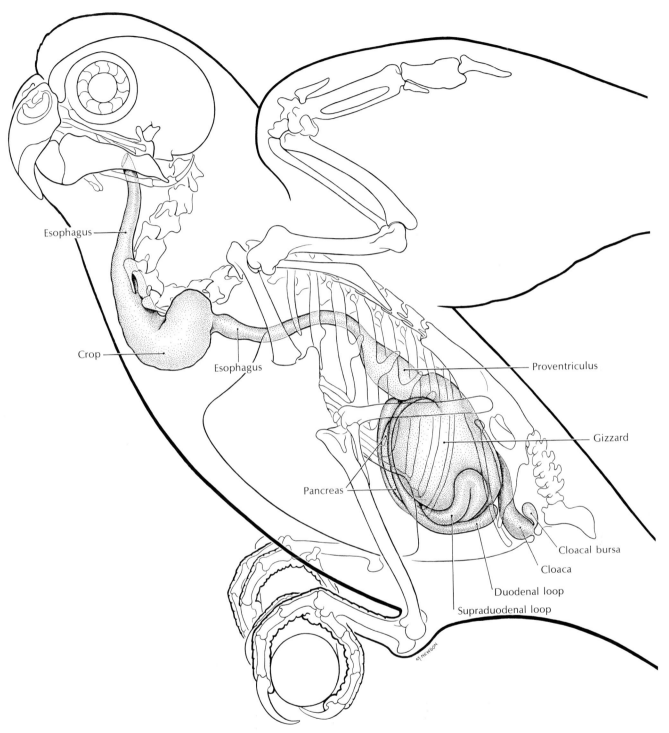

Fig. 5-18. *The digestive tract in relation to the skeleton.*

pubic space before turning back on itself. This duodenal loop, enclosing the pancreas, is the most caudally
located portion of the small intestine. The remainder
of the small intestine consists of four loops of ileum
tightly packed on the right side of the gizzard.

The large intestine, or rectum, is the short, straight
portion of the gut emptying into the cloaca. Since cecae

are lacking in the budgerigar, there is no indication
of the boundary between the small and the large
intestine. The cloaca receives the urinary and genital
ducts as well as the cloacal bursa (bursa of Fabricius),
which opens on its dorsal wall. The bursa is largest
in young birds.

Latimer and Osborn[86] were the first to describe the

topography of the viscera of the chicken with respect to the vertebral levels. They found a significant sex difference in the levels of the various organs, probably due to the greater development of the female reproductive tract.

MOUTH

The mouth is divided into an anterior oral cavity, bounded by the horny beak, and a posterior cavity, or pharynx, into which the nasal passages open. The angles of the mouth when formed by soft keratin are known as the rictus, and in some birds they exhibit a prominent fold which aids in prehension.

The *beak* is formed of modified skin sheathing the bones beneath. The epidermis is heavily keratinized and the dermis is fused with the periosteum. Numerous Pacinian corpuscles are present in the dermis of the beak. Although ancient cretaceous birds such as *Hesperornis* had teeth, no vestiges are found in modern birds. In the budgerigar the tip of the upper beak is sharp and composed of thicker keratin than the remainder of the beak. The lower beak, which is horseshoe-shaped and fits within the upper, also has a thick terminal portion which functions as an extension of the lower jaw. When the lower horny beak is lost in the prepared skull, one is apt to wonder how the jaws can function so efficiently with such an apparently poor fit.

The *palate* (Fig. 5-19) bears two prominent fleshy cushions, which are well vascularized and form a palatal notch against which the tongue can hold an object. The caudal margins of the palatal folds are fimbriated in the budgerigar, as they are in most birds.

The median *choana,* or opening of the nasal passageway, appears as a slit which begins between the palatal folds and continues along the roof of the pharynx. In the middle of the choana is the single median opening of the combined auditory tubes. The roof of the pharynx has several filiform papillae distributed primarily along the midline.

The floor of the mouth is occupied by the large blunt tongue and the glottis (Fig. 5-20). On the midline of the floor of the mouth, caudal to the tongue, is a prominent low papilla, through which a salivary duct opens (Fig. 5-20 A). Salivary glands of birds include several compound lobulated mucus-secreting glands distributed as lingual glands within the tongue, submaxillary glands in the inter-ramal region, angular glands beneath each zygomatic arch, palatine glands in the roof of the mouth, and occasionally other glands in the roof or floor of the pharynx.

The *tongue* in birds is usually narrow, pointed, and protrusible. It is heavily keratinized, and it contains

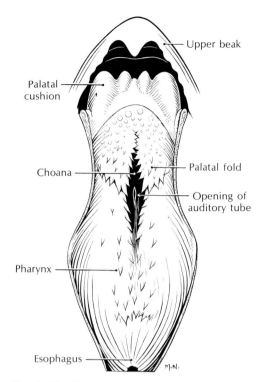

Fig. 5-19. *The palate and roof of the pharynx.*

little muscle and few if any taste buds. Tucker[154] pointed out that the mechanics of the avian and mammalian tongues differ greatly. He reviewed the kinetics of the avian tongue and studied the differentiation of epithelial and connective tissue components in the tongue of *Gallus.* Garrod[53] commented upon the tongues of several parrots. He noted that in all parrots the fleshy tongue ends anteriorly by a dilated portion supported on a narrower neck, and that the tip of the tongue is used much like a human finger tip to hold an object against the upper beak while the mandible is free to give another bite. In many parrots a nail-like plate appears on the lower margin of the anterior rounded surface of the tongue and is worn down by contact with food items. In typical parrots Garrod found this nail of the tongue is broader than long, horny in texture, and with the lateral margins extending up the sides and reaching the dorsal surface of the tongue. (The tongue of *Nestor* is smooth on top but has a fringe of "hairs" along the anterior tip of the nail plate; *Trichoglossus* has recurved papillae on the dorsal tip of the tongue.)

Although the tongue of the budgerigar is not very protrusible, it is mobile and is capable of manipulating objects with great dexterity. The tip of the tongue is smooth, except for several longitudinal creases. Within the tip of the tongue are the entoglossal bones (Fig. 5-20 B) and their associated muscles. The caudal boundary of the tongue bears a few filiform papillae

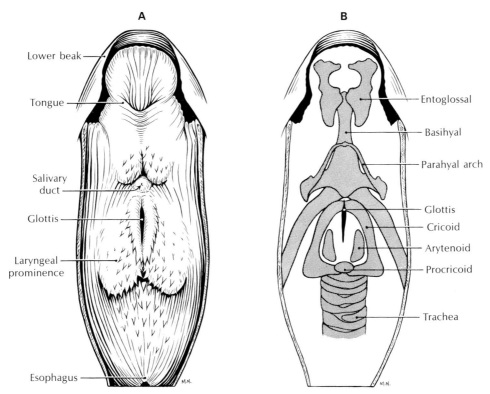

Fig. 5-20. *Structures of the floor of the mouth, dorsal view. A. The tongue and glottis. B. The hyoid bones and laryngeal skeleton.*

on its surface. Within the base of the tongue are the parahyal arch and associated muscles.

The *glottis*, or opening to the larynx, lies on the midline of the floor of the pharynx between the tongue and the opening of the esophagus. A few filiform papillae are distributed over the laryngeal prominence and posterior floor of the pharynx.

ESOPHAGUS

The esophagus is a muscular tube which originates from the pharynx caudo-dorsal to the glottis and trachea. It passes down the neck to the right of the trachea. At the level of the 6th cervical vertebra the esophagus widens to form the crop. The lining of the esophagus is characterized by presence of longitudinal ridges and mucus-secreting glands.

CROP

The crop is a dilatation of the esophagus that is present in gallinaceous birds, parrots, and a few others. Serving as a temporary storage chamber, it lies nestled in the thoracic inlet, lightly bound to the surrounding structures by fascia and conspicuous lobules of fat. It is very expansible and is lined by a mucous membrane provided with mucous glands. The greatest ex-

panse of the crop is in a transverse plane, with the inlet on the right, a saccular extension to the left, and the outlet on the midline (Fig. 7-21). Niethammer[118] saw the first indication of an esophageal dilatation in *Melopsittacus* on the 6th day of incubation.

The stomach consists of two portions, an elongated, thin-walled, glandular part, called the proventriculus, and a rounded, thick-walled, muscular portion, the ventriculus, or gizzard. The relative size of the gizzard is greatest in seed- or plant-eating birds, although parrots may have a proventriculus larger than the gizzard.

The proventriculus is characterized by the abundance of compound glands which lie embedded in the wall and compose most of its thickness. The glands are readily seen through the thin muscularis, and in the budgerigar they can be grossly teased apart after hydroxide maceration and removal of the tunica muscularis. The submucosal glands secrete both acid and enzyme. In injected specimens a rich arterial net is seen to envelop the bases of the proventricular glands. The development of these glands in *Melopsittacus* has been studied and illustrated by Joos[73] and reproduced by Romanoff.[132] The histochemistry of these submucosal glands of the proventriculus has been commented upon by Aitken[1] and Toner.[153] In some species of birds the proventricular glands are located as a band or patch in a particular part of the organ. More rarely they may be in crypts or diverticula.[8]

The gizzard is characterized by the great enlargement of its muscular walls, and the thick resilient, ridged lining traversed by simple tubular glands. This lining is often called keratin, but it is actually a combination of desquamated surface epithelium and proteinaceous rodlets with cementing mucin of glandular origin. Toner[153] has studied the fine structure of gizzard gland cells in the domestic fowl. In some birds, such as herons, the gizzard is soft-walled and bag-like. The openings of the proventriculus and duodenum are close together, so that food entering from the proventriculus that does not require further grinding can be passed immediately into the duodenum. To aid the gizzard in grinding food, grit or small pebbles are frequently swallowed and appear to remain for a time in the lumen of the gizzard. The pylorus is a valve-like fold between the gizzard and the duodenum.

SMALL INTESTINE

The intestinal convolutions and positional arrangements in birds have been the subject of several memoirs. Gadow[5] and Mitchell[108] described and illustrated the coils of the intestinal canal in many groups of birds. A review of Gadow's work appears in *A Dictionary of Birds* by Newton and Gadow,[117] and a review of Mitchell's work appears in *The Structure and Classification of Birds* by Beddard.[8]

There are three primary loops of the small intestine in the bird: (1) the duodenal loop, (2) the umbilical loop, and (3) the supraduodenal loop.

As development proceeds, the duodenal loop persists as a single elongated tube of the same diameter as the other portions of the small intestine. Its proximal portion begins at the pylorus and passes ventrally and caudally behind the gizzard, before turning cranially as the distal portion. The duodenum partially encircles the elongated pancreas, and lies ventral to the intestinal coils in contact with the body wall (Fig. 5-21). The distal portion of the duodenum receives one or two bile ducts from the liver and three pancreatic ducts, one from each lobe of the pancreas (see Fig. 5-27).

The umbilical and supraduodenal loops of the small intestine are equivalent to the jejunum and ileum, respectively, of mammals, and constitute the longest portion of the alimentary tract. Some authors refer to this entire portion of the small intestine as the ileum. In the budgerigar and several other birds the primary umbilical loop develops into three loops in the adult

(see Fig. 5-27), which may be referred to as the preumbilical, umbilical, and postumbilical loops. Each of these loops has a slightly spiral torsion. A remnant of the yolk sac, called Meckel's diverticulum, can often be observed near the apex of the umbilical loop. The terminal portion of the small intestine passes from right to left dorsal to the duodenum, as the supraduodenal loop, which is closely applied to the gizzard and then continues caudally as the large intestine.

LARGE INTESTINE

Cecae usually mark the junction of the small and the large intestine in mammals and birds. They are often large in herbivorous species, and are frequently distended with gas in the dead bird. Paired cecae are large and long in the chicken and owl, very small in the pigeon and passerine birds, and absent in the budgerigar and some others. A small unpaired cecum is said to be present in the heron.

The large intestine, or rectum, begins at the level of the gizzard and passes caudally parallel to the vertebral column. It is short and only slightly wider than the small intestine.

CLOACA

The cloaca is a terminal chamber of endodermal and ectodermal origin into which the digestive tract and the urogenital ducts empty. The rectum enters mid-ventrally into an area called the coprodeum. This is separated by a fold from a dorsal area, the urodeum, into which the ureters and the oviduct or, in the male, the deferent ducts enter. Both the coprodeum and urodeum are in open communication with a common chamber, the proctodeum, which opens to the outside by way of the vent. On the mid-dorsal wall of the proctodeum near the rim of the vent the opening to the cloacal bursa can be seen (Figs. 7-18, 7-28). The bursa is large and saccular in young birds but may be small and dense or absent in adults. This structure was first described and illustrated in the hen by Hieronymus Fabricius of Aquapendente in 1604. He assumed that it served as a reservoir for the storage of semen. Only within the past decade has the function of the bursa been elucidated as part of the antibody-production system of the bird. The bursa is similar to the thymus, in that both have masses of lymphocytes in early life.[113]

LIVER

The liver consists of right and left lobes of nearly equal size which lie caudal to the heart and partially surround its apex. Compared with that of the mammal

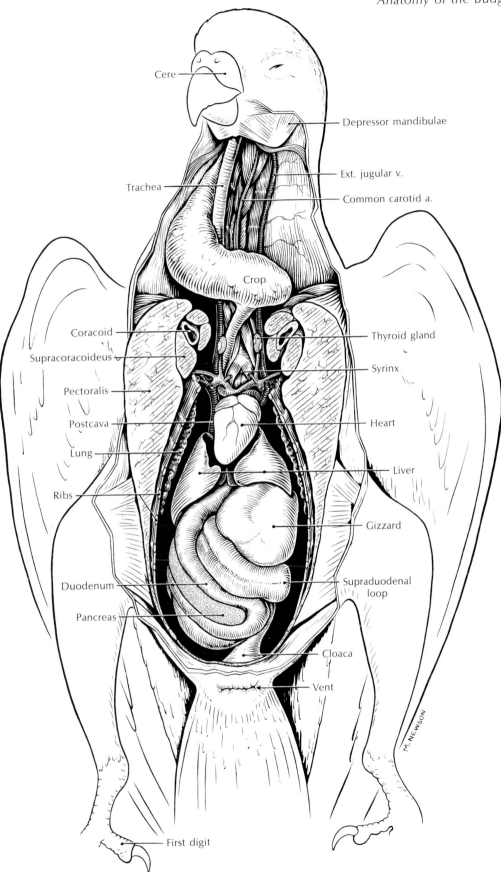

Fig. 5-21. *The viscera in situ, sternum and abdominal wall removed.*

the bird liver is relatively small and has little connective tissue, which possibly explains the paucity of septa and lack of extensive lobulation.

Peritoneal reflections over the liver connect it with various abdominal organs. A gastrohepatic ligament from the gizzard to the liver carries one or more small hepatic arteries from the aorta or left gastric artery to supply the liver parenchyma. The hepatoduodenal ligament between the base of the duodenal loop and the liver serves to carry the bile ducts from the liver to the duodenum. Although a gall bladder for the storage of bile is frequently present in birds (as in the chicken), it is lacking in the budgerigar. Within the parrot family some species lack a gall bladder, whereas in others it is present. A median falciform ligament which arises between the liver lobes unites with the apical part of the pericardial sac and with the ventral ligament of the gizzard before attaching to the sternum and linea alba. Within the falciform ligament remnants of the umbilical veins may occasionally be seen. This ventral mesentery partially divides the peritoneal cavity into a large right chamber and a smaller left chamber.

PANCREAS

The pancreas of the bird is usually located within or along the duodenal loop. In some species a pancreatic lobe may reach the spleen. In the budgerigar two pancreatic lobes are located within the duodenal loop, and one lies along the outside of the loop. However, the ducts from all three lobes (Fig. 5-27) open into the distal or ascending duodenum. Two of the ducts enter on the inner surface of the loop alongside the bile ducts, whereas the duct of the outer pancreatic lobe enters on the side of the duodenum opposite from the entrance of the bile ducts. The arterial supply to the pancreas is via the large pancreaticoduodenal artery, a branch of the celiac. As in the mammal, the pancreas of the bird consists of an exocrine and an endocrine portion.

Respiratory System

The respiratory system of birds is the most elaborately constructed of any found among vertebrates (Fig. 5-22). Interrelationships with the skeleton via air passageways into pneumatic bones and the proximity of air sacs to the abdominal viscera are unique features. The respiratory exchange surface within the lung is exceedingly compact, but the flow of air throughout the system is very rapid and efficient. Functional considerations have been reviewed by Akester,[2] Salt and Zeuthen,[135] Salt,[134] and King.[79a]

NOSE

The two external nares, or nostrils, at the base of the upper beak are surrounded in the budgerigar by a thick, soft cere. The paired nasal cavities are hidden from external view by a flap, and are separated from each other by an ossified septum. Within each nasal cavity there are cartilaginous turbinates which fill the antrum but allow inspired air to pass around and between them to reach the choana. Opening into the nasal antrum are the ducts of the paired nasal (salt) glands. Each gland lies within the orbit, beneath the supraorbital crest (see Fig. 5-30), and sends its duct across the hinge of the upper beak. The nasal gland of the budgerigar is comparatively large, considering the low-salt diet of the bird.

On the roof of the pharynx the slit-like median choana marks the location of the internal nares (see Fig. 5-19). The fimbriated end of the soft palate borders the opening. Inspired air crosses the pharynx to enter the glottis.

LARYNX

On the floor of the pharynx lies the larynx, or entrance to the trachea. The larynx is cradled on the hyoid apparatus (see Fig. 5-20) and covered with pharyngeal mucosa bearing a few filiform papillae. No vocal cords are present in the larynx of the bird.

The laryngeal skeleton consists of paired arytenoid cartilages, a trough-shaped cricoid cartilage, and a nodular procricoid cartilage. The fleshy laryngeal prominences, one on each side of the larynx, bound the glottis and function as a muscular sphincter (sphincter glottidis), stiffened by the arytenoid cartilages and capable of regulating the passage of air.

Caudal and dorsal to the larynx is the opening to the esophagus. Food passing from the oral cavity to the esophagus must cross the respiratory passageway from the choana to the glottis. This region where the two streams, air and food, cross in the pharynx is known as the pharyngeal chiasma. Birds killed by electric shock may "swallow" their larynx and thus have an intussusception. This occurs when the entrance of the esophagus engulfs the forward-lying floor of the pharynx because of violent muscular contraction caused by the electric shock.

The cricoid cartilage is the largest element of the larynx in the bird. In shape it rather resembles the mammalian thyroid cartilage. It forms the floor and side walls and is attached anteriorly to the hyoid apparatus below. In the budgerigar (see Fig. 5-20 B) the cricoid cartilage is horseshoe-shaped with the free ends almost meeting caudo-dorsally. Above the free ends of the cricoid cartilage is the nodular procricoid cartilage.

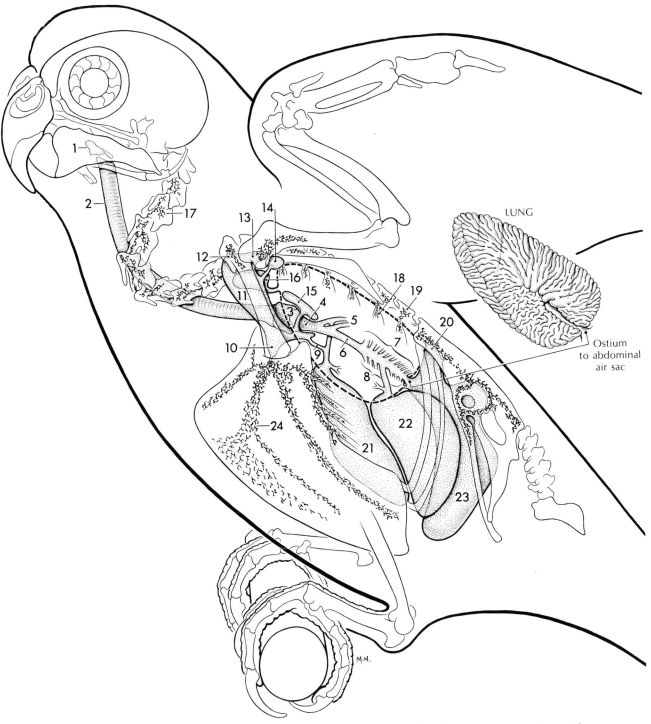

LUNG

Ostium
to abdominal
air sac

M.N.

Fig. 5-22. *Lateral view of the lung and respiratory passageways in relation to the skeleton. (Surface view of lung is displaced to show internal structures.) 1, Cricoid cartilage of larynx; 2, trachea; 3, syrinx; 4, left bronchus; 5, medial secondary bronchi (medibronchi); 6, mesobronchus; 7, dorsal secondary bronchi; 8, ventral secondary bronchi; 9, connection to interclavicular sac; 10, sternal diverticulum of interclavicular sac; 11, lateral diverticulum of interclavicular sac; 12, pneumatic foramen into coracoid bone; 13, subscapular diverticulum of interclavicular sac; 14, axillary diverticulum of interclavicular sac; 15, dorsal syringeal diverticulum of interclavicular sac; 16, cervical air sac; 17, pneumatic spaces in 4th cervical vertebra; 18, pneumatic spaces in rib; 19, pneumatized thoracic vertebra; 20, pneumatic diverticulum into the ilium from the abdominal sac; 21, cranial thoracic sac; 22, caudal thoracic sac; 23, abdominal sac; 24, pneumatic spaces within the carina of the sternum.*

Within the caudal margins of the glottis are the arytenoid cartilages, which presumably aid in the functioning of the sphincter glottidis.

TRACHEA

The trachea, or windpipe, is a very flexible tube, kept open by cartilaginous rings in its wall, and lined by a stratified squamous epithelium. It connects the larynx with the syrinx and lies to the left of the esophagus.

The tracheal rings are complete, calcified, and stain with Alizarine red dye, as do the tracheal rings of reptiles. In some species of birds the trachea is flattened dorso-ventrally or may have overlapping rings. In some swans and geese the trachea takes a serpentine course and may lie partly enclosed in the hollowed-out sternum.

The trachea of the budgerigar is about 2 mm. in diameter and consists of a series of cartilaginous rings, closed for the most part but occasionally open with overlapping ends. The beginning of the trachea at the larynx consists of several ventral semi-rings proximal to the first complete ring caudal to the larynx (see Fig. 5-10). Each ring is wide on one side and narrow on the other, alternating in series with the adjacent rings. This arrangement provides for a partial telescoping of the narrow portions of the rings within the alternating wide portions. (See McLelland[92] for an illustrated description.) The tracheal rings are composed of hyaline cartilage in the center and white fibro-cartilage along the edges. On each side of the trachea a thin band of muscle 1 mm. in width originates at the level of the larynx and passes to the region of the syrinx, where it enters into various relationships with the syringeal muscles.

SYRINX

The syrinx (see Fig. 5-16), a structure peculiar to birds, is the vocal organ formed by modified cartilages of the trachea or bronchi, or a combination of the two, with associated membranes and muscles. The muscles are capable of changing the shape of the cavity or the tension on the membranous parts of the organ.

Basically there are three types of syringes in birds: (1) tracheal (stork), (2) tracheo-bronchial (most passerine birds), and (3) bronchial (oilbird). The ancestral syrinx is believed to have been tracheo-bronchial. The budgerigar has a tracheo-bronchial syrinx and three pairs of associated muscles. The last few tracheal rings are fused to form a syringeal box; the first pair of bronchial semi-rings are much enlarged, articulate on

the syringeal box, and are free to move in one plane. A prominent membrane separates the second bronchial semi-ring from the enlarged first pair, and smaller membranes separate the subsequent bronchial semi-rings. It is this prominent membrane on each side which is tensed or relaxed by the tracheo-bronchial muscles.

Whereas in ducks and geese the syrinx may be greatly expanded and even form an osseous bulla, in the majority of birds it is the narrowest portion of the tracheo-bronchial tree. The median wall of the bronchial tubes is membranous and constitutes the internal tympaniform membrane.

For a description of the cartilages and muscles of the syrinx, refer to the discussion under Musculature, on pages 69–70, and see Ames.[4]

BRONCHI

Leading into either lung from the syrinx is a bronchus which has both an extra- and an intra-pulmonary portion. The extra-pulmonary bronchus, or main bronchus, has cartilaginous semi-rings on its lateral surface, whereas its medial surface is thin and elastic. The intra-pulmonary portion of each bronchus is called a mesobronchus, since it is surrounded by lung parenchyma.

The main bronchus enters the cranio-medial surface of the lung and courses caudo-laterally (Fig. 5-23). After entrance into the lung, the mesobronchus gives rise on the medial surface to several large secondary bronchi, which form dorsal and ventral arcades of smaller tubes called tertiary bronchi, or parabronchi. The ventral parabronchi turn under the cranio-ventral border of the lung and anastomose with a like number of parabronchi from large secondary bronchi on the

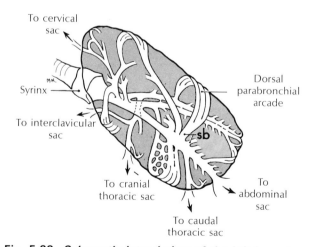

Fig. 5-23. *Schematic lateral view of the left lung showing the mesobronchus and a secondary bronchus (sb), which gives rise to a dorsal parabronchial arcade.*

lateral surface of the lung, forming the ventral parabronchial arcade.

Basically there are two large secondary bronchi which run longitudinally along the medial surface of the lung, while the mesobronchus runs obliquely through the lung to its caudolateral surface. Connecting these three primary longitudinal air channels (Fig. 5-23) are a series of secondary bronchi (dorso-bronchi and ventro-bronchi), which give rise to many tertiary bronchi (parabronchi), forming the arcades which are visible on the external surface of the lung.

On the caudolateral surface of the lung the mesobronchus gives rise to about eight dorsal and eight ventral secondary bronchi. The distribution of these secondary bronchi is as dorsal and ventral parabronchial arcades which pass around the margins of the lung to connect with the large medial secondary bronchi as indicated in Figure 5-23. The caudal continuation of the mesobronchus connects with the abdominal air sac. A more cranial ventral secondary bronchus exits from the medial ventral surface of the lung and supplies the caudal thoracic air sac.

LUNGS

The lungs are small and compact, and fit tightly against the dorsal wall of the thorax (see Fig. 5-22). The 2nd to 8th ribs indent and are enveloped by the dorsal margin of each lung, which prevents any change in the position of the lung. The lung consists of a mass of ramifying interconnected tubes visible to the naked eye. These are the tertiary bronchi (parabronchi), which arise from the secondary bronchi. Each parabronchial tube has numerous microscopic air capillaries which exit from it and lie in close apposition to blood capillaries in the lung parenchyma. When the air sac system is injected via the trachea some of these air capillaries fill with latex and give a fuzzy appearance to the cast of the parabronchial tubes. It is the air capillaries which represent the respiratory exchange site. Most of the air capillaries interconnect with other air capillaries from the same parabronchus, although they may also end blindly as Hazelhoff[61] noted in the fowl. The structure of the bird's lung has been described by Fischer,[44] Locy and Larsell,[88] Akester,[2] and King.[79a]

The diaphragm of birds is represented by thin membranous partitions in two planes. One portion, horizontal in position, is closely applied to the ventral surface of the lungs as it stretches from one side of the rib cage to the other with an anchorage on the ventral midline of the vertebral column. Delicate muscle strands from the body wall may pass onto this membrane but hardly appear to play a functional role. The other portion of the diaphragm is the oblique

septum. Huxley[69] coined the term oblique septum for the membranous partitions that extend from the midline between the lungs at the level of the base of the heart to the sternum and body wall and separate the abdominal from the pleural cavity. Although the oblique septum is usually membranous, it may be partially invaded by muscle fibers. Beddard[8] discussed the possible homologies of the oblique septum in birds and pointed out that as a general rule only the abdominal air sac projects through the oblique septum to lie in the abdominal cavity. The heart lies on the abdominal side of the cranial portion of the septum, which is unlike the situation in regard to the mammalian diaphragm.

AIR SACS

In most species of birds there are four paired air sacs and one median unpaired sac with several diverticula. Some authors consider the various diverticula as distinct air sacs, and this results in some confusion as to the number of air sacs said to be present in the different species. The sacs are thin-walled and lack blood vessels. Although they are in contact with one another, they do not communicate.

In the budgerigar (Figs. 5-22, 5-24) the four paired (cervical, two thoracic, and abdominal) and one unpaired (interclavicular) air sacs are large and fairly constant in morphology. Air sacs function as a bellows for receiving and then delivering a flow of air through the respiratory passageways. When the sternum is lowered and the thoraco-abdominal cavity is thus enlarged, air is drawn into the air sacs and parabronchial tubes simultaneously. The capacity of the air sacs is greater than the combined capacity in the various air tubes, and is such that on expiration they constitute a source of oxygen-rich air available to the parabronchial tubes. The mechanics and flow of air through the respiratory system of the bird is still a subject of considerable controversy and study. (See King[79a].)

INTERCLAVICULAR SAC. The interclavicular air sac is the most complicated of all the air sacs in its ramifications and connections. A median structure surrounding the syrinx and bronchi, it is supplied with air from both the right and the left mesobronchus (Fig. 5-24). The primary connection with the mesobronchus on each side consists of a large channel (*9*, Fig. 5-22) from a medial secondary bronchus which supplies the cranial thoracic sac. In addition there are two or more saccobronchi on each side, connecting the air sac with parabronchi on the craniomedial surface of the lung. These saccobronchi (formerly called recurrent bronchi),

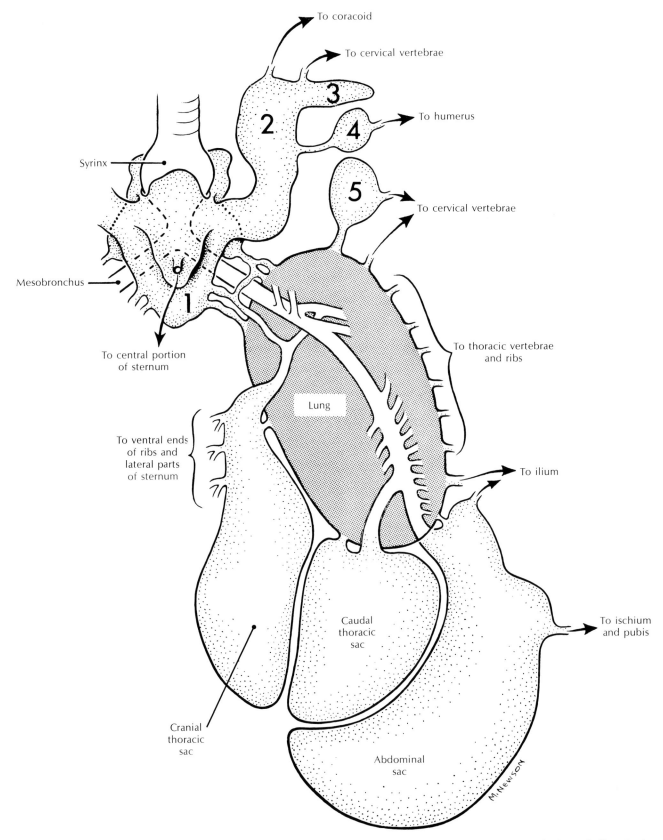

Fig. 5-24. *Schematic ventral view of the air sacs and their connections. 1, interclavicular sac; 2, lateral diverticulum of interclavicular sac; 3, subscapular diverticulum; 4, axillary diverticulum; 5, cervical sac.*

which are present on all air sacs except the cervical sacs, appear capable of conveying air in either direction. Akester[2] concluded that these channels in the lung of the fowl, duck, and pigeon are indistinguishable from tertiary bronchi, and the absence of valves leaves in doubt the recurrent flow concept that had been advanced earlier.

The ventral part of the interclavicular sac has a sternal diverticulum which lies behind the rostrum and between the coracoid bones. An air channel enters a median foramen to ramify within the sternum. At the points where the sternal ribs articulate there are communications of the sternal air channels with those of the ribs, and also connections with the cranial thoracic air sac. This arrangement permits the cranial thoracic air sac to supply the pneumatic spaces of both the ventral ribs and the lateral plate of the sternum.

A dorsal diverticulum of the interclavicular sac (*15*, Fig. 5-22) surrounds and is closely applied to the syrinx, covering the origin of the bronchi. It often has direct connections with parabronchi on the medial surface of the lung.

The largest parts of the interclavicular sac are the lateral portions which pass dorsally on each side of the trachea. Each gives rise to an axillary diverticulum beneath the shoulder joint which connects through the pneumatic foramen with the pneumatic spaces of the humerus of the same side. The most dorsal extension of the interclavicular sac on each side connects with pneumatic spaces within the coracoid bone and extends posteriorly as the subscapular diverticulum, which has connections with the pneumatic spaces of several vertebrae.

CERVICAL SACS. The paired cervical air sacs are small, and lie medial to the lateral diverticulum of the interclavicular sac at the base of the neck. Each cervical sac is supplied by a tertiary bronchus issuing from the cranial end of the lung rather than by a secondary bronchus. There are no saccobronchi connecting them with the lung as there are with all of the other air sacs. The cervical air sacs are, however, connected with the pneumatized cervical vertebrae, which in turn are connected with the lung by several parabronchi.

CRANIAL THORACIC SACS. The cranial thoracic air sacs are paired and each originates from the same large secondary bronchus that connects with the interclavicular sac. Each sac lies against the thoracic wall and has connections ventrally with the pneumatic spaces of the ribs and sternum (Fig. 5-22).

CAUDAL THORACIC SACS. The paired caudal thoracic air sacs arise from ventral secondary bronchi which emerge from the medial ventral surface of the lung. Each sac lies behind and somewhat medial to the cranial thoracic sac and lateral to the abdominal sac. The caudal thoracic air sac is the only sac which does not appear to have any connections with pneumatic bones.

ABDOMINAL SACS. The abdominal air sacs are the largest and most variable in shape since they must conform to the spaces around and between the viscera and abdominal wall. The left and right sacs differ from each other in shape and placement, but have similar origins and connections. The abdominal air sac originates at the caudo-lateral pole of the lung as a continuation of the mesobronchus. It is the only air sac connection that can be seen on the lateral surface of the lung when the thoracic wall is removed. Dorsally, the abdominal sac connects with pneumatic spaces in the ilium and more caudally with the ischium and pubis (Figs. 5-22, 5-24).

PNEUMATIC BONES

There are many pneumatic bones in the budgerigar, and several of them are supplied from more than one source. The function of such air spaces in bones is still open to conjecture, but their presence does help to keep the bones light. There is a detrimental feature of this extensive system of air passageways, in that it facilitates the rapid spread of air-borne diseases, and enhances the toxic effect of air pollutants. The vulnerability to traumatic hemorrhage of the airways often leads to sudden death.

The skull bones do not appear to be in communication with the respiratory system, although many of the bones consist of diploë enclosing open trabeculae. (Kaupp,[78] speaking of the chicken [p. 205] says the upper jaw and cranium receive air from the Eustachian tubes and the lower jaw receives air from the pneumatic foramen on each ramus behind the tympanic articulation and from an air cell which surrounds the joint.)

All vertebrae are pneumatic except the first two cervical and the free caudal vertebrae. The remaining cervical vertebrae are supplied by the interclavicular air sac, the cervical air sacs, and by some direct connections from the lungs. Thoracic vertebrae are supplied directly by tertiary bronchi from the lungs, which arise in the 2nd to 6th intercostal spaces. Lumbosacral vertebrae receive a few direct connections from the lungs, as well as from the abdominal air sacs via the ilium and ischium. The ilium, ischium, and pubis are all supplied by air passageways from the dorsal part of the ipsilateral abdominal air sac. In addition, the ilium receives direct parabronchi from the most caudo-dorsal portion of the lung. Each of the ribs receives dorsal air connections from the lung and ventral connections from the sternum and cranial thoracic sac (Fig. 5-22). The coracoid bone is pneumatized from the lateral diverticulum of the interclavicular air sac. The clavicle is so reduced it is non-pneumatic, and no evidence of air passageways can be seen in the scapula. The humerus is pneumatic for only half its length, and thus the more distal elements of the wing are non-pneumatic. The pelvic limb has no bones in communication with respiratory passageways, although a potential connection exists as a small protrusion from either abdominal air sac cranial to the acetabulum and the head of the femur. The sternum is well pneumatized throughout by means of connections from the sternal diverticulum of the interclavicular sac, as well as from the ventral border of the cranial thoracic sacs. The largest pneumatic channel within the sternum passes ventrally and can be identified externally as a perpendicular ridge on the carina (*24*, Fig. 5-22).

Circulatory System

The circulatory system functions to carry oxygen and nutrients to the tissues and transport metabolic end-products to the kidneys. Other functions include the distribution of body heat, the circulation of hormones, the combating of infection and repair of injury, and the support of growth.

The functional parts of the system consist of a muscular pump, the heart; a distribution system of arteries, arterioles, and capillaries; a collecting system of capillaries, venules, and veins; a lymphatic network for the return of tissue fluid; and a red, opaque, viscid fluid, the blood, consisting of plasma with red and white blood cells (see Lucas and Jamroz[89] and Sturkie[146]).

The embryonic development of the hematopoietic, vascular, and lymphatic systems in the bird has been reviewed and illustrated by Romanoff.[132]

Heart

The heart of a bird is comparatively larger and more elongate than that of the mammal. It is located on the midline in the anterior part of the thoracic cavity, immediately behind the syrinx (Fig. 5-25). Since the lungs are small and located dorsally, they do not surround the heart as they do in the mammal. Instead, the right and left lobes of the liver cradle the heart and partially hide it from ventral view. The base of the heart lies close to the hilus of the lung, and its

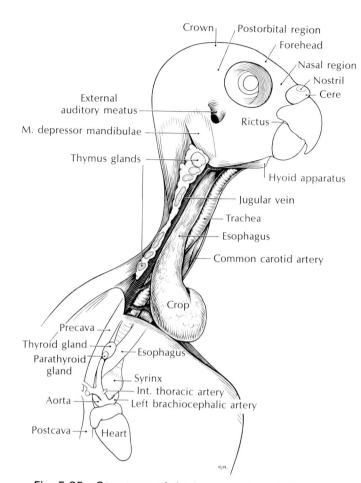

Fig. 5-25. *Structures of the head, neck, and thorax.*

apex extends caudo-ventrally. Kern[79] described the chicken's heart and included a bibliography.

Surrounding the heart is a fibrous pericardial sac attached to its base where the great vessels enter and leave. Within the pericardial sac there is a small amount of fluid, which acts as a lubricant.

The heart is four-chambered, as in the mammal, although the atria are small and externally somewhat indistinct from each other. The right atrium is larger than the left and receives the two precaval veins and one postcaval vein. The right atrium opens into the right ventricle via the right atrioventricular valve, which consists of two flaps. Internally the walls of the atria and ventricles are relatively smooth, compared with those of the mammalian heart. The right ventricle is smaller and thinner walled than the left and is closely applied to the convex septal wall formed primarily by the left ventricle. When cut in cross section the right ventricle appears as a crescentic cavity which does not extend as far as the apex of the heart. The right ventricle forms a conus arteriosus with a semilunar valve which leads to the pulmonary artery.

Immediately upon leaving the right ventricle of the

heart the pulmonary artery divides into right and left trunks which enter the dorsally lying lungs. Blood is returned from the lungs through the pulmonary veins and enters on the dorsal surface of the left atrium via short trunks which are hidden from view unless the apex of the heart is reflected cranially.

Arteries

ARCH OF AORTA

The aorta, as it leaves the base of the heart, gives rise to a right and a left brachiocephalic trunk (Figs. 5-25, 5-26). Unlike mammals, birds have retained the right aortic arch instead of the left. Glenny[56] has reviewed the literature on the morphology and development of the aortic arches in birds and has illustrated the adult patterns of many species, including the lorikeet *Trichoglossus*.

ARTERIES OF TRUNK, HEAD, AND WING

The aorta, as it emerges from the left ventricle, turns dorsally over the heart and is normally hidden from ventral view. It passes caudally below the vertebral column and above the lungs. Issuing from the aorta are dorsal segmental arteries to the musculature, and bronchial vessels to the lung.

The first dorsal segmental arteries leave the aorta at the level of the 6th thoracic vertebra, between the celiac and cranial mesenteric arteries. Small dorsal vessels from the aorta also arise at the 8th thoracic and the 1st lumbar vertebra. These dorsal vessels supply the axial musculature, vertebrae, and meninges.

The brachiocephalic arteries are almost as large as the aorta and lie on either side of the muscular syrinx. Each brachiocephalic artery divides into a large axillary artery and a smaller common carotid. The axillary artery gives rise to several large pectoral branches, a brachial artery, and an internal thoracic artery.

The pectoral arteries, three in number at their origin, enter the breast musculature where they ramify in the supracoracoideus and pectoralis. Some of the branches penetrate the pectoralis to supply the skin and feathers of the breast.

The brachial artery, called humeral by some authors, originates from the axillary artery between the pectoral and common carotid arteries. It passes laterally beneath the external jugular vein on its way into the wing. As the brachial artery enters the wing it supplies subscapular and coracoid twigs before giving rise to cranial and caudal circumflex humeral arteries. The brachial artery crosses the flexor surface of the elbow joint and divides into radial and ulnar arteries. Several

small arteries ramify in the contiguous muscles and in the patagial membrane. The radial artery continues along the leading edge of the wing; the ulnar artery courses along the trailing edge and continues into the terminal feathers at the tip of the wing.

The shoulder joint and dorsal shoulder musculature receive a large artery directly from the common carotid, rather than from the brachial.

The internal thoracic artery leaves the ventral surface of the brachiocephalic at the bifurcation of the common carotid and brachial arteries. It passes to the inner surface of the sternum and supplies the supracoracoideus muscle, the sternal ribs, and the intercostal muscles. After reaching the sternum each internal thoracic artery sends a branch along the coracoid bone to the shoulder joint.

The common carotid arteries (Fig. 5-26) are the largest branches of the brachiocephalic trunks. Each passes cranially medio-ventral to the external jugular vein. Leaving the dorsal surface of the common carotid artery, surrounded by the interclavicular air sac, is the costocervical-vertebral trunk. The costocervical artery passes between the heads of the ribs and supplies structures along the vertebral ends of the ribs; the vertebral artery passes cranially through the transverse foramina of cervical vertebrae to supply the neck vertebrae and associated structures.

According to Garrod,[53] who studied many species of parrots, there are three primary variations of the common carotid arteries in parrots: (1) right and left carotids side by side on the ventral surface of the cervical vertebrae (*Melopsittacus* and 18 others); (2) right carotid deep and left carotid superficial along the neck with the vagus nerve and jugular vein (*Ara* and 12 others); and (3) only the left carotid developed (*Kacatua*). Garrod believed the ancestral parrot possessed two carotids running symmetrically on the ventral surface of the neck. Glenny[56] has documented the arrangements of the carotid arteries in a great many birds and reviewed the literature.

About 2 cm. cranial to the heart, in contact with each common carotid artery, are the thyroid and parathyroid glands. Each thyroid gland is approximately 2 mm. long and 1.5 mm. wide. The number of parathyroid bodies varies from one to three (Fig. 5-26). Two arteries leave each common carotid artery in the region of the glands, and either one or both supply them. The arrangement of the vessels is asymmetrical. One of the two large arteries leaving the common carotid at the level of the glands turns medially to supply the syrinx and esophagus; the other passes laterally to reach the crop and muscles of the shoulder. The common carotids also supply the thyroid and parathyroid glands directly via short twigs on one or both

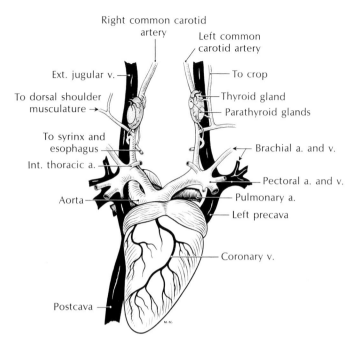

Right common carotid artery

Left common carotid artery

Ext. jugular v.

To dorsal shoulder musculature →

To syrinx and esophagus

Int. thoracic a.

Aorta

Postcava

To crop

Thyroid gland

Parathyroid glands

Brachial a. and v.

Pectoral a. and v.

Pulmonary a.

Left precava

Coronary v.

Fig. 5-26. *The heart and great vessels.*

sides before they converge on the midline to pass up the neck embedded in the ventral cervical muscles.

In the cranial third of the neck the carotid arteries emerge from the ventral neck musculature and diverge laterally to enter the head. It is at this point that the carotids are most accessible for injection of the arterial system.

As the carotid artery enters the head it divides into an external and an internal carotid. The external carotid artery supplies the upper and lower jaws, tongue, and occipital region. The internal carotid gives rise to cerebral arteries to the brain and an internal ophthalmic artery to the eye. References to the arteries of the brain in birds include Beddard,[9] Baumel,[7] and Vitums *et al.*,[158,159] who investigated the vascular supply of the hypothalamus in the white-crowned sparrow, with particular attention to the hypothalamic nuclei and portal systems. Kobayashi *et al.*[80] studied the hypothalamo-hypophyseal neurosecretory system of the budgerigar.

ABDOMINAL AORTA

The celiac artery, which is the first large branch of the abdominal aorta, supplies the proventriculus, gizzard, pancreas, duodenum, spleen, and liver (Fig. 5-27).

Near its origin from the aorta the celiac artery gives rise to an *esophageal branch,* which passes cranially onto the dorsal surface of the esophagus at the esophago-proventricular junction. Distally another large branch of the celiac artery, the proventricular artery, arborizes on the ventral surface of the proventriculus

and supplies the major portion of the glandular stomach. Many small capillaries can be seen to encircle the bases of the proventricular glands.

Upon reaching the cranial pole of the gizzard the celiac artery gives rise to a large left gastric artery, which supplies the left side and ventral surface of the gizzard. The left gastric artery also supplies one or two ascending branches to the glandular stomach, which anastomose with the proventricular artery. The largest branch of the left gastric artery supplies the mid-ventral region of the gizzard and sends twigs to both right and left sides.

Several short twigs may arise from the celiac artery, proximal to the origin of the left gastric artery, to supply the cranial pole of the gizzard. A long left hepatic artery arises from the left gastric or from the celiac artery. It is difficult to expose this branch to the liver without breaking it (*1,* Fig. 5-27).

The main continuation of the celiac artery passes to the right of the gizzard and to the left of the spleen, supplying two or three short splenic arteries before it bifurcates dorsal to the gastro-duodenal junction. One branch of the fork supplies the right side and caudal pole of the gizzard, whereas the other passes into the duodenal loop to become the pancreaticoduodenal artery. One of the proximal branches of this artery is the right hepatic artery to the liver, which parallels the bile ducts. Another major branch is the ileocolic artery, which passes onto the supraduodenal loop.

The small intestine forms five loops, three of which are supplied by branches of the cranial mesenteric artery and two by branches of the celiac artery (Fig. 5-27).

The first loop is the duodenal loop encircling the pancreas. It lies in the mid-plane of the bird caudal to the gizzard and is supplied by the pancreaticoduodenal artery. The second, third, and fourth loops lie on the right side of the bird and constitute the main "coils" of the intestinal mass. They are supplied by jejunal branches of the cranial mesenteric artery. The fifth loop is the supraduodenal loop which passes from right to left beneath the gizzard. This last loop of the small intestine lies on the left side of the gizzard caudal to the posterior thoracic air sac, and cranial to the duodenal loop. It is supplied by the ileocolic artery.

The second major branch of the abdominal aorta is the cranial mesenteric artery. It supplies jejunal branches to the three loops of the small intestine, a branch to the large intestine, and twigs to the duodenum. The cranial mesenteric artery leaves the aorta about 2 mm. caudal to the celiac artery and at the level of the spleen it trifurcates to supply the intestines.

One branch, the colic, passes dorsal to the intestinal loops and supplies the terminal straight portion of the

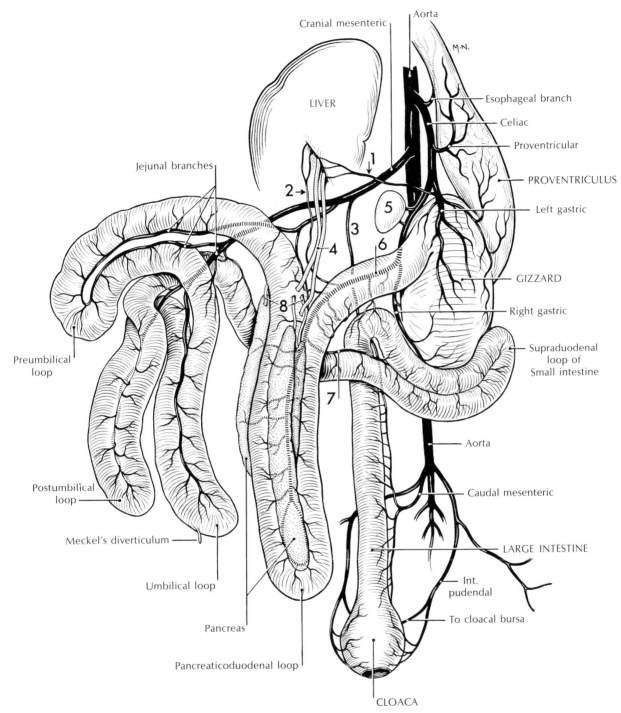

Fig. 5-27. *Arterial supply and structures of the digestive tract: 1 and 2, hepatic arteries; 3, colic artery; 4, bile ducts; 5, spleen; 6, pancreaticoduodenal artery; 7, ileocolic artery; 8, pancreatic ducts.*

intestine. Ceca are lacking in the budgerigar, but at the level where ceca would be expected to appear the colic artery anastomoses with the caudal mesenteric artery.

A larger branch of the cranial mesenteric artery anastomoses with the jejunal artery and supplies the distal limb of the duodenal loop. Its numerous twigs

anastomose with the pancreaticoduodenal artery and help supply the duodenum as well as the pancreas.

The main continuation of the cranial mesenteric artery supplies the three loops of the small intestine which lie between the first (duodenal) and the last (supraduodenal) portion of the small intestine.

The adrenal gland (see Fig. 5-29) is supplied by

small twigs directly from the aorta or from the most cranial renal artery. The gonads—the paired testes in the male and left ovary in the female—are supplied by a similar arrangement. The gonads partially or completely hide the adrenal glands from ventral view.

As the aorta courses between the lobes of the kidney it gives rise to paired renal arteries which pass into the cranial lobes, external iliac arteries emerging between the cranial and middle lobes, ischiatic arteries between the middle and caudal lobes, and renal arteries passing into the conjoined caudal lobes of the kidney. The external iliac artery supplies twigs to the kidney before it emerges to supply the abdominal wall and pelvic fat, and the ischiatic artery similarly supplies the kidney before it enters the pelvic limb (see Fig. 5-29).

ARTERIES OF THE PELVIC LIMB

The external iliac and ischiatic arteries are the major vessels of the pelvic limb. Szabó[148] and Nishida[119] have illustrated the vessels of the pelvic limb in the budgerigar and fowl, respectively.

The external iliac artery, which leaves the aorta between the cranial and middle lobes of the kidney, enters the limb in front of the acetabulum. It divides into cranial gluteal and circumflex femoral arteries which supply the sartorius and iliotibialis muscles, a femoral artery to the adductor and gastrocnemius, and a pelvic artery (umbilical of some authors), which runs along the pubis to supply the obturator muscles.

The ischiatic artery, which is the main vessel of the pelvic limb, after arising from the aorta between the middle and caudal lobes of the kidney passes through the ischiatic foramen and enters the leg. As the ischiatic artery leaves the pelvis, it gives rise to trochanteric and caudal gluteal arteries. More distally it supplies a nutrient artery to the femur and a deep femoral artery to the caudal thigh muscles. At the level of the knee the ischiatic artery gives rise to a genicular artery to the knee joint and a caudally directed branch into the shank muscles. Below the level of the knee the ischiatic artery divides into caudal, medial, and cranial tibial arteries. The cranial tibial artery passes over the lateral surface of the tibiotarsus and becomes the dorsal pedal artery on the cranial surface of the tibiotarsal joint. The dorsal pedal artery supplies the digital muscles and toes.

As the aorta emerges from the conjoined caudal lobes of the kidney in the budgerigar it gives rise to the internal pudendal arteries, the last large paired vessels to arise from it. These vessels supply the medial surface of the pelvis (internal obturator muscle included), continue on to supply the cloacal bursa (bursa of Fabricius), and terminate as numerous branches to the cloacal wall.

The caudal mesenteric artery (see Fig. 5-27) usually arises from the right internal pudendal artery rather than from the median sacral artery. Upon reaching the terminal portion of the digestive tract the caudal mesenteric artery divides into an ascending and a descending branch. The ascending branch supplies the terminal portion of the small intestine and anastomoses with the colic branch of the cranial mesenteric artery. The descending branch supplies the large intestine and anastomoses with the cloacal vessels (Fig. 5-29).

Distal to the origin of the internal pudendal arteries, the aorta is continued as the median sacral artery and terminates in the median coccygeal artery. One or more pairs of lateral coccygeal arteries supply the muscles and feathers of the uropygium.

Veins

Veins usually accompany arteries at more superficial levels but have distinctive main tributaries which are often unlike the arterial supply, particularly for the viscera and head.

VEINS OF HEAD

The head is drained by several large veins which enter the paired external jugular veins. These large superficial veins pass down the neck and are surrounded by fat and lobules of thymus gland (see Fig. 5-25). At the base of the neck one or two large tributary veins from the crop enter the jugular on each side. In some species of birds the left jugular vein is lost. Within the thoracic inlet the thyroid and parathyroid glands lie in contact with the ventral surface of the jugular vein and drain into it (Fig. 5-26). Closer to the heart the jugular veins on each side join the axillary veins to form the right and left precavae which enter the right atrium of the heart.

VEINS OF WING

The axillary vein is a short, wide vessel which receives the vertebral and costocervical veins from the neck, the brachial vein from the wing, and the pectoral vessels (internal and external thoracic veins) from the breast musculature.

The brachial vein of the wing is formed by a superficial and a deep radial vein on the leading edge, the ulnar vein on the trailing edge, and smaller tributaries from the patagial membrane, skin, and muscles.

VEINS OF PELVIC LIMB

The digital veins drain into two metatarsal veins which continue proximally as the cranial and caudal tibial veins. As they approach the back of the knee the tibial veins join in a single trunk and receive other smaller veins to form the popliteal vein. Above the level of the knee joint the popliteal vein becomes the femoral vein, which runs between the caudal thigh muscles and receives the deep femoral, nutrient, and pelvic veins. Draining the cranial thigh muscles are the branches of the cranial femoral vein, which join the femoral to form the external iliac vein.

VEINS OF DORSAL BODY WALL

The veins draining the kidney and dorsal body wall consist primarily of right and left superficial longitudinal veins on the surface of the kidney, and right and left deep longitudinal veins within the kidney (see Fig. 5-28). There are several connections between the superficial and deep longitudinal veins of the kidney and each receives tributaries from the pelvic limb and body wall. The superficial veins receive the external iliacs, and the deep veins receive the ischiatics as well as the external iliacs.

The deep longitudinal vein on each side, which drains into the external iliac vein, receives many small veins from the kidney and several major veins from the body wall. It is connected caudally with the renal portal vein, which is a remaining portion of the embryonic renal portal system. The renal portal system appears to be an early adaptation for allowing venous blood from the hind part of the body to pass through a capillary bed in the kidney in close proximity to the renal tubules. Sperber[140] demonstrated that venous blood from the leg flows in part through the intertubular capillary bed of the kidney on its way to the heart.

It can be seen from Figure 5-28 that the renal portal vein is continuous cranially with the postcava and caudally with the coccygeomesenteric vein on the large intestine. The coccygeomesenteric vein can thus drain either into the postcava and thence to the heart or into the hepatic portal vein which enters the liver. Ligation of the intestinal hepatic portal vein would result in a diversion of the flow of venous blood, through the renal portal vein to the postcava. Ranney et al.[129] described a procedure for producing an experimental functional hepatectomy in the bird by such a ligation.

VEINS OF VISCERA

The hepatic portal veins entering the liver receive venous blood from the stomach, spleen, pancreas, and intestines as well as from the liver itself. After ingestion of food, the portal blood shows a high concentration of glucose, amino acids, and fatty acids being transported to the liver. The portal veins break up into sinusoids within the liver before re-forming as hepatic veins which join the postcava.

The postcava receives blood from the posterior portion of the body, the pelvic limbs, and the viscera. As the largest venous trunk in the body it is formed by the confluence of the right and left common iliac veins at the level of the cranial poles of the kidneys (Fig. 5-28). The short adrenal and gonadal veins enter the postcava at its origin. The postcava passes dorsally through the right lobe of the liver and receives hepatic veins before it reaches the right atrium of the heart.

Lymphatic System

The lymphatic system consists of a closed capillary network and larger collecting vessels which return lymph or tissue fluid from all parts of the body to the venous system. Lymphatics in the bird terminate principally by two thoracic ducts which enter the right and left jugular veins by several orifices. There may also be lympho-venous anastomoses in other parts of the body. Lymphatics also carry absorbed fat from the intestine to the thoracic duct. Associated with lymphatic vessels are cell-producing lymph follicles, lymph nodes, thymus glands (Fig. 5-25), spleen, and the cloacal bursa, or bursa of Fabricius (Fig. 5-28).

Moore and Owen,[113] utilizing a chromosome marker technique in combination with various experimental procedures, concluded that the majority of bursal lymphocytes are derived not from primordial cells of the bursa but rather by proliferation of blood-borne progenitor cells which enter the bursal primordium during embryogenesis.

Lymph nodes are rare in birds, and when present usually lie at the root of the neck, in the axilla, or in the groin. In place of lymph nodes there are numerous interconnected lymph vessels forming plexuses around the major arteries and veins and on the various organs. These vessels are rarely visible without special preparations. Ducks and geese, according to Romanoff,[132] have cervical and lumbar lymph nodes. Owen[122] called attention to sacral or pelvic lymph vesicles on each side of the bird at the junction of the tail and thigh. These so-called "lymph hearts," which are present in reptiles, develop in the embryos of all birds. Not all species possess them as adults, but a few, such as the ostrich, have bean-shaped sacral lymph hearts which have a muscular coat and which pulsate in life.

Miller[104] studied the development of the jugular lymph sac in birds and referred to Sala, who in 1900 published an account of the development of lymphatics in the chick, particularly the posterior lymph hearts and thoracic duct. Kaupp[78] described the lymphatic system of the adult fowl and also noted the sacral lymph hearts.

Urogenital System

The development of the kidney and its excretory ducts is closely followed in time and location by development of the gonads. As a result, during early embryonic development parts of the mesonephric kidney and its ducts are modified in the male for sperm conduction. Thus the efferent ductules, epididymis, and deferent duct are components of the primitive urinary system remodeled to serve for genital purposes. In the female the embryonic kidney ducts degenerate and a new channel, the oviduct (Müllerian, or paramesonephric duct), develops.

Urinary Components

The kidneys of the bird are of the metanephric type and have numerous small glomeruli. They are homogeneous in cross section and it is difficult to distinguish between the cortex and medulla. They extend from the caudal margin of the lungs to the end of the synsacrum. Each is partially divided into three lobes as a result of being located in roughly three depressions and being traversed by two main blood vessels leaving the aorta on either side. The cranial lobe of the kidney lies on the ventral surface of the ilium between the 6th and 8th ribs, the middle lobe is more deeply recessed between the transverse processes of fused lumbar vertebrae, and the caudal lobe lies in the sacral region. The right and left kidneys of the budgerigar are often joined posteriorly, enclosing the aorta. Both broad and narrow connections have been seen. Figure 5-28 illustrates a typical broad connection.

In the budgerigar blood is supplied to the kidney from the aorta as well as from the renal portal veins. Studies of the avian renal portal system include those of Sperber[140] and Akester.[3] Blood from the large intestine, pelvic region, and pelvic limbs is brought to the kidney by the coccygeomesenteric, pelvic, and ischiatic veins. Some of this blood is passed through the capillary bed of the kidney to reach the postcava, but most of it reaches the postcava through larger connecting channels. Each lobe of the kidney is drained by several funnel-shaped urinary ducts which join the ureter (metanephric duct). The ureters, hidden at their origin by the renal veins, pass along the ventral sur-

face of the kidneys. A urinary bladder is lacking in almost all birds, and the ureters enter the cloaca medial to the deferent duct in the male and dorsal to the oviduct in the female (Figs. 5-28, 5-29). The ureter is capable of peristaltic movement, which aids the passage of urine. Normally urine and feces are voided from the cloaca at the same time. The characteristic "bull's-eye" appearance of the droppings of the budgerigar is the result of a white ring of uric acid surrounding the dark fecal material. During the time that excretions remain in the cloaca, some of the water is reabsorbed.

Other Excretory Organs

In addition to kidney function for maintaining water balance, many birds possess nasal salt-excreting glands which are highly efficient sodium excretors as well as osmoregulators. Some marine birds excrete more salt via the nasal gland than through the kidneys. Nasal salt secretion is not restricted to marine birds and reptiles, although few studies of terrestrial birds have been made. Marples[96] and Technau[150] described the anatomy of these glands in many species of birds. Owen[122] observed them in one or more species of every Order of birds. Schmidt-Nielsen et al.[136] and Fänge et al.[43] demonstrated the true function of these glands in marine birds.

Cade and Dybas[20] observed that the budgerigar was capable of living without drinking water for over four months. This is accomplished by reduction of activity and utilization of free water in the seed combined with metabolic water. They point out that wild budgerigars exist in large numbers in arid interior Australia, which suggests that this species may have special abilities to survive on a minimal intake of water. The fact that water is necessary under certain environmental conditions is shown by the thousands of budgerigars that drown while crowding the watering troughs during droughts in Australia. Cade and Greenwald[21] studied nasal secretions of falconiform birds and found high concentrations of sodium chloride, which presumably came from the nasal glands. They postulate the main adaptive value of a functional nasal salt gland is to permit a bird with its typically hypotonic urine to remain in water balance solely on the preformed and oxidative water associated with its food even when the evaporative loss of water is high.

The nasal gland of the budgerigar (see Fig. 5-30) lies above the eye in the rostro-dorsal quadrant of the orbit. It is pale yellow in color and has a prominent duct which passes forward through a foramen in the frontal bone beneath the fronto-nasal suture to enter the nasal cavity. Whether the nasal gland of the budgerigar can function for the excretion of salt is not known.

Genital Organs

MALE GENITAL ORGANS

The male genital tract consists of paired testes, epididymides, and deferent ducts. Accessory glands are lacking, and only a few species possess a penile structure.

The testes are oval or round, and lie close together on either side of the postcava closely attached to the dorsal body wall between the cranial poles of the kidneys (Fig. 5-28). Arterial blood reaches them by direct twigs from the aorta. Venous blood is returned either directly to the postcava or into the adrenal veins and thence into the postcava. The testes partially or completely hide the adrenal glands from ventral view, even in the nonbreeding state. In some birds the testes enlarge tremendously during the breeding cycle and often displace the viscera. Budgerigar testes do not exhibit such great cyclic change in size. The seminiferous tubules within the testis convey spermatozoa to the epididymis, which connects with the deferent duct. The epididymis is closely bound to the testis and is not seen without dissection.

The deferent duct arises from the epididymis on

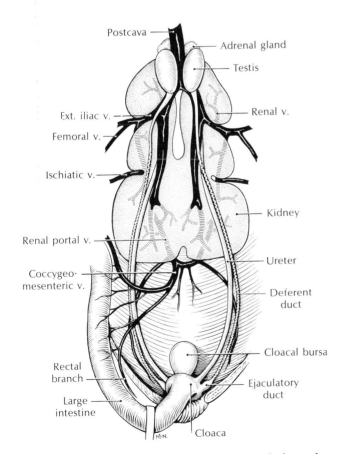

Fig. 5-28. *The male urogenital system and the veins of the trunk.*

Labels for Fig. 5-28:
Postcava
Adrenal gland
Testis
Ext. iliac v.
Femoral v.
Renal v.
Ischiatic v.
Kidney
Renal portal v.
Ureter
Coccygeo-mesenteric v.
Deferent duct
Rectal branch
Cloacal bursa
Large intestine
Ejaculatory duct
Cloaca

the caudo-dorsal pole of the testis, diverges laterally, and parallels the ureter for the remainder of its course. At the level of the middle lobe of the kidney the deferent duct becomes tightly pleated as it folds upon itself from side to side for the rest of its length, giving it a striated appearance. In several species of birds (sparrow, starling, and others) there is a "knot" of convoluted deferent duct close to the wall of the cloaca, known as the seminal glomus, which possibly functions for sperm storage. The budgerigar has no such structure, but it does have an enlargement of the terminal end of the deferent duct proximal to its entrance into the cloaca. This is the ejaculatory duct (Fig. 5-28) which, when forced against the cloacal wall by eversion of the cloaca, forms a slightly raised papilla which facilitates the transfer of semen to the everted orifice of the oviduct of the female during cloacal contact. Although a copulatory organ is lacking in most birds some, like the ostrich and goose, have developed a cloacal penis similar to that in reptiles. Identification of sex shortly after hatching in the chicken is based upon the appearance of the rudimentary copulatory organ on the ventral surface of the cloaca. An experienced sexer can determine the sex with over 95 per cent accuracy. (For plates showing sexual dimorphism of the cloaca in day-old chicks, see Canfield.[23]) Van Drimmelen[155] described the anatomical landmarks for the artificial insemination of the pigeon and fowl by the intraperitoneal injection of semen close to the infundibulum. He reported it was possible to obtain 14,000 chicks from a single cock in one season by artificial insemination. The average ejaculate of a rooster contains 3,200,000 spermatozoa per cubic millimeter.

FEMALE GENITAL ORGANS

The reproductive tract of the female consists of a left ovary attached by a short mesovarium to the dorsal body wall, and a left oviduct supported by a mesotubarium. Although the ovaries and oviducts of the bird develop as paired structures, they soon become asymmetrical in the embryo because for some unknown reason more primordial germ cells migrate into the left ovary. The right ovary and oviduct degenerate, but remnants are frequently present. Several species of hawks retain both right and left ovaries but only one oviduct. Some strains of domestic fowl show a high percentage of large persistent right oviducts, which often become cystic. A vestigial right oviduct 6 mm. long was present in the budgerigar chosen at random for illustration in Figure 5-29.

The ovary of the immature bird is an elongate, flattened mass of similarly sized small follicles tightly covered by a thin mesovarium that attaches it to the

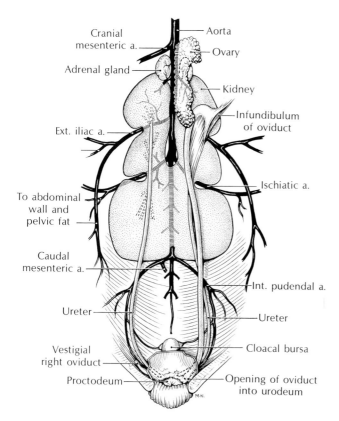

Cranial mesenteric a.

Aorta

Ovary

Adrenal gland

Kidney

Infundibulum of oviduct

Ext. iliac a.

Ischiatic a.

To abdominal wall and pelvic fat

Caudal mesenteric a.

Int. pudendal a.

Ureter

Ureter

Vestigial right oviduct

Cloacal bursa

Proctodeum

Opening of oviduct into urodeum

Fig. 5-29. *The female urogenital system and the arteries of the trunk.*

dorsal body wall. As the bird matures and the breeding season approaches, several of the follicles enlarge, become pedunculate, and give the ovary the appearance of a cluster of variously sized grapes. The thin-walled sac enclosing the growing ovum develops an extensive vascular plexus, which nourishes it. As the developing egg increases in size, a clear streak is seen to develop in the wall of the follicle enclosing the maturing ovum. This clear streak is the site of rupture during ovulation and is known as the stigma, or cicatrix. Although the stigma appears to be free of blood vessels, Nalbandov and James[116] have shown in the fowl that small vessels extend across it. The large-yolked ova of breeding birds occupy a considerable portion of the already crowded abdominal cavity. The base of the mature ovary still contains the many small ovarian follicles which will mature at a future time, and contains the cells responsible for elaboration of the three ovarian hormones—estrogen, androgen, and progesterone.

The number of ova that will mature during one reproductive cycle is a characteristic of the species and often of the individual. Most birds have a fairly constant clutch size, but many are capable of replacing eggs that are removed or damaged (indeterminate layers). The budgerigar, among others, lays 5 to 8 eggs, and does not replace eggs that are removed (deter-

minate layer). The maturation of eggs to be ovulated may be induced in birds by a variety of stimuli; these include increased light; sight of male or others; vocalizations of male or others; rainfall, related perhaps to food abundance; temperature; suitable nest site; and other factors. Van Tienhoven *et al.*[157] found that placing budgerigars in continuous darkness brought about development of the ovaries and egg laying in 7 to 14 days. Brockway[19] has identified the auditory signals that are important in budgerigar vocalizations for stimulation of egg development.

The oviduct of the nonbreeding bird is rather straight and uniform in diameter, with a funnel-like opening at its cranial end. The enlargement in size and changes in shape of the oviduct during the breeding cycle are very great. An increase in length causes a folding of the oviduct upon itself. Glandular development results in a thickening of its walls, which differentiates it into several functional regions associated with egg formation.

The opening into the oviduct, the infundibulum or ostium, provides the only communication between the peritoneal cavity and the outside. When it is not in the process of "swallowing" an egg, the infundibulum appears as a flattened funnel attached by a cranial ligament to the region of the last rib on the left side; a caudal ligament attaches to the length of the oviduct as far as the vagina. It is possible, with the abdomen opened surgically, to insert a capsule or a freshly ovulated egg into the infundibulum and observe its passage. The ovulated ovum has a strong vitelline membrane which permits considerable squeezing and deformation as it is engulfed and passed along by muscular contraction. Sperm have been seen at the infundibulum, and it is at this site that fertilization takes place.

The magnum is the cranial, glandular region of the oviduct, which secretes the thick albumen. It is the longest of the five regions of the oviduct; being about 25 cm. long in the fowl, about three hours is required for an egg to traverse it. Externally, the magnum appears wrinkled, folded, and light-colored. Internally, it has ridges and folds with tubular glands and goblet cells.

The isthmus is thinner walled than the magnum, and in the fowl there is characteristically a visible band at the junction of the two. In the fowl the isthmus is about 10 cm. long. The glands of its wall secrete the shell membranes, a process which requires about one hour.

The shell gland, or uterus, is a dilated portion of the oviduct with a well-developed muscle layer and an excellent blood supply.[48] The very conspicuous papillae or lamellae secrete the calcareous shell and thin albumen. This region, in the fowl, is about 10 cm. long and holds an egg for 20 hours.

The vagina is the short terminal portion of the oviduct proximal to its opening into the cloaca. It has a well-developed muscular wall and serves for the expulsion of the egg. Harris[60] published radiographs showing the rotation of the chicken's egg prior to laying, and points out that Fabricius in 1621 recognized that such rotation occurred and asked, "Why does the egg emerge blunt end first?"

The control of ovulation and the endocrinology of reproduction in birds has been the subject of considerable research. For an excellent review and summary of the literature with many references, see van Tienhoven.[156]

Nervous System and Sense Organs

The nervous system functions to regulate all of the body's internal organs as well as transmit external stimuli from sense organs or simple nerve endings to the spinal cord or brain to evoke an appropriate response.

The structural parts of the nervous system are similar in all vertebrates. Variously shaped neurons consisting of a cell body and a long or short axon interconnect via synapses to conduct impulses. Sensory neurons conduct impulses to the brain or spinal cord and form afferent tracts or nerves. Such sensory neurons may have their origin in the skin or skeletal muscles (somatic afferents), as well as in the viscera (visceral afferents). Motor neurons send their impulses away from the brain and spinal cord, to muscles, as efferent tracts or nerves. The skeletal muscles of the body receive somatic efferents, and the smooth muscles of the viscera and feathers receive visceral efferents. Supporting and protecting the impulse-conducting neurons are the neuroglial cells which form the glial feltwork and the Schwann cell sheaths with their myelin insulation. Surrounding the brain and spinal cord are vascularized membranes called the meninges. They consist of an outer fibrous dura and an inner pia-arachnoid tightly applied to the surface of the brain and cord.

A detailed account of the fiber tracts and nuclei of the bird is included under various section headings in the two-volume work of Kappers *et al., The Comparative Anatomy of the Nervous System of Vertebrates, Including Man.*[77] Romanoff[132] has reviewed the early development of the avian nervous system.

For purposes of discussion, the nervous system may be divided into various components (Table 5-2), based on functional, topographic, or developmental considerations.

Central Nervous System

Portmann and Stingelin[127] have reviewed the literature and summarized their studies of the gross features and cytoarchitecture of the central nervous system of birds. Several of their brain illustrations are of the budgerigar. Kalischer,[75] working with the parrot's brain, discussed the results of his experimental extirpations. Papez[123] described the morphology of the brain of the bird in relation to those of the reptile and mammal. He illustrated fiber tracts and nuclei of the brain with several cross sections. There is much current interest in functional studies of the brain of birds, and much remains to be learned about the anatomy of the central nervous system.

BRAIN

The brain of the bird is relatively large, when compared with that of reptiles, and it fills the skull very completely. Owing to the thinness of the roof of the skull the brain can be easily damaged. The position of the brain within the skull may vary considerably between Orders of birds. Most of the brain lies posterior to the orbits. Cobb[26] determined the brain-bill angle of various species of birds as one indication of the relative position of the brain within the skull. He plotted the cerebral axis (center of medulla to center of olfactory bulb) against the bill axis. An angle of 90 degrees indicates that the brain is perpendicular when the bill is horizontal. The angle in the budgerigar is 40 degrees; extremes include 15 degrees for the cormorant and 117 degrees for the woodcock.

Table 5-2. Components of Nervous System

Central Nervous System **Brain** **Spinal Cord**	**Peripheral Nervous System** **Cranial Nerves** **Spinal Nerves**
Autonomic Nervous System **Sympathetic** **Parasympathetic**	**Sensory Endings and Sense Organs** **Taste, Smell, Sight** **Equilibrium and Hearing**

The form of the brain is similar for the whole Class Aves, being narrow anteriorly where it tapers to the small olfactory lobes and wide posteriorly because of the expanded cerebral hemispheres. The bird brain has a shorter base than the reptile brain, which it resembles in several respects. Although the bird and mammal have evolved from reptilian ancestors, the brain of the bird is quite different from that of the mammal. The characteristic features of the bird brain are the large corpora striata of the forebrain, the large optic lobes of the midbrain, and the large median cerebellum of the hindbrain with its transverse folia.

FOREBRAIN, OR TELENCEPHALON.   The forebrain of the budgerigar is wider than it is long, and consists of two smooth hemispheres pointed at their anterior ends, where the small olfactory bulbs are located. (The hemispheres are separated by a deep longitudinal fissure.) The olfactory area in the nasal cavity is small and as a result the olfactory nerves are greatly reduced in number. The ventral surface of the forebrain is concave on each side, where it is in contact with the wall of the orbit. In some birds the olfactory bulbs are elongated and may enclose a ventricle which is continuous with the lateral ventricle. They may also fuse and appear as a single median bulb.

Cobb[27] lists the sizes of olfactory bulbs and cerebral hemispheres for 36 species of birds, including the budgerigar. The olfactory bulbs are relatively small in the seed-eating perching birds (Passeriformes and parrots), and relatively large in several families of water birds. The largest olfactory bulbs reported by Cobb were seen in the kiwi—that primitive, flightless, worm-eating ratite from New Zealand. Some representative percentages of olfactory bulb to hemisphere are: budgerigar 6%, canary 12%, vulture 17%, swan 21%, and kiwi 33%.

Haefelfinger[59] has shown that the developing cerebral hemisphere of the budgerigar on the 7th day of incubation has a large ventricle surrounded by a neopallium dorsally, a hyperstriatum plus neostriatum laterally, and a paleostriatum ventrally. On the dorsal midline is the archipallium, and on the ventral midline the eminentia basalis. By the 12th day of incubation the ventricle is quite reduced, because of the inward growth and enlargement of the striatal regions. In the adult forebrain cell differentiation results in the formation of layers or zones with the large neostriatum capping the hemisphere. The striatum in birds is a senso-motor correlation center having afferent connections with the tectum and thalamus, and efferent paths which reach the oculomotor, cerebellar, and masticatory centers of the brain. Functional considerations of the bird's hemispheres are reviewed by Portmann and Stingelin.[127]

INTERBRAIN, OR DIENCEPHALON.   The diencephalon is small in birds and serves to connect the forebrain with the midbrain and cerebellum. It consists of an epithalamus dorsally (epiphysis or pineal), a thalamus proper centrally (small nuclear masses and fiber tracts), and a hypothalamus ventrally (pituitary body and chiasma). The optic chiasma is large and most fibers enter the optic lobe of the midbrain. The thalamus is short and relatively small and, except for the optic tracts, is hidden from lateral view.

Krabbe[82] described the development of the epiphysis of the budgerigar and noted that it had a more eyelike parietal body than other bird embryos he examined.

The pituitary gland, or hypophysis, in the budgerigar is relatively large (1.75 mm. in diameter) and is located on the ventral surface of the brain between the optic chiasm and the medulla. It is tightly lodged in the sella turcica of the skull by a diaphragma sellae in which it usually remains when the brain is removed. Wingstrand,[163] in his monograph on the structure and development of the avian pituitary, discusses its relations to the vascular system and observes that it "may be correct to say that the pituitary is suspended in a mighty stream of venous blood which comes from the orbit and, in some species at least, from the forebrain, and leaves the sella through the vena carotis." Surgical approaches to the pituitary must take the extensive venous circulation into account. Vitums *et al.*[158,159] have described the vascularization of the hypothalamus in the white-crowned sparrow.

The bird's pituitary consists of a large adenohypophysis derived from Rathke's pouch and a smaller neurohypophysis derived from the diencephalon. The adenohypophysis is mainly pars distalis and is located anteroventral to the neurohypophysis. An intermedia is not present but the eminentia mediana is very large and serves to connect the pars tuberalis via the hypophysial stalk with the pars distalis.

Kobayashi *et al.*[80] studied the hypothalamo-hypophysial neurosecretory system of the budgerigar and the white-crowned sparrow with both light and electron microscopes. The neurosecretory centers consist of paired supraoptic and paraventricular nuclei, each of which is divisible into medial and lateral cell groups.

MIDBRAIN, OR MESENCEPHALON.   The midbrain of birds lies in close association with the diencephalon. It consists largely of the paired optic lobes (tecta, or corpora bigemina), which are displaced ventro-laterally by the large cerebral hemispheres and median cerebellum. In some birds the optic lobes are completely hidden from view by the enlarged hemispheres. Both the optic lobes and the diencephalon can be seen in the same cross section. The optic lobes can be seen in lateral view in the budgerigar. They receive afferent fibers from the retina and supply efferent fibers to the striatum. These nuclei and the fibers are an important part of the optico-sensory system. The midbrain also contains the oculo-motor centers and connections necessary for trans-mitting impulses to muscles involved in locomotion and flight.

METENCEPHALON. The cerebellum is characteris-tically large in birds, although it lacks the lateral lobes of the mammalian brain. It functions to regulate move-ments which maintain position and is thus of particular importance in birds.

In the budgerigar the cerebellum is longer than it is wide and has 10 well-developed transverse primary folia. Some authors[85,127] subdivide the cerebellum into anterior and posterior lobes, with a basal pars auric-ularis. Others consider the cerebellum to have an anterior, a medial, and a posterior lobe. The anterior lobe is hidden from view because the cerebellum is wedged between the cerebral hemispheres. The medial lobe includes the highest and most ventro-anterior portions, whereas the posterior lobe includes the nodulus and uvula on the ventral surface.

The auricle is a lateral extension from the basal por-tion of the caudal cerebellar region. The auricle of the nodulus on each side forms the flocculus, and a similar projection of the uvula forms the paraflocculus. The flocculus and paraflocculus on each side are so closely associated that they appear as a single, prominent blunt lobe, usually referred to as the flocculus.

MEDULLA, OR MYELENCEPHALON. The medulla contains several reflex centers necessary for maintaining life. It is directly continuous with the spinal cord, which it is generally agreed begins at the foramen magnum of the skull. Cranial nerves V through XII, with the exception of most of the fibers of XI, originate on the ventral surface of the medulla. The so-called brain stem, or lower brain, consists of the medulla, the pons, the midbrain, and the diencephalon. It does not include the cerebral hemispheres and basal ganglia (telencephalon).

SPINAL CORD

The spinal cord is a continuation of the medulla; beginning at the foramen magnum of the skull it ex-tends through the vertebral canal into the coccygeal region of the bird. Structurally, the cord is made up of an aggregation of cell bodies and fiber tracts en-closing a narrow fluid-filled lumen. The cell bodies are concentrated centrally to form the "gray matter" of the dorsal and ventral columns, whereas the fiber tracts lie peripherally as the "white matter" of the cord.

The simplest reflex arc through the spinal cord would be formed by sensory impulses entering the dorsal or afferent root of a spinal nerve and being transferred via a synapse in the cord to the ventral or efferent root of a spinal nerve. At the same time that this simple re-flex is occurring, other sensory (afferent) neurons in the spinal cord pick up the excitation and transmit it to the brain, which in turn routes the information to higher centers and then sends a "considered" response via a motor (efferent) neuron back to the appropriate level of the cord to produce or control movement.

The spinal cord of birds is distinguished by a long cervical region, a cervico-thoracic enlargement at the level of the brachial plexus, a short thoracic region, a lumbosacral enlargement, and, unlike mammals, a coccygeal region within the vertebral canal of the caudal vertebrae. In the lumbosacral region there is a dorsal cleft, the sinus rhomboidalis, filled with glycogen-rich cells. This structure, of unknown function, has been called the glycogen body. It is large in the embryo and persists in varying degrees in adults of some species.

Peripheral Nervous System

CRANIAL NERVES

There are 12 pairs of cranial nerves in birds, desig-nated by Roman numerals and named according to function or distribution. Some of these nerves are entirely sensory, some are entirely motor, and some are mixed.

I. The *olfactory nerve* is sensory and conducts im-pulses from the olfactory mucosa on the nasal turbi-nates to the olfactory bulb of the brain. It is small and passes through the dorsal portion of the orbit along the perpendicular plate of the ethmoid, where it enters the olfactory foramen of the skull. In birds, a sieve-like cribriform plate is lacking.

II. The *optic nerve* is sensory and conducts impulses from the retina to the optic lobe and thalamus. It is the largest cranial nerve and enters the skull through the optic foramen in the orbitosphenoid bone. Im-mediately after entering the cranial cavity the two optic nerves cross at the chiasma on the ventral sur-face of the diencephalon and enter the brain. Some authors say that not all fibers cross.

III. The *oculomotor nerve* from the midbrain is motor to all but two of the muscles which move the eyeball, innervating the dorsal, ventral, and medial rectus, and the ventral oblique muscles. In addition it innervates the palpebral muscles and Harder's gland. Within the skull, the oculomotor nerves are seen on each side of the pituitary body proximal to their exit behind the optic nerves. Visceral fibers from the ciliary ganglion accompany the oculomotor nerve to supply the choroid and iris.

IV. The *trochlear nerve* is motor to the dorsal oblique eye muscle. It is a small nerve which originates on the dorsal surface of the brain stem between the midbrain and cerebellum. After passing over the lateral surface of the midbrain the nerve enters the orbit via a small opening close to the optic foramen.

V. The *trigeminal nerve* is both motor and sensory to structures of the head. It is the second largest cranial nerve and leaves the antero-lateral surface of the brain stem at the ventro-caudal margin of the optic lobe. Close to its origin the trigeminal nerve has a prominent swelling, the Gasserian ganglion. Beyond this ganglion the nerve divides into three branches—the ophthalmic, maxillary, and mandibular nerves.

The *ophthalmic nerve* is the first to leave the parent trunk. It exits from the skull near the optic foramen and arches dorso-anteriorly through the orbit in contact with the medial surface of the eyeball. In its course through the orbit it passes over and under extrinsic eye muscles and may send a small nerve to the ciliary ganglion. At the anterior margin of the orbit the ophthalmic nerve passes close to the duct of Harder's gland and enters the upper beak as the nasal nerve. The ophthalmic branch is thought to be sensory from the nasal region, forehead, and upper beak. Slonaker[139] found that the long and short ciliary nerves in the sparrow were derived from the oculomotor and ophthalmic nerves. Stimulation of the ophthalmic nerve dilates the pupil.

The *maxillary nerve* leaves the skull through the oval foramen and enters the orbit, where it divides into supraorbital and infraorbital branches. The supraorbital branch receives afferent fibers from the skin of the dorsal region of the orbit. The infraorbital branch supplies the lacrimal gland and receives sensory fibers from the face, upper jaw, conjunctiva, and eyelids.

The *mandibular nerve*, which is both motor and sensory, is the largest of the three divisions of the trigeminal. It exits from the skull with the maxillary nerve through the oval foramen and passes ventrally to innervate the masticatory muscles and the skin of the lower jaw.

VI. The *abducens nerve* is motor to the lateral or external rectus muscle and the muscles of the nictitating membrane. This small nerve leaves the ventral surface of the medulla close to the midline, enters the orbit ventro-lateral to the optic foramen, and parallels the trochlear nerve for a short distance. Slonaker[139] found in the sparrow that at the level of the optic nerve within the orbit the abducens divides to send

twigs into the external rectus, quadratus, and pyramidalis muscles.

According to Kappers *et al.*,[77] the abducens root in most birds emerges partly anterior to the level of the facial roots, but in some (sparrow and cassowary) part or all of the sixth nerve emerges behind the seventh nerve.

VII. The *facial nerve* is motor to the constrictor colli, stapedius, depressor mandibulae (posterior belly, or digastricus), mylohyoideus, and some of the long hyoid muscles of the throat such as the serpihyoideus and stylohyoideus. The facial nerve also is said to have afferent fibers from taste buds which synapse in the geniculate ganglion before reaching the brain, and efferent secretory fibers which leave the medulla and pass to the salivary glands.

It has been pointed out by Black[12] that there is a close association of facial and trigeminal motor nuclei in birds due largely to the dominant influence of sensory trigeminal impulses upon the reflex action of both facial and trigeminal musculature. The anterior pterygoid muscle innervated by V acts to elevate the maxilla after the mandible is widely opened by the depressor mandibulae innervated by VII.

VIII. The *vestibulocochlear nerve* is sensory for hearing and positional orientation. It is short and thick and does not leave the skull since it enters the petrous temporal bone from the medial side. This nerve was formerly called the auditory, acoustic, or stato-acoustic nerve. Its two components are the *vestibular nerve* from the labyrinth and semicircular canals, and the *cochlear nerve* from the lagena, which is the simple cochlea of the bird.

IX. The *glossopharyngeal nerve* sends both motor and sensory fibers to the tongue, pharynx, esophagus, and throat both directly and through branches anastomosing with the vagus, spinal accessory, and hypoglossal nerves. The glossopharyngeal nerve also receives sympathetic fibers from the cranial cervical ganglion, which lies over the point of emergence of nerves IX and X. In the budgerigar nerves IX and X are so closely associated with each other that for a short distance they appear as one. A swelling close to the base of the combined nerves may represent the petrosal ganglion of the glossopharyngeal combined with the jugular ganglion of the vagus.

X. The *vagus nerve* originates from the medulla close to the origin of the glossopharyngeal nerve. In the budgerigar its exit from the skull is hidden by the large cranial cervical sympathetic ganglion.

Watanabe[161] found in the fowl that the vagus originates as 8 to 12 fine rootlets in series with the rootlets of nerves IX and XI. The vagus and spinal accessory nerves were enclosed in a common epineural sheath and fused as a single trunk at the ganglion radicis vagi. Below the vagal root ganglion the spinal accessory nerve separates from the common trunk and courses to superficial neck muscles. The main vagal trunk sends branches to the pharynx and larynx as well as anastomotic branches to the glossopharyngeal and hypoglossal nerves before continuing down the neck on the jugular vein.

Malinovsky[94] found in the pigeon that cranial nerves IX and X arise from the medulla by way of a common root ganglion, the ganglion radicis vagi of Cords[28] and Watanabe.[161] The vagus nerve in the pigeon emerges from the jugular foramen and sends a relatively long anastomotic branch into the glossopharyngeal nerve at the level of the petrosal ganglion. (This anastomosis is short or lacking in some birds.) Smaller branches of the vagus communicate with the cranial cervical ganglion and the hypoglossal nerve. From the ventrolateral aspect of the vagus, in the pigeon, arises the spinal accessory nerve. Lying within the loop resulting from the anastomosis of cranial nerves IX and X, the cranial cervical ganglion of the sympathetic system can always be seen.

In the budgerigar the vagus nerve emerges as a common trunk with the glossopharyngeal and spinal accessory nerves. On the lateral surface of this combined nerve trunk, the square-shaped cranial cervical ganglion is closely attached. It receives its fibers from the cervical sympathetic trunk.

The vagus nerve separates from the glossopharyngeal below the cranial cervical ganglion and passes caudally on the jugular vein medial to the hypoglossal nerve. At the base of the neck, caudal to the thyroid gland, the vagus nerve has a fusiform swelling, the nodose ganglion. Beyond the ganglion the vagus nerve leaves the jugular vein and sends branches to the heart, trachea, lungs, and proventriculus. The further course of the vagus nerve on the stomach has been described for the pigeon by Malinovsky.[95]

XI. The *spinal accessory nerve* arises mainly from the spinal cord at the level of the third cervical nerve, and runs anteriorly along the spinal cord through the foramen magnum into the cranium. Here it receives root fibers from the medulla, joins the root of the vagus, and emerges from the skull with the vagus and glossopharyngeal nerves. Since the spinal accessory is small and combined with the vagal trunk, it appears to be a branch of the vagus that passes ventrally to supply the constrictor colli muscles.

XII. The *hypoglossal nerve,* shortly after emerging from the cranium, is joined by branches from the first three cervical nerves. The combined trunk passes ventrally lateral to the vagus nerve and jugular vein. It divides into two branches, one of which supplies tongue muscles and the other descends on the trachea to the syrinx. Kappers *et al.*[77] state that the hypoglossal nucleus of birds supplies not only the poorly developed tongue musculature but also—and chiefly—the muscles of the syrinx via the ramus laryngeus. The musculature of the syrinx is believed to arise from the sternohyoideus, which is innervated in mammals by the ramus descendens hypoglossi.

The bulk of the tongue in the budgerigar and other parrots consists of intrinsic muscles which enable the bird to manipulate the tongue greatly and probably coordinate lingual action during phonation. Black[12] believed the large size and unique specialization of the nucleus intermedius XII in parrots was correlated with the large mass and complexity of their lingual musculature rather than with any syringeal peculiarities.

SPINAL NERVES

There are a pair of spinal nerves for each vertebral segment so that for different species the total number of spinal nerves varies with the number of vertebrae. Each spinal nerve has a dorsal, afferent or sensory root and a ventral, efferent or motor root. These roots join to form the spinal nerve which exits from the intervertebral foramen. After its emergence from the vertebral canal, the spinal nerve gives rise to a small dorsal branch, a large ventral branch, and a small communicating or visceral branch. The dorsal branch is particularly small, since it supplies the epaxial muscles and skin which are very reduced in the bird.

The spinal nerves are designated according to the vertebral regions in which they arise as cervical, thoracic, lumbar, sacral, and caudal. The type of nerve fibers contained in a nerve cannot be told by gross examination. Most nerves contain motor, sensory, and autonomic fibers. Many of the nerves in birds are striated in gross appearance, which aids in their identification.

CERVICAL REGION. There are 12 cervical nerves in the budgerigar, and all except the first one have large dorsal root ganglia. The first cervical nerve is small and has a dorsal root ganglion only half as large as the others. Cervical nerves 1, 2, and 3 anastomose with the hypoglossal nerve and supply hyoid as well as cervical muscles. The 4th to 9th cervicals have long ventral branches which pass external to the jugular vein and reach the ventral border of the neck. The 9th, 10th, 11th, and 12th cervicals and the 1st thoracic nerve join to form a brachial plexus which supplies the wing. The largest nerves of this plexus are the 11th and 12th cervicals and the 1st thoracic, whose fibers join totally, shortly after their emergence from the vertebral foramina, receive contributions from the other nerves, and then again separate to form the principal nerves of the wing.

THORACIC REGION.   There are eight thoracic nerves in the budgerigar. The 1st thoracic nerve divides equally to supply the brachial plexus and thoracic wall musculature. Thoracic nerves 2 through 7 parallel the ribs and innervate the intercostal muscles and overlying skin. The 8th thoracic nerve emerges from the intervertebral foramen at the level of the caudal tip of the lung and joins with the 1st and 2nd lumbar nerves to form the crural plexus described below.

LUMBAR-SACRAL-CAUDAL REGION.   The fusion of the last few thoracic vertebrae with the lumbar, sacral, and one or two caudal vertebrae to form a rigid synsacrum results in a loss of epaxial muscles and a diminution or loss of the dorsal branches of the spinal nerves. The ventral branches remain large, course through or above the kidneys, and supply the body wall, pelvic limbs, and tail. Yasuda[165] summarized the nerve supply of the pelvic limb in the fowl.

In the budgerigar a lumbosacral plexus is evident, although not all of the sacral nerves participate. On a topographic basis, one can distinguish, as did Imhof,[70] three nerve plexuses: (1) crural, (2) ischiatic, and (3) pudendal.

The crural plexus is made up of fibers of the 8th thoracic and 1st and 2nd lumbar, which join after emerging from their respective intervertebral foramina and then branch to supply part of the body wall, all of the muscles on the cranial aspect of the thigh, and the area along the elongate pubis. The major trunks of this plexus are the femoral and obturator nerves.

The ischiatic plexus consists of fibers from the 2nd to 5th lumbar nerves. The largest of these nerves is the 2nd, which also sends fibers into the crural plexus but is primarily the major contributor to the large ischiatic nerve of the limb. Distally, the peroneal and tibial nerves are formed.

The pudendal plexus is made up of the three sacral nerves and one or two coccygeal nerves which arise dorsal to the caudal lobe of the kidney and supply the oviduct, cloaca, and tail. Variable connections between these nerves constitute a minor plexus.

The nerves forming the crural and ischiatic plexuses have communicating rami to the sympathetic trunk. The pudendal plexus has no communicating ramus. Several small coccygeal nerves issue from the spinal cord between the free caudal vertebrae and innervate the uropygium.

Autonomic Nervous System

The nerves which innervate smooth muscles, blood vessels, and glands are either sympathetic or parasympathetic, depending on their physiological attributes and their place of exit from the central nervous system. Collectively, the sympathetic and parasympathetic nerves with their ganglia compose the autonomic nervous system, which is by definition an efferent or motor system. The cells of origin of autonomic nerves are located in the hypothalamus of the brain. Much of the viscera receives a dual innervation. The parasympathetic nerves slow the heart and enhance digestive processes, whereas the sympathetic nerves accelerate the heart, constrict blood vessels, and prepare the animal for fight or flight. Langley[84] described the anatomy and physiology of the sympathetic nervous system of birds and included a detailed consideration of the smooth muscles which move the feathers. Malinovsky[94] described the autonomic system in the neck and thorax of the pigeon. Both of these papers contain several references to early works on the sympathetic and parasympathetic nerves of birds.

PARASYMPATHETIC DIVISION

Fibers of the cranio-sacral or parasympathetic division leave the brain in cranial nerves III (oculomotor), VII (facial), IX (glossopharyngeal), and X (vagus), and also in sacral spinal nerves. The parasympathetic fibers of the oculomotor nerve innervate the ciliary muscle via the ciliary ganglion and cause constriction of the pupil. Those of the facial nerve pass into the lacrimal and salivary glands. The glossopharyngeal nerve innervates the pharynx and carries parasympathetic fibers to the salivary glands. The vagus nerve is the largest parasympathetic supply. It innervates the larynx, lungs, heart, and digestive tract to the level of the large intestine. Malinovsky[95] described the course of the vagal nerves on the pigeon's stomach and the pattern of the myogastric plexuses.

In the budgerigar the right and left vagal nerves accompany the jugular veins and are distinct until they reach the proventriculus, where they branch and overlap. At the hilus of the lung the vagal trunk divides into four branches. Two enter the lung and heart, one ascends the trachea, and one passes onto the proventriculus. A small twig from the recurrent branch to the trachea appears to innervate some syringeal structure. In the sacral region the parasympathetic nerves are distributed with fibers from the pudendal plexus to the terminal portion of the oviduct and the cloaca.

SYMPATHETIC DIVISION.   The thoraco-lumbar or sympathetic division of the autonomic nervous system arises as a series of communicating rami from thoracic and lumbar spinal nerves which course as a sympathetic trunk on each side of the vertebral column. The sympathetic trunks in the bird are not as regular in position or arrangement as they are in the mammal, but they can be seen to extend from the cranial cervical ganglion in the head to the ganglion impar or coalesced trunks on the ventral surface of the tail. Along the entire length of the sympathetic trunks, segmental ganglia are present. These ganglia are visible without dissection on the ventral surface of caudal, lumbar, and thoracic vertebrae, but are hidden from view at more cranial levels.

The sympathetic trunk in the neck of the budgerigar passes through the vertebral canal on each side and thus resembles the vertebral nerve of the mammal. However, unlike in the mammal, the sympathetic trunk in the bird possesses a ganglion at the level of each cervical spinal nerve. These sympathetic ganglia lie close to the intervertebral foramina and are partly hidden from view by the large dorsal root ganglion of each cervical nerve. Communicating rami are prominent on the last few cervical nerves (10th, 11th, and 12th), but at higher levels the close apposition of the sympathetic ganglia to the cervical nerves hides the short communicating rami. These cervical communicating rami probably contain only postganglionic fibers which run with the cervical spinal nerves to the blood vessels and feather muscles of the skin. Langley[84] found no preganglionic fibers in the cervical rami of the fowl except for the last cervical nerve.

A distinct sympathetic nerve which passes to the heart and lungs is formed by contributions from the sympathetic trunk at the 12th cervical and 1st thoracic ganglia. This nerve, which resembles the ansa subclavia of the mammal, crosses the vagus cranial to the heart and lung but does not appear to supply any fibers to accompany the vagus to the head. It is possible that some sympathetic fibers may turn cranially at the hilus of the lung and accompany the vagus nerve along the jugular vein, thus constituting a vago-sympathetic trunk as illustrated by Kappers[76] (reproduced by Ten Cate[151] on page 717).

The sympathetic trunk has a very small ganglion at the level of the 1st cervical nerve and then proceeds onto the head, where it forms the cranial cervical ganglion on the ventro-lateral surface of the skull. The cranial cervical ganglion is the largest sympathetic ganglion in the bird. It lies below the semicircular canals over the exit of the glossopharyngeal and vagus nerves. Sympathetic fibers leaving the ganglion accompany the large veins and arteries of the base of the skull. Several branches course over the medial surface of the eyeball and appear to supply the Harder and lacrimal glands.

In the thoracic region the sympathetic trunk may be double for a variable distance on one side or the other. One portion may pass between the rib heads and the other along the vertebral bodies. The chain ganglia of the thoracic trunk are located at the bases of the intercostal nerves between successive ribs. Leaving the sympathetic trunk from the ganglia located at thoracic nerves 2, 3, and 4 are the long splanchnic nerves.

The splanchnic nerves course caudoventrally and join to form a prominent ganglion on each side of the aorta at the origin of the cranial mesenteric artery. This cranial mesenteric ganglion is connected with the celiac ganglion on the celiac artery cranially and with the lumbar trunk caudally. From both the cranial mesenteric and the celiac ganglion a plexus is formed which sends sympathetic fibers to the viscera supplied by the respective blood vessels.

On the ventral surface of the 7th thoracic vertebra the sympathetic trunks converge to form paired ganglia which set the segmental pattern for the remainder of the trunk. Each of the chain ganglia is connected by a communicating ramus to its corresponding thoracic or lumbar spinal nerve. At the last lumbar level the two sympathetic trunks pass through the kidney parenchyma and join on the ventral surface of the 2nd free caudal vertebra. They continue into the tail with the termination of the aorta, the median coccygeal artery. A ganglion impar is usually present at the confluence of the sympathetic trunks.

Sensory Endings and Sense Organs

There are various receptors for external and internal stimuli, some of which are morphologically intricate and others which are quite simple. The various sense organs represent collections of similar sensory endings which are integrated for receiving stimuli producing a specific sensation, such as taste, smell, hearing, or sight. Birds have certain abilities of orientation for which no sensory organ is as yet apparent. The simplest sensory endings include free nerve terminations, branched arborizations, loops, and grape-like knobs such as are found in the skin, on tendons, or in mesenteries. More complicated yet solitary endings include Merkel's corpuscles of the skin and tongue, Grandry's corpuscles of the tongue, palate, and bill, and Herbst's corpuscles of the bill.[17] A review of avian sensory organs is provided by Portmann.[126]

SENSORY ENDINGS

TASTE. Although it is generally agreed that birds have few taste buds, there is no doubt that they are capable of taste discrimination. Similar instances are known in the mammal, where taste sensitivity may exist in the absence of taste buds. It is difficult to separate responses of taste, olfaction, and general chemical sense.[166]

Moore and Elliott[112] illustrated the distribution of the 27 to 59 taste buds on the base of the tongue of the pigeon and agreed with the findings of Botezat,[16] who described taste buds on the caudal soft portion of the tongue in the pigeon, sparrow, and duck. Bath[6] concluded that no taste buds were present on the tongue of the pigeon, sparrow, or budgerigar, but he did not consider the soft portion caudal to the tongue fold to be part of the tongue.

An examination of serial sections of the entire free portion of the tongue of a budgerigar did not reveal any taste buds, although many large nerve fibers and subepithelial tactile corpuscles were present. It is possible that taste buds are located around the base of the tongue or elsewhere in the oral cavity and pharynx.

SMELL.   The sense of smell in birds is believed to be relatively poorly developed, although contradictory experimental findings indicate that much is yet to be learned about olfactory structures. As was noted in the discussion of the brain, the olfactory bulbs are small in seed-eating birds, larger in aquatic birds, and largest in the kiwi. Matthews and Knight[99] called attention to the olfactory response of a parrot to cheese and of petrels to cooking fat. For a review of present knowledge concerning the olfactory system see Moulton and Beidler.[114]

EAR

The ear in birds, as in mammals, is the organ of hearing and balance. The apparatus for hearing consists of an external, a middle, and part of the inner ear. The external ear of the bird lacks the fleshy pinna so characteristic in mammals, the middle ear has only one bony ossicle instead of three, and the auditory portion of the inner ear is represented by a short lagena in place of a coiled cochlea. Stimuli perceived as sound are transmitted over the cochlear portion of the eighth nerve. The apparatus for balance consists of the semicircular canals and associated structures, the stimuli being transmitted over the vestibular portion of the eighth nerve.

EXTERNAL EAR.   The ear opening of the budgerigar, as in most birds, is hidden from external view by feathers. The skin surrounding the opening is loose and can be drawn forward by a dermo-osseus muscle located dorsal to the meatus (Fig. 5-17). When the skin is drawn forward, the oval-shaped meatus becomes a perpendicular slit limiting access to the auditory canal.

The auditory canal extends obliquely downward and backward so that the external orifice lies anterior and dorsal to the tympanic membrane and cavity. Near its external orifice the canal is narrowed by a bony shelf, which projects from its dorsal wall and appears to block easy access to the tympanic membrane.

MIDDLE EAR.   The middle ear cavity with its columella (stapes plus the extracolumella cartilage) transmits sound vibrations from the tympanic membrane to the oval window of the inner ear. The tympanic membrane is large and convex on its external surface. For a discussion of this apparatus and a functional interpretation of its elastic ligaments see Pohlman.[124]

The tripartite structure attached to the inner surface of the tympanic membrane is the extracolumella cartilage. Processes of this cartilage extend from the central area of the tympanum downward (intrastapedial), backward (extrastapedial), and toward the periphery (suprastapedial). Attaching to the suprastapedial process at the tympanic margin is a slender muscle. This muscle (Fig. 5-30) originates on the ventral surface of the occipital bone behind the middle ear cavity and pierces the posterior bony margin of the external auditory canal. It is the only muscle associated with the columella, and appears to be homologous with the mammalian stapedius muscle. Contraction of this muscle causes a backward and outward displacement of the extracolumella cartilage and a tightening of the tympanic membrane.

Passing anteriorly from the extracolumella cartilage

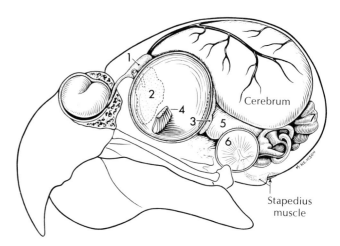

Fig. 5-30. *Lateral view of the head with the roof of the skull removed, the fundus of the eye in situ and the inner ear exposed: 1, nasal gland; 2, Harder's gland; 3, lacrimal gland; 4, pecten; 5, optic lobe; 6, tympanic membrane; and 7, cerebellum.*

across the tympanic cavity is a slender elastic ligament known as the columella-squamosal ligament. It extends from the suprastapedial process to the squamous temporal bone. Functionally this ligament opposes the action of the stapedius muscle. It is extremely delicate in the budgerigar and appears to stabilize the columella.

Connecting the middle ear cavity to the pharynx is the auditory tube. This passageway equalizes the pressure on both sides of the tympanic membrane. In birds, the auditory tubes open into the pharynx by a common median ostium rather than by an orifice on either side of the posterior nasopharynx as in mammals.

INNER EAR. The inner ear (Fig. 5-31) consists of three semicircular canals with their associated ampullae, connected to the sacculus, utriculus, and lagena.

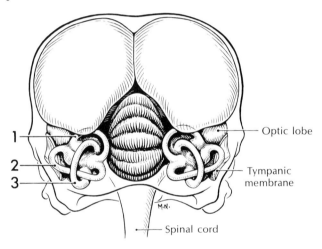

Fig. 5-31. *Posterior view of the head, with the skull removed and the inner ear exposed. Semicircular canals: 1, anterior, 2, lateral, and 3, posterior.*

The semicircular canals, consisting of an inner membranous and an outer bony portion, are very large and are housed in trabecular bone on either side of the cerebellum posterior to the cerebral hemispheres. They are filled with endolymphatic fluid, as are the other membranous parts of the inner ear, and function in registering movement and maintaining spatial orientation. The anterior semicircular canal is vertical and lies close to the cerebellum. The posterior canal is also vertical and arches external to the horizontal canal. The ampullae are swellings at one end of each semicircular canal, and the sacculus is a dilatation of the utriculus. All have sensory areas receiving stimuli which are transmitted over the vestibular portion of the eighth nerve. The short comma-shaped lagena, with a half-twist at most, is the homologue of the mammalian cochlea. Nerve fibers from the organ of Corti in the lagena join to form the cochlear portion of the eighth nerve.

EYE AND ADNEXA

The eye and its adnexa in the bird and mammal differ greatly in several structural and functional respects. The sense of vision in the bird is extremely well developed and the eye is relatively enormous. In a few birds the combined weight of the eyes is greater than the weight of the brain. The large size of the eyes necessitates large size of the orbits, with a consequent caudal displacement of the brain. Walls[160] points out that resolving power is particularly dependent upon absolute ocular size. Great speed, as in flight, demands high resolving power for the perception of movements and visual acuity for the avoidance of collisions. For a review of vision in birds see Pumphrey[28] and Tansley.[149] A very complete morphological and functional description of the eye and its accessory structures was given by Slonaker,[139] who used the English sparrow as a basis for comparison.

Several distinctive structures of the avian eye serve to enhance its functional capability. Such features include the nictitating membrane and its muscles, the Harder and lacrimal glands, the sclerotic ring in association with Brücke's muscle, the compressive mechanism of the ciliary body, the annular pad of the lens, the duplicate foveae of the retina, and the highly vascular, non-nervous pecten. Although the eye "sees," the brain must be capable of interpreting what is seen, and much research has been directed toward unraveling the visual mechanisms of the central nervous system. Cowan *et al.*[29] illustrated one approach through degeneration studies.

Birds are capable of color discrimination, pattern recognition, vision in bright and dim light, under-water accommodation, and sun orientation. Emlen[39] has shown that birds can probably recognize constellations for stellar orientation and navigation.

EYELIDS. There are three functional eyelids in birds. The upper and lower lids move vertically, and the nictitating membrane moves horizontally. When the eye is open the lids are retracted so as to produce a circular interpalpebral space. Both the upper and the lower lid of the budgerigar have short bristle-like lashes along their margins. These bristles are rudimentary feathers (filoplumes) without barbs. The lower lid is larger and more mobile than the upper.

At the medial canthus of the eye the "third eyelid," or nictitating membrane, is seen as a slight perpendicular fold resting on the rostral portion of the eyeball within the lids. It is drawn medio-laterally across the eyeball by contraction of the quadratus and pyramidalis muscles. The quadratus forms a pulley through which the pyramidalis redirects its force over a long tendon. The nictitating membrane forms a pocket into which the duct of Harder's gland (see Fig. 5-30) empties its secretion for lubricating the lids and cleansing the cornea. When drawn across the eye the membrane is translucent and the bird can see through it. The free margin is stiffened by a connective tissue fold which acts as a squeegee to draw fluid over the cornea and remove debris. Upon retraction of the nictitating membrane detritus and fluid are carried to the medial angle of the lids and either passed into the lacrimal ducts or expelled over the medial canthus.

LACRIMAL APPARATUS.   The glands of the eye function to lubricate the lids and nourish the cornea, while the lacrimal ducts drain the tears from the conjunctival sac into the lacrimal sac, lacrimal canal, and nasal cavity.

The lacrimal gland (Fig. 5-30) is flat, oblong, and closely applied to the caudal margin of the eyeball slightly below the equator. Its secretion enters the conjunctival sac at the lateral canthus via microscopic ducts.

Harder's gland is the largest gland of the orbit. It is irregular or boot-shaped and lies on the antero-medial surface of the eyeball, hidden from lateral view. The large duct of the gland can be seen to enter the space between the eyeball and the nictitating membrane. Judging by the large size of the gland in the budgerigar it must be the most important source of lacrimal secretions.

At the medial canthus of the eye there are two lacrimal puncta and ducts that drain into a large lacrimal sac. Leaving the sac is a wide lacrimal canal which turns inward and downward to enter the lower part of the nasal cavity dorsal to the choana.

Another gland within the orbit of the budgerigar is the nasal, or salt, gland, which lies dorso-medial to the eyeball. The duct of this ovoid, yellowish gland pierces the frontal bone and enters the nasal cavity where presumably the hypertonic salt solutions are excreted. Although this gland is not a part of the lacrimal apparatus, pathological involvement of the gland could affect the contents of the orbit.

EYEBALL.   The shape of the eyeball in birds varies greatly. In small birds it is hemi-spherical in the fundic half and flat in the external portion. Some larger birds have globose or tubular eyeballs. In all, the globe of the eye fits tightly in the orbit.

The lens consists of a dense central portion and a less dense ringlike peripheral region called the annular pad, or *ringwulst*. This annular pad is non-optic and is fused to the tips of the ciliary processes. Some authors maintain that the lens is constant in shape but altered

in position for accommodation, whereas most believe that it is capable of being altered in shape by ciliary muscle action. Perhaps a combination of the two actions is required for accommodation, namely, peripheral compression and rounding of the lens along with a lengthening of the optic axis.

There are three coats, or layers, of the eyeball as in mammals—an outer sclera, a middle choroid, and an inner retina.

The sclera, or fibrous coat, forms a strong, opaque cup within the orbit and has a clear external surface forming the cornea. The corneal curvature is greater then the fundic curvature. Within the orbit the sclera is stiffened by a hyaline cartilage cup. Encircling the cornea there are a series of bony scleral ossicles—the eyebones (see under Skeleton), which overlap each other and form a very rigid "floating" ring which can resist deformation of the eyeball when the ciliary muscles contract.

The choroid, or vascular coat, is thick and pigmented, and contains many blood vessels. The ciliary body, a part of the choroid, plays an important role in maintaining intraocular pressure and in accommodation. Included as parts of the ciliary body are the ciliary muscles (Crampton's and Brücke's muscles), the ciliary processes, and zonular fibers to the lens.

The iris, a thin diaphragm in front of the lens, has a pupil or opening which is controlled by circular constrictor fibers and radial dilator fibers. Fat droplets and pigment in the iris contribute to the beautiful color of the eyes of birds.

The retina is darkly pigmented and covers the entire fundus. In a preserved eye the retina appears white and wrinkled owing to the fixation of the many nerve fibers on its surface. The sensory part of the retina ends at the ora serrata, which is roughly behind the scleral ring, although pigmented non-nervous retina extends over the ciliary body and onto the inner surface of the iris. The entrance of the optic nerve is in the lower quadrant of the fundus, hidden by the pecten.

An area centralis of acute vision near the optic axis usually contains a groove or crater with a central depression, or fovea. Grain-eating birds may lack a fovea, whereas falconiform birds, swifts, swallows, and hummingbirds have, in addition to a central fovea, a temporal fovea. It is said that the temporal fovea of each eye can focus on the same object and thus confer binocular, stereoscopic vision. Several authors have noted that the cones outnumber the rods in day birds, whereas in night birds the rods predominate. Color vision is associated with cones, and there is no doubt that day birds have color vision. Tansley[149] cites work of Cinat-Tomson on the budgerigar showing that males will attack a female whose cere is painted blue (like that of a male) and court a male whose cere is painted brown (like that of a female).

Pecten. The pecten (Fig. 5-30) of the eye is a densely pigmented, pleated fan which projects into the vitreous chamber from the optic disc along an axis corresponding to the embryonic optic fissure. The gross form of the pecten and the fundus oculi in many species of birds has been described and well illustrated by Wood.[164] In the budgerigar the pecten is 2 mm. long at its base, slightly shorter along the flat apical bridge, 1 mm. high, and about 0.5 mm. thick. It is composed of nine folds which can be opened by microdissection after removal of the apical bridge.

Each fold of the pecten has a central artery and a marginal vein interconnected by fine capillaries which course through the pigmented intervascular tissue. There are no nerve fibers or nerve endings in the pecten. For a discussion of this interesting organ see Wood,[164] Slonaker,[139] and O'Rahilly and Meyer.[121]

Since the retina of the bird lacks its own blood supply it is generally assumed that the pecten functions to nourish the retina and assist in the diffusion of metabolites to and from the vitreous humor. Other functions which have been proposed are those of a heating element for the eye, a movement detector by means of perceiving small shadows,[30,31] a screen against bright light, a regulator of intraocular pressure, or a sensor of magnetic fields.

References

1. AITKEN, R. N. C.: A histochemical study of the stomach and intestine of the chicken. J. Anat., Lond. *92:*453–466, 1958.

2. AKESTER, A. R.: The comparative anatomy of the respiratory pathways in the domestic fowl (*Gallus domesticus*), pigeon (*Columba livia*) and domestic duck (*Anas platyrhyncha*). J. Anat., Lond. *94:*487–505, 1960.

3. AKESTER, A. R.: Radiographic studies of the renal portal system in the domestic fowl (*Gallus domesticus*). J. Anat., Lond. *98:*365–376, 1964.

4. AMES, P. L.: The morphology of the syrinx in passerine birds; its application to the classification of the order Passeriformes. Thesis, Yale University, 1965.

5. ANDERSON, R. M.: *Methods of Collecting and Preserving Vertebrate Animals,* 2nd ed. Bull. No. 69 Nat. Museum of Canada, Ottawa, 1948. 162 pp.

6. BATH, W.: Die Geschmacksorgane der Vögel und Krokodile. Arch. f. Biontol. *1:*1–47, 1906.

7. BAUMEL, J. J.: Asymmetry of encephalic arteries in the pigeon (*Columba livia*). Anat. Anz. *111:*91–102, 1962.

8. BEDDARD, F. E.: *The Structure and Classification of Birds.* London, Longmans, Green and Co., 1898. 548 pp.

9. BEDDARD, F. E.: A contribution to the knowledge of the arteries of the brain in the class Aves. Proc. Zool. Soc. Lond. 1905, pp. 102–117.

10. BEECHER, W. J.: Adaptations for food getting in the American blackbirds. Auk *68:*411–440, 1951.

11. BEECHER, W. J.: The bio-mechanics of the bird skull. Bull. Chicago Acad. Sci. *11:*10–33, 1962.

12. BLACK, D.: The motor nuclei of the cerebral nerves in phylogeny. A study of the phenomena of neurobiotaxis. IV. Aves. J. Comp. Neurol. *34:*233–275, 1922.

13. BLOOM, M. A., DOMM, L. V., NALBANDOV, A. V., and BLOOM, W.: Medullary bone of laying chickens. Am. J. Anat. *102:*411–453, 1958.

14. BOCK, W. J.: Secondary articulation of the avian mandible, Auk *77:*19–55, 1960.

15. BOCK, W. J.: Kinetics of the avian skull. J. Morphol. *114:*1–41, 1964.

16. BOTEZAT, E.: Geschmacksorgane und andere nervöse Endapparate im Schnabel der Vögel. Biol. Centralbl. *24:*722–736, 1904.

17. BOTEZAT, E.: Die Nervenendapparate in den Mundteilen der Vögel und die einheitliche Endigungsweise der peripheren Nerven bei den Wirlbeltieren. Z. f. wiss. Zool. *84:*205–360, 1906.

18. BRADLEY, O. C.: *The Structure of the Fowl,* 4th ed., revised by T. Grahame. Edinburgh, Oliver and Boyd, 1960. 143 pp.

19. BROCKWAY, B. F.: Investigations of the auditory stimuli for laying in Budgerigars (*Melopsittacus undulatus*). Am. Zoologist *2:*508–509, 1962 (Abst.).

20. CADE, T. J., and DYBAS, J. A., Jr.: Water economy of the budgerygah. Auk *79:*345–364, 1962.

21. CADE, T. J., and GREENWALD, L.: Nasal salt secretion in falconiform birds. Condor *68:*338–350, 1966.

22. CALHOUN, M. L.: *Microscopic Anatomy of the Digestive System of the Chicken.* Ames, Iowa State University Press, 1954. 108 pp.

23. CANFIELD, T. H.: Sex determination of day-old chicks. II. Type variations. Poultry Sci. *20:*327–328, 1941.

24. CHAMBERLAIN, F. W.: *Atlas of Avian Anatomy, Osteology-Arthrology-Myology.* East Lansing, Michigan State College, 1943. 45 pp., 95 plates.

25. CHANDLER, A. C.: A study of the structure of feathers, with reference to their taxonomic significance. Univ. Calif. Pub. Zool. *13:*243–446, 1916.

26. COBB, S.: On the angle of the cerebral axis in the American woodcock. Auk *76:*55–59, 1959.

27. COBB, S.: Observations on the comparative anatomy of the avian brain. Perspectives in Biol. & Med. *3:*383–408, 1960.

28. CORDS, E.: Beiträge zur Lehre vom Kopfnervensystem der Vögel. Anat. Hefte *26:*49–100, 1904.

29. COWAN, W. M., ADAMSON, L., and POWELL, T. P. S.: An experimental study of the avian visual system. J. Anat., Lond. *95:*545–563, 1961.

30. CROZIER, W. J., and WOLF, E.: Theory and measurement of visual mechanisms: X. Modifications of the flicker response contour and the significance .of the avian pecten. J. Gen. Physiol. *27:*287–313, 1944.

31. CROZIER, W. J., and WOLF, E.: Flicker response contours for the sparrow, and the theory of the avian pecten. J. Gen. Physiol. *27:*315–324, 1944.

32. CURTIS, E. L., and MILLER, R. C.: The sclerotic ring in North American birds. Auk *55:*225–243, 1938.

33. DARLING, L., and DARLING, L.: *Bird.* Boston, Houghton Mifflin Company, 1962. 261 pp.

34. DE BEER, G. R.: *The Development of the Vertebrate Skull.* London, Oxford University Press, 1937. 552 pp.

35. EDE, D. A.: *Bird Structure, an Approach through Evolution, Development and Function in the Fowl.* Essex, Hutchinson, 1964. 120 pp.

36. EDWARDS, J. J., and EDWARDS, M. J.: *Medical Museum Technology.* London, Oxford University Press, 1959, 172 pp.

37. ELDER, W. H.: The oil gland of birds. Wilson Bull. *66:*6–31, 1954.

38. ELLENBERGER, W., and BAUM, H.: Handbuch der vergleichenden Anatomie der Haustiere, 18th ed. Berlin, Springer-Verlag, 1943, 1155 pp.

39. EMLEN, S.: Migratory orientation in the Indigo bunting *Passerina cyanea.* Part I. Evidence for use of celestial cues. Part II. Mechanism of celestial orientation and navigation. Auk *84:*309–342, 463–489, 1967.

40. ENGELS, W. L.: Tongue musculature of passerine birds. Auk *55:*642–650, 1938.

41. ENGELS, W. L.: Structural adaptations in thrashers (Mimidae: Genus Toxostoma) with comments on interspecific relationships. Univ. Calif. Publ. Zool. *42:*341–400, 1940.

42. EVANS, H. E.: Clearing and staining vertebrates, in toto, for demonstrating ossification. Turtox News *26:*42–47, 1948.

43. FÄNGE, R., SCHMIDT-NIELSEN, K., and OSAKI, H.: The salt gland of the herring gull. Biol. Bull. *115:*161–171, 1958.

44. FISCHER, G.: Vergleichend-anatomische Untersuchungen über den Bronchialbaum der Vögel. Zoologica Stuttgart 19 (Heft 45), 1905. 45 pp.

45. FISHER, H. I.: Adaptations and comparative anatomy of the locomotor apparatus of New World vultures. Am. Midl. Nat. *35:*545–727, 1946.

46. FISHER, H. I., and GOODMAN, D. C.: The myology of the whooping crane, *Grus americana.* Ill. Biol. Monographs *24*(2):1–127, 1955.

47. FOX, D. L.: *Animal Biochromes and Structural Colors.* Cambridge University Press, 1953. 190 pp.

48. FREEDMAN, S. L., and STURKIE, P. D.: Blood vessels of the chicken's uterus (shell gland). Am. J. Anat. *113:*1–7, 1963.

49. FRIEDMAN, H.: The birds of North and Middle America. Part II. Bull. U. S. National Museum, 1950.

50. FÜRBRINGER, M.: Untersuchungen zur Morphologie und Systematik der Vögel, zugleich ein Beitrag zur Anatomie der Stütz- und Bewegungsorgane. Amsterdam, T. van Holkema, 1888. 2 vols., 1751 pp. plus 30 plates.

51. GADOW, H.: On the taxonomic value of the intestinal convolutions in birds. Proc. Zool. Soc. Lond. 1889, pp. 303–316.

52. GADOW, H., and SELENKA, E.: Vögel. In Bronn's *Klassen und Ordnungen der Thier-reichs,* 1891. Vol. 6, 1008 pp.

53. GARROD, A. H.: On some points in the anatomy of the parrots which bear on the classification of the suborder. Proc. Zool. Soc. Lond. 1874, pp. 586–598.

54. GEORGE, J. C., and BERGER, A. J.: *Avian Myology.* New York, Academic Press, 1966. 500 pp.

55. GIEBEL, C.: Die Zunge der Vögel und ihr Gerüst. Z. f. Naturwiss. *11:*19–51, 1858.

56. GLENNY, F. H.: Modifications of pattern in the aortic arch system of birds and their phylogenetic significance. Proc. U.S. Nat. Museum *104:*525–621, 1955.

57. GOODMAN, D. C., and FISHER, H. I.: Functional anatomy of the feeding apparatus in waterfowl. Aves: Anatidae. Carbondale, Southern Illinois University Press, 1962.

58. GRASSÉ, P. P., ed.: *Traité de Zoologie.* Vol. 15. Oiseaux. Paris, Masson et Cie., 1950. 1164 pp.

59. HAEFELFINGER, H. R.: *Beitrage zur vergleichenden Ontogenese des Vorderhirns bei Vögeln.* Basel, Helbing & Lichtenhahn, 1958.

60. HARRIS, H. A.: De formatione ovi et pulli. Brit. Med. J. *1:*585–586, 1948.

61. HAZELHOFF, E. H.: Structure and function of the lung of birds. Poultry Sci. *30:*3–10, 1951.

62. HOLMGREN, N.: Studies on the phylogeny of birds. Acta Zool. *36:*243–328, 1955.

63. HOWARD, H.: The avifauna of Emeryville shellmound. Univ. Calif. Publ. Zool. *32:*301–394, 1929.

64. HOWELL, A. B.: Morphogenesis of the shoulder architecture: Aves. Auk *54:*364–375, 1937.

65. HOWELL, A. B.: Muscles of the avian hip and thigh. Auk *55:*71–81, 1938.

66. HUDSON, G. E.: Studies on the muscles of the pelvic appendage in birds. Am. Midl. Nat. *18:*1–108, 1937.

67. HUDSON, G. E., and LANZILLOTTI, P. J.: Gross anatomy of the wing muscles in the family Corvidae. Am. Midl. Nat. *53:*1–44, 1955.

68. HUDSON, G. E., and LANZILLOTTI, P. J.: Muscles of the pectoral limb in galliform birds. Am. Midl. Nat. *71:*1–113, 1964.

69. HUXLEY, T. H.: On the respiratory organs of *Apteryx*. Proc. Zool. Soc. Lond. 1882, pp. 560–569.

70. IMHOF, G.: Anatomie und Entwicklungsgeschichte des Lumbalmarks bei den Vögeln. Arch. mikroskop. Anat. u. Entwicklungsges. *65:*498–610, 1905.

71. INTERNATIONAL ANATOMICAL NOMENCLATURE COMMITTEE: *Nomina Anatomica,* 3rd ed. Amsterdam, Excerpta Medica Foundation, 1966. 112 pp.

72. JOLLIE, M. T.: The head skeleton of the chicken and remarks on the anatomy of this region in other birds. J. Morph. *100:*389–436, 1957.

73. JOOS, C.: Vergleichende Untersuchungen über die Ontogenese des Darmtraktus von *Melopsittacus undulatus* Gould. Verhandl. naturforsch. Ges. Basel *53:*15–70, 1941.

74. KADONO, H., OKADA, T., and ONO, K.: Electromyographic studies on the respiratory muscles of the chicken. Poultry Sci. *42:*121–128, 1963.

75. KALISCHER, O.: Das Grosshirn der Papageien in anatomisher und physiologischer Beziehung. Abh. IV d. Königl. Preuss. Akademie d. Wiss. (Berlin), 1905. 105 pp.

76. KAPPERS, C. U. ARIENS: *Anatomie Comparée du Systéme Nerveux.* Päris, Masson et Cie., 1947. (Fig. 174 Autonomic system of the pigeon.)

77. KAPPERS, C. U. ARIËNS, HUBER, G. C., and CROSBY, E. C.: *The Comparative Anatomy of the Nervous System of Vertebrates, Including Man.* New York, Macmillan Co., 1936. 2 vols. 1845 pp.

78. KAUPP, B. F.: *The Anatomy of the Domestic Fowl.* Philadelphia, W. B. Saunders Co., 1918. 373 pp.

79. KERN, A.: Das Vogelherz. Untersuchungen an *Gallus domesticus.* Gegenbaurs Morph. Jahrb. *56:*264–315, 1926.

79a. KING, A. S.: Structural and Functional Aspects of the Avian Lungs and Air Sacs. In *International Review of General and Experimental Zoology,* W. J. L. Felts and R. J. Harrison, eds. New York, Academic Press, 1966. Vol. 2, pp. 171–267.

80. KOBAYASHI, H., BERN, H. A., NISHIOKA, R. S., and HYODO, Y.: The hypothalamo-hypophyseal neurosecretory system of the parakeet, *Melopsittacus undulatus.* Gen. & Comp. Endocrinol. *1:*545–564, 1961.

81. KOMARÉK, V.: Krajing tela husy a kura (Regiones corporis der Gans und des Huhnes). Acta universitatis agriculturae et sylviculturae, Brno. VI(XXVII): 1–19, 1958.

82. KRABBE, K. H.: Development of the pineal organ and a rudimentary parietal eye in some birds. J. Comp. Neurol. *103:*139–149, 1955.

83. LAFEBER, T. J.: Bird clinic. The Budgerigar. Animal Hospital *1:*122–132, 1965.

84. LANGLEY, J. N.: On the sympathetic system of birds and on the muscles which move the feathers. J. Physiol. *30:*221–252, 1903.

85. LARSELL, O.: The development and subdivisions of the cerebellum of birds. J. Comp. Neurol. *89:*123–189, 1948.

86. LATIMER, H. B., and OSBORN, J. L.: The topography of the viscera of the chicken. Anat. Rec. *26:*275–289, 1923.

87. LEMMRICH, W.: Der Skleralring der Vogel. Jena. Z. f. Naturwiss. *65:*513–586, 1931.

88. LOCY, W. A., and LARSELL, O.: The embryology of the bird's lung. Am. J. Anat. (Part I) *19:*447–504; (Part II) *ibid. 20:*1–44, 1916.

89. LUCAS, A. M., and JAMROZ, C.: *Atlas of Avian Hematology.* Agriculture Monograph *25.* Washington, D.C., United States Department of Agriculture, 1961. 271 pp.

90. LUCAS, A. M., and STETTENHEIM, P. R.: Avian Anatomy. In *Diseases of Poultry,* 5th ed., H. E. Biester and L. H. Schwarte, eds. Ames, Iowa State University Press, 1965. Pp. 1–59.

91. LUCAS, A. M., and STETTENHEIM, P. R.: Avian Anatomy. United States Department of Agriculture. (In Press)

92. MCLELLAND, J.: The anatomy of the rings and muscles of the trachea of *Gallus domesticus.* J. Anat. Lond. *99:*651–656, 1965.

93. MCLEOD, W. M., TROTTER, D. M., and LUMB, J. W.: *Avian Anatomy.* Minneapolis, Burgess Press, 1964. 143 pp.

94. MALINOVSKY, L.: Contribution to the anatomy of the vegetative nervous system in the neck and thorax of the domestic pigeon. Acta Anat. *50:*326–347, 1962.

95. MALINOVSKY, L.: The nerve supply of the stomach in the domestic pigeon (*Columba domestica*). Morfologie *11*:16–27, 1963.

96. MARPLES, B. J.: The structure and development of the nasal glands of birds. Proc. Zool. Soc. Lond. 1932, pp. 829–844.

97. MARSHALL, A. J., ed.: *Biology and Comparative Physiology of Birds.* New York, Academic Press. Vol. I, 1960, 518 pp.; Vol. II, 1961, 468 pp.

98. MASON, C. W.: Structural colors in feathers. J. Phys. Chem. *27*:201–251, 1923.

99. MATTHEWS, L. H., and KNIGHT, M.: *The Senses of Animals.* New York, Philosophical Library, 1963. 240 pp.

100. MAYNARD, C. J.: *Vocal Organs of Talking Birds and Some Other Species.* Publ. by author, West Newton, Mass., 1928. 380 pp.

101. MEISTER, W.: Changes in histological structure of the long bones of birds during the molt. Anat. Rec. *111*:1–21, 1951.

102. MERYMAN, H. T.: The preparation of biological museum specimens by freeze-drying. Curator *3*:5-19, 1960.

103. MILLER, A. H.: The vocal apparatus of some North American owls. Condor *36*:204–213, 1934.

104. MILLER, A. M.: The development of the jugular lymph sac in birds. Am. J. Anat. *12*:473–491, 1912.

105. MILLER, W. DeW.: Further notes on ptilosis. Bull. Am. Mus. Nat. Hist. *50*:305–331, 1924.

106. MISKIMEN, M.: Sound production in passerine birds. Auk *68*:493–504, 1951.

107. MISKIMEN, M.: The syrinx in certain Tyrant Flycatchers. Auk *80*:156–165, 1963.

108. MITCHELL, P. C.: On the intestinal tract of birds. Proc. Zool. Soc. Lond. 1896, pp. 136–159.

109. MIVART, ST. G.: On the hyoid bone of certain parrots. Proc. Zool. Soc. Lond. 1895, pp. 162–174.

110. MIVART, ST. G.: The skeleton of *Lorius flavopalliatus* compared with that of *Psittacus erithacus.* Proc. Zool. Soc. Lond. 1895, pp. 312–337 (part I), 363–399 (part II).

111. MONTAGNA, W.: A re-investigation of the development of the wing of the fowl. J. Morph. *76*:87–113, 1945.

112. MOORE, C. A., and ELLIOTT, R.: Numerical and regional distribution of taste buds on the tongue of the bird. J. Comp. Neurol. *84*:119–131, 1946.

113. MOORE, M. A. S., and OWEN, J. J. T.: Experimental studies on the development of the bursa of Fabricius. Develop. Biol. *14*:40–51, 1966.

114. MOULTON, D. G., and BEIDLER, L. M.: Structure and function in the peripheral olfactory system. Physiol. Rev. *47*:1–52, 1967.

115. MUDGE, G. P.: On the myology of the tongue of parrots, with a classification of the Order, based upon the structure of the tongue. Trans. Zool. Soc. Lond. *16*:211–278, 1902.

116. NALBANDOV, A. V., and JAMES, M. F.: The bloodvascular system of the chicken ovary. Am. J. Anat. *85*:347–377, 1949.

117. NEWTON, A., and GADOW, H.: *A Dictionary of Birds.* London, Adam and Charles Black. In four parts, 1893–1896. 1088 pp.

118. NIETHAMMER, G.: Anatomisch-Histologische und Physiologische Untersuchungen über die Kropfbildungen der Vögel. Mit besonderer Berücksichtigung der Umbildungen im Kropfe brütender Tauben. Z. f. wiss. Zool. *144*:12–101, 1933.

119. NISHIDA, T.: Comparative and topographical anatomy of the fowl. X. The blood vascular system of the hind limb in the fowl. Part 1. The artery (In Japanese and English.) Jap. J. Vet. Sci. *25*:93–106, 1963.

120. NITZSCH, C. L.: *Pterylography*, P. L. Sclater, ed.; translated from German to English by W. S. Dallas. London, The Ray Society, 1867. 181 pp.

121. O'RAHILLY, R., and MEYER, D. B.: The Development and Histochemistry of the Pecten Oculi. In *The Structure of the Eye*, G. K. Smelser, ed. New York, Academic Press, 1961. Pp. 207–219.

122. OWEN, R.: *On the Anatomy of Vertebrates.* London, Longmans, Green and Co., 1866. Vol. 2, Birds and Mammals, pp. 14–259.

123. PAPEZ, J. W.: *Comparative Neurology.* New York, Thomas Y. Crowell Company, 1929. 518 pp.

124. POHLMAN, A. G.: The position and functional interpretation of the elastic ligaments in the middle-ear region of *Gallus.* J. Morphol. *35*:229–262, 1921.

125. PORTMANN, A.: *Animal Forms and Patterns. A Study of the Appearance of Animals.* (Translated from *Die Tiergestalt* by H. Czech.) London, Faber & Faber, 1952. 246 pp.

126. PORTMANN, A.: Sensory Organs: Part I. Skin, Taste and Olfaction; Part II. Equilibration. In *Biology and Comparative Physiology of Birds*, A. J. Marshall, ed. New York, Academic Press, 1961. Vol. II, pp. 37–54.

127. PORTMANN, A., and STINGELIN, W.: The Central Nervous System. In *Biology and Comparative Physiology of Birds*, A. J. Marshall, ed. New York, Academic Press, 1961. Vol. II, pp. 1–36.

128. PUMPHREY, R. J.: Sensory Organs: Vision. In *Biology and Comparative Physiology of Birds*, A. J. Marshall,

ed. New York, Academic Press, 1961, Vol. II, pp. 55–68.

129. RANNEY, R. E., CHAIKOFF, I. L., and DOBSON, E. L.: A procedure for functional hepatectomy of the unanesthetized fowl. Am. J. Physiol. *165:*588–595, 1951.

130. RAWLES, M. E.: Tissue interactions in scale and feather development as studied in dermal-epidermal recombinations. J. Embryol. Exp. Morphol. *11:*765–789, 1963.

131. RAWLES, M. E.: Tissue Interactions in the Morphogenesis of the Feather. In *Biology of the Skin and Hair Growth,* A. G. Lyne and B. F. Short, eds. New York, American Elsevier Publishing Company, Inc., 1965. Pp. 105–128.

132. ROMANOFF, A. L.: *The Avian Embryo. Structural and Functional Development.* New York, The Macmillan Company, 1960. 1305 pp.

133. ROWLEY, J.: *Taxidermy and Museum Exhibition.* New York, D. Appleton and Company, 1925. 331 pp.

134. SALT, G. W.: Respiratory evaporation in birds. Biol. Rev. *39:*113–136, 1964.

135. SALT, G. W., and ZEUTHEN, E.: The Respiratory System. In *Biology and Comparative Physiology of Birds,* A. J. Marshall, ed. New York, Academic Press, 1960. Vol. I, pp. 363–409.

136. SCHMIDT-NIELSEN, K., JÖRGENSEN, C. B., and OSAKI, H.: Extrarenal salt excretion in birds. Am. J. Physiol. *193:*101–107, 1958.

137. SENGEL, P.: The Determinism of the Differentiation of the Skin and the Cutaneous Appendages of the Chick Embryo. In *The Epidermis,* W. Montagna and W. C. Lobitz, Jr., eds. New York, Academic Press, 1964. Pp. 15–34.

138. SHUFELDT, R. W.: *The Myology of the Raven* (Corvus corax sinuatus). *A Guide to the Study of the Muscular System in Birds.* London, Macmillan and Co., 1890. 343 pp.

139. SLONAKER, J. R.: A physiological study of the anatomy of the eye and its accessory parts of the English sparrow (*Passer domesticus*). J. Morph. *31:*351–459, 1918.

140. SPERBER, I.: Investigations on the circulatory system of the avian kidney. Zool. Bidrag. Uppsala *27:*429–448, 1949.

141. SPRING, L. W.: Climbing and pecking adaptations in some North American woodpeckers. Condor *67:*457–488, 1965.

142. STEINER, H.: Das Problem der Diastataxie des Vogelflügels. Jena. Z. f. Naturwiss. *55:*221–496, 1918.

143. STORER, R. W.: Adaptive Radiation in Birds. In *Biology and Comparative Physiology of Birds,* A. J. Marshall,

ed. New York, Academic Press, 1960. Vol. I, pp. 15–55.

144. STRESEMANN, E.: Aves. In *Handbuch der Zoologie,* W. Kükenthal and T. Krumbach, eds. Berlin, Walter de Gruyter & Co. Vol. 7, Part 2, 1934. 899 pp.

145. STRONG, R. M.: *A Bibliography of Birds.* Chicago Field Mus. Nat. Hist., Zool. Ser. Vol. 25: 1939 Part 1 Author catalog A–J, pp. 1–464; 1939 Part 2 Author catalog K–Z, pp. 469–937; 1946 Part 3 Subject Index, pp. 1–528; 1959 Part 4 Finding Index, pp. 1–185.

146. STURKIE, P. D.: *Avian Physiology,* 2nd ed. Ithaca, N.Y., Comstock Publishing Associates, 1965. 766 pp.

147. SWINEBROAD, J.: A comparative study of the wing myology of certain passerines. Am. Midl. Nat. *51:*488–514, 1954.

148. SZABÓ, L.: A hullámos papagáj (*Melopsittacus undulatus*) érrendszere. Thesis, Budapest, 1958.

149. TANSLEY, K.: *Vision in Vertebrates.* London, Chapman & Hall Ltd., 1965. 132 pp.

150. TECHNAU, G.: Die Nasendrüse der Vögel. J. Ornithol. *84:*511–617, 1936.

151. TEN CATE, J.: The Nervous System of Birds. In *Avian Physiology,* 2nd ed., P. D. Sturkie, ed. Ithaca, N.Y., Comstock Publishing Associates, 1965. Pp. 697–751.

152. TOMPSETT, D. H.: *Anatomical Techniques.* Edinburgh, Livingston, 1956. 240 pp.

153. TONER, P. G.: The fine structure of gizzard gland cells in the domestic fowl. J. Anat., Lond. *98:*77–85, 1964.

154. TUCKER, R.: Differentiation of epithelial and connective tissue components in the tongue of *Gallus domesticus.* Res. Vet. Sci. *7:*1–16, 1966.

155. VAN DRIMMELEN, G. C.: Artificial insemination of birds by the intraperitoneal route. Onderstepoort J. Vet. Res. Supplement No. 1, pp. 1–212, 1951.

156. VAN TIENHOVEN, A.: Endocrinology of Reproduction in Birds. In *Sex and Internal Secretions,* 3rd ed., W. C. Young, ed. Baltimore, Williams & Wilkins Co., 1961. Pp. 1088–1169.

157. VAN TIENHOVEN, A., SUTHERLAND, C., and SAATMAN, R. R.: The effects of exposure to darkness on the reproductive and hypothalamo-hypophysial systems of budgerigars, *Melopsittacus undulatus.* Gen. & Comp. Endocrinol. *6:*420–427, 1966.

158. VITUMS, A., MIKAMI, S.-I., OKSCHE, A., and FARNER, D. S.: Vascularization of the hypothalamo-hypophysial complex in the white-crowned sparrow, *Zonotrichia leucophrys gambelii.* Z. Zellforsch. *64:*541–569, 1964.

159. VITUMS, A., ONO, K., OKSCHE, A., FARNER, D. S., and KING, J. R.: The development of the hypo-

physial portal system in the white-crowned sparrow, *Zonotrichia leucophrys gambelii.* Z. Zellforsch. *73:*335–366, 1966.

160. WALLS, G. L.: *The Vertebrate Eye and Its Adaptive Radiation.* Bloomfield Hills, Mich., Cranbrook Institute of Science, 1942. 785 pp.

161. WATANABE, T.: Comparative and topographical anatomy of the fowl. VII. On the peripheral course of the vagus nerve in the fowl. (In Japanese and English.) Jap. J. Vet. Sci. *22:*145–154, 1960.

162. WATSON, G. E.: Feather replacement in birds. Science *139:*50–51, 1963.

163. WINGSTRAND, K. G.: *The Structure and Development of the Avian Pituitary.* CWK Gleerup/Lund, 1951. 316 pp.

164. WOOD, C. A.: *The Fundus Oculi of Birds Especially As Viewed by the Ophthalmoscope. A Study in Comparative Anatomy and Physiology.* Chicago, The Lakeside Press, 1917. 181 pp.

165. YASUDA, M.: Comparative and topographical anatomy of the fowl. XI. On the nervous supply of the hind-limb. (In Japanese and English.) Jap. J. Vet. Sci. *23:*145–156, 1961.

166. ZOTTERMAN, Y., ed.: *Olfaction and Taste,* Proceedings of the First International Symposium held at the Wenner-Gren Center, Stockholm, September 1962. London, Pergamon Press, Ltd., 1963. 396 pp.

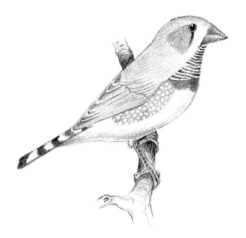

6

Some Physiological Attributes of Small Birds

Donald S. Farner

Although many species of medium-sized and small birds have been maintained in captivity as pets, knowledge of their physiology is strikingly fragmentary. All too frequently inferences regarding their physiology are based on information derived from study of larger domestic birds, a practice that involves obvious hazards. Attention in this Chapter is directed primarily to psittaciform and passeriform birds, since most species of birds that are maintained as pets belong to these Orders. Emphasis is placed on the physiological attributes that are characteristic of small birds. More extensive treatments of these and other aspects of the biology and physiology of small birds may be found in *Biology and Comparative Physiology of Birds.*[107]

The striking physiological attributes common to small birds are associated primarily with adaptation to flight and with provision of the great amount of energy required for maintenance of homeothermy in a body of such small size. The principal physiological differences among small birds are associated with adaptations in feeding and nutrition, with adaptations to different conditions of temperature and availability of water, and with the evolution of a diversity of systems for the control of such functions as reproduction, molt, and migration.

FOOD INTAKE AND DIGESTION

The distinctive features of the feeding apparatus and the process of digestion in birds are associated with the evolution of flight and high metabolic rates. (For a more extensive discussion of avian digestion, see

Farner.[51]) The cephalic portion of the alimentary apparatus is reduced to the minimum required for procurement of food. It is characterized by a light horny bill, with relatively light jaw structure and musculature, and the absence of teeth. The bill and tongue vary greatly in form, the result of adaptation to various nutritional regimens.[172] Beyond functioning in the procurement of food, the bill may be involved to a limited extent in the initial mechanical processes of alimentation, such as seed-cracking in some granivores and tearing and shearing functions in some frugivores. The buccal cavity functions primarily as a passageway for food from the mouth to the pharynx.

Although they vary considerably in form and number, seven groups of salivary glands can be recognized.[2] The glands are mucigenic and are thus important primarily in the lubrication of the food. Although a salivary amylase has been reported for some finches, existence of such an enzyme still remains uncertain. Actually, since an amylase cannot function extensively until the food has reached the small intestine, the question of its occurrence in the saliva is relatively unimportant. The secretory activity of the salivary glands increases during feeding.

The process of deglutition is not adequately understood and may vary among members of different taxonomic groups. In general, however, birds propel food posteriorly into the pharynx by raising the head and/ or by quick forward thrust of the head, and by raising the tongue. At least in some species of parrots and parrot-like birds the tongue has a more active role in moving food posteriorly into the pharynx. The choanal slit is closed reflexively, as is also the glottis, by forward movement of the larynx against the base of the tongue. Once it is in the posterior pharynx, the food is caught up by peristaltic action and is moved thereby through the esophagus. In drinking, most species of birds must allow water to flow passively into the buccal cavity. The mouth is then closed and the head is raised, thereby permitting flow of the water to the esophagus by gravity. Presumably this also involves reflexive closure of the choanal slit and glottis. However, some species, including pigeons, doves, hummingbirds, and some parrots, can drink actively without raising the head.

The esophagus serves primarily as a passageway for food between the pharynx and stomach. In many species, including some of the finches, it also has a storage function. Performance of this function may involve a simple expansion of a morphologically unmodified tube, or it may be achieved by a morphologically differentiated expansion or diverticulum, the crop. A fusiform crop occurs in many finches such as the canary (*Serinus canarius*). The fusiform crop, when filled, may occupy a position dorsal to the vertebral column. In some species, such as the redpoll (*Acanthis flammea*) and the zebra finch (*Poephila castanotis*), the crop is a diverticulum which, when filled, has two lobes and extends dorsally to the vertebral column. Although the crop functions primarily as a place for the storage of food, in granivores the softening of food by the uptake of water while in the crop is an important preliminary digestive process. Also among those granivores, such as the zebra finch, that feed seeds to the young, an important preliminary softening of the seeds may occur in the crop of the adult. The movements of the crop are controlled through parasympathetic fibers from the vagus, sympathetic fibers, and fibers of the myenteric nervous system. Crop glands, when present, are mucigenic.

The mucosa of the crop of pigeons and doves becomes thickened and glandular during the reproductive season, when it produces the crop milk that is fed the young. In pigeons and doves it appears that the crop may have a limited role in carbohydrate digestion; the crop glands have serous and mucous elements, and have been reported to produce amylase and sucrase.

The gastric apparatus of birds usually consists of an anterior glandular stomach, or proventriculus, and a posterior muscular stomach (ventriculus), or gizzard.

The proventriculus functions as a passageway from the esophagus to the gizzard, and secretes the acid gastric juice. The simple tubular glands are probably involved only in the production of mucus. The compound glands produce the acid gastric juice and pepsin. In some groups of birds the proventriculus is expansible and serves as a storage chamber. Both neural and hormonal mechanisms are involved in the secretion of gastric juice. It appears probable that a control system similar to that in which gastrin is involved in mammals is also present in birds. Although there is a cephalic phase in the neural control of gastric secretion in ducks and chickens, it is not yet known whether or not this is generally true among birds.

In most birds the gizzard acts as an organ both of trituration and of acid proteolysis. Variations in the degree of development of the smooth musculature and in the thickness and hardness of the koilin, the scleroproteinaceous lining of the organ,[34,68,89] occur as adaptations to the nutritional regimen among species[45,51] and occur also to a lesser extent among individuals of the same species. Among seed-eating birds a pH (hydrogen ion concentration) of about 2 to 3, due to hydrochloric acid from the proventriculus, is maintained in the gizzard during periods of digestion. The activity of the musculature of the gizzard is characterized by rhythmic contractions of varying amplitudes and frequencies. In the chicken, at least, the cycle appears to involve first a contraction of the lateral muscles causing a narrowing of the lumen, followed by asymmetrical contractions of the intermediate muscles, resulting in a rubbing or grinding effect.[106] Basically the motor activity of the gastric apparatus is a function of an intrinsic myenteric nervous system,[77,124-128] which can be modified by impulses transmitted by the vagus and celiac fibers.

Many species of granivores, herbivores, and omnivores retain grit in the gizzard, thereby enhancing its triturating function. The period of retention of food varies greatly, from a few minutes to a few hours, depending on the nature of the food and the physiologic state of the digestive system.

The principal organ for chemical digestion and for absorption is the small intestine. Here the chyme from the gizzard is neutralized by the highly buffered bile, pancreatic juice, and succus entericus so that the pH, especially in the ileum, usually is between 6 and 8.[51] The chemical digestion of starch is effected largely in the small intestine through the actions of pancreatic amylase and of intestinal and pancreatic maltase. The reported occurrence of amylase in the succus entericus remains to be verified. Lactose and sucrose are hydrolyzed by the lactase and "sucrase" (maltase), respectively, of the succus entericus. Although microbial digestion and fermentation of cellulose occur in the ceca of at least some of the galliform species, the frequently repeated suggestion that these processes also occur in the small intestine of herbivorous, frugivorous, and granivorous species, such as parrots, doves, and finches which have no functional ceca, still requires experimental verification.

Whole protein and protein hydrolysates produced by peptic digestion are hydrolyzed to amino acids by the action of pancreatic trypsin and as yet largely uncharacterized peptidases from the succus entericus and possibly also from the pancreatic juice. Although our knowledge is meager, it appears that the small intestine produces an enterokinase that catalyzes the conversion of inactive pancreatic trypsinogen to trypsin. The principal lipolytic enzyme is pancreatic lipase; the occurrence of lipase in the succus entericus remains to be verified.

The principal functions of the bile include the neutralization of chyme and emulsification of fat; however, at least in the chicken, the bile contains a significant amount of amylase. The gall bladder, when present, has both storage and reabsorbing functions. Gall bladder bile has a greater emulsifying but less neutralizing effect than does hepatic bile. The gall bladder is lacking, however, in many species, including some doves and pigeons, many parrots, and some passerine birds.

The movements of the small intestine, and their control, have been studied only to a limited extent and almost exclusively in the chicken. Both peristaltic and segmenting movements are obviously involved.[193] Peristaltic waves travel at the rate of several centimeters per second. Intestinal motility is a complex function of the rhythmicity of smooth muscle, the intrinsic functions of the myenteric nervous system, extrinsic neural control, hormonal control, and the effects of local chemical and mechanical stimuli.

The myenteric nervous system, including the myenteric plexus (Auerbach) and submucosal plexus (Meissner), is conspicuously developed.[192,135] The extrinsic nerve supply consists of parasympathetic fibers from the vagus and sympathetic fibers which reach the intestine via the celiac plexus and, in part, then through Remak's nerve, and via the mesenteric plexus.[123] The celiac and mesenteric nerves contain parasympathetic fibers; Remak's nerve consists of fibers of celiac and sacral origin and is a source of extrinsic innervation of the ileum.[123]

The enteric nervous system consists of an assemblage of neurons arranged in two layers, *central* and *peripheral*. The cells of the central layer are in synaptic organization for conduction aborally and connect synaptically with the functionally inhibitory and stimulatory fibers of the peripheral layer which, in turn, connect with the muscle cells. The enteric nervous system also contains afferent fibers that are parts of reflex arcs with their "central" synapses in the ganglia of the enteric plexus.

The enteric nervous system of the small intestine, especially that of the upper part, is intimately associated with that of the gizzard[125]; the stimulatory effect of the vagus on the upper small intestine apparently operates primarily through this connection. The lower ileum tends to have its own rhythm. The extrinsic nerves contain both preganglionic and postganglionic fibers, the latter being sympathetic fibers that exert an inhibiting effect on intestinal movement. The preganglionic fibers are both sympathetic and parasympathetic (vagal) and operate only via synapses with the connector neurons of the enteric ganglionic chain. In general parasympathetic impulses cause increased motility.

As the posterior extension of the small intestine, from the level of the ceca, the large intestine has little function as a digestive organ although it appears to have a role in absorption of water. The cloaca is a common chamber for the digestive, reproductive, and excretory systems. The musculature of the caudal part, including the anal sphincter, has striated fibers. There is some evidence that the cloaca also has a water-reabsorbing function.

There is typically in young birds, at the junction of the large intestine and the cloaca, a dorsal diverticulum, the bursa of Fabricius, or cloacal bursa, which eventually loses its lumen and becomes lymphoid in nature (see discussion of this structure later in the Chapter).

RESPIRATION

Although external respiration and the transport of respiratory gases in birds do not differ, in principle, from those of other air-breathers, it is clear from the anatomy of the respiratory system (Fig. 6-1) that the process of ventilation of the avian lung is unique. The tidal volume, even in a resting bird, exceeds very substantially the maximal capacity of the lungs. This is possible only because of a movement into and out of the air-sac system during each cycle of ventilation. Although the details of the air-flow patterns are not yet understood, it appears that air must be almost continually in motion in the parabronchi so that a stagnation period, such as is characteristic of the ventilation cycle of the mammalian lung, does not occur.

Since the stresses on the body during flight and during standing are very different, it follows that the ventilation movements may also show important differences. The information available concerns ventilation movements as they have been studied in standing birds. It should be noted that, in a bird held upside down, the shift in position of the viscera may result in a markedly abnormal pattern of ventilation movements.

The following account is derived primarily from the treatise of Soum,[162] the reviews of Salt and Zeuthen[149] and King and Farner,[86] and the discussion of King and Payne.[83]

In the standing bird, contraction of the inspiratory muscles (*M. scalenus, Mm. levatores costarum, Mm. intercostales externi, Mm. costosternales, Mm. serratus, M. sternocoracoideus*) increases the angle between the vertebral and sternal segments of the ribs; the sternum is thus thrust forward and downward, causing it and the coracoid bones to rotate around the shoulder. The thoracoabdominal space is thus enlarged dorsoventrally. In expiration these movements are actively reversed by contraction of the expiratory muscles (*M. obliquus externus, M. obliquus abdominis internus, M. rectus abdominis, Mm. intercostales interni, Mm. iliocostales, M. transverso-analis, M. transversus abdominis*). Thus ventilation is entirely active and normally without interruption between the inspiratory and expiratory phases. The ventilation movements affect both the lungs and the air sacs. By enlarging the thoracoabdominal cavity a negative pressure is created in the air sacs and air is drawn into the system. Air is then driven out of the system by reduction of the size of the thoracoabdominal cavity. Thus ventilation is accomplished basically by a bellows action. However, in most medium-sized and small birds, ventilation continues by increased rib action even after the action of the posterior air sacs is eliminated. This can be explained by the fact that the ribs are embedded dorsomedially in the lungs and thus impart directly to the lungs a degree of change in volume through the course of each cycle. This passive movement of the lungs, imposed by the

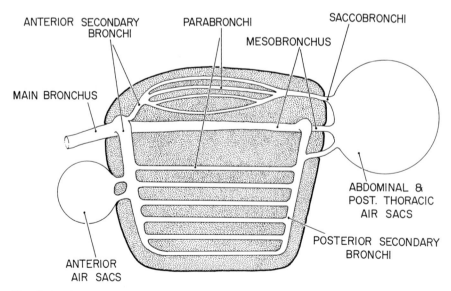

Fig. 6-1. *Schematic diagram of the avian respiratory system.* (*From King and Farner,*[86] *modified from Zeuthen, 1942, in* Handbook of Physiology *Section 4, 1964; courtesy of the American Physiological Society.*)

ribs, is essential in ventilation, since freeing of both lungs from the ribs results in immediate suffocation.[104] The abdominal diaphragm has no active role in ventilation. The pulmonary diaphragm, however, does have muscle slips whose contraction during expiration increases the tension on the diaphragm, perhaps thereby reducing the changes in pulmonary volume.

Air enters the respiratory system via the external nares, and from the nasal cavities continues posteriorly, through the choanal slit into the pharynx, through the glottis, and into the trachea. It then passes the length of the trachea into the syrinx, the sound-producing organ. Beyond the syrinx paired bronchi lead to the lungs. Since the air sacs were first described early in the 17th Century by Coitier and a few decades later by Harvey, the pattern or patterns of air flow through them and through the lungs have been the subject of almost continuous controversy. (For review, see Salt and Zeuthen.[149]) Almost all hypotheses and most of the pertinent data and observations suggest that the system provides a continuous movement of air through the parabronchi, thereby maintaining relatively constant concentration gradients in the air capillaries and across the respiratory surfaces. Thus it is possible to account for the much smaller size of the lungs of birds in relation to the lungs of mammals of comparable size.

The air sacs appear to serve at least three functions: (*a*) as air reservoirs in the bellows-type ventilation system, (*b*) as surfaces for evaporative cooling and thus as an element in the thermoregulatory system, and (*c*) as surfaces through which a limited amount of CO_2 diffuses into the respiratory air.

There are remarkably few quantitative data on the performance of the respiratory system of small birds. Ventilation rate, of course, varies widely with the state of activity and with environmental temperature.

Thus Kendeigh[81] found that the ventilation rate in the house sparrow (*Passer domesticus*) at rest varied from over 90 cycles per minute at $-40°C.$ to about 60 per minute at $+30°C.$ and then to as much as 200 per minute at $+45°C.$ (Fig. 6-2). The rapid rate at high temperature is, of course, a thermoregulatory response that increases the rate of evaporative cooling. In the house wren (*Troglodytes aedon*) (body weight 8–10 grams) the ventilation rate within normal limits of body temperature ranges from approximately 100 to 300 cycles per minute. In general it can be said that caged finch-sized birds at ordinary room temperatures have ventilation rates of the order of 70 to 100 cycles per minute. There has been no adequate study of tidal volumes and composition of expired air in small birds. In the resting domestic pigeon with a ventilation rate of 30–50 cycles per minute, the tidal volume is of the order of 4 to 8 cc.[148,152,162] The increase in ventilation rate that comes with hyperthermia is accompanied by a decrease in tidal volume and an increase in minute volume[148]; under these circumstances it appears probable that much of the air, both in inspiration and expiration, is shunted directly between the trachea and the air sacs without passing through the parabronchial system, thus providing an increase in evaporative cooling without the danger of apnea due to respiratory alkalosis.[86,148,149,201] The role of the respiratory system in the regulation of body temperature is discussed in a subsequent section of this Chapter.

The mechanisms involved in the regulation of ventilation rate and tidal volume in birds are still poorly understood. The available information has been obtained from the larger species of domestic birds. Consequently the summary in Table 6-1, based largely on the analyses of Salt and Zeuthen,[149] must be regarded as extremely tentative. According to Salt and Zeuthen,[149] the respiratory center is basically automatic although

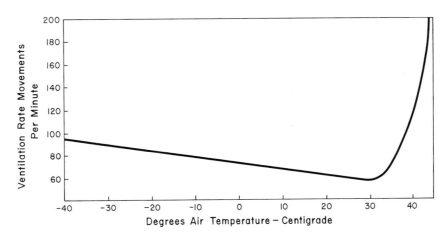

Fig. 6-2. *The rate of ventilation movements as a function of ambient temperature in the house sparrow,* **Passer domesticus.** (*From Kendeigh.*[81])

Table 6-1. Mechanisms Involved in Ventilation and Its Control in Birds*

| Peripheral Input | | Central Mediation | Output | Function |
Type	Route			
————	————	inspiratory center (medulla)	automatic discharge of low-frequency bursts to inspiratory muscles the same to expiratory muscles	generation of slow basic automatic ventilation cycle
————	————	expiratory center		
impulses from pulmonary stretch receptors	vagal afferents	stretch stimulates expiratory center	motor discharge to expiratory muscles and inhibition of inspiratory center	provides normal inspiration-expiration pattern
(?) impulses from pulmonary stretch receptors	vagal afferents	collapse stimulates inspiratory center	increases motor discharge to inspiratory muscles	increases tidal volume
impulses from receptors in tracheal mucosa	vagal afferents	expiratory center	increases motor discharge to expiratory muscles	probably a part of normal expiratory pattern
low O_2 high CO_2	blood to head	inspiratory center	increases motor discharge to inspiratory muscles	increases tidal volume
increase in temperature	blood to head	inspiratory and expiratory centers via panting center (midbrain)	shortens duration of motor discharge and increases frequency of discharges	increases rate of ventilation and reduces tidal volume (panting)

*Based largely on analyses of Salt and Zeuthen.[149]

the rate of discharge is much lower than the natural ventilation rate. Salt and Zeuthen also plausibly suggest that there are separate inspiratory and expiratory centers which alternately discharge bursts of motor impulses to the inspiratory and expiratory muscles, respectively. The necessarily reciprocal functional relationships between these centers have not yet been characterized.

Although information is extremely limited, there is no reason to assume that the mechanisms of transport of respiratory gases in the blood of birds differ in any very significant way from those in mammals. The available data,[32,117,199,200] all for larger birds, suggest that avian hemoglobin has a somewhat lower affinity for oxygen than has mammalian hemoglobin, and therefore it releases oxygen more readily in the systemic capillaries. The high percentage of oxygen saturation in avian arterial blood (usually 90–98% saturated; O_2 tension 90–110 mm. Hg; 12–20 volume %), despite this lower O_2 affinity, correlates with the more favorable diffusion gradients for O_2 in the avian lung. Venous blood is approximately 40% saturated with O_2 (O_2

tension 35–55 mm. Hg; 5–8 volume %). In larger birds, again, arterial CO_2 content is of the order of 35 to 45 volume % (CO_2 tension 35–55 mm. Hg); venous CO_2 content is of the order of 40 to 55 volume % (CO_2 tension 45–70 mm. Hg). The utilization of O_2 by tissues (removal from blood) is high, more than 50 per cent usually being removed from the blood in its passage through systemic capillaries. This reflects both the high metabolic rate and the relatively lower affinity of avian hemoglobin for oxygen. The hemoglobin concentration in small birds is of the order of 13 to 16%,[56] perhaps slightly higher than that of larger species.[56,101,150,206] Adult birds of the smaller passerine species have erythrocyte counts of the order of 4 to 6 million per cu. mm.[122,150] At the time the bird develops the ability to fly there is a conspicuous increase in erythrocyte count and hemoglobin content of the blood.[150]

CIRCULATION

Except for the presence of a functional renal portal system, the functions and processes of avian circulatory systems do not differ in principle from those in mammals. However, the hemodynamics in small birds with heart rates of several hundred to a thousand per minute represent a challenging and virgin area for research. Despite numerous exceptions, heart size generally is inversely related to body size; in small birds the mass of cardiac tissue constitutes 0.9–2 per cent of body weight. The relatively large size of the avian heart is doubtless a part of the complex of adaptations to flight.

The flow pattern and the function of the cardiac valves during the cardiac cycles are generally similar to those in mammals and need not be discussed in detail here. It should be noted that the right atrioventricular valve is muscular and probably closes actively at the beginning of ventricular systole. There appears to be no useful information available on intracardiac pressures, volume changes, and stroke volumes for small birds.

The following description of the conducting system is based primarily on the pigeon and domestic duck.[36–38] The sinu-atrial node, at the junction of the right precaval vein with the right atrium, extends through the entire thickness of the atrial wall. The nodal fibers are continuous with the Purkinje fibers that ramify throughout the atria to connect with ordinary myocardial fibers. The atrioventricular node lies in the connective tissue in the lower and posterior part of the atrial septum, as in mammals. The atrioventricular bundle extends caudally and ventrally into

the interior of the ventricular septum and subsequently divides into right and left limbs which ramify into a plexus of Purkinje fibers that extend throughout the myocardium of the right and left ventricles. A separate division of the right branch of the atrioventricular bundle passes directly to the right atrioventricular valve. Davies and Francis[38] suggest that the greater profusion in birds than in mammals of Purkinje fibers in both atria and ventricles may provide the basis for the relatively higher cardiac rates in birds. According to Davies,[36] the atrioventricular node is probably derived from the sinu-atrial ring; the right vagal and right sympathetic fibers are associated with the sinu-atrial ring, whereas the left vagal and left sympathetic fibers are associated with the atrioventricular node.

In the cardiac cycle the wave of electrical excitation slightly precedes the actual contraction. In larger birds, at least, it spreads from the sinu-atrial node through the atria, after which the excitation of the atrioventricular node spreads throughout the myocardium of the ventricles[87,88,98,105,174]; activation of the epicardial surface of the ventricle occurs before that of the endocardial surface.[88]

The normal electrocardiograms of the larger birds that have been studied exhibit P, S, and T waves,[88,105,174,176] but no Q wave. (For a discussion of the avian electrocardiogram, see Sturkie.[175])

For a 10-gram tit with a cardiac rate of about 1,000 per minute, the periods of atrial systole and diastole have been calculated to be 0.014 and 0.046 second, respectively; for ventricular systole and diastole, 0.024 and 0.036 second.[157]

The cardiac rates of birds are generally higher than those of mammals of the same body weight; smaller species usually have higher rates than larger species (Table 6-2). Rates following exercise or excitement may be two or three times as great as basal rates.[129,130]

Although the extent of the effect varies considerably among species, the role of the vagal efferents is generally cardio-inhibitory. Bilateral vagotomy is usually followed by an acceleration of heart rate; also atropine usually causes an increase in cardiac rate. Stübel[173] has suggested that the cardio-inhibitory effect is more pronounced in species in which the heart is relatively large in comparison with body size. Sympathetic afferents, from the cervical and upper thoracic spinal nerves, are cardio-accelerators.[134,173]

There are very few quantitative data bearing on the hemodynamics of the circulatory systems of small birds. Table 6-3 indicates the approximate range of systemic arterial blood pressures for a few species. Pulmonary arterial pressure is much lower; in the domestic fowl systolic and diastolic pressures of 20 and 8 mm. Hg,

Table 6-2. Observed Cardiac Rates in Selected Species of Small Birds*

Species	Weight (grams)	Resting Cardiac Rate (cycles per minute)
Zenaidura macroura (Mourning dove)	ca. 130	135–570
Sturnus vulgaris (Starling)	ca. 75	375–500
Turdus migratorius (American robin)	ca. 75	500–600
Passer domesticus (House sparrow)	25–30	350–900
Chloris chloris (Greenfinch)	22–27	700–850
Melospiza melodia (Song sparrow)	20	450–1,000
Domestic canary	16	500–1,000
Carduelis carduelis (European goldfinch)	13–16	750–900
Parus major (Great tit)	16	800
Parus ater (Coal tit)	8	1,000
Troglodytes aedon (House wren)	11	450–950
Estrilda troglodytes (Black-rumped waxbill)	6–7	500–1,000

*From Buchanan,[24] Odum,[129,130] Woodbury and Hamilton,[213] Stübel,[173] Sergeev and Skvortsova,[157] Lasiewski *et al.*[96] When a range in rates is given, the lower is basal or near basal, and the upper is maximal or near maximal.

respectively, have been reported.[146] The fragmentary information available on vasomotor controls suggests that they are similar to those of mammals.

Circulating blood in birds constitutes about 10 per cent of the total body weight. Published venous hematocrit values for a variety of domestic species range from 30 to 50 per cent. Although avian hematology has been studied extensively, most attention has been directed to the domestic fowl. However, the monographs of Sandreuter[150] and of Lucas and Jamroz,[101] the latter profusely illustrated, contain considerable information on other species. Small birds, as noted above, usually have erythrocyte counts within the range of 4 to 6 million per cu. mm., which is somewhat higher

than the range for larger birds. The elliptical avian erythrocyte is nucleated and therefore, compared with the mammalian erythrocyte, is metabolically much more active. Among the white cells the lymphocytes and heterophils (neutrophils) are normally the most abundant. There are conspicuous interspecies differences in differential white-cell counts. The data for the starling (*Sturnus vulgaris*) (Table 6-4) are presented as illustrative for a small passerine species. The data in Table 6-4 must be accepted cautiously, however, because of the large number of factors, such as time of day and season,[150] that affect the cell counts. In general, the erythrocytes of passerine birds are somewhat smaller ($11–14 \times 4–6$ microns) than those of larger species. The nucleated thrombocytes have the same function as the blood platelets of mammals and, like the mammalian platelets, are extremely fragile. Superficially the characteristics of clotting of avian blood resemble those of mammalian blood. However, research has not proceeded far enough to permit an effective comparison.

ENERGY METABOLISM, BODY TEMPERATURE, AND THERMOREGULATION

With the exception of hummingbirds, some goatsuckers, some swifts, and perhaps a few additional species, birds are true homeotherms. Small birds, with their high surface-volume ratios, have high metabolic rates. At relatively high environmental temperatures and mild or greater activity, the heat generated in motor activity may exceed that required to maintain body temperature. Under such conditions thermoregulatory mechanisms increase the rate of heat loss. With lower environmental temperatures during sleep, or relatively low motor activity, thermogenesis may become inadequate for maintenance of body temperature. Under such conditions the thermoregulatory apparatus first causes adjustments to reduce heat loss; if these adjustments are not sufficient to maintain the body temperature, thermogenesis is increased by acceleration of metabolic rate.

The chemical energy obtained in food is expended in a variety of energy-requiring functions. The chemical reactions involved in the metabolic processes and the physicochemical and chemical functions for which energy is expended involve the loss of varying amounts of energy as heat. The general history of energy derived from food is outlined in Figure 6-3. Since the metabolizable energy, which excludes the energy of the nonmetabolizable amino groups, is eventually converted

Table 6-3. Systemic Arterial Pressure in Small Birds*

Species	Number of Individuals	Arterial Blood Pressure (mm. Hg)	
		Systolic	Diastolic
Columba livia (Domestic pigeon)	4	120-140	100-115
Turdus migratorius (American robin)	2	110-125	80
Sturnus vulgaris (Starling)	2	150-210	100-160
Serinus canarius (Domestic canary)	4	200-250	150-160

*From Woodbury and Hamilton.[213]

Table 6-4. Blood Cell Counts: A Comparison between a Galliform and a Passerine Species

	Domestic Fowl				Starling (*Sturnus vulgaris*)	
	♂		♀		♂	♀
	Lucas and Jamroz[101]	Sandreuter[150]	Lucas and Jamroz[101]	Sandreuter[150]	Sandreuter[150]	
Erythrocytes (millions per cu. mm.)	3.8	4.4	3.0	3.2	3.2	5.8
Thrombocytes (thousands per cu. mm.)	28		31			
Leukocytes (thousands per cu. mm.)	17		29			
Leukocytes (distribution %)						
Lymphocytes	64.0	56.7	76.1	73.0	61.5	58.6
Monocytes	6.4	10.9	5.7	7.5	8.7	9.2
Heterophils (neutrophils)	25.8	26.0	13.3	14.2	20.0	22.4
Eosinophils	1.4	2.2	2.5	2.8	3.5	4.3
Basophils	2.4	4.2	2.4	2.5	6.3	5.5

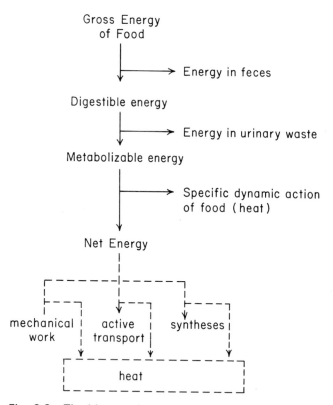

Fig. 6-3. *The history of energy derived from food.*

entirely, or almost entirely, into heat, the rate of energy metabolism for a bird in caloric steady state can be measured either by determination of the net daily intake of metabolizable energy or by determination of the rate of heat loss. Because metabolic rate is affected by motor activity, environmental temperature, and other factors, comparisons among species, and among individuals within species, require the use of standard conditions. Standard metabolism is therefore the metabolic rate of a bird in post-absorptive condition (*i.e.*, not digesting or absorbing food) in a thermoneutral environment (*i.e.*, not having to generate heat to maintain body temperature), and as completely as possible at rest. The examination of data obtained under these conditions for a large number of species indicates that the standard metabolic rate (expressed as kilocalories per bird per day) is a function of the logarithm of body weight (Fig. 6-4). The metabolic rate per unit mass decreases as body size increases. This relationship, as shown in Figure 6-4, may be expressed approximately by the following equation:

$$\log_{10}M = 1.90 + 0.66 \log_{10}W \pm 0.07,$$

where M is standard metabolic rate in kilocalories per day and W is body weight in grams. For a more extensive discussion of this relationship, King and Farner[85] may be consulted. Standard metabolic rates for a few selected small species are given in Table 6-5.

The maintenance of a stable body temperature requires a constant balance between heat production and heat loss. The thermoregulatory control mechanisms acting in birds are shown schematically in Figure 6-5. The rate of heat loss from the surface of the body is a function of the difference between the surface temperature and the ambient temperature. Were the thermolytic behavior of a small bird identical with that of an ideal physical object, the metabolic rate would necessarily be increased uniformly as a function of the difference between surface and environmental temperature in order to maintain a constant body temperature.

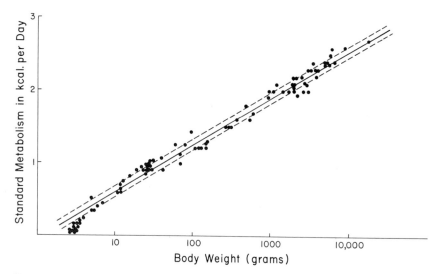

Fig. 6-4. *Standard metabolic rate as a function of body weight. The cluster of points at about 5 grams is for hummingbirds.*

Table 6-5. Standard Metabolic Rate for Selected Species of Small Finches

Species	Weight (grams)	Standard Metabolic Rate (kcal. per day)	Reference
Poephila castanotis	*ca.* 12	4.5	Calder[28]
(Zebra finch)		5.1	Cade *et al.*[27]
Estrilda troglodytes	*ca.* 6.5	2.6	Lasiewski *et al.*[96]
(Black-rumped waxbill)		2.7	Cade *et al.*[27]
Vidua paradisea	10.5	4.0	Terroine and Trautmann[183]
(Paradise whydah)			
Zonotrichia leucophrys gambelii	28.6	8.0	King[84]
(White-crowned sparrow)			
Passer domesticus	*ca.* 27	7.0	Kendeigh[81]
(House sparrow)		8.5	Steen[170]
Emberiza hortulana	22	8.7	Wallgren[197]
(Ortolan bunting)			

An examination of Figure 6-6 shows that this is clearly not the case for a live bird over the range of environmental temperatures that it encounters. In all species that have been studied carefully, there is a range of environmental temperature in which there is relatively little change in metabolic rate. Within this so-called thermoneutral range the bird regulates body temperature by physical thermoregulation, that is, by control of the heat loss from the external body surface (Fig. 6-7) primarily through conduction and convection, and from the surfaces of the lungs and air sacs (Fig. 6-8) primarily through evaporation and convection.

The control of heat loss from the external body surface is effected primarily by control of the temperature gradient of the shell (*i.e.,* feathers, skin, and vari-

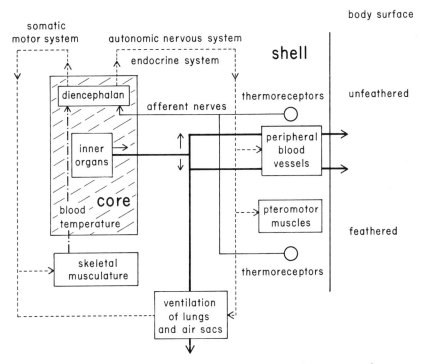

Fig. 6-5. *Schematic representation of the thermoregulatory control system in birds. Modified from Precht* **et al.**[138] *and King and Farner.*[85]

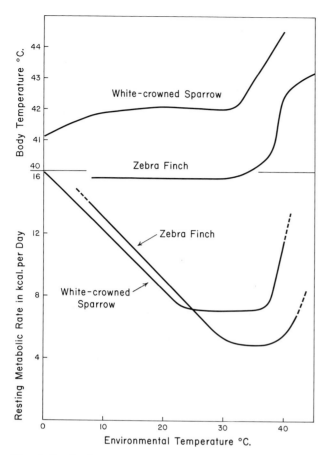

Fig. 6-6. *Body temperature and resting metabolic rate as functions of environmental temperature in the zebra finch,* Poephila castanotis (*Calder*[28]) *and the white-crowned sparrow,* Zonotrichia leucophrys gambelii (*King*[84]). *The thermoneutral range for the zebra finch lies at approximately 32–40°C., for the white-crowned sparrow at approximately 25–37°C.*

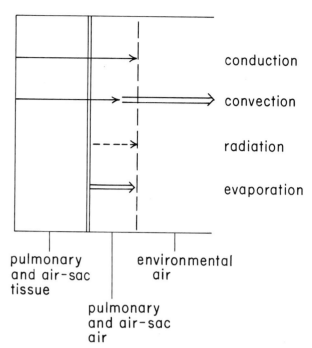

Fig. 6-8. *Representation of mechanisms of heat loss through respiratory system of birds.*

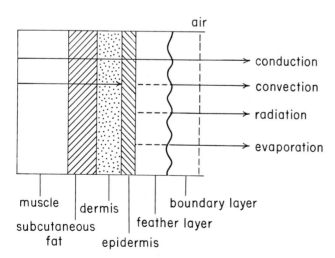

Fig. 6-7. *Representation of mechanisms of heat loss through the outer body surface of birds in contact with air.*

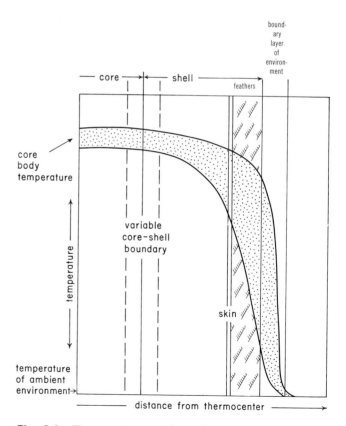

Fig. 6-9. *Temperature gradients in the shell in thermo-regulation. Note the wide range of gradients that may occur in the feather layer of the shell.*

able amount of subcutaneous tissue) through alteration of the insulative characteristics of the feather cover and through changes in the rate of delivery of blood to the skin and subcutaneous tissues (Figs. 6-5, 6-9). The rate of loss of heat from the surfaces of the lungs and air sacs is primarily a function of the rate of ventilation.

As environmental temperature decreases to the lower limit of the thermoneutral range (the lower critical temperature), physical adjustments for reduction of heat loss have essentially reached their limit; at environmental temperatures below the lower critical temperature, body temperature can be maintained only by an increase in the rate of metabolism (Fig. 6-6). Therefore the metabolic rate of a resting bird at environmental temperatures below the lower critical temperature is a regular inverse function of environmental temperature throughout the range in which it can remain homeothermal. As environmental temperature is increased above the upper limit of the thermoneutral range (the upper critical temperature) the bird can lose additional heat, and thereby maintain body temperature, primarily only by increasing the rate of evaporation (Fig. 6-10). This requires an increase in rate of ventilation movements (Fig. 6-2) and therefore an increase in rate of energy expenditure (Fig. 6-6). Obviously, the effectiveness of increased ventilation in thermoregulation is an inverse function of the relative humidity of the environmental air. For more detailed discussions of thermoregulation and thermoregulatory processes, the reader is referred to King and Farner.[85,86] To a limited extent, some small species of birds are able to tolerate, at least temporarily, hyperthermia occasioned by elevated environmental temperatures.

Within limits, cold resistance may be an adaptive phenomenon involving changes in the insulative properties of the shell (denser plumage) and adjustments in metabolism, the former obviously being the more important,[39,57,79,80,85,86,155] although Hudson and Kimzey[74] have shown that a southeast-Texas population of house sparrows does in fact have a standard metabolic rate lower than that of more northern populations.

It should be noted that the thermoneutral range for small birds is relatively high. For the black-rumped waxbill (*Estrilda troglodytes*), body weight 5–7 grams, it is approximately 32 to 40°C.[27,96] For the zebra finch (Fig. 6-6), weight 10–12 grams, the range is approximately 32 to 40°C.[27,28] For the larger white-crowned sparrow (Fig. 6-6), weighing 26–30 grams, it is approximately 25 to 37°C.[84] These findings indicate that the intake of metabolizable energy required by small birds at room temperatures and lower is a distinct, inverse function of the ambient temperature.

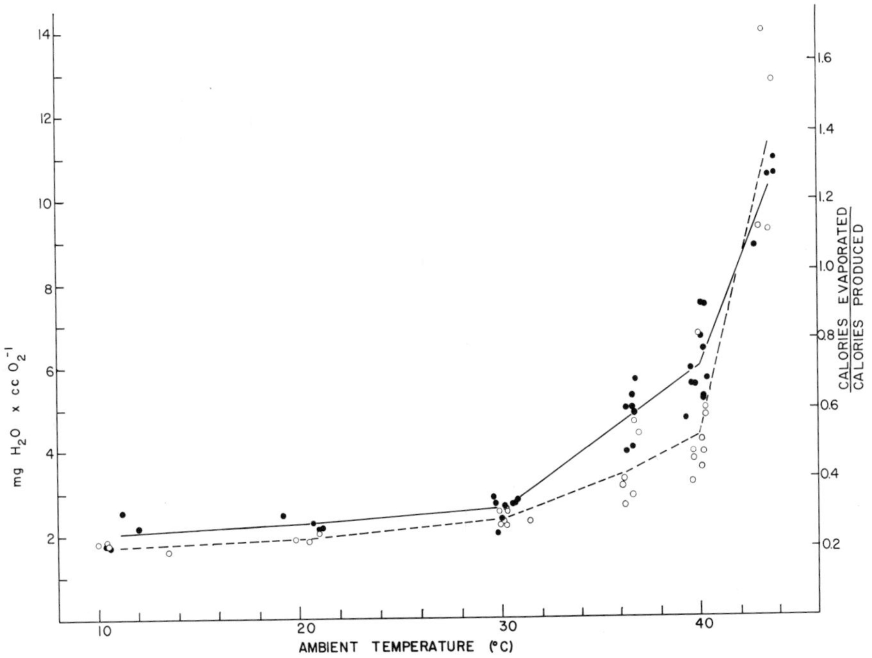

Fig. 6-10. *Pulmocutaneous water loss and evaporative cooling as functions of ambient temperature. Birds receiving water ad libitum indicated by* **solid circles and** **line**, *birds on restricted-water regimen by* **open circles** *and* **broken line**. *Lines pass through mean values for each temperature. (From Calder[28]; courtesy of University of Chicago Press.)*

Surprisingly little attention has been given to the metabolic cost of molting. The hypothetical calculations of King and Farner[85] suggest that if the molt is extended over several weeks the increase in metabolic rate probably does not exceed 10 per cent. This, however, does not take into account the additional energy that may be lost because of defective insulation during the molt.

Unlike the precocial chicks of galliform species, which become homeothermal very soon after hatching, the altricial young of psittacine and passerine species are poikilothermal for a substantial portion of the nestling period. For example, young budgerigars do not have good thermoregulation until at least eleven days after hatching.[20] By the ninth day budgerigar chicks have developed the ability to pant as a mechanism that can prevent hyperthermia.

With the exception of species in which temporary hypothermia is a normal phenomenon, it is now clear that the deep body temperature of adult birds has a normal range of variation of the order of 6 or 7 degrees. There are well-established differences among species, the functional basis and significance of which are not known. Comparison of body temperatures among species is difficult because of differences apparent even among individuals of the same species, the lability of body temperature in individual birds, differences in temperature at different sites within the same bird,[78,171] diurnal variations,[12,85] and differences in methods of measurement.[85] Deep body temperatures of active non-flying adult birds of some selected species are recorded in Table 6-6.

In most species the deep body temperature appears to have a rather pronounced daily cycle, with the higher temperature occurring during the part of the day when the bird is active and the lower during the period when it is inactive. The order of difference is apparent from an examination of Table 6-7. The daily cycle in body temperature has an obvious endogenous component, probably associated in some way with the endogenous component of the daily activity cycle, since it can be shifted in phase, but only slightly if at all in frequency. The magnitude of variation in the daily cycle in body temperature is functionally related to environmental temperature, since it is suppressed by elevated, constant environmental temperatures.[15,40,202]

EXCRETION AND OSMOREGULATION

The affinities of birds and reptiles are nowhere more evident than in nitrogen metabolism and renal function. Most of the amino nitrogen and all of the purine nitrogen is excreted as uric acid. The avian kidney itself is characteristically reptilian, with a functional renal portal system, small glomeruli, and a rather substantial fraction of cortical nephrons. The discussion

Table 6-6. Deep Body Temperature of Active Non-flying Adults of Selected Species of Small Birds

Species	Site	Body temperature (°C.)	Method	Reference
Melopsittacus undulatus (Budgerigar)	cloaca	40-42	thermocouple	Böni[20]
Poephila castanotis (Zebra finch)	cloaca	40-42	thermocouple	Calder[28]
	cloaca	40-42	thermometer	Cade *et al.*[27]
Estrilda troglodytes (Black-rumped waxbill)	cloaca	39.5-41.5	thermometer	Cade *et al.*[27]
Passer domesticus (House sparrow)	proventriculus	41-44	thermometer	Bernard *et al.*[19]
Serinus canarius (Canary)	cloaca	41-42		Gelineo[57]
Zonotrichia leucophrys (White-crowned sparrow)	cloaca	41-43	thermocouple	King[84]
	proventriculus	41.5-44	thermometer	Bernard *et al.*[19]
Richmondena cardinalis (Cardinal)	cloaca	41-42.5	thermometer	Dawson[41]
	proventriculus	41.5-43	thermometer	Wetmore[203]
Pica pica (Black-billed magpie)	proventriculus	41-43	thermometer	Wetmore[203]

Table 6-7. Diurnal Cycles in Body Temperature for Selected Species of Small Birds

Species	Body Temperature (°C.)			Reference
	Day	*Night*	*Difference*	
Turdus merula (European blackbird)	42.7	38.5	4.2	Simpson and Galbraith[160]
Sturnus vulgaris (Starling)	–	–	3.3	Simpson and Galbraith[160]
Passer domesticus (House sparrow)	43	39	4	Hudson and Kimzey[74]
Richmondena cardinalis (Cardinal)	41.5–42.5	38.5–40.0	2.0–3.0	Dawson[41]
Hesperiphona vespertina (Evening grosbeak)	41.5	38.0	3.5	West[202]
Pipilo aberti (Abert's towhee)	42.0	39.2	2.8	Dawson[40]

of renal physiology presented herein is based extensively on the review of Sperber,[167] which should be consulted for further details.

The basic functions of glomerular filtration, tubular excretion, and tubular resorption are involved in the formation of urine in birds. The importance of cloacal reabsorption of water remains to be ascertained; it may vary considerably among species. An analysis of the roles of these processes in the formation of urine is usefully preceded by consideration of certain anatomical features. The avian kidney has two afferent blood supplies: arterial and renal portal. The latter is represented by the ischiatic, external iliac, hypogastric, and coccygeo-mesenteric veins, among which there are numerous anastomoses. The interlobular veins conduct portal blood to the intertubular capillaries, which also receive blood from the afferent arterioles of the glomeruli. The external iliac vein anastomoses with the afferent renal vein; at the anastomosing junction there is a well-innervated muscular valve,[60,120,142,163,164] which controls the rate of flow of renal-portal blood to the capillaries of the kidney. The arterial flow to the renal capillaries is subject to vasomotor control in the afferent and efferent arterioles. Thus, although the full significance of the system is not apparent, it is obvious that the rates of flow of portal and arterial blood, and the ratios of the mixing of the two in the renal capillaries, can be varied over a wide range. It should also be noted that a rather small fraction of the nephrons have thin loops extending into the cortex. In the domestic fowl, and perhaps in many other species, this may be related to the normal production of hypotonic urine and a limit of concentrating capacity usually

not exceeding 600 milliosmols (*i.e.,* twice the osmolarity of blood).[31] This, however, cannot be stated generally for all birds, for a salt-marsh race of savannah sparrow (*Passerculus sandwichensis beldingi*), given hypertonic sodium chloride solution to drink, can produce a hypertonic urine with a concentration of the order of 2,000 milliosmols when the blood-plasma concentration is about 500 milliosmols.[137] A similar concentration may occur in the zebra finch, which tolerates well the intake of hypertonic salt solutions.[27,131,153]

Beyond the estimation of rates of glomerular filtration in the domestic fowl based on studies using various substances,[136,158,167] there are few useful quantitative data on glomerular filtration in birds. The available data suggest, however, that the process differs in no significant way from that in the other vertebrates. The water in avian urine is derived solely from the filtrate.[33] Normally more than 90 per cent of the water of the original glomerular filtrate is reabsorbed by the tubule. In zebra finches and budgerigars this percentage can be substantially greater, since these birds can survive for protracted periods on a dry diet and with no water intake.[26,27,131] The resorption of sodium chloride and bicarbonate ions can be extensive in view of normal production of hypotonic urine. Resorption of glucose, which is normally complete, can be blocked with phlorizin.

Tubular excretion is of relatively great importance in birds because it is by this means that uric acid, normally accounting for more than 60 per cent of the urinary nitrogen, is excreted.[59,93,109,158,177] A wide variety of compounds, including serotonin, creatine, choline, riboflavin, epinephrine, glucuronides, guanidine, and histamine, are removed by tubular excretion.[99,140,141,144,151,165–167,178,192] There is substantial evidence also that there is active tubular excretion of potassium ions[18,133,143] and phosphate,[35] excretion of phosphate being at least partially controlled by the parathyroid glands.

Although the osmolarity of avian urine, except in salt-loading or dehydration in some species, is relatively low, its nitrogen content is high because of the high concentration of colloidal uric acid. In the domestic fowl the concentration may be as high as 22 grams per 100 cc.[59]

It has long been known that uric acid is formed in the liver of at least some species.[95,116] In the pigeon, the liver lacks xanthine oxidase, the hypoxanthine produced in the liver being converted to uric acid by the xanthine oxidase of the kidney.[95]

The avian neurohypophysial antidiuretic hormone is arginine vasotocin.[17,121] It is not clear whether its antidiuretic effect is due to a double action of reducing glomerular filtration and increasing tubular resorption of water[25] or to the single action of increasing tubular resorption.[161] Epinephrine increases the rate of filtration but increases the volume-rate of urine formation only slightly and irregularly.[58,93,109,159]

The kidney plays an important role in regulation of the acid-base balance. The formation of substantial quantities of uric acid places an additional load on the avian kidney in the retention of sodium ions. Depletion of alkali reserve is accompanied by increase in hydrogen ion concentration and in titratable acid in the urine. The latter increase is the result of excretion of acid phosphate and uric acid, both of which are important as buffers at the pH of the urine.[211] Uric acid is the major component of the titratable acid. Excretion of ammonia is increased as a base-conserving mechanism.

In addition to its functions in excretion and acid-base regulation, the kidney has an important osmoregulatory role in which, of course, the removal of nitrogenous waste is an important feature. The avian kidney displays a wide range of interspecific differences with respect to water conservation. As noted above, wild zebra finches, when brought into captivity, can be maintained in good health on a dry diet and without water,[131,153] whereas domestic zebra finches appear to have a reduced ability in this respect.[27] As noted above, the osmolality of avian urine is rarely twice as great as that of the plasma although it is clear that this ratio is exceeded in some species. In experiments with a salt-marsh race of the savannah sparrow, mentioned above, birds were found to maintain body weight while drinking 600 or 700 mM sodium chloride solution, producing urine with an osmotic pressure more than four times that of the plasma.[137]

The performances described above for zebra finches and budgerigars, of course, represent extreme conditions. Without temperature stress, and with water available *ad libitum*, the daily intakes of these species are of the order of 25 per cent and 5 per cent of body weight, respectively.[14] The daily water intake of small birds in cages, under ordinary conditions, can be expected to vary from as little as 5 per cent of body weight per day to as much as 100 per cent (Table 6-8).

A substantial number of species of marine birds can remove excess salt via the nasal gland. However, no such mechanism has been definitely demonstrated in passerine or psittacine birds. The remarkable ability of budgerigars and zebra finches to handle hypertonic drinking solutions appears to be associated entirely with adaptation in renal function. The kidney is involved in the regulation of total osmotic concentration of the body fluids and also in the regulation of the relative concentrations of different ions by controlling the volume of water and concentrations of ions that enter the urine. The very substantial interspecies differences that can exist with respect to the removal of ions is illustrated by comparison of the house finch (*Carpodacus mexicanus*) and the savannah sparrow (*Passerculus sandwichensis beldingi*) when they are given sodium chloride solutions to drink. The savannah sparrow can produce urine with over 900 milliequivalents of chloride ion per liter from a blood plasma that probably contains no more than 200 milliequivalents per liter; the house finch can produce a urine with a chloride concentration no greater than approximately 350 milliequivalents per liter from a blood plasma containing approximately 150 milliequivalents per liter. Thus the house finch cannot elevate the chloride level in urine more than about 2.4 times that in its plasma, whereas the savannah sparrow can produce urine with a chloride concentration approximately 5 times that of its plasma.[14]

THE ENDOCRINE SYSTEM

Although the endocrine system of birds is of the typical vertebrate pattern, it has characteristics and functions that are uniquely avian. Primary emphasis here is placed on those features that are unique to the Class.

PITUITARY GLAND

The anterior pituitary, or pars distalis, consists of cytologically distinct rostral and caudal lobes.[115,185,205] Tixier-Vidal,[185] primarily on the basis of investigations on the domestic mallard, has recognized two cell types, alpha and gamma, that are restricted to the caudal

Table 6-8. Consumption of Water in Selected Species of Small Birds in the Absence of Temperature Stress

Species	Mean Body Wt. (grams)	Daily Intake of Water (Supplied ad libitum) in % Body Wt.		Reference
		Mean	Minimum	
Zenaidoura macroura (Mourning dove)	100	10	3	MacMillen[103]
Melopsittacus undulatus (Budgerigar)	30	5	<1	Cade and Dybas[26]
Carpodacus mexicanus (House finch)	21	16	10	Bartholomew and Cade[13]
Passerculus sandwichensis beldingi (Savannah sparrow)	17	100	46	Poulson and Bartholomew[137]
Poephila castanotis (Zebra finch)	12	24	<1	Cade et al.[27]
		17	<1	Farner and Serventy (unpublished)
		25	<1	Calder[28]
Estrilda troglodytes (Black-rumped waxbill)	6.5	42	–	Cade et al.[27]

lobe; the gamma cells are thought to produce a luteotropic hormone. Four cell types apparently occur exclusively in the rostral lobe—beta, eta, epsilon, and kappa. She has concluded that the beta cells produce follicle-stimulating hormone and that the eta and epsilon cells produce prolactin and corticotropin, respectively. Delta cells occur in both lobes and are thought to produce thyrotropin.

The avian pituitary also produces a melanophore-stimulating hormone.[114] The existence of a specific pituitary growth hormone in birds is still an open question, although Tixier-Vidal[185,186] has demonstrated the presence of cells in the pars distalis of the duck that appear to be homologous with the somatotropin-producing cells of mammals. The production of luteinizing and follicle-stimulating hormones, which may not be homologous with the corresponding mammalian hormones,[54,189] appears to be closely controlled by the hypothalamus.[6,7,8,10,54,102] The anterior pituitary can produce thyrotropin independently of hypothalamic control, although it appears that maximal production is dependent on hypothalamic stimulation.[6,7,102,187] The production of corticotropin appears to be even more independent of hypothalamic control.[6,7,102,188] Unlike the situation in mammals, in which the hypothalamus actively inhibits production of prolactin, the production of this hormone in birds is controlled through a stimulatory neurohormone from the hypothalamus.[9,94]

Because purified avian gonadotropins have not been available for experimental investigations, their precise functions are still not definitely understood. It is clear, however, that luteinizing hormone promotes the endocrine activity of the cells of Leydig. Its role in the control of the endocrine functions of the ovary is much less clear; in some species, at least, it may be involved in ovulation. (For review and discussion, see van Tienhoven.[189]) Luteinizing hormone causes the development of the male nuptial plumage of some species of weaver finches,[154,184,207–209] although it now seems clear that this is not by way of a direct effect on the feather follicles.[139] Follicle-stimulating hormone promotes growth and development of the seminiferous tubules and the initiation of spermatogenesis; in a way that is clearly more complex it is involved in the development of the ovary and in oogenesis. There are certainly very distinct differences occurring between species.

Prolactin, which is produced by the anterior pituitary glands of both sexes, has several functions. Interacting with estrogen, and possibly also with progesterone, it causes the development of the incubation patch. (See Eisner,[46] Lehrman,[97] Selander and Kuich,[156] and Steel and Hinde,[168,169] for discussion.) The role of prolactin in the induction of incubation behavior is obscure. Possibly it contributes through its antigonadal effect. This would be consistent with the fairly general observation that incubation is associated with a phase of reduced gonadal activity. (See Lehrman[97] and Eisner,[46] for discussion.) There is some evidence that prolactin, probably in interaction with other hormones, has a role in the development of parental behavior. The role of prolactin in causing proliferation of crop epithelium and the production of milk in both sexes of pigeons and doves is well established. In the white-crowned sparrow (*Zonotrichia leucophrys gambelii*), prolactin appears to have a role in the induction of migratory fattening and behavior.[110,111]

Although corticotropin is clearly involved in the control of synthesis and release of corticosterone,[42,43,73] there is evidence that the adrenal cortex has considerable autonomy. (For discussion, see deRoos.[44])

The role of thyrotropin in birds is very similar to its role in mammals. Hypophysectomy decreases iodine uptake by the thyroid and reduces the synthesis of thyroxine.[187]

The hormones known to be produced by the avian pars nervosa, or posterior pituitary, are arginine vasotocin and oxytocin. Arginine vasotocin is the avian antidiuretic hormone. It has been suggested that in the domestic fowl it may be involved in oviposition, since its concentration in the pars nervosa is reduced at the time of ovipositing,[181,182] and since posterior-lobe extracts induce ovulation. However, Opel[132] has shown that removal of the pars nervosa does not prevent ovulation. The function of oxytocin in the bird is unknown.

PINEAL GLAND

The function of the avian pineal gland has been the subject of an extensive and controversial literature. A number of investigations produced evidence of an antigonadotropic function. (See Benoit[16] and Moszkowska,[119] for review and discussion.) Contrariwise, it has been suggested[11] that the gonadotropic effect of long daily photoperiods, at least in the domestic fowl, may be mediated by alteration in the rate of melatonin synthesis in the pineal body.

THYROID GLAND

Our knowledge of the functions of the avian thyroid gland is based largely on investigations of the domestic fowl, domestic mallard, and domestic turkey. (See Ringer,[145] Tixier-Vidal and Assenmacher,[187] and Tixier-Vidal *et al.*,[188] for discussion.) It can only be assumed that the species investigated are generally representative of the entire class. Both thyroxine and triiodothyronine occur in the blood. The major function of the thyroid gland appears to be its role, as a component of the hypothalamo-hypophysio-thyroid axis, in thermoregulation by which the rate of thermogenesis is altered by alteration of the metabolic rate. Histologic studies on

wild species, however, suggest that there are annually periodic (circennial) changes in thyroid activity that may deviate significantly from cycles occurring in birds kept in artificial environments.[204] Although molt can be induced readily by the administration of desiccated thyroid tissue, thyroid hormone, or thyroid-stimulating hormone, and although thyroidectomy delays or prevents molt,[7,72,191,195,196] it is by no means clear that the thyroid gland is actually involved in the normal control of molt.[180] Rather, it seems that normal thyroid activity is essential for molt and feather growth, but that molting and re-growth of feathers are actually initiated and controlled by other mechanisms. (For an extensive discussion of endocrine mechanisms in molt, see Assenmacher[6] and Voitkevich.[191])

PARATHYROID GLANDS

Since the parathyroid glands arise from the third and fourth branchial pouches, there are typically two pairs, although in some species subsequent fusion may result in existence of only one pair. Our scanty knowledge of the function of the avian parathyroids suggests that, as in mammals, they produce a hormone that mobilizes calcium by releasing it from bones, and promotes retention of phosphate by the kidney. It should be noted here that the extensive mobilization of calcium and the high levels of calcium in the blood during egg laying are induced by estrogens. Although parathyroid hormone is probably involved also, the nature of the interrelationship is at present not clear.

ADRENAL GLANDS

The avian adrenal gland has only recently become a subject of extensive experimental investigation. (For a critical review, see deRoos.[44]) Unlike the adrenal gland of the eutherian mammals, the gland in birds is not discretely divided into cortex and medulla. Rather, the "cortical" (interrenal) and "medullary" (chromaffin) tissues are extensively intermingled, the interrenal tissue occurring in cords, and the chromaffin tissue in islets. The major corticoid hormone is corticosterone; aldosterone is also produced, and possibly cortisol in small amounts. Corticosterone is probably the principal glucocorticoid, and aldosterone the principal mineralocorticoid. Birds show no condition similar to the familiar stress syndrome of mammals, although it is clear that certain forms of stress alter adrenal activity and lymphoid tissue. Annual cycles in adrenal activity have been reported from several wild species.[55,69,100]

So far as is known, the endocrine function of the avian chromaffin tissue is similar to that of the corresponding tissue in mammals.

PANCREAS

The hormones of the endocrine pancreas of birds are glucagon, produced by the alpha cells, and insulin, produced by the beta cells.[48,49,113] Truly total pancreatectomy in birds is usually followed by hypoglycemia, but confusion has been created by reports of investigations in which the splenic lobe, which contains most of the alpha cells, was not removed.[113] The avian pancreas contains, and probably secretes, relatively greater amounts of glucagon than does the mammalian pancreas.[194] The higher blood-glucose levels of birds (150–250 mg. per 100 ml., or somewhat higher[50,65]) are doubtless a reflection of the glucose-mobilizing effect of the high glucagon output,[113] whereas the lower blood-glucose levels in mammals are the result of the glycogen-synthesizing effect of a relatively greater output of insulin. Birds in general are relatively resistant to exogenous insulin (perhaps, at least in part, because of its rapid destruction in the liver) and, as a rule, are far less sensitive to alloxan than are mammals.

GONADS

OVARY. In addition to its gametogenic functions the ovary is also an endocrine organ, although the actual sites of production or types of cells that produce the various steroid hormones have not been identified with certainty. Estriol, 17β-estradiol, and estrone have been identified in the ovary of the domestic fowl. However, the identities of estrogens circulating in the blood of birds in general are still not known. Estrogens are involved in the induction of numerous secondary female sex characteristics, such as the change in bill color during the breeding season in some species (*e.g.*, budgerigar and the red-billed weaver, *Quelea quelea*), development of the incubation patch by interaction with prolactin and possibly with progesterone,[168,169] the plumage typical of the female of many species, development of the oviduct by interaction with progesterone and possibly with prolactin,[168] nest-building behavior,[198] and the mobilization of calcium in egg-shell production, probably by some interaction with the parathyroid glands or with their hormone. (See Marshall[108] and van Tienhoven,[189] for reviews and discussion.)

The avian ovary also produces androgen, the functions of which are not as well known, although it is clear that the growth of the comb during egg production in the female domestic fowl is androgen-induced. The yellow bill of the breeding female starling is also androgen-induced.[210] Progesterone plays a role in the ovulatory cycle, at least in the chicken; it is involved synergistically with estrogen in development of the oviduct, and it may have some role in the develop-

ment of incubation behavior. (See Lehrman,[97] for review and discussion.)

TESTIS. The testis also has a dual role as a gametogenic and an endocrine organ. It now is quite clear that the interstitial cells (cells of Leydig) are the endocrine elements of the testes. The principal avian androgen is probably testosterone. Androgens in male birds are responsible for a variety of secondary sex characteristics, such as male sexual behavior (including song), development of combs and wattles, change in bill color during the breeding season in some species (*e.g.*, house sparrow, and weaver finches of the genus *Euplectes*), and development of nuptial plumage in some species. Testosterone has been reported to restore spermatogenesis in the inactive testes in some species; in others it is effective only if spermatocytes are present. In still other species it seems to have no role in spermatogenesis.[189] Testosterone is required also for the final phase of development of the Wolffian duct. Although there is some evidence that the testes may normally produce estrogens, no conclusions or generalizations can be made at the present incomplete state of our knowledge. In general our knowledge of the function of testicular progesterone is similarly inadequate, although van Tienhoven[189] has proposed an ingenious hypothesis involving a role for progesterone in the males of species in which both sexes incubate.

Control of Reproduction

The processes of spermatogenesis and oogenesis have been reviewed extensively and very adequately by Benoit,[16] Marshall,[108] and van Tienhoven,[189] and therefore will not be discussed here. Rather, attention will be given to the factors involved in control of reproductive activity.

Reproductive activity in birds is intermittent. During the course of the evolution of natural species control mechanisms have developed that cause reproduction to occur at times when the probability of survival of young is maximal. For most temperate zone species the optimal season is spring and/or early summer. In some desert species, such as the budgerigar and zebra finch, reproductive activity is adjusted to rainy periods, even in areas where the rains are aperiodic.

Despite the wide variety of reproductive patterns among birds it is clear that all control systems have some elements in common (Figs. 6-11, 6-12). The hypothalamus, because of its unique dual role as an organ of both the endocrine and the nervous system, occupies a central position in the mechanism that controls reproductive activity. The currently available

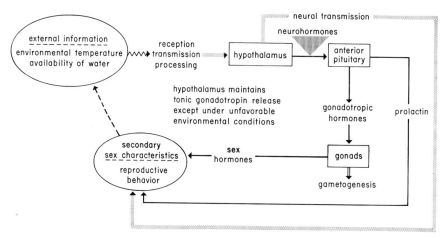

Fig. 6-11. *Schematic representation of factors involved in the control of reproductive periods in opportunistic desert species such as the zebra finch,* Poephila castanotis. *The hypothalamus tonically stimulates gonadotropic activity of the anterior pituitary unless unfavorable environmental conditions* (e.g., *low temperature, lack of water*) *intervene.*

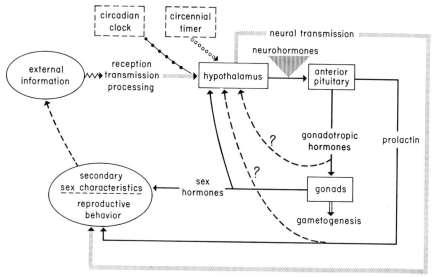

Fig. 6-12. *A general schematic representation of the major functional relationships involved in the timing of reproductive periods in birds. The role of hormonal feedbacks on the hypothalamus in the termination of the reproductive period is not yet understood; it doubtless differs among species.*

evidence suggests that the control schemes—from the level of hypothalamic output of neurohormones, which control the gonadotropic activity of the anterior pituitary, to the gonads and their functions—probably differ only in minor details among the various species of birds. The great array of adaptive differences among these species is associated primarily with the sources of information, both external and internal, used by the hypothalamus, and with the ways in which such information is processed therein.[52,54] The evidence now available suggests that there are two basic patterns

of hypothalamic activity with respect to the control of the gonadotropic function of the anterior pituitary. At one extreme is the pattern in which the hypothalamus appears to be tonic with respect to stimulation of pituitary gonadotropic activity except when it is inhibited by unvariable environmental conditions (Fig. 6-11). The zebra finch and the budgerigar, at least under their native conditions, are examples of this type. Fundamentally these species are reproductively active as long as environmental conditions (water, temperature, and food) are adequate; the hypothalamus appears to be inhibited by low temperatures or lack of adequate water. Superimposed on this pattern of control, of course, are requirements with respect to nesting sites, availability of mates, and the like. It seems obvious that this type of hypothalamic control of reproductive activity contributes to the relative ease with which these species can be induced to breed in captivity. At the other extreme is the pattern of hypothalamic activity in which the hypothalamus is inactive gonadotropically except during periods in which the system is receiving specific environmental information (Fig. 6-12). The most conspicuous examples of this type are the photoperiodic species of the mid and high latitudes in which the basic timing of the reproductive cycle is rigidly controlled by day length. The white-crowned sparrow (*Zonotrichia leucophrys gambelii*), for example, remains reproductively inactive as long as it is maintained on short days; on the other hand, reproductive activity can be induced experimentally in midwinter by artificially lengthening the daily period of illumination.[52] The domestic canary, although by no means completely photoperiodically controlled, also uses photoperiodic information in the control of its annual reproductive cycle.[66,90,91,179,190] Among the species showing photoperiodicity there is considerable variation as to the extent to which day length is the dominant source of information for the control system. In most, if not all, photoperiodic species, the female requires additional environmental information (*e.g.*, singing male, availability of nesting material, and the like) to achieve complete reproductive activity. Among the photoperiodic species there occurs, apparently always, some sort of mechanism that causes the bird to become photorefractory, with a consequent regression of the gonads, while the days are still long in mid or late summer. This is clearly an adaptation that causes discontinuation of reproductive activity in time to permit the annual molt and, in migratory species, to allow preparation for migration to occur under favorable environmental conditions. It must be emphasized that many periodically breeding species are not photoperiodic, but rather use other sources of environmental information. This clearly must be the case for periodic breeders of the equatorial regions. (For review and discussion, see Marshall[108] and Farner and Follett.[54])

The final development of the complex of reproductive functions involves an intricate, species-characteristic pattern of behavior.[46,66,67] This behavior pattern includes interactions between male and female of the pair and, in some species (*e.g.*, the budgerigar), interactions with other individuals. Such behavior is especially necessary for the final stages of reproductive development in the female. Such essential sexual and reproductive behavior has been analyzed and described in some detail for various species, for example, for the zebra finch,[75,76,118] for the budgerigar,[21-23] and for the domestic canary.[66]

THYMUS, BURSA OF FABRICIUS, AND UROPYGIAL GLAND

THYMUS

The avian thymus, which consists of a variable number of paired bodies, contains predominantly lymphoid tissue with some reticular and epithelioid cells. In at least some birds the epithelioid cells are arranged in Hassall's corpuscles. In many species the thymus undergoes rapid involution with sexual maturity. However, Höhn[70,71] has demonstrated in a variety of species that the thymus returns to its early size and type of microscopic structure for a period of time following the first sexual cycle, and possibly also after later ones. The significance of this is unknown. Apparently the role of the thymus is primarily that of an organ of lymphocyte formation. Höhn[72] has pointed out that some forms of stress cause atrophy of the thymus in birds. This and other observations indicate that the thymus is doubtless under hormonal control, although details and information on the significance of such control are still lacking.

BURSA OF FABRICIUS

The bursa of Fabricius, or cloacal bursa, is a dorsal evagination of the proctodeum, occurring in most, if not all, species of birds. It reaches its maximal development early in life and then diminishes gradually in size as sexual maturity approaches. It is a lymphoid structure and, in many ways, can be regarded as analogous with the thymus. (For a general description of the organ, see Benoit.[16]) Its regression can be hastened experimentally by administration of adrenal corticoids, estrogens, and testosterone. It is now clear that this organ is important as a site of antibody formation in the domestic fowl[29,30,61] and in the ring-necked pheasant.[82]

UROPYGIAL GLAND

The uropygial gland (also known as the oil, or preen, gland) has been the subject of a very extensive literature and, with respect to its function, the center of intermittent controversy for more than two centuries. From a careful review of the literature, and from the results of experiments on three species of ducks, Elder[47] concluded that the oil gland secretes a mixture containing much fatty acid, some fat, and some wax. Apparently preening induces reflexively the flow of the secretion onto the nipple of the gland or onto the surrounding feathers, from which it is transferred by the bill and the head plumage to the plumage of the body. In waterfowl, at least, the secretion contributes to waterproofing, either directly or through maintenance of feather structure. The secretion appears to be necessary also for maintaining the normal surface of the bill and the skin of the legs. Later experiments by Gomot[62] on the domestic mallard led to similar conclusions with respect to maintenance of the plumage.

CIRCADIAN PERIODICITIES

As in most if not all animals, many functions in birds show circadian periodicities, or endogenous rhythms having natural periods of approximately 24 hours. Normally such periodicities are entrained to periods of 24 hours by the natural 24-hour light-dark cycle. When the light time in the 24-hour light-dark cycle is changed the circadian periodicity is re-entrained through the course of a few to several days, depending on the magnitude of the shift of light time. Among the most conspicuous endogenous periodicities are those observed in motor activity. In conditions of continuous light the frequency of the periods of motor activity is directly proportional to intensity of the light.[3,4] For example, Aschoff *et al.*[5] reported that motor activity in chaffinches (*Fringilla coelebs*) in constant light showed a periodicity of about 25 hours when the intensity was 0.4 lux, and periodicity of about 22 hours with an intensity of 120 lux. It is well known that body temperature in mammals has a circadian periodicity. This has been demonstrated also in the house sparrow, together with a related circadian periodicity in metabolic rate.[74] It is reasonable to expect that these phenomena will be found to be common among birds. It now seems clear that some sort of circadian periodicity in sensitivity to light is basic to the "measurement" of the duration of the daily light period in the photostimulated gonadal growth of photoperiodic species.[52,53,63,64,112,212] It is clear that good avicultural practice and therapeutic management must take into account the nature and pervasiveness of circadian periodicities.

References

1. ABRAHÁM, A.: Beiträge zur Kenntnis der Innervation des Vogeldarmes. Z. Zellforsch. mikr. Anat. *23:*737–745, 1936.

2. ANTONY, M.: Über die Speicheldrüsen der Vögel. Zool. Jahrb. Abt., Anat. Ontog. Tiere *41:*547–660, 1920.

3. ASCHOFF, J.: Exogenous and endogenous components in circadian rhythms. Cold Spring Harbor Symp. Quant. Biol. *25:*11–28, 1960.

4. ASCHOFF, J.: Die Tagesperiodik licht- und dunkelaktiver Tiere. Rev. suisse Zool. *71:*528–558. 1964.

5. ASCHOFF J., DIEHL, I., GERECKE, U., and WEVER, R.: Aktivitätsperiodik von Buchfinken (*Fringilla coelebs* L.) unter konstanten Bedingungen. Z. vergleich. Physiol. *45:*605–617, 1962.

6. ASSENMACHER, I.: La mue des oiseaux et son déterminisme endocrinien. Alauda *26:*241–289, 1958.

7. ASSENMACHER, I.: Recherches sur le contrôle hypothalamique de la fonction gonadotrope préhypophysaire chez le Canard. Arch. Anat. microscop. Morphol. exp. *47:*447–572, 1958.

8. ASSENMACHER, I.: Les régulations hypothalamiques de la fonction gonadotrope. Acta Neuroveget. *25:* 339–382, 1963.

9. ASSENMACHER, I., and BAYLÉ, J.-D.: Répercussions endocriniennes de la greffe hypophysaire ectopique chez le Canard mâle. Compt. Rend. Acad. Sci. Paris *259:*3848–3850, 1964.

10. ASSENMACHER, I., and TIXIER-VIDAL, A.: Hypothalamic-pituitary relations. Proc. 2nd Intern. Cong. Endocrinol., London, 1964. Part I, pp. 131–145.

11. AXELROD, J., and WURTMAN, R. J.: Melatonin synthesis in the hen pineal gland and its control by light. Nature *201:*1134, 1964.

12. BALDWIN, S. P., and KENDEIGH, S. C.: Physiology of the temperature of birds. Sci. Pub. Cleveland Mus. Nat. Hist. *3:*1–196, 1932.

13. BARTHOLOMEW, G. A., and CADE, T. J.: Water consumption of house finches. Condor *58:*406–412, 1956.

14. BARTHOLOMEW, G. A., and CADE, T. J.: The water economy of land birds. Auk *80:*504–539, 1963.

15. BARTHOLOMEW, G. A., Jr., and DAWSON, W. R.: Body temperature and water requirements in the mourning dove, *Zenaidura macroura marginella.* Ecology *35:*181–187, 1954.

16. BENOIT, J.: Reproduction. Caractères sexuels et hormones. Déterminisme du cycle sexuel saisonnier. In *Traité de Zoologie*, P.-P. Grassé, ed. Paris, Masson et Cie., 1950. Vol. 15, Oiseaux, pp. 384–478.

17. BENTLEY, P. J.: Neurohypophysial function in amphibians, reptiles and birds. Symposia of the Zoological Society of London *9*:141–152, 1963.

18. BERLINER, R. W.: Some Aspects of Ion Exchange in Electrolyte Transport by the Renal Tubules. In *Metabolic Aspects of Transport across Cell Membranes*, Q. R. Murphy, ed. Madison, University of Wisconsin Press, 1957. Pp. 203–220.

19. BERNARD, R., CAYOUETTE, R., and BRASSARD, J.-A.: Mesure de la température normale des oiseaux au moyen de thermomètres à mercure. Rev. can. biol. *3*:251–277, 1944.

20. BÖNI, A.: Über die Entwicklung der Temperaturregulation bei verschiedenen Nesthockern (Wellensittich, Neuntöter und Wendehals). Arch. suisses d'Ornithol. *2*:1–56, 1942.

21. BROCKWAY, B. F.: The effects of nest-entrance positions and male vocalizations on reproduction in Budgerigars. Living Bird *1*:93–101, 1962.

22. BROCKWAY, B. F.: Ethological studies of the Budgerigar: Reproductive behavior. Behaviour *23*:295–324, 1964.

23. BROCKWAY, B. F.: Social influences on reproductive physiology and ethology of budgerigars (*Melopsittacus undulatus*). Animal Behavior *12*:493–501, 1964.

24. BUCHANAN, F.: The frequency of the heart-beat and the form of the electrocardiogram in birds. J. Physiol. *38*:lxii–lxvi, 1909.

25. BURGESS, W. W., HARVEY, A. M., and MARSHALL, E. K., Jr.: The site of the antidiuretic action of pituitary extract. J. Pharmacol. Exp. Therap. *49*:237–249, 1933.

26. CADE, T. J., and DYBAS, J. A., Jr.: Water economy of the budgerygah. Auk *79*:345–364, 1962.

27. CADE, T. J., TOBIN, C. A., and GOLD, A.: Water economy and metabolism of two estrildine finches. Physiol. Zool. *38*:9–33, 1965.

28. CALDER, W. A.: Gaseous metabolism and water relations of the zebra finch, *Taeniopygia castanotis*. Physiol. Zool. *37*:400–413, 1964.

29. CHANG, T. S., RHEINS, M. S., and WINTER, A. R.: The significance of the bursa of Fabricius in antibody production in chickens: 1. Age of chickens. Poultry Sci. *36*:735–738, 1957.

30. CHANG, T. S., RHEINS, M. S., and WINTER, A. R.: The significance of the bursa of Fabricius of chickens in antibody production: 2. Spleen relationship. Poultry Sci. *37*:1091–1093, 1958.

31. CHEW, R. M.: Water metabolism of desert-inhabiting vertebrates. Biol. Rev. *36*:1–31, 1961.

32. CHRISTENSEN, E. H., and DILL, D. B.: Oxygen dissociation curves of bird blood. J. Biol. Chem. *109*:443–448, 1935.

33. CUYPERS, Y.: Étude de la sécrétion urinaire chez le coq. Arch. intern. Physiol. Biochim. *67*:35–42, 1959.

34. DAM, H., FUNCH, J. P., HANSEN, P. W., PRANGE, I., and SØNDERGAARD, E.: Investigations on the gizzard lining of the chick. Acta Physiol. Scand. *44*:322–335, 1958.

35. DAVIDSON, D. G., and LEVINSKY, N.: Effect of parathyroid extract on renal excretion of phosphate in the chicken. Fed. Proc. *16*:28, 1957.

36. DAVIES, F.: The conducting system of the bird's heart. J. Anat. *64*:129–146, 1930.

37. DAVIES, F.: Further studies on the conducting system of the bird's heart. J. Anat. *64*:319–323, 1930.

38. DAVIES, F., and FRANCIS, E. T. B.: The conducting system of the vertebrate heart. Biol. Rev. *21*:173–188, 1946.

39. DAVIS, E. A., Jr.: Seasonal changes in the energy balance of the English Sparrow. Auk *72*:385–411, 1955.

40. DAWSON, W. R.: Temperature regulation and water requirements of the Brown and Abert Towhees, *Pipilo fuscus* and *Pipilo aberti*. Univ. Cal. Publ. Zool. *59*:81–124, 1954.

41. DAWSON, W. R.: Relation of oxygen consumption and evaporative water loss to temperature in the cardinal. Physiol. Zool. *31*:37–48, 1958.

42. DEROOS, R.: The corticoids of the avian adrenal gland. Gen. Comp. Endocrinol. *1*:494–512, 1961.

43. DEROOS, R.: *In vitro* corticoid production by the adrenal of the brown towhee, *Pipilo fuscus*. Am. Zoologist *1*:445, 1961.

44. DEROOS, R.: The physiology of the avian interrenal gland: A review. Proc. XIII Intern. Ornithol. Cong., vol. 2, pp. 1041–1058, 1963.

45. EBER, G.: Vergleichende Untersuchungen über die Ernährung einiger Finkenvögel. Biologische Abhandlungen *13/14*:1–60, 1956.

46. EISNER, E.: The relationship of hormones to the reproductive behaviour of birds, referring especially to parental behaviour: A review. Animal Behaviour *8*:155–179, 1960.

47. ELDER, W. H.: The oil gland of birds. Wilson Bull. *66*:6–31, 1954.

48. EPPLE, A.: Über Beziehungen zwischen Feinbau und Jahresperiodik des Inselorgans von Vögeln. Z. Zellforsch. *53*:731–758, 1961.

49. EPPLE, A.: Zur vergleichenden Zytologie des Inselorgans. Verhandlungen der Deutschen Zoologischen Gesellschaft in Müchen, *1963*, 461–470. 1963.

50. ERLENBACH, F.: Experimentelle Untersuchungen über den Blutzucker bei Vögeln. Z. vergleich. Physiol. *26:*121–161, 1938.

51. FARNER, D. S.: Digestion and the Digestive System. In *Biology and Comparative Physiology of Birds,* A. J. Marshall, ed. New York, Academic Press, 1960. Vol. 1, pp. 411–467.

52. FARNER, D. S.: Annual endocrine cycles in temperate-zone birds with special attention to the white-crowned sparrow, *Zonotrichia leucophrys gambelii.* Proc. 2nd Intern. Cong. Endocrinol., London, 1964. Part I, pp. 114–118.

53. FARNER, D. S.: Circadian Systems in the Photoperiodic Responses of Vertebrates. In *Circadian Clocks,* Proceedings of the Feldafing Summer School, 7–18 September 1964, J. Aschoff, ed. Amsterdam, North-Holland Publishing Company, 1965. Pp. 357–369.

54. FARNER, D. S., and FOLLETT, B. K.: Light and other environmental factors affecting avian reproduction. J. Animal Sci. *25*(Suppl.):90–118, 1966.

55. FROMME-BOUMAN, H.: Jahresperiodische Untersuchungen an der Nebennierenrinde der Amsel (*Turdus merula* L.). Vogelwarte *21:*188–198, 1962.

56. GELINEO, A., RAIEVSKAIA, T., and GELINEO, S.: La concentration de l'hémoglobine dans le sang chez quelques Oiseaux. Compt. Rend. Soc. Biol. Paris *149:*1411–1413, 1955.

57. GELINEO, S.: Température d'adaptation et production de chaleur chez les oiseaux de petite taille. Arch. sci. physiol. *9:*225–243, 1955.

58. GIBBS, O. S.: The renal blood-flow of the bird. J. Pharmacol. Exp. Therap. *34:*277–291, 1928.

59. GIBBS, O. S.: The secretion of uric acid by the fowl. Am. J. Physiol. *88:*87–100, 1929.

60. GILBERT, A. B.: The innervation of the renal portal valve of the domestic fowl. J. Anat. *95:*594–598, 1961.

61. GLICK, B., CHANG, T. S., and JAAP, R. G.: The bursa of Fabricius and antibody production. Poultry Sci. *35:*224–225, 1956.

62. GOMOT, L.: Effects de l'ablation de la glande uropygienne chez le Canard. Ann. sci. Univ. Besançon, 2e Série, Zool. *17:*61–66, 1962.

63. HAMNER, W. M.: Diurnal rhythm and photoperiodism in testicular recrudescence of the house finch. Science *142:*1294–1295, 1963.

64. HAMNER, W. M.: Avian Photoperiodic Response—Rhythms: Evidence and Inference. In *Circadian Clocks,* Proceedings of the Feldafing Summer School, 7–18 September 1964, J. Aschoff, ed. Amsterdam, North-Holland Publishing Company, 1965. Pp. 379–384.

65. HAZELWOOD, R. L.: Carbohydrate Metabolism. In *Avian Physiology,* 2nd ed., by P. D. Sturkie. Ithaca, N.Y., Comstock Publishing Associates, 1965. Pp. 313–371.

66. HINDE, R. A.: Interaction of internal and external factors in integration of canary reproduction. In *Sex and Behavior,* F. A. Beach, ed. New York, John Wiley & Sons, Inc., 1965. Pp. 381–415.

67. HINDE, R. A., and WARREN, R. P.: The effect of nest building on later reproductive behavior in domesticated canaries. Animal Behaviour *7:*35–41, 1959.

68. HOFMANN, K. B., and PREGL, F.: Über Koilin. Hoppe-Seyler's Z. physiol. Chem. *52:*448–471, 1907.

69. HÖHN, E. O.: Sexual behaviour and seasonal changes in the gonads and adrenals of the Mallard. Proc. Zool. Soc. London *117:*281–304, 1947.

70. HÖHN, E. O.: Seasonal cyclical changes in the thymus of the mallard. J. Exp. Biol. *24:*184–191, 1947.

71. HÖHN, E. O.: Seasonal recrudescence of the thymus in adult birds. Can. J. Biochem. Physiol. *34:*90–101, 1956.

72. HÖHN, E. O.: Endocrine Glands, Thymus and Pineal Body. In *Biology and Comparative Physiology of Birds,* A. J. Marshall, ed. New York, Academic Press, 1961. Vol. 2, pp. 87–114.

73. HOLMES, W. N., and PHILLIPS, J. G.: Adrenocortical hormones and electrolyte metabolism in birds. Proc. 2nd Intern. Cong. Endocrinol., London, 1964. Part I, pp. 158–161.

74. HUDSON, J. W., and KIMZEY, S. L.: Temperature regulation and metabolic rhythms in populations of the house sparrow, *Passer domesticus.* Comp. Biochem. Physiol. *17:*203–217, 1966.

75. IMMELMANN, K.: Experimentelle Untersuchungen über die biologische Bedeutung artspezifischer Merkmale beim Zebrafinken (*Taeniopygia castanotis* Gould). Zool. Jahrb., Abt. für Systematik, Ökologie und Geographie der Tiere *86:*437–592, 1959.

76. IMMELMANN, K.: Beiträge zu einer vergleichenden Biologie australischer Prachtfinken (Spermestidae). Zool. Jahrb., Abt. für Systematik, Ökologie und Geographie der Tiere *90:*1–196, 1962.

77. IWANOW, I. F.: Die sympathische Innervation des Verdauungstraktes einiger Vogelarten (*Columba livia* L., *Anser cinereus* L., und *Gallus domesticus* L.). Z. mikroskop.-anatom. Forschung. *22:*469–492, 1930.

78. KALLIR, E.: Temperaturtopographie einiger Vögel: Experimentelle Untersuchungen. Z. vergleich. Physiol. *13:*231–248, 1930.

79. KENDEIGH, S. C.: The role of environment in the life of birds. Ecol. Monographs *4:*299–417, 1934.

80. KENDEIGH, S. C.: The relation of metabolism to the development of temperature regulation in birds. J. Exp. Zool. *82*:419–438, 1939.

81. KENDEIGH, S. C.: Effect of air temperature on the rate of energy metabolism in the English sparrow. J. Exp. Zool. *96*:1–16, 1944.

82. KERSTETTER, T. H., Jr., BUSS, I. O., and WENT, H. A.: Antibody-producing function of the bursa of Fabricius of the ring-necked pheasant. J. Exp. Zool. *149*:233–237, 1962.

83. KING, A. S., and PAYNE, D. C.: Normal breathing and the effects of posture in *Gallus domesticus*. J. Physiol. *174*:340–347, 1964.

84. KING, J. R.: Oxygen consumption and body temperature in relation to ambient temperature in the White-crowned Sparrow. Comp. Biochem. Physiol. *12*:13–24, 1964.

85. KING, J. R., and FARNER, D. S.: Energy Metabolism, Thermoregulation, and Body Temperature. In *Biology and Comparative Physiology of Birds*, A. J. Marshall, ed. New York, Academic Press, 1961. Vol. 2, pp. 215–288.

86. KING, J. R., and FARNER, D. S.: Terrestrial Animals in Humid Heat: Birds. In *Handbook of Physiology*, Sect. 4 "Adaptation to the Environment," D. B. Dill, E. F. Adolph, and C. G. Wilber, eds., Washington, D.C., American Physiological Society, 1964. Pp. 603–624.

87. KISCH, B.: Observations on the haematology of fishes and birds. Exp. Med. Surg. *7*:318–326, 1949.

88. KISCH, B.: The electrocardiogram of birds (chicken, duck, pigeon). Exp. Med. Surg. *9*:103–124, 1951.

89. VON KNAFFL-LENZ, E.: Über die Diaminosäuren des Koilins. Hoppe-Seyler's Z. Physiol. Chem. *52*:472–473, 1907.

90. KOBAYASHI, H.: Acceleration of molting in the canary by reducing the daily light period. Annot. Zool. Japon. *26*:156–161, 1953.

91. KOBAYASHI, H.: Physiological nature of refractoriness of ovary to the stimulus of light in the canary. Annot. Zool. Japon. *30*:8–18, 1957.

92. KOLOSSOW, N. G., SABUSSOW, G. H., and IWANOW, J. F.: Zur Innervation des Verdauungskanales der Vögel. Z. mikroskop.-anatom. Forschung. *30*:257–294, 1932.

93. KORR, I. M.: The osmotic function of the chicken kidney. J. Cell. Comp. Physiol. *13*:175–193, 1939.

94. KRAGT, C. L., and MEITES, J.: Stimulation of pigeon pituitary prolactin release by pigeon hypothalamic extract *in vitro*. Endocrinology *76*:1169–1176, 1965.

95. KREBS, H. A.: Metabolism of amino acids and related substances. Ann. Rev. Biochem. *5*:247–270, 1936.

96. LASIEWSKI, R. C., HUBBARD, S. H., and MOBERLY, W. R.: Energetic relationships of a very small passerine bird. Condor *66*:212–220, 1964.

97. LEHRMAN, D. S.: Hormonal Regulation of Parental Behavior in Birds and Infrahuman Mammals. In *Sex and Internal Secretions*, 3rd ed., W. C. Young, ed. Baltimore, Williams & Wilkins Co., 1961. Pp. 1268–1382.

98. LEWIS, T.: The spread of the excitatory process in the vertebrate heart. V. The bird's heart. Phil. Trans. Roy. Soc. London, Ser. B. *207*:298–310, 1916.

99. LINDAHL, K. M., and SPERBER, I.: Tubular excretion of histamine in the hen. Acta Physiol. Scand. *36*:13–16, 1956.

100. LORENZEN, L. C., and FARNER, D. S.: An annual cycle in the interrenal tissue of the adrenal gland of the white-crowned sparrow, *Zonotrichia leucophrys gambelii*. Gen. Comp. Endocrinol. *4*:253–263, 1964.

101. LUCAS, A. M., and JAMROZ, C.: *Atlas of Avian Hematology*. Agriculture Monograph *25*. Washington, D.C., United States Department of Agriculture, 1961. 271 pp.

102. MA, R. C. S., and NALBANDOV, A. V.: Discussion on "Physiology of the Pituitary Gland as Affected by Transplantation or Stalk Transection," by J. W. Everett and M. Nikitovitch-Winer. In *Advances in Neuroendocrinology*, A. V. Nalbandov, ed. Urbana, University of Illinois Press, 1963. Pp. 306–311.

103. MACMILLEN, R. E.: The minimum water requirements of Mourning Doves. Condor *64*:165–166, 1962.

104. MAKOWSKI, J.: Beitrag zur Klärung des Atmungsmechanismus der Vögel. Pflüger's Arch. ges. Physiol. *240*:407–418, 1938.

105. MANGOLD, E.: Erregungsursprung und -leitung im Herzen der Vögel und niederen Wirbeltiere. Deutsch. med. Wchschr. *40*:1035–1036, 1914.

106. MANGOLD, E.: Die Verdauung bei den Nutztieren. Berlin, Akademie-Verlag, 1950. 108 pp.

107. MARSHALL, A. J., ed.: *Biology and Comparative Physiology of Birds*. New York, Academic Press. Vol. 1, 1960, 518 pp.; Vol. 2, 1961, 468 pp.

108. MARSHALL, A. J.: Reproduction. In *Biology and Comparative Physiology of Birds*, A. J. Marshall, ed. New York, Academic Press, 1961. Vol. 2, pp. 169–213.

109. MAYRS, E. B.: Secretion as a factor in elimination by the bird's kidney. J. Physiol. *58*:276–287, 1924.

110. MEIER, A. H., and FARNER, D. S.: A possible endocrine basis for premigratory fattening in the white-crowned sparrow, *Zonotrichia leucophrys gambelii* (Nuttall). Gen. Comp. Endocrinol. *4*:584–595, 1964.

138   *Diseases of Cage and Aviary Birds*

111.   MEIER, A. H., FARNER, D. S., and KING, J. R.: A possible endocrine basis for migratory behaviour in the White-crowned Sparrow, *Zonotrichia leucophrys gambelii*. Animal Behaviour *13:*453–465, 1965.

112.   MENAKER, M.: Circadian Rhythms and Photoperiodism in *Passer domesticus*. In *Circadian Clocks*, Proceedings of the Feldafing Summer School, 7–18 September 1964, J. Aschoff, ed. Amsterdam, North-Holland Publishing Company, 1965. Pp. 385–395.

113.   MIALHE, P.: Glucagon, insuline et régulation endocrine de la glycémie chez le canard. Acta Endocrinol., Suppl. *36:*1–134, 1958.

114.   MIALHE-VOLOSS, C., and BENOIT, J.: L'intermedine dans l'hypophyse et l'hypothalamus du Canard. Compt. Rend. Soc. Biol. Paris *148:*56–59, 1954.

115.   MIKAMI, S. I.: The cytological significance of regional patterns in the adenohypophysis of the fowl. J. Fac. Agric. Iwate Univ. *3:*473–545, 1958.

116.   MINKOWSKI, O.: Beiträge zur Pathologie der Leber und des Icterus: III. Ueber den Einfluss der Leberexstirpation auf den Stoffwechsel. Arch. exp. Pathol. Pharmakol. *21:*41–87, 1886.

117.   MORGAN, V. E., and CHICHESTER, D. F.: Properties of the blood of the domestic fowl. J. Biol. Chem. *110:*285–298, 1935.

118.   MORRIS, D.: The reproductive behaviour of the Zebra Finch (*Poephila guttata*), with special reference to pseudofemale behaviour and displacement activities. Behaviour *6:*271–322, 1954.

119.   MOSZKOWSKA, A.: L'antagonisme epiphysohypophysaire. Rev. suisse Zool. *62*(Suppl.):198–213, 1955.

120.   MOUCHETTE, R., and CUYPERS, Y.: Étude de la vascularisation du rein de Coq. Arch. Biol. (Liege) *69:*577–589, 1958.

121.   MUNSICK, R. A., SAWYER, W. H., and VAN DYKE, H. B.: Avian neurohypophysial hormones: Pharmacological properties and tentative identification. Endocrinology *66:*860–871, 1960.

122.   NICE, L. B., NICE, M. M., and KRAFT, R. M.: Erythrocytes and hemoglobin in the blood of some American birds. Wilson Bull. *47:*120–124, 1935.

123.   NOLF, P.: Les nerfs extrinsèques de l'intestin chez l'oiseau. II. Les nerfs coeliaques et mésentériques. Arch. intern. Physiol. *39:*165–226, 1934.

124.   NOLF, P.: De la longue durée des effets chronotrope et inotrope exercés par les nerfs gastro-intestinaux et de la possibilité de les obtenir séparément. Arch. intern. Physiol. *44:*38–111, 1936.

125.   NOLF, P.: Le système nerveux gastro-entérique. Ann. Physiol. Physicochimie biol. *14:*293–320, 1938.

126.   NOLF, P.: L'appareil nerveux de l'automatisme gastrique de l'oiseau. II. Étude des effets causés par

une ou plusieurs sections de l'anneau nerveux du gésier. Arch. intern. Physiol. *46:*441–559, 1938.

127.   NOLF, P.: The intrinsic gastro-intestinal fibres are connecting fibres. J. Physiol. *91:*1–2P, 1938.

128.   NOLF, P.: Les éléments intrinsèques de l'anneau nerveux du gésier de l'oiseau granivore. Part 1. Arch. intern. Physiol. *47:*453–518, 1938.

129.   ODUM, E. P.: Variations in the heart rate of birds: A study in physiological ecology. Ecol. Monographs *11:*299–326, 1941.

130.   ODUM, E. P.: The heart rate of small birds. Science *101:*153–154, 1945.

131.   OKSCHE, A., FARNER, D. S., SERVENTY, D. L., WOLFF, F., and NICHOLLS, C. A.: The hypothalamo-hypophysial neurosecretory system of the Zebra Finch, *Taeniopygia castanotis*. Z. Zellforsch. *58:*846–914, 1963.

132.   OPEL, H.: Oviposition in chickens after removal of the posterior lobe of the pituitary by an improved method. Endocrinology *76:*673–677, 1965.

133.   ORLOFF, J., and DAVIDSON, D. G.: Mechanism of potassium excretion in the chicken. Fed. Proc. *15:*139, 1956.

134.   PATON, D. N.: On the extrinsic nerves of the heart of the bird. J. Physiol. *45:*106–114, 1912.

135.   PATZELT, V.: Der Darm. In Wilhelm von Mollendorf, *Handbuch der mikroskopischen Anatomie des Menschen*, Teil III, Bd. *5*, pp. 1–448, 1936.

136.   PITTS, R. F.: The excretion of phenol red by the chicken. J. Cell. Comp. Physiol. *11:*99–115, 1938.

137.   POULSON, T. L., and BARTHOLOMEW, G. A.: Salt balance in the savannah sparrow. Physiol. Zool. *35:*109–119, 1962.

138.   PRECHT, H., CHRISTOPHERSON, J., and HENSEL, H.: *Temperatur und Leben*. Berlin, Springer-Verlag, 1955. 514 pp.

139.   RALPH, C. L., HALL, P. F., and GRINWICH, D. L.: Failure to demonstrate a direct action of luteinizing hormone (LH or ICSH) on regenerating feathers in African weaver birds. Am. Zoologist *5:*212–213, 1965.

140.   RENNICK, B. R.: The renal tubular excretion of choline and thiamine in the chicken. J. Pharmacol. Exp. Therap. *122:*449–456, 1958.

141.   RENNICK, B. R.: Renal tubular excretion of riboflavin in the chicken. Proc. Soc. Exp. Biol. Med. *103:*241–243, 1960.

142.   RENNICK, B. R., and GANDIA, H.: Pharmacology of smooth muscle valve in renal portal circulation of birds. Proc. Soc. Exp. Biol. Med. *85:*234–236, 1954.

143.   RENNICK, B. R., LATIMER, C., and MOE, G.: Excretion

of potassium by the chicken kidney. Fed. Proc. *11:*384–385, 1952.

144. RENNICK, B. R., and YOSS, N.: Renal tubular excretion of *dl*-epinephrine-2-C¹⁴ in the chicken. J. Pharmacol. Exp. Therap. *138:*347–350, 1962.

145. RINGER, R. K.: Thyroids. In *Avian Physiology,* 2nd ed., by P. D. Sturkie. Ithaca, N. Y., Comstock Publishing Associates, 1965. Pp. 592–648.

146. RODBARD, S., and TOLPIN, M.: A relationship between the body temperature and the blood pressure in the chicken. Am. J. Physiol. *151:*509–515, 1947.

147. VON SAALFELD, E.: Untersuchungen über das Hacheln bei Tauben. Z. vergleich. Physiol. *23:*727–743, 1936.

148. SALT, G. W.: Respiratory evaporation in birds. Biol. Rev. *39:*113–136, 1964.

149. SALT, G. W., and ZEUTHEN, E.: The Respiratory System. In *Biology and Comparative Physiology of Birds,* A. J. Marshall, ed. New York, Academic Press, 1960. Vol. 1, pp. 363–409.

150. SANDREUTER, A.: Vergleichende Untersuchungen über die Blutbildung in der Ontogenese von Haushuhn (*Gallus gallus* L.) und Star (*Sturnus v. vulgaris* L.). Acta Anat. *11*(Suppl. 14):1–72, 1951.

151. SANNER, E., and WORTMAN, B.: Tubular excretion of serotonin (5-hydroxytryptamine) in the chicken. Acta Physiol. Scand. *55:*319–324, 1962.

152. SCHARNKE, H.: Experimentelle Beiträge zur Kenntnis der Vogelatmung. Z. vergleich. Physiol. *25:*548–583, 1938.

153. SCHMIDT-NIELSEN, K.: Desert Birds. In *Desert Animals,* K. Schmidt-Nielsen, ed. London, Oxford University Press, 1964. Pp. 204–224.

154. SEGAL, S. J.: Response of weaver finch to chorionic gonadotrophin and hypophysial luteinizing hormone. Science *126:*1242–1243, 1957.

155. SEIBERT, H. C.: Differences between migrant and non-migrant birds in food and water intake at various temperatures and photoperiods. Auk *66:*128–153, 1949.

156. SELANDER, R. K., and KUICH, L. L.: Hormonal control and development of the incubation patch in icterids, with notes on behavior of cowbirds. Condor *65:*73–90, 1963.

157. SERGEEV, P. M., and SKVORTSOVA, T. A.: Rabota sredtsa y melkikh ptits. Priroda *1957,* pp. 97–99.

158. SHANNON, J. A.: The excretion of exogenous creatinine by the chicken. J. Cell. Comp. Physiol. *11:*123–134, 1938.

159. SHARPE, N. C.: On the secretion of urine in birds. Am. J. Physiol. *31:*75–84, 1912.

160. SIMPSON, S., and GALBRAITH, J. J.: An investigation into the diurnal variation of the body temperature of nocturnal and other birds, and a few mammals. J. Physiol. (London) *33:*225–238, 1905.

161. SKADHAUGE, E.: Effects of unilateral infusion of arginine-vasotocin into the portal circulation of the avian kidney. Acta Endocrinol. *47:*321–330, 1964.

162. SOUM, J. M.: Recherches physiologiques sur l'appareil respiratoire des oiseaux. Ann. Univ. Lyon *28:*1–126, 1896.

163. SPANNER, R.: Der Pfortaderkreislauf in der Vogelniere. Gegenbaurs morph. Jahrb. *54:*560–632, 1925.

164. SPANNER, R.: Die Drosselklappe der veno-venösen Anastomose und ihre Bedeutung für den Abkürzungskreislauf im porto-cavalen System des Vogels; zugleich ein Beitrag zur Kenntnis der epitheloiden Zellen. Z. Anat. Entwicklungsgesch. *109:*443–492, 1939.

165. SPERBER, I.: A new method for the study of renal tubular excretion in birds. Nature *158:*131, 1946.

166. SPERBER, I.: The excretion of some glucoronic acid derivatives and phenol sulphuric esters in the chicken. Ann. Roy. Agric. Coll. Sweden *15:*317–349, 1948.

167. SPERBER, I.: Excretion. In *Biology and Comparative Physiology of Birds,* A. J. Marshall, ed. New York, Academic Press, 1960. Vol. 1, pp. 469–492.

168. STEEL, E. A., and HINDE, R. A.: Hormonal control of brood patch and oviduct development in domesticated canaries. J. Endocrinol. *26:*11–24, 1963.

169. STEEL, E. A., and HINDE, R. A.: Effect of exogenous oestrogen on brood patch development of intact and ovariectomized canaries. Nature *202:*718–719, 1964.

170. STEEN, J.: Climatic adaptation in some small northern birds. Ecology *39:*625–629, 1958.

171. STEEN, J., and ENGER, P. S.: Muscular heat production in pigeons during exposure to cold. Am. J. Physiol. *191:*157–158, 1957.

172. STRESEMANN, E.: Aves. In *Handbuch der Zoologie,* W. Kükenthal and T. Krumbach, eds. Berlin, Walter de Gruyter & Co. Vol. 7, Part 2, 1934, 899 pp.

173. STÜBEL, H.: Beiträge zur Kenntnis der Physiologie des Blutkreislaufes bei verschiedenen Vogelarten. Pfluger's Arch. ges. Physiol. *135:*249–365, 1910.

174. STURKIE, P. D.: The electrocardiogram of the chicken. Am. J. Vet. Res. *10:*168–175, 1949.

175. STURKIE, P. D.: *Avian Physiology,* 2nd ed. Ithaca, N.Y., Comstock Publishing Associates, 1965. Pp. 133–151.

176. STURKIE, P. D., and HUNSAKER, W. G.: Role of estrogen in sex difference of the electrocardiogram of

the chicken. Proc. Soc. Exp. Biol. Med. *94:*731–733, 1957.

177. SYKES, A. H.: The renal clearance of uric acid and p-amino-hippurate in the fowl. Res. Vet. Sci. *1:*308–314, 1960.

178. SYKES, A. H.: The excretion of inulin, creatinine and ferrocyanide by the fowl. Res. Vet. Sci. *1:*315–320, 1960.

179. TAKEWAKI, K., and MORI, H.: Mechanism of molting in the canary. J. Fac. Sci., Univ. Tokyo, Section IV, *6:*547–575, 1944.

180. TANABE, Y., and KATSURAGI, T.: Thyroxine secretion rates of molting and laying hens, and general discussion on the hormonal induction of molting in hens. Bull. Nat. Inst. Agr. Sci. (Japan), Series G, *21:*49–59, 1962.

181. TANAKA, K., and NAKAJO, S.: Participation of neurohypophysial homone in oviposition in the hen. Endocrinology *70:*453–458, 1962.

182. TANAKA, K., and NAKAJO, S.: Difference in the neurohypophysial hormone content between the laying and the non-laying hen. Poultry Sci. *42:*729–731, 1963.

183. TERROINE, E.-E., and TRAUTMANN, S.: Influence de la température extérieure sur la production calorique des homéothermes et loi des surfaces. Ann. physiol. physicochim. biol. *3:*422–457, 1927.

184. THAPLIYAL, J. P., and SAXENA, R. N.: Plumage control in Indian weaver bird (*Ploceus philippinus*). Naturwissenschaften *48:*741–742, 1961.

185. TIXIER-VIDAL, A.: Histophysiologie de l'adénohypophyse des oiseaux. In *Cytologie de l'adénohypophyse,* J. Benoit and C. DaLage, eds. Colloq. Intern. Centre Nat. Rech. Sci. (Paris), No. 128, 1963. Pp. 255–274.

186. TIXIER-VIDAL, A.: Caractères ultrastructuraux des types cellulaires de l'adénohypophyse de Canard mâle. Arch. Anat. microscop. Morphol. exp. *54:*719–780, 1965.

187. TIXIER-VIDAL, A., and ASSENMACHER, I.: The effect of anterior hypophysectomy on thyroid metabolism of radioactive iodine (I^{131}) in male ducks. Gen. Comp. Endocrinol. *2:*574–585, 1962.

188. TIXIER-VIDAL, A., ASSENMACHER, I., and BAYLE, J.-D.: Étude cytologique de greffes hypophysaires ectopiques chez le Canard mâle. Compt. Rend. Acad. Sci. Paris *260:*310–312, 1965.

189. VAN TIENHOVEN, A.: Endocrinology of Reproduction in Birds. In *Sex and Internal Secretions,* 3rd ed., W. C. Young, ed. Baltimore, Williams & Wilkins Co., 1961. Pp. 1088–1169.

190. VAUGIEN, L.: Mue, activité thyroïdienne cyclique et

cycle des gonades chez les Oiseaux passeriformes. Compt. Rend. Acad. Sci. Paris *226:*353–354, 1948.

191. VÓITKEVICH, A. A.: Pero ptitsy. Akademii Nauk USSR. 1962. 285 pp.

192. VOLLE, R. L., GREEN, R. E., PETERS, L., HANDSCHUMACHER, R. E., and WELCH, A. D.: Renal tubular excretion studies with pyrimidine derivatives and analogs. J. Pharmacol. Exp. Therap. *136:*353–360, 1962.

193. VONK, H. J., and POSTMA, N.: X-ray studies on the movements of the hen's intestine. Physiologia Comparata et Oecologia *1:*15–23, 1949.

194. VUYLSTEKE, C. A., and DE DUVE, C.: Le contenu en glucagon du pancréas aviaire. Arch. Intern. Physiol. *61:*273–274, 1953.

195. WAGNER, H. O.: Schilddrüse und Federausfall. Z. vergleich. Physiol. *44:*565–575, 1961.

196. WAGNER, H. O.: Der Einfluss endo- und exogener Faktoren auf die Mauser gekäfigter Vögel. Z. vergleich. Physiol. *45:*337–354, 1962.

197. WALLGREN, H.: Energy metabolism of two species of the genus *Emberiza* as correlated with distribution and migration. Acta zool. Fennica *84:*1–110, 1954.

198. WARREN, R. P., and HINDE, R. A.: The effect of oestrogen and progesterone on the nest-building of domesticated canaries. Animal Behaviour *7:*209–213, 1959.

199. WASTL, H., and LEINER, G.: Beobachtungen über die Blutgase bei Vögeln. I. Mitteilung. Pflüger's Arch. ges. Physiol. *227:*367–420, 1931.

200. WASTL, H., and LEINER, G.: Beobachtungen über die Blutgase bei Vögeln. II. Mitteilung. Pflüger's Arch. ges. Physiol. *227:*421–459, 1931.

201. WEIS-FOGH, T.: Functional design of the tracheal system of flying insects as compared with the avian lung. J. Exp. Biol. *41:*207–227, 1964.

202. WEST, G. C.: Responses and Adaptations of Wild Birds to Environmental Temperature. In *Comparative Physiology of Temperature Regulation,* J. P. Hannon and E. G. Viereck, eds. Proceedings, Symposia on Arctic Biology and Medicine, Arctic Aeromedical Laboratory, Fort Wainwright, Alaska, 1962. Pp. 291–333.

203. WETMORE, A.: A study of the body temperature of birds. Smithsonian Misc. Coll., Vol. 72, No. 12, December 30, 1921. 52 pp.

204. WILSON, A. C., and FARNER, D. S.: The annual cycle of thyroid activity in White-crowned Sparrows of Eastern Washington. Condor *62:*414–425, 1960.

205. WINGSTRAND, K. G.: *The Structure and Development of the Avian Pituitary.* C. W. K. Gleerup/Lund, 1951. 316 pp.

206. WINTROBE, M. M.: Variations in the size and hemoglobin content of erythrocytes in the blood of various vertebrates. Folia Haematol. *51:*32–49, 1933.

207. WITSCHI, E.: Comparative physiology of the vertebrate hypophysis (anterior and intermediate lobes). Cold Spring Harbor Symp. Quant. Biol. *5:*180–190, 1937.

208. WITSCHI, E.: Vertebrate gonadotrophins. Mem. Soc. Endocrinol. *4:*149–163, 1955.

209. WITSCHI, E.: Sex and Secondary Sexual Characters. In *Biology and Comparative Physiology of Birds,* A. J. Marshall, ed. New York, Academic Press, 1961. Vol. 2, pp. 115–168.

210. WITSCHI, E., and FUGO, N. W.: Response of sex characters of the adult female starling to synthetic hormones. Proc. Soc. Exp. Biol. Med. *45:*10–14, 1940.

211. WOLBACH, R. A.: Renal regulation of acid-base balance in the chicken. Am. J. Physiol. *181:*149–156, 1955.

212. WOLFSON, A.: Circadian Rhythm and the Photoperiodic Regulation of the Annual Reproductive Cycle in Birds. In *Circadian Clocks,* Proceedings of the Feldafing Summer School, 7–18 September 1964, J. Aschoff, ed. Amsterdam, North-Holland Publishing Company, 1965. Pp. 370–378.

213. WOODBURY, R. A., and HAMILTON, W. F.: Blood pressure studies in small animals. Am. J. Physiol. *119:*663–674, 1937.

Suggested Reading

ASCHOFF, J., ed.: *Circadian Clocks,* Proceedings of the Feldafing Summer School, 7–18 September 1964. Amsterdam, North-Holland Publishing Co., 1965. 479 pp.

GRASSÉ, P.-P., ed.: *Traité de Zoologie,* Vol. 15, *Oiseaux.* Paris, Masson et Cie., 1950. 1164 pp.

MARSHALL, A. J., ed: *Biology and Comparative Physiology of Birds.* New York, Academic Press. Vol. 1, 1960, 518 pp.; Vol. 2, 1961, 468 pp.

STRESEMANN, E.: Aves. In *Handbuch der Zoologie,* W. Kükenthal and T. Krumbach, eds. Berlin, Walter de Gruyter & Co. Vol. 7, Part 2, 1934. 899 pp.

STURKIE, P. D.: *Avian Physiology,* 2nd ed. Ithaca, N.Y., Comstock Publishing Associates, 1965. 766 pp.

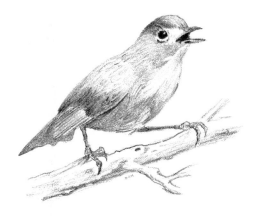

7

Nutrition

C. Ivar Tollefson

Birds have been raised in captivity for hundreds of years, with reasons for raising them being many and varied. They have been raised (*a*) as a source of meat and eggs; (*b*) as an interesting hobby: for their color, shape, pattern, song, or powers of mimicry; (*c*) for hunting and sport: falcons, game cocks; (*d*) for means of communication: pigeons, frigate birds; (*e*) for use in detection of gas in mines; (*f*) for their scientific value: as laboratory animals for studies in genetics, nutrition, and behavior, and for medical research; (*g*) for their therapeutic value in correctional institutions; (*h*) for their ornamental value in parks and zoos; (*i*) for use in religious ceremonies; and (*j*) for their feathers: ostrich farms.

However, despite their long history of being raised in captivity, little is known of the actual nutritive requirements of birds other than commercial poultry.[50] In general, knowledge of the dietary requirements of many species of birds is based on observations of their eating habits in the wild, examination of the crop and stomach contents of wild birds, and a "trial-and-error" approach to feeding in captivity. By this means, more or less satisfactory diets have been developed in most cases, and there is a large volume of popular literature on the care and feeding of different species.

Availability of food is an important factor in determining a bird's diet in the wild. Within limits, a bird will eat what is available. For instance, the American robin (*Turdus migratorius*) may eat earthworms in the spring, cherries in the summer, and palmetto buds in the winter.[58] In turn, the availability of suitable foods may determine the geographical distribution of various types of birds and be partly responsible for migration patterns.

The selection of food is influenced by certain physical attributes of the bird that enable it to capture or to utilize different foods. During the course of evolution, various adaptations have fitted different birds to seek foods in certain habitats or to eat certain types of foods.[58,73]

Adaptations of the feet and wings are associated with methods of obtaining food in certain habitats. For example, swifts (Apodidae) catch insects on the wing, ducks (Anatidae) dive for food under water, and quail (Phasianidae) grub for food on the ground. In other birds, adaptations of the tongue are associated with the type of food eaten and the method of obtaining it. Woodpeckers (Picidae) have long tongues with barbed tips which can be extended beyond the bill to extract grubs from burrows. Hummingbirds (Trochilidae), sunbirds (Nectariniidae), and honey-eaters (Meliphagidae) have tubular tongues, brushy at the tips, which aid in getting nectar out of flowers. Lories or brush-tongued parrots (Psittacidae) have fleshy tongues that open into a brush when extended, for collecting nectar and fruit juices. Ducks and flamingos (Phoenicopteridae) use the tongue to force water out of the mouth through strainers on the edge of the bill.

Adaptations of the bill are associated with methods of food gathering and are often correlated with the type of food taken. The bill of the crow (Corvidae) is strong enough to kill small mammals or to open nuts but is fine enough at the tip to pick up small insects. Many song birds have slender bills for picking insects off leaves or out of cracks; others have broad flat bills for catching flies or strong thick bills for cracking shells of seeds. Woodpeckers have a chisel-like bill for cutting holes in trees in search for wood-boring insects, and the hooked bill of birds of prey is designed for tearing flesh. A definite correlation between bill size and size of seed selected by finches (Estrildidae and Fringillidae) was observed, although there was almost no correlation between body size and size of seed selected.[43] There also appears to be an association between the size of the bill in parrots and the size of the seed selected as food.[25]

Adaptations of the digestive system as related to nutrition are well described by Farner.[29] In some birds, the crop serves merely as an organ for storage, but in others it may act as a digestive organ; in pigeons and doves, it produces a "milk" for feeding the young. The glandular stomach (proventriculus) may function merely in production of gastric juices or, in addition, may serve as a storage organ or as an organ of digestion. The gizzard (muscular stomach, or ventriculus) shows a high degree of variation, which correlates with

type of nutrition: the musculature of the gizzard shows greatest development in seed-eating and herbivorous species, but in fruit-eaters the gizzard may be reduced to an insignificant band between the proventriculus and the intestine. Variations in the intestines also relate to the type of nutrition. Thus, in view of the anatomic differences in the digestive system of different species of birds it is not surprising that they have different food requirements and habits.

The diet should supply proper amounts of all the nutrients required for vigorous growth, normal development, reproduction, and resistance to diseases and parasites. Growth is manifested by an increase in size but it also involves continuous multiplication of cells and their differentiation to perform the different functions of the organism. Maximal size of the animal may be limited by heredity, but maximal development can be achieved only by continuous realization of the full growth potential, which requires a high level of nutrition throughout the growing period. Additional dietary stresses are imposed on adult birds during periods of reproduction and feeding the young. Many studies have also shown that malnutrition is accompanied by decreased resistance to parasites and disease. Thus it would appear that diet is the most important single factor in ensuring a long, healthy life and complete physiological efficiency.

FOODS AND THEIR FUNCTIONS

All natural foods contain many different chemical constituents, which may be classified into a number of groups having certain common properties: carbohydrates, fats, proteins, vitamins, minerals, and water. Whenever a serious deficiency of any of these essential substances occurs, there may be characteristic symptoms of deficiency as well as non-specific symptoms such as retarded growth, poor feather development, decreased egg production, and low hatchability of eggs. When the deficiency is mild, only the non-specific symptoms may be seen; this makes it difficult to pinpoint the problem, since the non-specific symptoms can result from a number of nutritional deficiencies as well as from disease.[51]

Energy is required for all body movements and for maintaining body temperature. The energy level of the diet governs the feed intake—that is, a bird will consume smaller amounts of a high-energy feed than of a low-energy feed. Thus the dietary requirements for protein, vitamins, and minerals should not be expressed as a percentage of the diet except at a specified energy level. In the case of protein, the situation is further complicated by the fact that proteins are not completely balanced and utilization of protein as such is limited by the essential amino acid present at the lowest percentage of the bird's requirement—excess protein is metabolized as a source of energy. As the ratio of energy to protein increases, protein intake may be restricted so that growth rate of young birds is limited. During periods of hot weather, birds tend to consume less, thereby reducing their protein intake and increasing the need for protein supplements at such times.

Classes of Food Elements

CARBOHYDRATES

Carbohydrates include sugars and starches, which function mainly as sources of energy and heat. Fiber, including fibrous husks, is also "carbohydrate," but since it is generally not digested by birds, it is not a good source of energy or heat. In fact, many birds remove the husks before they swallow the seeds.

FATS

Fats, like carbohydrates, are used to furnish heat and energy. They also serve as sources of some essential fatty acids, and aid in the absorption of the fat-soluble vitamins. Because excess foods are generally stored in the body as fats, insufficient exercise and too much food will lead to obesity with all its attendant dangers.

PROTEINS

Proteins are a highly important class of foods since muscle, most of the body organs, feathers, skin, beak, claws, and eggs contain large amounts of protein. Although proteins are very complicated in structure, they are composed of relatively simple units called amino acids. During digestion, proteins are broken down into these simpler compounds, which are then absorbed and rebuilt into protein as needed. The efficiency with which a given protein can be utilized for synthesis of tissue protein is called its biological value. Besides being needed for growth, maintenance and repair of body tissues, and production of eggs, some amino acids have other functions. Tyrosine is used in formation of the hormone thyroxine; methionine is a source of methyl groups for methylation processes and may be involved in choline synthesis; tryptophan can partially replace the vitamin niacin; lysine and tyrosine seem to be involved in formation of some feather pigments.

Some of the amino acids cannot be manufactured by the bird; they are therefore called "essential" amino acids and must be supplied in the diet, in contrast to the "non-essential" amino acids, which can be manufactured by the bird. Plant proteins tend to be deficient in certain essential amino acids such as lysine, methionine, and tryptophan, and hence have lower biological value than animal proteins. Since the protein content of cereal grains is relatively low, as well as the proteins being of lower biological value, it should be evident that young seed-eating birds need protein supplements in order to achieve optimal growth. Because various proteins differ in amino acid composition, the use of a wide variety of protein supplements increases the assurance of adequate amounts of all the essential amino acids in the diet.

VITAMINS

Vitamins are required in very small amounts, but deficiencies of them result in major disturbances of metabolism because they function as integral parts of enzyme systems.[67] A marked deficiency of a single vitamin in the diet results in the breakdown of the metabolic process in which the particular vitamin is concerned. In some instances, a deficiency of any one of several vitamins can result in a particular symptom. For example, perosis in chicks occurs when the diet is deficient in choline, niacin, biotin, or folic acid, or in the mineral manganese. Uncomplicated deficiency of a single vitamin seldom, if ever, occurs on practical diets.

Symptoms of vitamin deficiency are frequently observed in young birds shipped from breeders to dealers. At this time, the birds require a highly nutritive diet, but they are sometimes maintained only on millet or antibiotic-treated millet. They are crowded in dark shipping boxes with little feed available. Frequently, such birds respond remarkably to vitamin supplements and proper supplementary feeds. It is possible for indiscriminate use of antibiotics to induce vitamin deficiencies owing to alterations in the intestinal flora, and it is recommended that during antibiotic treatment the birds be supported by vitamin therapy. The economic aspects of treatment of pet birds or valuable zoo birds differ greatly from the considerations involved in treatment of flocks of domestic fowl.

There are many different vitamins, and undoubtedly most of them are essential for birds. The vitamins are sometimes classed as fat-soluble (A, D, E, and K) and water-soluble (the B complex and C). The functions of and requirements for various vitamins have been intensively studied only in domestic chickens (*Gallus gallus*), but it may be assumed that the same principles formulated in those studies would apply also to cage birds.

VITAMIN A is a dietary essential for all birds and is stored in the liver. This vitamin does not occur as such in plants, but certain plant parts contain carotene, which can be converted in the body to vitamin A. Seeds, however, are generally deficient in carotene. Deficiency of vitamin A may result in epithelial changes in the respiratory, alimentary, and reproductive tracts, as well as in the eye. This lowers resistance of the epithelial tissues to the entrance of pathogenic organisms, with the result that respiratory troubles and sinus infections tend to be more severe in vitamin A–deficient birds.[52] Vitamin A has commonly been supplied to cage birds by adding cod liver oil to seeds at a rate of about 1 teaspoonful per pound of seed. However, cod liver oil is liable to become rancid and promote destruction of vitamin E.

Evidence has been presented[80] that excess vitamin A may be one of the factors involved in development of French Molt in budgerigars. The proportion of those who used cod liver oil was higher among breeders who had serious French Molt trouble than among breeders who were free from it. Cod liver oil may not only supply excess vitamin A but may also contribute to the destruction and hence deficiency of vitamin E, which also may be involved in the syndrome.

VITAMIN D is required for normal calcification of bones in young birds. The amount needed varies with the calcium and phosphorus content of the diet, more being needed if the amount of calcium or phosphorus or the ratio between them is suboptimal. The most effective form of this nutrient for birds is vitamin D_3. Vitamin D promotes net retention of calcium and phosphorus in the body by increasing absorption or decreasing excretion of these elements. It helps maintain normal blood levels of the two minerals and has some specific action in connection with deposition of calcium salts in the bone, these effects possibly being related to alkaline phosphatase activity. Vitamin D deficiency may cause soft-shelled eggs, which can result in egg binding. Severe deficiency in young birds can result in rickets.

It has been suggested that the secretion of the uropygial (oil or preen) gland is converted to vitamin D through action of sunlight on the feathers and that the bird consumes small but important amounts of vitamin D from this source during preening.[27] The cage bird, being deprived of the action of sunlight on its skin, has a greater need for a dietary source of this vitamin than has its counterpart in the wild. There is some storage of vitamin D in the liver.

VITAMIN E serves many functions, but it is difficult to demonstrate effects of deficiency in seed-eating birds since the seed germs are good sources of this vitamin. Vitamin E deficiency may be precipitated by excessive use of cod liver oil, the unsaturated fatty acids of which cause oxidation of vitamin E.

VITAMIN K is involved in the formation of prothrombin in the liver and hence affects blood coagulation time. Since the vitamin is synthesized by microorganisms in the digestive tract, a dietary source is not generally necessary. Deficiency of vitamin K could result from changes in intestinal flora caused by indiscriminate use of antibiotics.

VITAMIN B_1, or **THIAMINE,** functions as a constituent of cocarboxylase, a coenzyme for several enzyme systems involved in the utilization of carbohydrate to provide energy. Vitamin B_1 deficiency results in loss of appetite, impairment of digestion, general weakness, and frequently in convulsions; in acute polyneuritis, the head may be retracted (opisthotonos). Paresis and paralysis of one or both legs are the most common results of vitamin B_1 deficiency. Paresis is manifested by reduced clutching ability, weakness of leg muscles, and lack of sureness on the perch. Paralysis is manifested by rigid extension of the leg and tightly clenched toes, symptoms that may occur also in adenocarcinoma of the kidney (particularly in budgerigars), fibrosarcoma of the femoral region, and femoral fractures. If the bird has normal thighs and has had adequate vitamin B_1 in its diet, it may have adenocarcinoma of the kidney.[47] In any case, the first step in treatment should be administration of supplementary vitamin B. If the condition has not persisted long enough to result in irreversible degeneration of the nervous system, response to additional vitamin B is frequently dramatic. There is little storage of thiamine in the body, so its provision in the diet is essential at all times. Cereal seeds are fairly good sources of this vitamin.

VITAMIN B_2, or **RIBOFLAVIN,** functions as a constituent of the flavoprotein enzymes and the amino acid oxidase and xanthine oxidase systems, so that it is involved in release of energy as well as in metabolism of protein and purine. A deficiency of riboflavin is reflected in a wide variety of symptoms, with curly toe paralysis being perhaps the most characteristic symptom.[67]

NIACIN functions as a component of two coenzymes, diphosphopyridine nucleotide (DPN) and triphosphopyridine nucleotide (TPN), which act in conjunction with flavoprotein enzymes in cell respiration. A deficiency of niacin results in poor growth, poor feathering, perosis, and scaly dermatitis. Tryptophan can partially compensate for a niacin deficiency, indicating some conversion of tryptophan to niacin.

VITAMIN B$_6$, or **PYRIDOXINE,** functions in several enzyme systems concerned in metabolism of protein and fat. A severe deficiency of this vitamin results in loss of appetite, followed by rapid loss of weight and death. Production and hatchability of eggs are markedly reduced by even mild deficiencies of this vitamin.

PANTOTHENIC ACID is a constituent of coenzyme A, which functions in the acetylation of choline and other compounds, as well as in the synthesis of cholesterol. Deficiency of this vitamin results in retardation of growth and feather development, dermatitis, granulation of the eyelids, necrosis around the mouth and on the feet, liver damage, changes in the spinal cord, and decreased hatchability of eggs.

BIOTIN seems to be required for good hatchability of eggs and apparently is one of the nutrients useful in prevention of perosis.

CHOLINE is a constituent of the phospholipid lecithin. It is also involved in fat metabolism, preventing abnormal accumulation of fat in the liver. It is essential for formation of acetylcholine, a source of labile methyl groups, and plays a specific role in prevention of perosis.

FOLIC ACID is an antianemia factor. A deficiency of folic acid in young chicks results in perosis, retarded growth, poor feathering, depigmentation of feathers, and development of anemia characterized by reduction in red blood cells and hemoglobin.

VITAMIN B$_{12}$ functions in synthesis of nucleic acids and of methyl groups. It may be involved in metabolism of carbohydrate, protein, and fat. Deficiency results in poor hatchability of eggs and bone abnormalities. Vitamin B$_{12}$ is not present in higher green plants or cereals; it is found in meat, milk, cheese, yeast, and fermentation products. It is synthesized by intestinal microorganisms and a dietary source is not necessary, since the bird may obtain it through coprophagy. However, provision of supplementary vitamin B$_{12}$ seems justified, particularly for breeding birds.

VITAMIN C, or **ASCORBIC ACID,** is not generally considered a dietary essential for birds. However, the red-vented bulbul (*Pycnonotus cafer*) has been reported to lack an enzyme necessary for conversion of glucose to vitamin C in the liver, and therefore must have preformed vitamin C in the diet. It is possible that other fruit- and nectar-eating birds may also require dietary vitamin C.

MINERALS

Minerals have many functions and are as necessary to life as any other class of foods. They are important as structural elements, particularly for skeletal development; in the regulation of osmotic activity and pH, and provision of the proper ionic environment for normal functioning of protoplasm; in transport of oxygen; and for activation of many enzyme systems. Mineral deficiencies may be manifested by leg weakness, loss of feathers, and by feather picking and feather eating.[5]

CALCIUM is the chief mineral constituent of the body and of the whole egg. It is required in the diet in larger amounts than any other mineral. Because most seeds are deficient in calcium, some supplementary form of the mineral is nearly always added to diets for seed-eating birds. This is generally in the form of cuttle-fish bone or crushed oyster shell. When cuttlefish bone is used, it is important that it be placed with the soft side toward the bird. The metabolism of calcium is linked with that of phosphorus and vitamin D, so that adequate amounts of these nutrients are necessary for proper utilization of calcium. The normal calcium/phosphorus ratio for chickens is about 1.5/1.0, or the diet should contain about 1 per cent calcium and 0.7 per cent phosphorus, depending somewhat on the energy level of the diet.

PHOSPHORUS is not only a constituent of bone, but it is also an important constituent of the proteins of the cell nucleus. It is associated with transfer and release of energy and is involved in the metabolism of carbohydrates and fats.

MAGNESIUM is associated with calcium and phosphorus metabolism. It is present in bone and egg shell; it is necessary for the activation of some enzymes; and it is involved in carbohydrate metabolism. The magnesium provided by the ordinary diet is generally sufficient, so that supplementary amounts are not needed.

SODIUM and **CHLORINE** are usually added to poultry diets in the form of common salt at a level of about 0.5 per cent of the diet. These elements are important in the osmotic relationships of the body tissue and fluids. Sodium is involved in acid-base equilibrium and regulation of pH of the blood. Chlorine is necessary for the synthesis of the gastric acids.

MANGANESE is essential in the feeding of poultry. Deficiency of this element may result in failure to maintain weight, decrease in egg production, reduction of strength of egg shells and hatchability of eggs, and in muscular incoordination and perosis.

ZINC, required in trace amounts, appears to be intimately concerned with synthesis of protein at the cellular level.[41] It apparently is required for activity of an enzyme involved in synthesis of pyrimidine.[62]

IRON is essential for the formation of hemoglobin. A deficiency of iron results in a characteristic form of anemia.

SELENIUM appears to aid in prevention of muscular dystrophy in chicks by helping in retention of vitamin E.[65]

IODINE is necessary for normal activity of the thyroid gland. Many seeds are deficient in iodine, and it is recommended that supplemental iodine be given in the drinking water. This is particularly necessary for budgerigars, which appear to have a species-susceptibility to thyroid problems. Deficiency of iodine results in enlargement of the thyroid gland, which may be accompanied by difficulty in breathing, regurgitation of food (not to be confused with normal courtship feeding behavior), lack of activity, feather problems, and other symptoms. Schlumberger[63] found thyroid glands 23 mm. long in budgerigars, in contrast to the normal maximum of 2 mm. The stress of breeding and caring for the young appeared to be a factor in development of these goiters. (For further discussion, see Chapter 22, Diseases of the Endocrine System.)

GRIT

All seed-eaters need a source of gravel or grit. The grit aids in grinding food in the gizzard, and therefore should be a hard and insoluble material with sharp edges (such as quartz), to give good grinding action. Some commercial grits contain charcoal, but the value of this is questionable since charcoal has been reported to adsorb vitamins A, B_2, and K from the intestinal tract, thus creating vitamin deficiencies.[1] Grit should not be considered a source of minerals, but rather the minerals should be supplied separately. It seems possible that use of mineralized grits could result in excessive intake of minerals, with possible damage to the kidneys. Some authors state that grit should be kept in a cup rather than on the floor of the cage, where it can become contaminated with droppings; others believe that grit on the floor of the cage serves a useful purpose in keeping the bird's feet clean.

WATER

Besides food, birds require water, which may be obtained by drinking or by eating succulent foods. Water is an essential constituent of living organisms. It is the solvent in which biochemical reactions of metabolism occur; it is the medium by which nutrients and products of metabolism are transported; and it is important in the regulation of body temperature.[51] Physiologically birds are less dependent than mammals on drinking water, because they eliminate their nitrogenous wastes in the form of insoluble uric acid. Although birds do not perspire as a means of controlling body heat, considerable water is lost through respiration, which is essentially the only method for dissipating body heat through evaporative cooling when ambient temperatures approach or exceed skin temperature. According to King and Farner,[39] evaporative cooling can account for loss of about 40 per cent of the resting heat production. The water lost, including excretory loss, exceeds that produced in the metabolic processes; this water deficit is especially pronounced in small birds, since they lose proportionately more water in the process of breathing than large birds do. The avian species for which a water supply is most critical are small sparrows and finches that live on a diet of dry seeds which provide little free water.[15] It is frequently stated that birds can live much longer without food than they can without water. Canaries may die within about 48 hours if they are deprived of water. Many seed-eating birds do not seem to have evolved physiological mechanisms for conserving water that could allow them to live on "metabolic water." However, budgerigars seem to have special abilities to survive on minimal intake of water. Two birds were reported in good health after 130 days without drinking, a phenomenon attributed to reduced activity and an intrinsically low basal metabolic rate.[15] Despite this finding, it is recommended that fresh water be available for budgerigars at all times.

In all cases, containers for food and water should be kept scrupulously clean. Contamination of the food or water by droppings may cause spread of intestinal diseases. Besides this, molds and fungi grow readily in dirty food containers. Not all molds are toxic, but there is no easy way to differentiate between toxic and non-toxic molds other than by feeding. The toxic factor aflatoxin, elaborated by *Aspergillus flavus*, has an LD_{50} of 20 micrograms for day-old ducklings.[54] The first symptoms of aflatoxin poisoning are lack of appetite and reduced growth rate. Non-specific but characteristic changes occur shortly before death, the most important being damage to the liver. Ergot, a fungus of certain cereals, can cause a number of symptoms, including dry gangrene, when consumed by birds. Symptoms of ergot poisoning in chickens were reported to include blackening of the nails, toes, shanks, beak, and comb.[3] We have seen a few budgerigars with similar symptoms (legs and toes black and brittle), and have had numerous letters describing such symptoms plus sloughing of toes. Although it was never proved that ergotism was involved, the symptoms were suggestive.

GENERAL NUTRITIVE REQUIREMENTS OF BIRDS

In general, the nutritive requirements of all birds for energy, proteins, vitamins, and minerals tend to be similar. Some restrictions on type of food suitable for a given species are imposed by the various adaptations of the bill and of the digestive system mentioned earlier in the Chapter. In the wild, a bird is free to select a varied diet of suitable foods within the limits of availability. The cage bird, by contrast, is limited to the diet with which it is supplied; all too frequently the bird is maintained on a suboptimal diet through lack of knowledge rather than lack of interest. In addition, the bird's well-being depends not only on what food is offered, but also on whether or not the food is accepted.

Factors Influencing Choice of Food

It has been suggested[40] that three factors influence a bird's choice of food:

Habit is possibly the strongest factor affecting food selection. The earliest influence comes from the food fed to the chick by its parent. The variety of foods available during the impressionable period after the chick leaves the nest is also highly important in the development of food selection habits.

Appearance is the second factor influencing food selection. A bird has keen eyesight but rather poorly developed senses of taste and smell. Thus it will eat what looks like the food to which it is accustomed. New foods may be regarded with suspicion as potentially dangerous objects. Color may play a part in this judgment. Whatever the cause, most birds have ultraconservative eating habits and do not readily change them.

"Personality" may be the third factor influencing food selection. There are definite differences in the ease with which different birds of the same species accept new foods. These personality differences may result from the combined effects of heredity and experience.

Factors Influencing Nutrient Requirements

Nutrient requirements of birds are dependent on their stage of life, activity, and reproductive status. These may be considered under four categories: (1) nonbreeding adults; (2) breeding birds (*a*) during egg production or (*b*) during parental feeding of the young; and (3) the growing chick.

NONBREEDING HEALTHY ADULT BIRDS have only maintenance requirements for protein, energy, vitamins, and minerals. Energy requirements depend on their activity and the environmental temperature. A bird allowed freedom of flight expends more energy and can be fed foods with higher energy value than one that is continually caged. Protein requirements are somewhat higher during the molt because of new feather growth. Normally, nonbreeding seed-eating birds remain healthy on a diet consisting of little except seeds; since all cereal grains are deficient in vitamins A, D, B_2, and B_{12}, it must be concluded that the birds' requirements for these vitamins are extremely low. Nevertheless, it seems a wise precaution to supply these birds with supplementary vitamins, which may be done by feeding some of the commercially available "Condition" foods or by administering a proprietary multivitamin preparation in the drinking water. The latter method may not always be successful, since some birds refuse to drink medicated water.

DURING EGG PRODUCTION the dietary requirements of breeding birds are increased. Mild deficiencies of vitamins or minerals may manifest themselves by low hatchability of eggs and high chick mortality without any characteristic symptoms of disease. The breeding female requires larger amounts of protein, minerals, and vitamins for the production of eggs.

The egg of the domestic hen (*Gallus gallus*) is approximately 58% white, 31% yolk, and 11% shell.[57] The composition of egg shell on a dry basis is approximately 85% calcium carbonate, 1.4% magnesium carbonate, 0.76% phosphate, and 4% organic matter. These values are fairly close to the composition of cuttlefish bone. Cuttlefish (*Sepia* spp.) bone contains about 85% calcium carbonate and 4% protein; spectrographic assays also show about 1% magnesium, 0.1% manganese, and trace amounts (less than 0.01%) of silicon, titanium, iron, copper, nickel, chromium, vanadium, zinc, barium, lithium, zirconium, aluminum, and molybdenum.

On a low calcium diet, a laying hen is in negative calcium balance and the supply of skeletal calcium, which is only sufficient for a few egg shells, is soon exhausted so that the shells become progressively thinner. On an adequate calcium intake, the calcium drawn from the bones is replaced by the calcium ingested. Just prior to ovulation, blood calcium is increased by the activity of hormones secreted by the anterior pituitary, parathyroid, ovary, and perhaps other endocrine glands. Since egg shell is mainly calcium carbonate, poor shell structure is usually ascribed to dietary deficiencies of calcium and vitamin D. The ability to produce strong shells is an inherited characteristic. However, hens able to produce strong shells are likely to produce a few weak shells when just coming into or going out of production, and the shells tend to become thinner after prolonged laying or with advancing age of the bird.

Environmental temperatures have a pronounced effect on shell thickness; blood calcium begins to drop and the shells become thinner as the air temperature rises above 73°F. Any or all of these factors may play some part in the production of egg binding. Not only is the nutritive value of the bird's diet important for the production of eggs, but it also markedly affects development of the embryo and viability of the chick after hatching.

WHILE FEEDING THE YOUNG the parent birds also have increased dietary requirements. Parental feeding of young birds takes many different forms. The young songbird at hatching is naked (or nearly so) and blind, and for some days its activities are limited to gaping for food which the parents thrust into its mouth.[58] Young hatched in this condition are called altricial. In contrast, a newly hatched duckling is covered with down and as soon as it is dry it can walk about and pick up its own food. This type of bird is called precocial.

Many songbirds bring food in the bill and simply stuff it into the gaping maw of the young bird. Baby hawks and owls nibble bits of meat held in the parent's bill, but soon learn to tear to pieces the whole carcasses of small animals that the parents bring to the nest. Gulls regurgitate food in front of the young, which help themselves to it. The female hummingbird inserts its long bill and injects nectar and tiny insects into the gullet of the young.

More completely processed food is provided by pigeons, which in the early days provide the nestlings with "pigeon milk," secreted by glands of the crop of both parents.[16] The secretion, which is controlled by a hormone from the anterior pituitary gland,[60] contains about 28% solids, composed of 33.8% fat, 58.6% protein, and 4.6% ash, the fat containing considerable amounts of lecithin, possibly in loose combination with protein.[19]

After the first week, the "pigeon milk" is gradually mixed with grain, and after the second week the bulk of the material fed to the young is grain.[18]

The young of the parrot family are altricial, and they are fed by regurgitation by the parent birds. The newly hatched budgerigar is fed on a material sometimes improperly called "crop milk," which appears to be a secretion from the proventriculus of the hen.[77] This secretion is very rich in protein. The newly hatched chicks are fed on almost pure "crop milk," but as they grow older they receive less "crop milk" and more seeds.[77] Obviously the type of diet supplied by the parent might be expected to have a bearing on the type of foods most readily accepted by the young when they begin to feed themselves. The rate of growth and the well-being of the young are directly dependent on the type of food supplied by the parents. Since this is a period when the rate of growth (skeletal development and growth of muscles, organs, and feathers) is greatest, it is imperative that the parents have a diet containing adequate amounts of energy-supplying foods, protein and essential amino acids, and vitamins and minerals. Maximal development of the young can be achieved only if full growth potential is continuously realized.

Since the young generally are entirely dependent on the parents for at least two weeks after hatching, the parents require food for their own maintenance, plus the additional amounts needed for the young and for the additional activity involved in obtaining and carrying food to the young. Even after the young leave the nest, they may be partially fed by the parents. If the parents start another nest immediately, this further increases the need for a good diet for the parents.

YOUNG BIRDS have a continuing need for a high quality diet if optimal development is to be achieved. They may reach adult weight in a few weeks (about six weeks for the budgerigar), but ossification of the skeleton may not be complete, and the nervous and muscular systems continue to develop. During the early impressionable period, the food selection habits of young birds are reinforced and the habits acquired then will affect the bird throughout its entire life.

CLASSIFICATION OF BIRDS ACCORDING TO EATING HABITS

Aviculturists classify cage birds on the basis of their food preferences or requirements. *Seed-eaters,* or *hard-bills,* include finchlike birds (canaries, waxbills, parrot finches, mannikins, diamond and Java sparrows, buntings, grosbeaks, whydahs, weavers, cardinals, bullfinches) and parrot-like birds (parrots, conures, macaws, lovebirds, parakeets, budgerigars, cockatoos, cockatiels). *Insect-eaters,* or *softbills,* include mynahs, babblers, warblers, thrushes, flycatchers, mockingbirds, orioles, starlings, pittas, woodpeckers, and doves. *Fruit-* and *nectar-eaters* include lories or brush-tongued parrots, toucans, hummingbirds, sunbirds, honey-eaters, white-eyes, and other birds that live primarily on fruit and nectar produced in the corollas of flowers. Although most seed-eaters primarily eat seeds, many species, especially during the nesting season, will eat insects. Similarly, many of the insect-eaters live primarily on insects but will also eat seeds; this is particularly true of the larger species, such as pigeons and doves.[61]

Generally, insect-eaters require a great deal of care in feeding, whereas seed-eaters are easily fed. The basic diets for both soft-billed and hard-billed birds may be purchased in pet stores or supermarkets. Foods for soft-billed birds are likely to be more expensive and somewhat more messy to feed. The commercial food mixtures may differ considerably in nutritive values, so that more or less supplementation may be necessary for optimal health. Many of the diets used by fanciers seem to be unnecessarily complicated, but perhaps this is part of the fun of keeping birds.

Although many different kinds of birds can be kept in captivity, as mentioned in Chapter 1, the most popular have been species from three large groups: (1) the parrot family, Psittacidae, which includes budgerigars; (2) the finch families: (*a*) Fringillidae—canaries, siskins, bullfinches, goldfinches, cardinals, and buntings; (*b*) Estrildidae*—waxbills, mannikins, avadavats, Java sparrows, and fire finches; (*c*) Ploceidae—weavers, house sparrows, and whydahs; and (3) the starling family, Sturnidae, which includes mynahs. By far the most numerous cage birds, at least in the U.S.A., are budgerigars and canaries.

FEEDING OF SEED-EATERS, OR HARDBILLS

BUDGERIGARS (*Melopsittacus undulatus*)

Budgerigars are primarily seed-eaters, although there have been reports that in the wild they eat some insects.[86]

Canary seed (*Phalaris canariensis*) and millet (*Panicum miliaceum*) are the basic components of most diets for budgerigars. The seeds are dehusked in a characteristic fashion and swallowed whole—the discarded husk

is not eaten, even when the birds are hungry. Many birds suffer from malnutrition because the owner does not realize that the seed cup is filled with an accumulation of empty husks rather than with whole seeds. The safest way to assure adequate nutrition is to empty the feed cup and refill it with fresh seeds each day.

In laboratory feeding tests (unpublished) budgerigars consumed approximately normal amounts of decorticated canary seed, millet, rape, sesame, and oats when these were fed in the absence of whole seeds. However, when whole and decorticated seeds were supplied simultaneously, the budgerigars showed a distinct preference for the whole seeds.

In free-choice feeding studies over a period of four months, nonbreeding adult budgerigars consumed about 6 gm. of seed and 3 ml. of water per day.[9] The average composition of the diet selected was: 31.7% canary seed, 21.7% red proso millet, 20.7% yellow proso millet, 19.3% white proso millet, and 6.6% chopped oat groats. The seed cups containing the different seeds were rotated throughout the test, because of the known effect of position on food selection. Similar results regarding quantities consumed and seeds selected were reported by Worden.[86]

Although canary seed and millet appear to be preferred, budgerigars will select a variety of other seeds if given the opportunity. In free-choice tests using 12 different seeds and wheat germ, nonbreeding adult budgerigars selected diets which contained 80% canary seed and millet, or 20% of seeds other than canary and millet.[9]

In addition to seeds, budgerigars will consume small amounts of supplementary foods such as greens, vegetables, and mashes. In a two-year study 50 adult nonbreeding budgerigars were maintained in excellent condition on a diet composed of the basic canary seed–millet mix, a supplementary seeds mixture, and a mash supplement.[9] The mash supplement contained dried egg yolk, dried bakery product, alfalfa leaf meal, milk protein, iodized salt, parsley flakes, wheat germ, yeast, vitamins A, D_3, and B_{12}, plus a little canary seed and millet to give the product an appearance more familiar to the birds. The amount of mash supplement consumed was approximately 14 per cent of the total food consumption. The same rations were also fed to flights of budgerigars for several months in preparation for breeding trials; pairs were then selected and consumption data recorded through laying, incubation of eggs, and rearing of the young. Consumption of the canary seed–millet mixture decreased during laying and incubation, with concurrently increased consumption of the mash supplement. While the nestlings were being fed, consumption of all dietary items was considerably above the level for nonbreeding adult birds. The data suggest

---

*The family Estrildidae has also been considered a subfamily (Estrildinae) of the family Ploceidae.

an increased need for extra protein, vitamins, and other elements from the mash supplement during the breeding period.

In other tests in our aviary (unpublished), the breeding performance on the diets described above was compared with performance on a simple canary seed–millet mixture. On the "complete" diet, as many as 14 consecutive nests were produced by a single pair in a period of two years without decrease in egg production, hatchability of eggs, or in viability or rate of growth of the young. By contrast, birds on the canary seed–millet mixture alone performed very poorly. Some pairs failed to breed; others produced only a few nests with low egg production, poor hatchability, high chick mortality, and poor growth rate for the young that survived.

Although nonbreeding adults can apparently remain in satisfactory condition for long periods on a canary seed–millet mixture, for optimal health it is recommended that supplementary foods be supplied at all times. "Treat" and "Condition Food" products (similar to the supplementary seeds mix and the mash supplement described above), which supply the required protein, vitamin, and mineral supplements, are available in supermarkets and other stores. They are easily fed and are thus more likely to be administered regularly than are those supplements that require considerable effort for their preparation. New owners should be advised to feed budgerigars the packaged seed mixtures prepared by reliable birdseed firms.[68] This not only ensures a variety of seeds, with greater probability of a good diet than if the owner chooses a diet based on fancy, but also provides a better nutritional background in event of illness. Cage birds should not be fed at the table; if necessary, they should be locked in the cage at mealtime. Well-meaning owners often tend to "treat" their pets with cake, candy, and alcoholic beverages, thereby causing them to lose their appetite for natural foods.

The basic commercial seed mixture for budgerigars is usually millet and canary seed in a ratio ranging from 60/40 to 40/60.[86] The composition of the different brands of "Treat" and "Condition Food" products may differ considerably—some are merely mixtures of seeds, whereas others may contain supplements of high quality protein, vitamins, and minerals. For example, one brand of "Parakeet Condition Food" lists the following ingredients: millet, oats, canary seed, flax, soy grits, teazle, and anise seed. The list of ingredients of another brand includes: oats, millet, niger, canary seed, caraway, flax, and sesame seeds, dried bakery product, dried egg yolk, vegetable oil, oyster shell, iodized salt, wheat germ meal, dried whey, alfalfa leaf meal, parsley flakes, Torula dried yeast, vitamin A palmitate, D-activated

animal sterol, and vitamin B_{12}. Obviously, these two products are quite different in nutritive value, even though both are labeled "Parakeet Condition Food." A careful study of the label should indicate the preparation that would supply the most vitamin, mineral, and protein supplements to a normal seed diet. As applied to some commercial products, the terms "Treat" and "Condition Food" are really misnomers, for they carry the connotation that these foods are basically non-essential and need be provided only occasionally, as a sweet dessert would be, or when the bird is "out of condition." Actually, these mixtures are necessary sources of nutrition and should be fed as regularly as the basic mixture.[40]

In some cases, seed mixtures have been treated with vitamins and minerals. Actually, such mixtures may not provide the nutritional values claimed since the birds remove the husks before they swallow the kernels. Statements of ingredients and guaranteed analysis values provide useful information, but the values refer to the whole mixture, including husks, whereas the portion actually selected and swallowed by the bird may be quite different from the whole mix. The husk may account for about 20 per cent of the weight of the seed in some millets, and over 50 per cent in sunflower seed.

If the owner does not wish to use commercial supplemental foods, a number of useful dietary items are available. Greens such as chickweed, dandelion, spinach, carrot tops, and the like are valuable sources of vitamins and minerals. Greens should be washed to remove residues of herbicides and pesticides, and care should be exercised regarding the amount fed, since excessive amounts will cause diarrhea. Vegetables and fruits such as carrots, celery, and apple may be relished by the birds. Some authors caution against the use of green or tart fruits. Vitamins may also be supplied by adding pediatric vitamin preparations (such as Upjohn's Zymadrops) to the drinking water. This may not be successful, because of refusal of some birds to drink medicated water. Also, the dosage received depends on the amount of water consumed; sick birds may not drink normal amounts of water, and therefore do not receive adequate amounts of the supplemental vitamins when they are most needed. Milk and eggs are valuable sources of protein. Breeders frequently give breeding stock milk or diluted milk (equal parts of milk and water) in place of water. Crumbled hard-cooked egg is a commonly used supplemental food. In some cases, a soft food made from precooked cereal, egg, and milk is valuable for young birds, birds in poor condition, or sick birds, as well as for breeding birds.

The baby budgerigar, as mentioned earlier, is fed a nutritive "milk," commonly called "crop milk," which appears to be secreted by the proventriculus of the hen. Taylor[77] reported that the crop contents of chicks from "good rearing parents" contained 24–26 per cent protein on a dry matter basis, compared with 19.2 per cent protein in the seed fed to the parents. By contrast, the crop contents of chicks from French Molt producers contained only 20–22 per cent protein. These figures indicate there is a difference in the chemical composition of the "milk" from different hens, regardless of whether or not the incidence of French Molt is related to protein level.

After they leave the nest, baby budgerigars may have difficulty finding seed in the seed cup. There should be plenty of feed in a flat dish on the floor of the cage; after a few days, the baby finds the feed cup and the dish may be removed from the floor. During this period it is important that supplementary foods as well as the seed mix be supplied at all times—not only because of the high nutritive requirements, but also to strengthen good habits in selection of foods. Some birds seem to prefer to eat from a feed cup in a certain location. One bird, supplied with three feed cups containing three different foods, would eat whatever was placed in the cups in two of the locations, but completely ignored the third cup, regardless of what it contained. In such cases, it would be desirable to mix the seed and supplementary foods, or to rotate positions of the feed cups regularly.

Excessive amounts of food and lack of exercise will result in obesity. Increased exercise (freedom of flight) is the best means of preventing this condition. Altman and Altman[2] recommended feeding obese budgerigars only white millet with water-soluble vitamins supplied in the drinking water.

PARROTS OTHER THAN BUDGERIGARS

The parrot family (Psittacidae) includes about 325 species.[24] Fortunately, the food requirements for all except the subfamily Loriinae are similar. Nearly all parrots, macaws, and cockatoos may be fed a seed mixture as follows[53]:

> one part sunflower seed
> one part hemp seed
> two parts canary seed
> one part large millet seed
> one-half part white millet seed
> one part peanuts

Fruits such as grapes, apples, and pears should be given in moderation and, in addition, other nuts and green food should be supplied.

Bates and Busenbark[6] suggest that small parrots such as lovebirds (*Agapornis*), parrotlets (*Forpus*), and cocka-

tiels (*Nymphicus hollandicus*) be fed the same diet as that used for budgerigars. Some sunflower seed may also be given. Medium-sized parrots, such as conures and some parakeets, may also be given the same diet, with the addition of sunflower seed, and a variety of fresh fruits and vegetables. Large parrots, such as amazons, cockatoos, and macaws, can be fed the same diet as the medium-sized parrots, with the addition of peanuts, pumpkin seed, pigeon feed, chillies, and a little raw meat or mealworms occasionally.

The feeding of lories and lorikeets, of the subfamily Loriinae, family Psittacidae, is discussed later under the heading, "Feeding of Fruit- and Nectar-Eaters."

Some species of birds may have unusual dietary requirements for breeding. The thick-billed parrot (*Rhynchopsitta pachyrhyncha*) has been kept at the San Diego Zoo for a number of years, but this species did not breed until the birds were supplied with piñon nuts obtained from pine cones from the Chiricahua Mountains of Arizona.[4]

Whenever new birds are acquired, they should be isolated from other birds for a time to be reasonably certain that the new stock is healthy. Imported parrots are usually given an antibiotic prophylactically as a safeguard against psittacosis. Buckley[14] reported the loss of a number of blue-crowned hanging parrots (*Loriculus galgulus*) from candidiasis after treatment with chlortetracycline hydrochloride,* whereas treatment with an antimycotic combined with tetracycline† was apparently safe and successful. Other imported parrots (*Agapornis* spp.) had been lost under similar circumstances.

In another case, the weights of *Agapornis* decreased steadily after chlortetracycline hydrochloride treatment was instituted in the quarantine period.[25] When *Lactobacillus acidophilus*‡ was added to the diet, weights increased, even though the antibiotic treatment was continued. It would appear that changes in intestinal flora resulting from antibiotic administration can have serious consequences.

CANARIES (*Serinus canarius*)

Canary seed (*Phalaris canariensis*), rape seed (*Brassica rapa*), and millet seed (*Panicum miliaceum*) are the basic components of most canary diets. Many other seeds are also used by fanciers to bring the birds into breeding condition, to tighten and gloss the plumage for exhibition, or to improve color. Like other seed-eaters, canaries remove the husk and swallow the ker-

---

*Aureomycin: American Cyanamid Co., Princeton, N.J.
†Mysteclin F: E. R. Squibb & Sons, New York, N.Y.
‡Lactinex—a standardized viable mixed culture of *Lactobacillus acidophilus* and *L. bulgaricus:* Hynson, Westcott and Dunning, Inc., Baltimore, Maryland.

nel whole. Grit, cuttlefish bone, and water should be supplied at all times.

In free-choice feeding studies over a period of four months, nonbreeding adult canaries consumed about 3.4 gm. of seeds and 5.4 ml. of water per day.[8] The average composition of the diet selected was: 47% canary seed, 27.7% rape seed, 5.6% red proso millet, 5.4% white proso millet, and 14.3% yellow proso millet. In similar studies with 25 young canaries just removed from the nesting cages, the percentages of seeds selected and the quantities consumed per day over a period of four months were essentially the same as for the nonbreeding adult canaries. In all studies, seed cups were rotated regularly to eliminate biased selection due to feed cup position.

In addition to seeds, canaries will consume small quantities of supplementary foods such as greens, vegetables, and mashes. In the study with young canaries,[8] the birds were found to consume an average of 0.34 gm. of a mash supplement per day, this amounting to approximately 10 per cent of the total food consumption. The mash supplement contained bakery crumbs, dried egg yolk, dried milk protein product, wheat germ meal, alfalfa leaf meal, dried yeast, parsley flakes, soy grits, vegetable oil, iodized salt, and supplements of vitamins A, D_3, and B_{12}.

In another free-choice feeding study in the R. T. French Company laboratory (unpublished), six pairs of adult canaries were offered eight different seeds plus a supplemental mash. The average composition of the diet selected over a period of five weeks was: 26.1% niger, 16% canary seed, 15.7% oat groats, 10.1% rape seed, 9.9% sesame seed, 8% yellow proso millet, 7.3% mash supplement, 5.4% flax seed, and 1.5% blue poppy seed. In this study, with a larger variety of oil seeds available, the birds selected a diet containing over 50 per cent of oil seeds compared with 28 per cent of oil seeds in a previous test. By contrast, budgerigars and most small finches tend to select mainly carbohydrate seeds.

Many nonbreeding adult canaries receive nothing but a seeds mixture and appear to remain in satisfactory condition. However, for optimal health, it is recommended that supplementary foods be supplied at all times. There are various commercially available "Condition Food," "Song Food," and "Molting Food" products which will supply the required protein, vitamin, and mineral supplements. As with budgerigars, Siegmund[68] suggests that new owners of finch-type birds be advised to feed the packaged products of reliable birdseed firms.

Fanciers use many special foods for bringing birds into breeding condition and while they are rearing the young. A variety of seeds, such as niger, poppy (maw), teazle, and lettuce, are used for these purposes, and the feeding methods may vary considerably. For example, some feed niger during the breeding season only; others feed it the year around. Some feed niger only to the hens; others feed it to both sexes. In some instances soaked or sprouted seeds are advocated; Brooks[13] recommended that soaked seed and soft food be given to young canaries until the age of 7 weeks, and cautioned against the use of hard seed before 6 weeks of age. On the other hand, Douglas[26] claimed better results were obtained by feeding only hard seed and greens—no soaked seed, egg food, or soft food.

Flowers and Flowers[31] suggest that nonbreeding adult canaries should be fed only a seed mixture and green food, considering that egg food is too fattening for such birds. Egg food, however, is considered the most important item for successful rearing of young birds. It is prepared by boiling an egg 20–30 minutes, mashing it as finely as possible, and mixing it with 2 tablespoonfuls of cracker crumbs or toasted stale bread crumbs. If necessary, a little water may be added. A commercial nestling food may be used instead of the cracker crumbs. "Milk sop" (crackers soaked in milk) is often fed every second day.

Blythe[11] suggested the following formula for a soft food for breeding finches:

> 1 lb. bread rusk
> 2 oz. non-fat dry milk
> 1 oz. wheat germ (Bemax)
> 1 oz. bran
> 1 oz. peanut oil
> 1 oz. cod liver oil

The mixture is moistened with water until it is crumbly, and it is fed with seed mix and green food. For soft-billed birds 1 oz. dried yeast and 2 oz. fish meal can also be added.

The color of canary plumage is affected by the diet. If one wishes to color-feed birds, it must be done during the molting season. Red pepper has customarily been used as a color food for canaries, with green food given in addition because it "helps set the color."[31] However, red factor canary fanciers are not allowed to use red pepper,[81] even though, according to Dean,[21] red pepper does not intensify the color of red factors.

Canaries have the ability to convert xanthophyll into the yellow pigment of feathers, and the hooded siskin produces red color from carotene. Red factors have the ability to convert both xanthophyll and carotene into the feather colors, the net effect depending on the relative amounts of each consumed. Since red pepper does not contain carotene, Dean[21] maintains it cannot intensify the red color of red factors; for maximal plumage color he[22] suggests feeding 75% niger and 25% groats or oatmeal, plus carrot.

Swallow[74] recommended feeding red factor canaries as follows: 1 hopper canary seed, 2 hoppers niger, and 1 hopper oat groats, plus plenty of green food and sliced carrots, and a little soft food once a week. The soft food contained sausage rusk (or commercial conditioning food), baby cereal, raw egg, milk, and carrot.

On the other hand, Murray[46] states that it is taboo for red factor fanciers to feed carrot to bring out the natural color of their stock, although it apparently is in order for non-color-fed varieties of canaries to be given lutein to help bring out their natural color.

Depth-of-color potential appears to be genetically controlled, but proper diet is required for its full expression. The question of what constitutes color-feeding seems somewhat controversial.

FINCHES OTHER THAN CANARIES

Like canaries, other members of the finch families are mainly seed-eaters, although some species also eat live food on a daily basis, and many others require it at breeding time. The basic diet should therefore consist of a seed mix, dietary supplements, cuttlefish bone, grit, and water.

The seed mix for finches generally contains millets, canary seed, and occasionally oats. Thus most finches do well on a budgerigar seed mix.[23] Morris[43] found a definite correlation between size of seed selected and beak size of finches, whereas there was almost no correlation between size of seed selected and body size. In Morris's studies the Cuban finch (*Tiaris canora*) selected about 9% canary seed (*Phalaris canariensis*), 10% white proso millet (*Panicum miliaceum*), and 81% small yellow millet (*Setaria italica*). Goodwin,[35] however, found the amounts selected were 60% proso millet and 32% canary seed, the remainder being Condition Food, rape, flax, and niger. The difference between the findings in the two studies undoubtedly reflects the preference of this species for the smaller-sized seeds (*Setaria italica*) when they are available. Goodwin also recorded that these finches took small amounts of green food and large numbers of cluster flies (*Pollenia*) when they were available. Most finches, except canaries and possibly some other members of the family Fringillidae, consume very little rape seed. A mixed collection of small finches (lavender, society, zebra, cutthroat and pintail whydah) selected a diet composed of 14.1% canary seed, 0.6% rape seed, 31.8% red proso millet, 23.2% white proso millet, and 30.3% yellow proso millet.[8]

By contrast, canaries selected about 47% canary seed, 27.7% rape seed, 5.6% red proso millet, 5.4% white proso millet, and 14.3% yellow proso millet.

The dietary supplements may include commercial "Parakeet" or "Canary Condition Food," green food, fruits, and live food. "Mockingbird Food" or softbill meal (see section on "Feeding of Softbills, or Insect-Eaters") may be used to supply the insect requirements of many finches. Outdoor flight spaces are often planted with shrubs to attract insects as well as to beautify the space. Bates and Busenbark[7] suggest the following as satisfactory for aviary use: olive trees, bottle bushes, *Pittosporum*, privets, *Euonymus*, *Forsythia*, *Cotoneaster*, magnolia, honeysuckle, small bamboo, and *Pyracantha*. Other plants recommended by Murphy[45] include *Escallonia*, *Viburnum*, azaleas, clematis, roses, and spiraea. Poisonous plants, such as oleander and castor bean, should be avoided. Plants can be placed in tubs, which makes it easier to remove them from the aviary for cleaning or for restoration of vitality.

The family Fringillidae contains the subfamilies Carduelinae (goldfinch, canary, siskin, linnet, hawfinch, greenfinch, bullfinch), Emberizinae (buntings), and Richmondeninae (cardinals, some buntings, and a few finches). Members of the emberizine group are said to be decidedly more insectivorous than other finches.[36] Insects are a necessity for breeding birds, and soft food should be available at all times. Live food is also required by richmondenine and some cardueline species while breeding and rearing young.

The family Estrildidae includes waxbills (*Estrilda* and *Pytilia* spp.), grassfinches (*Zonaeginthus*, *Poephila*, and *Erythrura* spp.), and mannikins (*Padda*, *Amadina*, and *Lonchura* spp.). The term "mannikin" must be distinguished from the term "manakin"; "manakin" refers to species of the family Pipridae, which are allied to the Cotingidae and Tyrannidae and are largely insect- and fruit-eaters. The members of the family Estrildidae are generally seed-eaters, and most species prefer small yellow or spray millet. Small insects are very useful dietary items, especially during breeding. Small mealworms, gentles (maggots of the blowfly or bluebottle fly), spiders, and small flies are generally accepted readily. A fine-textured softbill meal is also very valuable. The Java sparrow (*Padda oryzivora*), one of the largest of the estrildines, does not show the marked preference for spray millet which is exhibited by the smaller species. In free-choice tests, Java sparrows chose 30.6% canary seed, 26.3% white proso millet, and 43.1% small yellow millet.[43] Similar results were obtained by Bice,[8] who reported consumption of 34.2% canary seed, 3.6% rape seed, 15.7% red proso millet,

23.7% white proso millet, and 22.8% yellow proso millet.

The family Ploceidae includes two subfamilies: Ploceinae (weavers, house sparrows, and bishops) and Viduinae (combassous and whydahs). The weavers eat mainly canary seed, millet, and green food. In captivity the red color of some weavers tends to fade, presumably because of dietary deficiencies. Ant eggs and grated raw carrot are supposedly of value in enabling them to retain good color. Egg and biscuit food is also recommended. While breeding, the birds require live food or softbill meal. Whydahs feed almost exclusively on seed; a few will accept insects, but very few show any interest in green food.[71]

There is still much to be learned about the exact food requirements of finches. It would seem that a varied diet, with provision of an ample supply of high quality protein, vitamins, and minerals, would be the best means of ensuring health and longevity of the birds.

FEEDING OF SOFTBILLS OR INSECT-EATERS

Different species of soft-billed birds vary in their food requirements. Swallows (Hirundinidae) eat practically nothing but insects; tanagers (Thraupidae) eat mainly fruit and some insects; thrushes (Turdidae) and larks (Alaudidae) eat small fruits, insects, and seeds; pigeons and doves (Columbidae) feed almost entirely on seeds.

Aviculturists have repeatedly stressed the desirability of feeding insectivorous birds large quantities of a variety of live foods, such as flies, spiders, worms, moths, snails, butterflies, beetles, and cockroaches. Insectivorous birds obviously are adapted physiologically to the nutritional elements composing insects which render the natural items more valuable than the most elaborate laboratory foods. The insects are generally swallowed whole, with any chitinous parts being cast up as pellets.

Many methods of capturing insects that have been developed by entomologists can be used by aviculturists.[30] However, these methods may be of little value during the winter, when very few insects are to be found. At such times, methods of culturing a variety of insects will be useful. Methods have been described for culturing crickets, wax moths, house flies, and blowflies,[30] locusts,[34] bluebottle maggots,[20] mealworms,[70] and moths and beetles.[42]

If the birds are maintained in an outdoor aviary, insects may be attracted by ripe fruit, meat, or various types of shrubbery. It is desirable to use dwarf shrubs planted in tubs that can be removed from the aviary for cleaning. Softbills do not eat the leaves of shrub-

bery, and many types of shrubs are suitable for use in aviaries.

Mealworms (*Tenebrio* spp.) have been widely used by fanciers of soft-billed birds. They can be purchased in some pet shops or they may be raised in a simple culture of bran with a little apple or lettuce added to provide moisture. Mealworms are considered a highly concentrated food, and it is recommended that only limited quantities be fed. Too many worms will make the bird fat, and its appetite for other foods will be diminished. A thrush-sized bird might be given 3 to 6 worms per day during the off season, with the amount being doubled or tripled when the bird is in full song. For small soft-billed birds, small mealworms should be used, or large mealworms should be placed in boiling water for a few minutes to soften the skin and then they should be cut into small pieces.[48]

Bee larvae (*Apis mellifera*) are considered excellent food for softbills. They were readily accepted by American goldfinch fledglings (*Spinus tristis*), and were used as a base for hand-rearing of Traills' flycatchers (*Empidonax traillii*). Methods of culturing bee larvae were described by Gary *et al.*[32]

Although it may be possible to purchase, capture, or culture some live food, it will generally be necessary to use an "insectile food" as partial or complete replacement for live food. Various commercial preparations known as mockingbird food, softbill meal, or insectile food are available in some areas. Such products may contain dried insects, ant eggs, ground seeds, suet, and other materials suitable for softbills. The mix is usually moistened with freshly grated carrot or apple to make a crumbly, but not wet, mass before it is fed to the birds. Some finely ground boiled beef or hard-boiled egg may be added. Various fresh fruits in season are usually given separately.[48]

For those who wish to mix their own insectile foods, a number of formulas are available. Ficken and Dilger[30] kept several species of thrush (Turdidae) in perfect condition on an inexpensive mixture consisting of equal parts of dog meal, dried flies, and turkey or chick starter mash. The three components were mixed with cottonseed oil until slightly moist, which greatly increased palatability of the mixture. After it is mixed the food should be used in a few days, because the unsaturated fatty acids of the cottonseed oil cause oxidation of vitamin E and to a lesser extent of vitamin A; this oxidizing tendency may be essentially eliminated by addition of an antioxidant.

The following formula by T. G. Taylor was reported by Carr[17]:

3½ lb. fine biscuit meal or sausage rusk
8 oz. dry whole milk

8 oz. wheat germ
8 oz. white fish meal
4 oz. dried yeast
½ oz. Adexolin (vitamins A and D) in 5 oz. peanut oil

The whole mixture should have a crumbly consistency when fed.

Another formula, reported by Tanner,[75] consists of the combination of two mixtures:

A. Combine 4 oz. ant eggs
           4 oz. dried flies or shrimp meal
           3 oz. melted drippings
B. Combine 8 oz. powdered rich tea biscuits
           3 oz. melted honey
           3 oz. egg powder

Mix A and B. A little cod liver oil and Bemax cereal may be added. A useful but perishable addition to this mixture is finely scraped raw meat made into small pellets.

Woodward[85] recommended the following in place of live food: one third of the ration should be minced raw lean meat, the balance being composed of equal parts of soft food, poultry crumbs and fine puppy meal which have been soaked with hot water until soft. Grated carrot, finely chopped lettuce, soaked raisins, and shrimp or tinned sardines may also be added.

In the wild, insectivorous birds search continually for food; they must capture it or starve. They seem to be psychologically adapted to eating whenever food is available. When such birds are given food *ad libitum,* they tend to overeat and quickly become obese. This problem is much more serious in birds kept in cages than in those kept in aviaries. According to Dilger (see Chapter 3), the only solution seems to be restriction of the amount of food made available to the bird. Woodward[84] also observed that aviary life is too easy, and that soft-billed birds in captivity have a great tendency to overeat and become obese.

In addition to live food and "insectile mix," there are many food items which may be used to give variety in the menu. Hard-boiled egg may be mashed and mixed with the insectile food or fed separately. Peanut butter is relished by many softbills. Precooked baby cereal or sponge cake can be mixed with milk to form a nutritious thick mush. Fruits of various kinds form an essential element in the daily diet of nearly every softbill.[48] Some authors recommend using only sweet, ripe fruits, and caution against the use of tart or unripe fruits.

Most softbills can be fed a basic diet consisting of a standard insectile mix plus fresh fruit and some live food if available. Additions to this basic diet can be made as needed. The basic diet should be satisfactory

for bulbuls (Pycnonotidae), mynahs and starlings (Sturnidae), mockingbirds (Mimidae), and robins or thrushes (Turdidae). A few softbills will eat some seeds in addition to the basic diet. Included in this group are larks (Alaudidae), tits (Paridae), and the Pekin robin or Pekin nightingale (*Leiothrix lutea*, family Timaliidae). Others that are largely fruit- and insect-eaters include flycatchers (Muscicapidae), fruit-suckers (Aegithinidae), orioles (Oriolidae), quetzals and trogons (Trogonidae), solitaires or clarinos (Turdidae), sugar-birds or honeycreepers (Coerebidae), tanagers (Thraupidae), and troupials or hangnests (Icteridae). The fruit-eaters relish a honeyed milk sop which is composed of a sponge cake or Farina moistened with milk and sweetened with honey.

FEEDING OF FRUIT- AND NECTAR-EATERS

This group of birds includes lories and lorikeets (Psittacidae), toucans, toucanettes, and aracaris (Ramphastidae), hummingbirds (Trochilidae), sunbirds (Nectariniidae), honey-eaters (Meliphagidae), white-eyes (Zosteropidae), honeycreepers (Coerebidae), and flower-peckers (Dicaeidae). These birds feed on the sugary liquids (nectar) found in the corolla of flowers and on the insects found in or with the nectar. In addition, sweet ripe fruit is an important part of their diet.

Lories and lorikeets of the subfamily Loriinae of the family Psittacidae and other nectar-feeding species may be fed nectar composed of Mellin's Food,* evaporated milk, and honey (1 teaspoonful of each in 1 cup of water), plus sweet fruit. In addition, some species will eat canary seed and sunflower seed.[53] For lories and lorikeets Bronson[12] suggests brown or wild rice boiled in milk, with brown sugar or honey added. Fruits may be mixed with mashed potato. Fruit cake, sponge cake, or whole wheat bread soaked in milk and sweetened with honey is valuable. Fresh fruits, berries, canned baby food, and canned fruit salad are also recommended. The food dishes should be washed daily and refilled with fresh material.

There are a number of formulas for nectar, many of them being based on Mellin's Food, condensed milk, and honey. The New York Zoological Park uses two different formulas for feeding hummingbirds:

Formula A:

Mellin's Food	4 teaspoons
Honey	5 teaspoons
Condensed milk	1 teaspoon
Beef extract	5 ml.

*Mellin's Food: a maltose dextrin mixture with added thiamine mononitrate, ferric glycerol phosphate, and potassium bicarbonate.

	Vitamins (Multiple)	4 drops
	Warm water	1 quart
Formula B:	Honey	5 teaspoons
	Beef extract	5 ml.
	Vitamins (Multiple)	4 drops
	Warm water	1 quart

A ruby-throated hummingbird (*Archilocus colubris*) weighing 2.5 gm. consumed 121.8 ml. of formula in 7 days: 112 ml. of formula A fed in the morning and 9.8 ml. of formula B fed in the evening.[72]

Sunbirds were fed the following diet at the London Zoo[76]: nectar food, grapes, and a few mealworms. The nectar food was made by mixing 1 level dessertspoonful of baby food, 1 heaped dessertspoonful of sweetened condensed milk, and 1½ dessertspoonfuls of honey with ¾ pint of boiling water. (A dessertspoonful equals 8 ml.)

Honey milk sop (sponge cake or precooked cereal moistened with milk and sweetened with honey) is a valuable dietary item for some members of this group. Fresh fruit, berries, canned baby food, or canned fruit salad may also be used.

If the fruit- and nectar-eaters can be kept in a large, well-planted aviary, some nectar may be available from the flowers, which will also attract insects. Ripe fruit is often used to attract insects, such as fruit flies (*Drosophila* spp.)

FEEDING OF ZOO BIRDS

The general principles outlined above for feeding seed-eaters, insect-eaters, and nectar-feeders would naturally apply also to feeding birds of these classes in zoos. Food requirements for a number of species are tabulated by Siegmund.[69]

In addition to birds that may be kept in cages, a number of species are frequently kept in aviaries or other enclosures. These include game birds, the most common types of which belong to the order of gallinaceous birds, such as pheasants, partridges, quail, peafowl, guinea fowl, guans, and turkeys. Others that adapt to enclosures are cranes, trumpeters, rails, bustards, tinamous, rheas, and emus. All of these are essentially grain-eaters, and they may be fed various commercial poultry feeds. They may also pick up insects, which constitute an important supplement during breeding. Cranes and rails may require a protein supplement such as fish meal to keep them in optimal condition.[58]

Starter and breeder diets for pheasants were reported by Scott,[64] who found that the amino acid requirements of ring-necked pheasants and bobwhite quail were similar to those of turkey poults when the requirements were expressed as percentages of the dietary protein. Diets for wild waterfowl under game farm conditions were reported by Scott and Holm.[66] These diets were similar to those that produced excellent growth in domestic ducks. The protein requirement of wild ducklings of several species was found to be no greater than 19 per cent of the diet.

Ratcliffe[59] reported on two basic diets that had been used successfully for omnivores and carnivores at the Philadelphia Zoological Gardens for five years.

The ration for omnivores was made up of 1 part of ground boiled horsemeat and 9 parts of a mixture of the following ingredients:

Rolled oats	20%
Whole wheat meal	20%
Soybean oil meal	20%
Peanut oil meal	10%
Yellow corn meal	10%
Dry buttermilk	5%
Dried brewer's yeast	5%
Alfalfa leaf meal (dehyd.)	5%
Oyster shell flour	2%
Iodized salt	2%
Cod liver oil conc.	1%

These materials were mixed in bulk and the mixture was used as needed. The ground meat was blended later with the dry ingredients and enough meat broth was added to form a stiff mash. The mash was pressed into shallow pans, refrigerated overnight, and cut into pieces appropriate to the size of the animal. A large number of species of Passeriformes, Psittaciformes, Columbiformes, Galliformes, and Anseriformes were fed this diet (which made up about 70 per cent of their intake), supplemented with green vegetables, fruits, and sprouted grains. During the five-year period reported, the birds showed noteworthy improvement in plumage colors and lessened morbidity and mortality.

Carnivores received a ration containing 60% ground raw horsemeat, 10% ground green vegetables, and 30% of a mixture of the following:

Soybean oil meal	30%
Peanut oil meal	25%
Dry buttermilk	25%
Oyster shell flour	6%
Alfalfa leaf meal (dehyd.)	4%
Dried brewer's yeast	4%
Cod liver oil conc.	4%
Iodized salt	2%

This ration was fed to hawks (Accipitriformes) and owls (Strigiformes). These birds did not have an opportunity for breeding, but the drop in mortality rate in comparison with that occurring previously on other diets was so pronounced that it warranted special mention.

Naether[49] reported a basic ration, composed of many ingredients which supplement one another, used by Hans Wackernagel at the Basel Zoological Gardens for feeding many species of birds. The composition of the basic ration is as follows:

Ground corn	18%
Ground wheat	11%
Ground barley	10%
Rolled oats	10%
Peanut meal	8%
Soybean meal	10%
Nettle leaf meal	6%
Dried yeast	8%
Skimmed milk powder	10%
Stabilized fat	5%
Bone meal	2%
Iodized salt	0.9%
Trace mineral mixture	0.1%
Vitamin mixture (including vitamin C)	1%

This basic ration is mixed with other ingredients as follows:

Basic ration	50%
Minced cooked meat	20%
Ground carrots	20%
Ground hard-boiled eggs with shells	7%
Supplement (one part Aurofac,* one part fat-soluble extract of alfalfa, four parts dried yeast)	3%

The composition of the final mixture is approximately:

Crude protein	19%
Crude fat	6%
Crude fiber	2%
Calcium	0.6%
Phosphorus	0.4%
Aureomycin	20 mg./kg.
Vitamin C	150 mg./kg.

The moist, friable mixture is supplemented with seeds or minced meat to satisfy the requirements of different species. The ration has proved its worth for both maintenance and rearing. Ducks, geese, fowl, ostriches, ibises, plovers, avocets, kookaburras, and various parrots are among the birds that have been fed this ration; Naether states that the rearing of bolectus parrots (= eclectus?) is proof of the suitability of the ration.

Most of the red, orange, and yellow colors in birds' feathers are the result of carotenoids, which apparently are not synthesized by the birds but must be present

in the food and are merely deposited unchanged or transformed by oxidation. Maintaining natural coloration is a major problem in captive birds; the brilliant colors tend to fade, possibly from lack of specific carotenoids in the diet. Many different substances have been used to improve the color of feathers, including ground carrots, carrot juice, fresh beets, Scottish seaweed meal, and ground shells of lobsters and shrimp. Naether[49] reported marked intensification of plumage color in the scarlet ibis (*Eudocimus ruber*) and scarlet cock-of-the-rock (*Rupicola peruviana sanguinolenta*) on the diet described in the foregoing paragraph.

Poulsen[55] obtained good results from feeding paprika (*Capsicum annuum*) to flamingos (Phoenicopteridae) at the Copenhagen Zoo. Beginning a month before the molt, a handful of ground sweet peppers was added daily to a pail of soupy food mixture. The red portions of the skin on the legs and bill retained their natural color, and the feather color was practically the same as that in wild flamingos. Improvement was also visible in scarlet ibis, scarlet cock-of-the-rock, and scarlet tanagers (*Ramphocelus brasilius*).

Wackernagel[82] reported improvement of the colors of sunbirds (Nectariniidae) resulting from addition to the diet of a synthetic carotenoid, canthaxanthin. Spectacular results also occurred in a hybrid canary (*Serinus canarius* × *Spinus cucullatus*, or red siskin). The scarlet ibis and scarlet cock-of-the-rock responded to a fat-soluble extract of alfalfa with marked deepening of red color, although full development of natural color was not obtained.

Quackenbush *et al.*[56] found that in skin pigmentation of birds the xanthophylls of yellow corn are utilized more efficiently than those of alfalfa.

Touracos (Musophagidae) are unusual in having a true green pigment in the plumage and in having a red pigment which is due to uroporphyrin and its copper salt, turacin, rather than to carotenoids.[28] The green pigment, turacoverdin, is an oxidized form of turacin. Possibly the coloration of touraco feathers is influenced by the mineral content of the diet. In the wild, touracos eat mainly fruit, tree buds, shoots, green leaves, and insects.

MOLTING AND FEATHER PROBLEMS IN RELATION TO NUTRITION

Molting is a process of renewing the protective feather coating. During molting, a new feather grows in the skin under the old one, emerging after the old feather falls out. A single papilla may produce different sorts of feathers, depending on age of the bird and the time of year, as illustrated by the inconspicu-

---

*Aurofac—Aureomycin food additive compound: American Cyanamid Co., Princeton, N.J.

ous plumage in winter contrasted with the display or summer plumage of certain birds.

Most birds keep the whole plumage for a year, although some renew it twice yearly. In some cases the small body feathers are molted twice while the large wing and tail feathers are molted only once a year. A few birds keep the wing feathers two years.[37] Juvenal plumage is frequently molted after a few weeks and replaced by feathers more like those of the adults; the wing and tail feathers usually are not involved in this first molt.

During the molt, the bird generally leads a quiet life. Since feathers are largely protein in nature, there is an increased need for high quality dietary protein at this time. Kendeigh[38] studied the effect of the protein level of the diet on molting in house sparrows. The birds were on a 10-hour light period per day and were given isocaloric diets containing different amounts of protein. In birds on the 3% protein diet molting was repressed in both intensity and duration; birds on the 5% protein diet molted at an intermediate level, and those on 9% protein had a normal extensive molt. There was no consistent difference in body weight of birds on the different levels of protein, nor did the energy metabolized at the same temperature show differences related to the level of protein in the diet.

It is not unusual for canaries to stop singing during the molt and to be slow at regaining song after the molt, especially if the diet is suboptimal.

Deficiencies of several vitamins produce alterations of skin and feathers; deficiencies of some amino acids and minerals have also been implicated in such disorders. The first step in treatment of these problems should be to ensure an adequate diet. Some of the commercial "Condition Foods" will provide the necessary high quality protein, vitamin, and mineral supplements; however, they are of no value unless they are consumed. Because of the ultraconservative feeding habits of birds, their reluctance to eat new foods, and the known effect of feed cup position on feed selection, it may be necessary to interchange feed cup positions regularly and/or mix the supplemental foods with the basic fare. In some instances feather picking has been controlled by adding salt to the diet for a few days—about 2% salt to an all-mash diet, or 4% to a mash fed with grain.[10]

IDENTIFICATION AND COMPOSITION OF VARIOUS SEEDS

Birds eat a wide variety of seeds, particularly seeds of the cereal or grass family (Gramineae). The grain or kernel of a cereal is a nutlike fruit, or caryopsis. The fruit contains only one seed, and, as it ripens, the ovary wall or pericarp becomes rather firmly attached to the wall of the seed proper and forms the outer tissue, or the bran. The floral envelopes, or chaffy parts, within which the caryopsis develops, persist to maturity. In some cereals such as rice, oats, and barley, some of the chaffy structures envelop the caryopsis so closely that they remain attached when the grain is threshed. These structures constitute the hull of such grains, which are said to be "covered." In the common wheats, rye, hull-less barley, and corn, the caryopsis separates readily from the floral envelopes when the grain is threshed. Such grains are said to be "naked."[33]

Physical Characteristics of Various Seeds

The more common seeds used in feeding cage birds are described below, and most of them are illustrated in Figure 7-1. The descriptions are based on Winton and Winton[83] and Geddes.[33] The numbers on the paragraphs correspond to those of the pictures of the respective seeds in the Figure.

THE GRASS FAMILY (GRAMINEAE)

1–3. **COMMON,** or **PROSO, MILLET** (*Panicum miliaceum* L.). There are three common varieties of millets, differing mainly in the color of the husk, which may be white, yellow, or red. The seed is about 3 mm. long × 2 mm. wide, flattened and ovoid in shape, and tightly enclosed in a smooth, lustrous, hard and coriaceous lemma (flowering glume) and palea (or palet).

4. **SPRAY,** or **FOXTAIL, MILLET** (*Setaria italica* Beauv.). There are several varieties, differing chiefly in color of the grain (yellowish, reddish, or blackish). The seed is enclosed in envelopes which have fine transverse wrinkles (evident under a lens) except on the wings of the palea, which are smooth. At maturity the envelopes are dark-colored and tightly applied to the fruit. The kernel is a flattened ovoid shape, about 2 × 1.5 × 1 mm.

5. **CANARY SEED** (*Phalaris canariensis* L.). The fruit is brown, and tightly enveloped by lustrous, light buff-colored lemma and palea. It has a flattened, ovoid shape, about 5 × 2 mm. Occasionally there may be two boat-shaped clasping empty glumes attached. Under a lens, stiff hairs may be seen on both sides of the tip of the five-nerved shiny lemma and along the back of the palea.

6. **WHEAT** (*Triticum vulgare* Vill.). The kernel varies in color from light buff or yellow to red-brown and in shape from blunt spindle-shaped to ovate. It may be rounded or somewhat triangular in cross section, the dorsal side generally being rounded, and the ventral side having a deep groove or crease extending the entire length of the kernel. At the apex, which is commonly narrower than the base, is a tuft of fine, short hairs. The kernel may vary in size from 4 × 6 mm. to 3 × 9 mm.

7. **OATS** (*Avena sativa* L.). The kernels are tightly clasped by the yellowish, seven-nerved lemma and the two-keeled palea. Separated from the hull, the kernels (groats) are seen to be clothed with hairs which, being longer than those of wheat and not confined to the apex, give the kernels a more downy appearance. The kernel is longer and narrower than that of wheat, being about 12 × 3 mm., and it is softer than the wheat

kernel. The hulls may comprise 20–45 per cent of the weight of the grain.

8. **RICE** (*Oryza sativa* L.). The seeds are characterized by several shallow longitudinal grooves, which are formed by close contact of the caryopsis with the ridges on the inner surface of the lemma and palea. The kernel is generally about 10 × 3 mm.

9. **MILO** and **KAFIR** (*Andropogon sorghum* [L.] Brot.). These grains are related varieties of the non-saccharine sorghums. The kernel is naked, nearly globular, and about 4 mm. in diameter. Sorghum seeds occur in many different colors, but the types most commonly fed to birds are white or red.

10. **CORN,** or **MAIZE** (*Zea mays* L.). The kernel is wedge- or tooth-shaped, broader at the apex than at the point of attachment to the cob, flattened, and with a dent at the top.

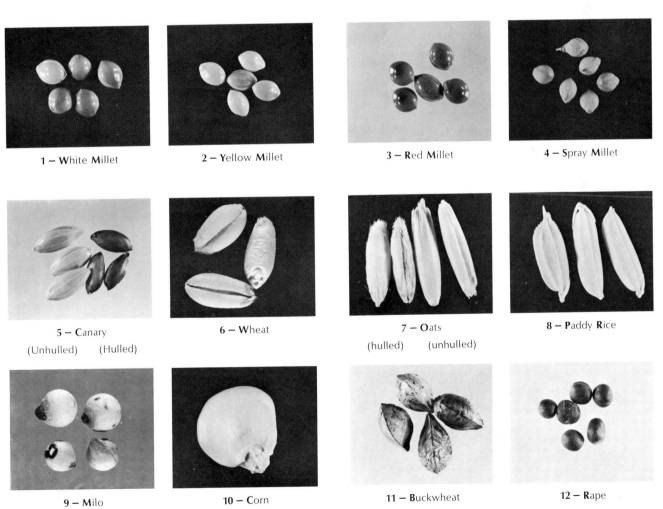

1 – White Millet 2 – Yellow Millet 3 – Red Millet 4 – Spray Millet

5 – Canary (Unhulled) (Hulled) 6 – Wheat 7 – Oats (hulled) (unhulled) 8 – Paddy Rice

9 – Milo 10 – Corn 11 – Buckwheat 12 – Rape

Fig. 7-1. *Common seeds used in feeding cage birds.*

THE FAMILY POLYGONACEAE

11. **BUCKWHEAT** (*Fagopyrum esculentum* Mönch). The three-sided, sharply angled, pointed, dry fruit is an achene about 4 to 6 mm. long. It may occur in various shades of brown or grey, or be streaked with both. The kernels are covered with a thick fibrous pericarp which is not fused to the seed. Pinnately arranged striations proceed diagonally from the midrib on each face to the angles. A portion of the calyx often remains attached to the base of the fruit. The kernels of wild buckwheat are similar in shape but smaller in size and almost black in color.

THE MUSTARD FAMILY (CRUCIFERAE)

12. **RAPE** (*Brassica rapa* L. var. *oleifera* D.C.). The seed is spherical and up to 2.5 mm. in diameter. The surface is dull, with very fine reticulations evident under magnification. The husk may be reddish or blackish, and the kernel is yellowish.

13. **GOLD OF PLEASURE,** or **FALSE FLAX** (*Camelina sativa* L.). The seeds are oblong, about 2 × 1 mm., with a longitudinal ridge on the ventral surface and a crease on each side of the ridge, reddish brown in color, with a granular surface; the kernel is yellow. The seed looks somewhat like a miniature wheat kernel.

THE FAMILY LINACEAE

14. **FLAX SEED** (*Linum usitatissimum* L.). The seed is flattened, ellipsoidal, lustrous, brown or yellow, anatropous, and up to 6 mm. long.

THE FAMILY COMPOSITAE

15. **NIGER** (*Guizotia abyssinica* [L.] Cass.). The fruit is a lustrous black achene of sunflower type, about 5 × 1.5 mm., the plant being a member of the sunflower tribe, Helianthoideae. Thistles and burdock belong to the widely separated thistle tribe (Cynaroideae) of the Compositae family.

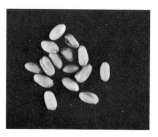
13 – Gold of Pleasure

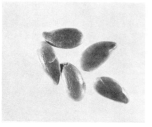
14 – Flax

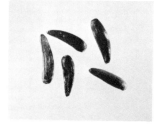
15 – Niger

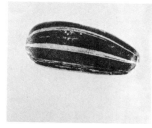
16 – Sunflower

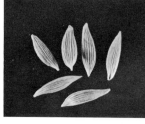
17 – Lettuce

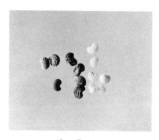
18 – Poppy
(Blue)   (White)

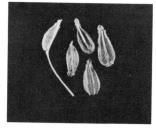
19 – Anise

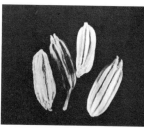
20 – Fennel

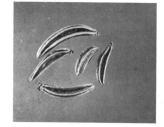
21 – Caraway

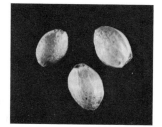
22 – Hemp

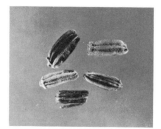
23 – Teazle

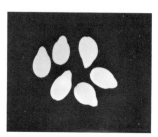
24 – Sesame

Fig. 7-1. *Common seeds used in feeding cage birds* (continued).

16. **SUNFLOWER** (*Helianthus annuus* L.). The achenes are obovate, flattened, more or less diamond-shaped in cross section, and up to 19 mm. long. They are white, black, or white-and-black striped. The pericarp is leathery, with a paper-like lining within which is a thin spermoderm and endosperm.

17. **LETTUCE** (*Lactuca sativa* L.). The seed is about 5 × 1 mm., flattened, and sharp-pointed; it has about seven longitudinal ribs on each side, and is greyish in color.

THE FAMILY PAPAVERACEAE

18. **POPPY,** or **MAW** (*Papaver somniferum* L.). There are two common varieties of poppy seeds: white (var. *album* D.C.) and blue (var. *nigrum* D.C.). The minute, half anatropous seeds are kidney-shaped, with one end broader than the other and with a marked notch in which are both the hilum and chalaza, connected by a short raphe. The seeds range in color from white through blue, grey, and brown to nearly black. Under a lens, the surface is beautifully reticulated. Poppy seeds are entirely free from opium.

THE FAMILY UMBELLIFERAE

19. **ANISE** (*Pimpinella anisum* L.). The seeds are small, ovoid, slightly elongated (4–6 mm. long), hairy, ridged cremocarps, each usually bearing a small portion of its stem. The seed has five ribs.

20. **FENNEL** (*Foeniculum vulgare* Miller). The fruit is a green or yellow cremocarp composed of two narrow, slightly curved carpels which look like miniature bananas. The carpels are usually separated and may be 10–12 mm. long. The epicarp is smooth, the mesocarp reticulated. Each carpel has five ribs.

21. **CARAWAY** (*Carum carvi* L.). The fruit is shorter than that of fennel, being about 5 mm. long. It consists of two carpels, which are almost regularly pentagonal in cross section. The carpels, which usually become separated during threshing, are dark brown, compressed at the sides, occasionally curved, and longitudinally striated.

THE MULBERRY FAMILY, CANNABINACEAE

22. **HEMP** (*Cannabis sativa* L.). The fruit is an oval, somewhat flattened achene, up to 5 mm. long, with a rib on each of the narrow sides. Except for the ribs and base, which are white, the sur-face is brown, with delicate white veins. The pericarp is hard and shell-like.

THE FAMILY DIPSACACEAE

23. **TEAZLE** (*Dipsacus* spp. L.). The seed is about 4 mm. long, roughly square in cross section, and about 1–1.5 mm. wide, with a longitudinal ridge on the center of each side. The pericarp is covered with fine hairs, is grey to brown in color, and appears striated owing to ridges at corners and on the sides.

THE FAMILY PEDALIACEAE

24. **SESAME** (*Sesamum indicum* [L.] D.C.). The seed is flattened, pear-shaped, and up to 3 mm. long. The color varies from light straw color to dark brown. An indistinct longitudinal ridge through the center of one side marks the position of the raphe. Other ridges run around each side near the edge.

THE FAMILY LEGUMINOSAE

25. **PEANUT** (*Arachis hypogaea* L.). The nut grows in a one- to several-seeded pod which, after fertilization, is forced underground by downward growth of the fruit stalk. The pericarp is brittle, pale yellow, buff, or orange in color; a number of longitudinal ridges, connected here and there by branches, form reticulations on the surface. Adjoining ends of the seeds are flattened, usually obliquely. The seed is enveloped in a thin skin, copper-colored, brown, or purple on the outer side, and yellow or white on the inner side. The elongated cotyledons are about 6 mm. in diameter × 15 mm. long; each has a longitudinal groove through the middle of the inner side.

OTHER TYPES OF SEEDS

Besides the seeds described above, many other types of seeds, including wild seeds, are relished by birds. Some of these are described by Morse.[44]

COMPOSITION OF VARIOUS SEEDS

Seeds are sometimes classified as starch (carbohydrate) seeds or oil seeds. Starch seeds include the cereal or grass seeds and buckwheat; oil seeds include rape, flax, niger, poppy, sesame, hemp, and peanut. Starch seeds generally contain less protein than the oil seeds, as shown by the analytical values presented in Table 7–1.

The values for any given sample of seed may vary,

Table 7-1. Percentage Composition of Some Common Seeds[83]

Seed	Moisture	Protein	Fat	Fiber	Ash	N.F.E.*
Common millet	8.93	12.77	3.27	8.95	3.78	62.30
Spray millet	11.76	14.50	5.56	11.24	5.50	51.44
Canary seed	14.30	13.67	3.52	21.29	9.99	37.23
Wheat	10.52	11.87	2.09	1.79	1.83	71.90
Oats	9.96	12.07	4.42	11.92	3.35	58.28
Rice	11.68	8.09	1.80	8.89	5.02	64.52
Milo	12.36	12.11	3.63	2.39	1.43	68.08
Corn	13.06	8.61	3.84	1.93	1.31	71.25
Buckwheat	12.62	10.02	2.24	8.67	2.02	64.43
Rape	7.30	19.54	45.00	5.95	4.21	17.99
Gold of pleasure	8.7	22.2	30.6	11.1	6.8	21.6
Flax	7.06	24.28	36.50	6.30	3.75	22.10
Niger	7.02	19.37	43.22	14.33	3.48	12.37
Sunflower	6.88	15.19	28.29	28.54	3.20	17.36
Anise	12.78	18.12	11.60	13.35	8.20	33.45
Fennel	17.19	16.28	11.75	13.74	8.60	32.34
Caraway	8.90	21.45	16.53	16.34	7.39	29.39
Poppy	4.22	21.10	50.02	5.40	6.86	9.96
Hemp	8.75	21.51	30.41	18.84	4.60	15.89
Sesame	5.61	21.12	46.78	5.08	6.02	18.63
Peanut	13.15	27.95	35.77	3.04	2.36	17.73

*N.F.E., or nitrogen-free extract, is the difference between 100 per cent and the sum of the percentages of moisture, protein, fat, fiber, and ash. It is considered to represent the carbohydrate other than fiber.

depending on type of soil on which it was produced, fertilizers used, growing conditions (e.g., precipitation and temperature), harvesting conditions, storage conditions, and possibly other factors. The percentages shown in the table should not be considered absolute but only as indicative of the comparative values for the different types of seeds. Furthermore, the values given relate to the composition of the whole seed, including the husk, which many birds discard before they swallow the kernel.

Not only do cereal grains contain less protein than do the oil seeds, but the biological value of their protein is lower than that of the oil seeds. Cereal grains contain vitamins of the B group, but they are completely lacking in vitamin C (unless the grain is sprouted) and vitamin D. Yellow corn differs from white corn and the other cereal grains in containing carotenoid pigments, which are convertible in the body to vitamin A. The oils of the embryos of cereal grains, particularly of wheat, are rich sources of vitamin E. All varieties of millet used for feeding cage birds are low in protein. In common with the other cereal grains, such as canary seed, they are low in the essential amino acid lysine.[79] Common millet (*Panicum miliaceum*) is deficient in tryptophan, and spray millet (*Setaria italica*) is somewhat low in arginine. Canary seed (*Phalaris canariensis*) is a fairly good source of arginine and tryptophan but is low in methionine, hence the proteins of millet and canary seed tend to supplement each other with respect to their amino acids.[78]

There has been considerable prejudice among fanciers against the use of red millet for feeding birds—a prejudice which Bice[8] showed to be without scientific basis. It has also been stated that canaries will not eat millet unless they are starved, yet in free-choice feeding tests conducted over a four-month period, nonbreeding canaries chose a diet consisting of approximately 25% millet, 28% rape, and 47% canary seed.[8]

"TOXIC" AND "WEBBY" SEEDS

TOXIC SEEDS. When disease of unknown origin appears among birds, or an apparently healthy bird dies suddenly, the first impulse of the owner is to blame the feed. The experience of many laboratories shows that nearly all samples of feed which was alleged to have killed chickens proved to be perfectly harmless.[10] For many years samples of such feed have been tested in our aviary by supplying them as the sole source of food to a bird for a period of at least a week, if a sufficient amount was available; in no instance have adverse effects resulted.

WEBBY SEED. Occasionally seeds become infested with insects, sometimes resulting in the formation of webs in the seed. The insects are not harmful to the birds; on the contrary, the birds may derive valuable protein supplements from them. In the wild, such insects would be a natural part of the bird's diet.[6]

References

1. ALMQUIST, H. J., and ZANDER, D.: Adsorbing charcoals in chick diets. Proc. Soc. Exp. Biol. Med. *45:*303–305, 1940.

2. ALTMAN, I., and ALTMAN, R.: Nutritional guide for aviaries. All-Pets Magazine *31*(12):34, 36, December, 1960.

3. ANON.: Feeds Illustrated *16*(11):30, 1965.

4. AVIS: On the wing—nuts for Ringo. Cage & Aviary Birds *128:*330, 1965.

5. BACHRACH, A.: Strictly for the birds. Budgerigar Bulletin No. 113, pp. 41–45, 1956.

6. BATES, H., and BUSENBARK, R.: *Parrots and Related Birds.* Jersey City, T.F.H. Publications, Inc., 1959. Pp. 15–21.

7. BATES, H., and BUSENBARK, R.: *Cage Birds.* Jersey City, T.F.H. Publications, Inc., 1964. P. 10.

8. BICE, C. W.: Millets for cage birds. All-Pets Magazine *26*(3):72–84 and *26*(4):109–126, 1955.

9. BICE, C. W.: Observations on budgie feeding. Budgerigar Bulletin No. 113, pp. 19–27, 1956.

10. BIRD, H. R.: *Nutritive Requirements and Feed Formulas for Chickens.* U.S.D.A. Circular No. 788, 1950. P. 9.

11. BLYTHE, H.: A feeding method for breeding finches. Avic. Mag. *63:*65, 1957.

12. BRONSON, J. L.: *Parrot Family Birds,* rev. 3rd ed. Fond du Lac, Wis., All-Pets Books, Inc., 1953. P. 36.

13. BROOKS, W. E.: Why maw seed. Cage Birds *111:*720, 1957.

14. BUCKLEY, F. G.: The occurrence and treatment of candidiasis in the Blue-crowned Hanging Parrot (*Loriculus galgulus*). Avic. Mag. *71:*143–145, 1965.

15. CADE, T. J., and DYBAS, J. A., JR.: Water economy of the budgerygah. Auk *79:*345–364, 1962.

16. CARR, R. H., and JAMES, C. M.: Synthesis of adequate protein in the glands of the pigeon crop. Am. J. Physiol. *97:*227–231, 1931.

17. CARR, V. A. V.: Topical comment. Cage & Aviary Birds *127:*512, 1965.

18. CLARKSON, T. B., PRICHARD, R. W., LOFLAND, H. B., and GOODMAN, H. O.: The pigeon as a laboratory animal. Laboratory Animal Care *13:*767–780, 1963.

19. DAVIES, W. L.: The composition of the crop milk of pigeons. Biochem. J. *33:*898–901, 1939.

20. DAVIS, SIR GODFREY: The succulent maggot. Avic. Mag. *72:*3–5, 1966.

21. DEAN, W.: Red pepper does not intensify colour in Red Factors. Cage & Aviary Birds *128:*63, 1965.

22. DEAN, W.: Replies to queries—moulting problem. Cage & Aviary Birds *128:*65, 1965.

23. DILGER, W. C.: Personal communication, 1963.

24. DILGER, W. C.: *Finding Out About Birds.* New York, Home Library Press, 1963. P. 8.

25. DILGER, W. C.: Personal communication, 1966.

26. DOUGLAS, A.: Feeding your young canaries properly. Cage & Aviary Birds *127:*456, 1965.

27. ELDER, W. H.: The oil gland of birds. Wilson Bull. *66:*6–31, 1954.

28. EVERITT, C.: Rearing White-cheeked Touracos. Cage & Aviary Birds *127:*455, 1965.

29. FARNER, D. S.: Digestion and the Digestive System. In *Biology and Comparative Physiology of Birds,* A. J. Marshall, ed. New York, Academic Press, 1960. Vol. 1, pp. 411–467.

30. FICKEN, R. W., and DILGER, W. C.: Insects and food mixtures for insectivorous birds. Avic. Mag. *67:*46–55, 1961.

31. FLOWERS, M. L., and FLOWERS, F.: *Aviary and Cage Birds, Part 3, Canaries,* Reseda, Bird Haven, 1941. Pp. 21–37.

32. GARY, N. E., FICKEN, R. W., and STEIN, R. C.: Honey bee larvae (*Apis mellifera* L.) for bird food. Avic. Mag. *67:*27–32, 1961.

33. GEDDES, W. F.: Cereal Grains. In *The Chemistry and Technology of Food and Food Products,* 2nd ed., M. B. Jacobs, ed. New York, Interscience Publishers, Inc., 1951. Vol. 2, pp. 1022–1133.

34. GILPIN, H. G. P.: Locusts as live food. Cage & Aviary Birds *128:*21, 1965.

35. GOODWIN, R.: Grassquits—birds for cage and aviary. All-Pets Magazine *31*(10):66–67, October, 1960.

36. HARMAN, I.: *Finches.* Fond du Lac, Wis., All-Pets Books, Inc., 1955. P. 43.

37. HEINROTH, O., and HEINROTH, K.: *The Birds.* Ann Arbor, Univ. of Michigan Press, 1958.

38. KENDEIGH, S. C.: Personal communication, 1962.

39. KING, J. R., and FARNER, D. S.: Energy Metabolism, Thermoregulation and Body Temperature. In *Biology and Comparative Physiology of Birds,* A. J. Marshall, ed. New York, Academic Press, 1961. Vol. 2, pp. 215–288.

40. LAFEBER, T. J.: Nutrition of the budgerigar (*Melopsittacus undulatus*). Animal Hospital 1:276–287, 1965.

41. LUECKE, R. W.: The significance of zinc in nutrition. Borden's Rev. of Nutrition Res. 26(4):45–53, Oct.-Dec., 1965.

42. MEADEN, F.: Insect culturing for softbills. Avic. Mag. 67:120–122, 1961.

43. MORRIS, D.: Seed preferences of certain finches under controlled conditions. Avic. Mag. 61:271–287, 1955.

44. MORSE, R.: *Wild Plants and Seeds for Birds.* London, Link House, 1926.

45. MURPHY, T.: Plants in aviaries. Cage & Aviary Birds 128:312, 1965.

46. MURRAY, J. P.: Type standards for new colours? Cage & Aviary Birds 128:345–346, 1965.

47. MVP REDBOOK: A handbook on cage birds. Mod. Vet. Pract. 46(12):176–198, Oct. 15, 1965.

48. NAETHER, C.: *Soft-Billed Birds.* Fond du Lac, Wis., All-Pets Books, Inc., 1955.

49. NAETHER, C.: Feeding birds—a nutritional guide to health and vigor. All-Pets Magazine 32(12):34–35, December, 1961.

50. NATIONAL RESEARCH COUNCIL: *Nutritive Requirements for Domestic Animals.* No. 1. Nutrient requirements for poultry, NRC Publication 301, 1960.

51. NORRIS, L. C., and SCOTT, M. L.: Proteins, Carbohydrates, Fats, Fiber, Minerals and Water in Poultry Feeding. In *Diseases of Poultry,* 4th ed., H. E. Biester and L. H. Schwarte, eds. Ames, Iowa State University Press, 1959. Pp. 93–125.

52. PFIZER, CHAS., & CO., INC.: Nutrition and egg production. Agradata 2(1):1–18, January, 1958.

53. PLATH, K., and DAVIS, M.: *Parrots Exclusively.* Fond du Lac, Wis., All-Pets Books Inc., 1957. P. 9.

54. POMERANZ, Y.: Formation of toxic compounds in storage-damaged foods and feedstuffs. Cereal Science Today 9(4):93–96, 150, 1964.

55. POULSEN, H.: Colour feeding of flamingos. Avic. Mag. 66:48–51, 1960.

56. QUACKENBUSH, F. W., KVAKOVSZKY, S., HOOVER, T., and ROGLER, J. C.: Deposition of individual carotenoids in avian skin. J. Assoc. Off. Agric. Chem. 48:1241–1244, 1965.

57. RALSTON PURINA: Thin shelled eggs—a problem. Ralston Purina News Bull. 13(4), 1957.

58. RAND, A. L.: Bird. In *Encyclopedia Brittanica,* W. E. Preece, ed. Chicago, William Benton, 1965. Vol. 3, pp. 674–690.

59. RATCLIFFE, H. L.: Diets for a zoological garden: Some results during a test period of five years. Zoologica 25:463–472, 1940.

60. RIDDLE, O., and BRAUCHER, P. F.: Studies on the physiology of reproduction in birds: Control of the special secretion of the crop-gland in pigeons by an anterior pituitary hormone. Am. J. Physiol. 97:617–625, 1931.

61. RIPLEY, S. D., II: Aviary and Aviculture. In *Encyclopedia Brittanica,* W. E. Preece, ed. Chicago, William Benton, 1965. Vol. 2, pp. 894–896.

62. SANDER, E. G., WRIGHT, L. D., and MCCORMICK, D. B.: Evidence for function of a metal ion in the activity of dihydroorotase from *Zymobacterium oroticum.* J. Biol. Chem. 240:3628–3630, 1965.

63. SCHLUMBERGER, H. G.: Spontaneous goiter and cancer of the thyroid in animals. Ohio J. Sci. 55:23–43, 1955.

64. SCOTT, M. L.: The Nutrition of Pheasants and Quail. Proceedings 1963 Cornell Nutrition Conference for Feed Manufacturers, 1963. Pp. 127–130.

65. SCOTT, M. L.: Comparative biological effectiveness of *d-, dl-,* and *l-* forms of α-tocopherol for prevention of muscular dystrophy in chicks. Fed. Proc. 24:901–905, 1965.

66. SCOTT, M. L., and HOLM, E. R.: Nutrition of Wild Waterfowl. Proceedings 1964 Cornell Nutrition Conference for Feed Manufacturers, 1964. Pp. 149–155.

67. SCOTT, M. L., and NORRIS, L. C.: Vitamins and Vitamin Deficiencies. In *Diseases of Poultry,* 4th ed., H. E. Biester and L. H. Schwarte, eds. Ames, Iowa State University Press, 1959. Pp. 126–161.

68. SIEGMUND, O. H., ed.: *The Merck Veterinary Manual,* 2nd ed. Rahway, N.J., Merck & Co., Inc., 1961. Management of Caged Birds, pp. 1394–1399.

69. SIEGMUND, O. H., ed.: *The Merck Veterinary Manual,* 2nd ed. Rahway, N.J., Merck & Co., Inc., 1961. Zoo Animal Nutrition (Birds), pp. 806–809; Poultry Nutrition, pp. 813–846.

70. SILVER, A.: Breeding mealworms. Cage & Aviary Birds 127:502, 1965.

71. SODERBERG, P. M.: *Foreign Birds for Cage and Aviary— Waxbills, Weavers and Whydahs.* Jersey City, T.F.H. Publications, Inc., 1963.

72. SPECTOR, W. S., ed.: *Handbook of Biological Data.* Philadelphia, W. B. Saunders Co., 1956. P. 213.

73. STORER, R. W.: Adaptive Radiation in Birds. In *Biology and Comparative Physiology of Birds,* A. J. Marshall, ed. New York, Academic Press, 1960. Vol. 1, pp. 15–55.

74. SWALLOW, J. W.: Red Factor Canaries. Cage & Aviary Birds *126:*616, 1964.

75. TANNER, E. B.: Breeding foreign softbills. Cage & Aviary Birds *125:*313, 1964.

76. TANNER, E. B.: Old World gems. Cage & Aviary Birds *129:*225–226, 1966.

77. TAYLOR, T. G.: *Feeding Exhibition Budgerigars,* 2nd ed. London, Iliffe Press, 1958.

78. TAYLOR, T. G.: We are not so very wide of the mark. Cage Birds *116:*167, 1959.

79. TAYLOR, T. G.: Nutrient requirements of budgerigars. Mod. Vet. Pract. *46*(9):60, 66, August, 1965.

80. TAYLOR, T. G.: Vitamins and French Moult incidence. Cage & Aviary Birds *129:*104, 1966.

81. ULYATT, B.: Red Factor Canaries and colour-feeding. Cage & Aviary Birds *128:*108, 1965.

82. WACKERNAGEL, H.: Some results with colour feeding of carotenoids in birds at the Basel Zoological Gardens. Avic. Mag. *65:*20–21, 1959.

83. WINTON, A. L., and WINTON, K. B.: *The Structure and Composition of Foods.* Vol. 1. *Cereals, Nuts, Oil Seeds* (1932); Vol. 2. *Vegetables, Legumes, Fruits* (1935); Vol. 4. *Sugar, Cocoa, Coffee, Tea, Spice Leaves* (1939). New York, John Wiley & Sons.

84. WOODWARD, I. D.: Catering for softbills. Cage & Aviary Birds *127:*497, 1965.

85. WOODWARD, I. D.: Catering for softbills. Cage & Aviary Birds *128:*6, 1965.

86. WORDEN, A. N.: Focus on budgerigar nutrition. Cage Birds *116:*145–147, 1959.

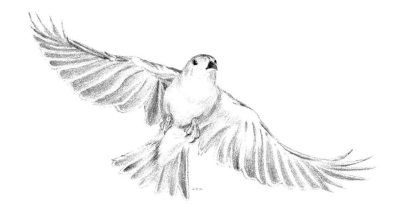

8

Orphan Birds

Katharine Tottenham

There are certain basic principles which apply to the rearing of all young animals. A regular routine, observation of principles of cleanliness, and provision of digestible nutrient material are equally important, but, although normally mammals of any species will instinctively suck to obtain nourishment, young birds will feed only if the correct stimulus is given. For this reason, raising orphan birds is sometimes very difficult.

The main difficulty arises from the common assumption that a young bird should be fed by forcing morsels into its beak—a practice that increases the bird's fear amid unfamiliar surroundings and reduces its chances of survival. Success depends on voluntary food intake, triggered by the manner in which the food is offered. Finding the correct method may be a matter of trial and error, and in such a case each action must be a concise one so that when the bird reacts the stimulus is known and the correct procedure may be adopted in future attempts.

TYPES OF YOUNG BIRDS BASED ON CONDITION AT HATCHING

Young birds are of two main types: nidicolous chicks, which hatch at an early stage of development and are generally blind, helpless, and more or less naked (nestlings); the second type, nidifugous chicks, have a longer incubation period; they leave the shell clad in down feathers and have the ability to run about and pick up food for themselves. Chicks of both types require warmth, but this is all that they have in common. Table 8-1 lists various cage and wild birds classified according to behavioral type of the newly hatched chick and gives appropriate dietary items for the nidicolous species.

169

Table 8-1. Classification of Cage and Wild Birds According to Behavioral Type and Diet of Chicks

Nidicolous Insectivores **(Insects)** Flycatchers Swallows Tufted titmouse Chickadee Nuthatches Dippers Wrens Waxwings Orioles Meadowlarks Bobolinks Cuckoos Tanagers Roadrunners	***Nidicolous Carnivores*** **(Fish)** Kingfishers Darters Herons Bitterns
Nidicolous Mixed Feeders **(Egg and biscuit meal plus live foods)** Thrashers Mockingbirds Catbirds Thrushes Robins Bluebirds Cardinals Grosbeaks Buntings Sparrows Finches Canaries	***Nidicolous Carnivores*** **(Meat, insects)** Owls Hawks Shrikes ***"Milk" Feeders*** Pigeons Doves Parrot family ***Nidifugous Self-feeders*** Grouse (N. Am.) inc. prairie chickens Pheasants Partridges Quail Turkeys Ducks Geese
Nidicolous Omnivores **(Insects, fruit, cereal, egg)** Crows Magpies Bluejays Starlings Mynah birds	***Nidifugous Beak-feeders*** Gallinules Coots Rails Cranes Grebes Great northern diver (loon)

MANAGEMENT OF NIDICOLOUS CHICKS

Nidicolous chicks include all passerine birds, the parrot family, swallows, birds of prey, and kingfishers. These may be grouped on the basis of their usual diet, as seed-eaters, insectivores, and carnivores.

The situation with seed-eaters is unlike that of other species with more obvious dietary demands. In most cases, the chicks are naturally fed on insects until the beak hardens sufficiently to allow the bird to husk seeds for itself. Finches and buntings are in this cate-

gory and, except for parrots, most birds that crack seeds will require a proportion of insects in their food at the chick stage. Clearly then, if the species of a helpless orphan nestling is in doubt, no harm will be done if it is fed on insects or an equivalent kind of food.

Foods To Be Used

A number of foods manufactured to suit various species of cage birds and their young are on the market, and these may be used for both tame and wild species, but an additional amount of fresh food is essential. Fishermen's maggots, mealworms, and fruit flies, which are ideal live foods for birds, can be purchased or cultured. In the country, further supplies of mixed insects may be obtained by using a muslin sweep-net among rough herbage, but it is urgent to be sure that insecticides have not been sprayed over the area during the preceding twelve months.

Egg is a useful food and may be the only item used for finches and insectivores when alternatives are not available. An egg should be hard-boiled or, better still, scrambled, and mashed or sieved before feeding. Hen and pigeon eggs are best for this purpose; duck eggs are too rich for small birds.

Large passerine birds, such as crows, will thrive on poultry meal mixed with milk and rolled into pellets; as this food has balanced ingredients of proteins and carbohydrates, no additives are necessary.

Foods suitable for pigeons and doves and for parrot-like birds are so specialized that these are dealt with under separate headings later in the Chapter.

Young birds of prey need fresh meat in the form of large insects and small mammals and birds. Useful foods include mealworms, beetles, and large grubs (larvae), dead mice and sparrows, rabbit meat, and poultry giblets (heart, liver, and gizzard).

Of all nestlings, kingfishers are the most demanding, as they must have frequent feedings of freshly-killed small fish, and it is possible to rear them only if a constant supply of minnows or guppies is available.

Cages and Enclosures

Nidicolous chicks should be kept in a simulated nest inside a cage so that the birds are safe and quiet. At feeding times the nest can be brought out to a table or the food may be given within the cage. Warmth is important, and if a number of chicks are to be maintained for a period of time it is worth obtaining a hospital cage, designed for use by keepers of cage birds. Such cages consist of a glass-fronted box fitted with a thermostatically controlled electric heater, and provided with air-inlets so arranged as to avoid both stuffiness and drafts. Lacking the real thing, it is quite possible to have a carpenter construct a hospital cage which can be warmed with the aid of an electric light bulb, but in this case the level of heat must be watched carefully; 70°F. is the correct temperature.

When a bird has acquired flight plumage and leaves the nest it can be transferred to a wire-fronted box cage, provided with low perches and with containers for food and water. The size of the cage is a matter of common sense; a small finch will be content in a cage 2 feet long, but a young crow will need an aviary.

Feeding

The majority of young birds "freeze" at unaccustomed sights or sounds, and in this state they obviously will refuse to accept food, but quietness and steady movements will do much to prevent fright.

The initial feed is the most difficult. Once a young bird has taken food, it is likely to feed readily at each subsequent meal, but at first extreme patience may be needed. There are nestlings which feed the instant the beak is touched, but these are few; consequently, when the first touch has failed to stimulate feeding, the only thing to do is to follow a series of movements until the right one is discovered. Touch the beak at the tip, on the sides, and at the base where it joins the head, then the chin, the crown of the head, and the back of the body at the shoulders, and finally the sides of the nest as if a parent bird were alighting there. If the chick's eyes are open it may respond to food raised and lowered in front of the beak. If this series of movements fails, try the movements again until the bird gapes, however slightly, and then insert the food into its beak at once.

For small birds the best feeder is a thin, round-tipped wooden spatula cut from a match stick, as this allows the food to be pushed to the back of the bird's tongue and the entrance to the gullet. It is important not to clog the mouth with food, as this may block the windpipe and cause suffocation.

All young passerine birds gape for food, which the parents place right in the gullet (Fig. 8-1). If the species of a nestling is not known, then the presence of "lips" at the sides of the beak will confirm that it is a gaping type. These lips shrivel when the bird becomes self-supporting.

Mynah birds that are to be taught to talk are usually purchased at the gaping stage, but these are easily managed as they are tame and ready to take food from anyone.

The amount of food to give is sometimes a problem; it is generally safe to continue feeding until the bird ceases to gape. Hand-raised young birds are more likely to die of starvation than of a surfeit of food, because the rate of digestion is so fast. As an example, a young mynah bird fed on blackberries passed purple-colored feces three minutes later.

The chicks of seed-eating species may be fed on a proportion of commercial rearing food intended for canaries. This is made from dried egg and biscuit meal and forms a good staple diet, to which small insects

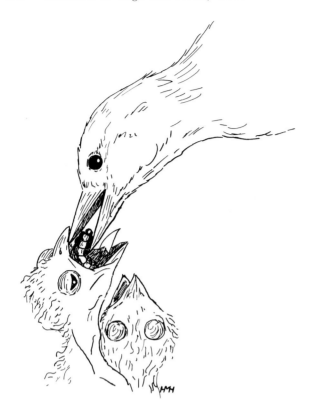

Fig. 8-1. *Gaping young receiving food from parent bird.*

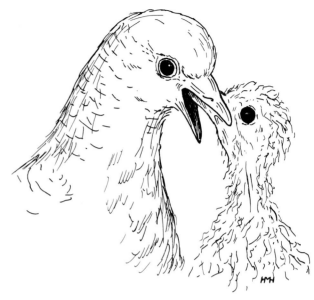

Fig. 8-2. *Parent dove feeding young by regurgitation.*

and larvae and freshly prepared cooked egg should be added.

Insectivorous birds of the passerine group have gaping chicks which require quantities of live food. Small species, such as warblers, will thrive on maggots, fruit flies, and netted insects. An important point in feeding live foods is that the creature must be killed before it is given to a chick—adult birds will be seen to kill insects before taking them to the nest—and this may be done by pinching the heads of larvae and flies with forceps. The same instrument can be used on earthworms to pinch the body along its length. Fresh but dead food is needed, because if a chick swallows a wriggling animal it is likely to die itself.

Fledgling insectivores will learn to eat insectile mixtures sold for cage birds if some of their accustomed fresh food is placed over it in the dish.

Feeding of Nestling Pigeons and Doves

Nestling pigeons and doves feed naturally by thrusting their soft, pliable beak into the parent's gullet to drink a gruel-like liquid secreted from the lining of the adult bird's crop (Fig. 8-2). Such chicks present great difficulty when being raised by hand because they will never accept offered food.

There are two alternative methods for solving this problem: the bird may be trained to drink a milky

fluid from a small vessel, such as an egg-cup, or it can be force-fed. This is the only situation in which force pays, as it is simpler and surer; but efforts to establish feeding by the first method are worth while if a very tame bird is desired.

Force-feeding involves prising open the chick's beak between finger and thumb and inserting pellets of bread soaked in creamy milk well down the gullet with the forefinger of the other hand. The bread should be thoroughly soaked but not dripping milk, as the liquid could enter the trachea and cause drowning.

This system prevents the bird from indicating when it has had enough, making the only guide the condition of the crop. It should be well filled but by no means taut; the condition of the crop will also act as a guide to the frequency of feeding, as when it begins to sag another feeding is due.

Pigeons and doves very quickly acquire the plumage necessary for flight, and grow at an equal rate, so that they soon need additional foods in the form of soaked corn (maize) and maple peas, various berries, and green garden peas of a size suited to the species. The beak gradually hardens, and the bird begins to pick up corn for itself when it is about a month old.

In all cases involving the use of fingers for hand-feeding it is important to be sure that the hands are clean and the nails pared smoothly, because damage to the delicate membranes of the chick's mouth or throat may result in inflammation followed by infection.

Feeding of Baby Parrots

Birds of the parrot family feed their young on a substance rather similar to "pigeon milk," but pass the food from beak to beak. South American Indians, who raise large numbers of parrot chicks, feed the birds chewed cereals from their own mouths, but it is quite possible to feed orphan parrots in a less personal manner by giving a mixture of milk-soaked bread between finger and thumb, gently squeezing the beak at either side and allowing the bird to gobble morsels one at a time. Banana and soft fruit may also be given, but in small amounts.

When the parrot chick begins to feather it may be given soaked corn (maize) until the beak is strong enough to crack hard seeds.

Parakeets, including budgerigars, can be raised in the same way, but on smaller seeds. Ground and winnowed millet seed is the best food; this is prepared by scalding it in hot water, draining, and allowing it to cool before feeding. Fresh supplies must be made for each feed, which means a lot of work with a pestle and mortar; it is certainly easier to use a manufactured canary-rearing food, although the results may not be as good.

A very small amount of clean earth can be added to foods for baby parrots. This is not essential, but it is noticeable that breeding birds kept in an aviary with an earth floor have a better record of producing fledged young.

Feeding of Birds of Prey

Birds of prey bring whole animals to the nest and there rip them up, giving small pieces to the young from their beaks. An owl or hawk chick will often feed if a mouse or bird is dismembered in front of it, but should this procedure fail it will almost certainly accept meat that is raised and lowered slowly a few inches from its face, leaning forward to take the food which should then be pushed gently into the side of the hooked beak.

These birds are equipped with sensitive bristle-like feathers on each side of the beak, and a weak specimen that fails to respond to visual temptation will bite at small pieces of meat rubbed gently across the tips of the bristles.

Once they have begun to feed, the chicks will call when they are hungry. They require about six small meals a day at first, and then graduate to consuming larger chunks at longer intervals.

Young birds of prey alter their mode of accepting food when they are about 4 weeks old, refusing it in the beak but taking pieces placed in the talons. At this age they may be given small mice whole and larger pieces of other animals, until they gain enough strength to tear up dead sparrows, mice, and chicken or rabbit heads. A young eagle or vulture will tackle sheep heads.

Birds of prey regurgitate pellets of indigestible matter, such as bones and feathers, in the normal course of digesting their natural foods, and it is often assumed that roughage must be given to young owls and hawks if they are to thrive. This is not necessary, and such action may even be the cause of so many failures in hand-rearing of these birds. Plenty of flesh food is the important point, and if this consists of mice and sparrows so much the better, but strips of beef steak will be just as nourishing for a fast-growing chick.

Carnivores are liable to suffer from thirst and as water cannot be given until the bird is capable of drinking from a dish, part of the meat in each meal should be dipped in water immediately before it is offered.

Young birds of prey do not need a heated cage in normal summer weather.

Feeding of Kingfishers

Kingfishers feed their young on small whole fish. Guppies form an ideal food for hand-raised chicks, but a daunting number is required daily to satisfy these birds, which will take up to six an hour from dawn until dusk. No alternative diet has proved successful.

MANAGEMENT OF NIDIFUGOUS CHICKS

The management of young birds that hatch as fluffy chicks, able to run about as soon as they are dry, differs from that of nidicolous species. Apart from a few exceptions, nidifugous chicks are of two kinds: those that are self-feeding and those that take food which is dangled from a parent bird's beak.

Nutritional and Other Needs

The first group includes pheasants, partridges, quail, ducklings, and goslings, all of which will feed from a trough on foods manufactured for young poultry. Game chicks will eat a crumb feed intended for turkey chicks but require some live food in the form of maggots as well; they should also have access to a turf, as scratching gives them strengthening exercise and they obtain grit from the earth adhering to their feet.

Water is essential, but this must be supplied in a way that prevents the chicks from getting wet. The old-fashioned inverted jampot drinker is as good as anything for the purpose.

Sometimes pheasants and other chicks will not feed,

but this problem is usually solved by sprinkling eye-catching maggots on the dry food and prodding among the food with a forefinger. If this method fails, the alternative is to introduce, as a "teacher," a farmyard chick of the same age.

Young wildfowl can be managed similarly, but they may be given chicken crumb feed, which has a lower protein content than the turkey crumb feed. Goslings will thrive on a finely pelleted chicken feed. The smaller ducks, like wood ducks, need a proportion of live food, such as maggots, and a ration of chopped lettuce or juicy waterweed.

Water birds that are deprived of their natural mother lack sufficient oil in their plumage to render them waterproof, and so they must be prevented from bathing, let alone swimming. At the same time, because it is essential for them to be able to immerse their heads in water at least once a day if the eyes are not to become inflamed, the best water container is a narrow trough of suitable depth.

Water birds should be handled as little as possible, as disturbance of the plumage retards waterproofing and development of buoyancy.

Self-feeding chicks are comparatively easy to manage for, if they are provided with a source of heat and supplies of food and water, they can be left without attention for a day if necessary. This is not true of beak-fed nidifugous chicks, which require constant care. Examples of this type of chick are gallinules and rails, species that are difficult to rear without extreme patience and a good measure of luck.

Parent birds of these species feed their young by offering morsels of insects, seeds, and weeds dangling from the beak, which the young bird takes for itself. This method can be simulated by holding such morsels with tapering, round-tipped forceps, which should be moved gently up and down in imitation of the bobbing of a bird's head. These chicks need feeding at least once an hour, but otherwise they will thrive under the same conditions as game birds and wildfowl.

Young gulls are occasionally orphaned and may be reared by beak-feeding with a mush made from flaked raw fish, a teaspoonful of cod liver oil, bread, and enough milk to make a wet but not sloppy mixture.

In all cases where hand-feeding is necessary, an obvious point is sometimes forgotten: the parent bird is bigger than the chick, and so a chick will expect food to be presented from an angle above its head. Finally, some young birds will ignore every method of presenting food and then respond surprisingly to a human attempt, however ludicrous, at imitating the adult bird's call.

Meeting Heat Requirements

Nidifugous chicks are mobile from the first, but require a source of heat as a central point from which they can venture to feed and take exercise. Most such chicks can be fostered by a bantam or small farmyard fowl, if a reliable one is readily available.

Pheasants, partridges, quail, ducklings, and goslings are all suitable for fostering, as they are self-feeders by nature and require only warmth and protection from the mother hen.

If a broody bird is not available, another solution is use of an artificial brooder, which may be a real brooder made for chicken farmers or a makeshift devised from a wooden crate and a 60-watt electric light bulb protected by a sleeve of wire mesh. An artificial brooder must be used for beak-fed nidifugous chicks, as they have to be fed by hand.

When the chicks are feathered and no longer need heat, they may be kept in a wire-netting enclosure on grass, with access to a vermin-proof house. Rats and other predators will take chicks in preference to other foods, making it necessary for the birds to be shut in at night.

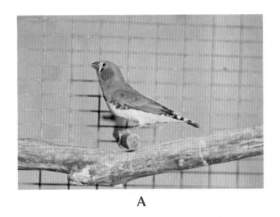

A

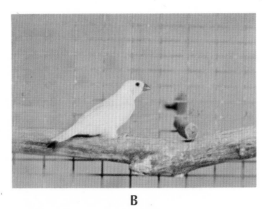

B

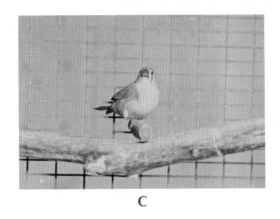

C

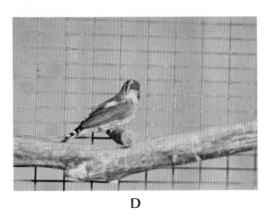

D

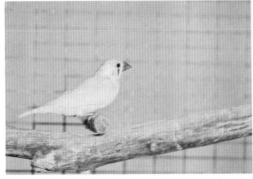

E

Plate 1. *Leucism in zebra finch. A, Normal male. B, Complete leucism. C, Partial leucism in female. D, Fawn variant, female. E, Dilute variant, female.*

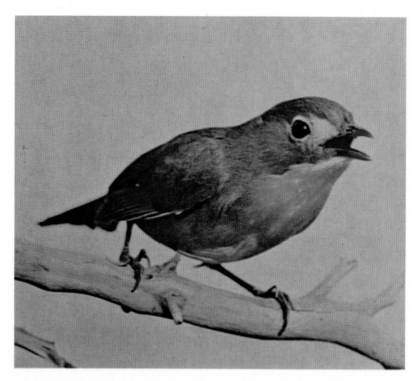

Plate 2. *The Pekin nightingale is one of the most popular and inexpensive of all soft-billed birds. Its cheerful song and perky liveliness are just as important as its hardiness and attractive coloring. (Courtesy of Bates and Busenbark: Finches and Soft-Billed Birds. Jersey City, N.J., T.F.H. Publications, Inc., 1963.)*

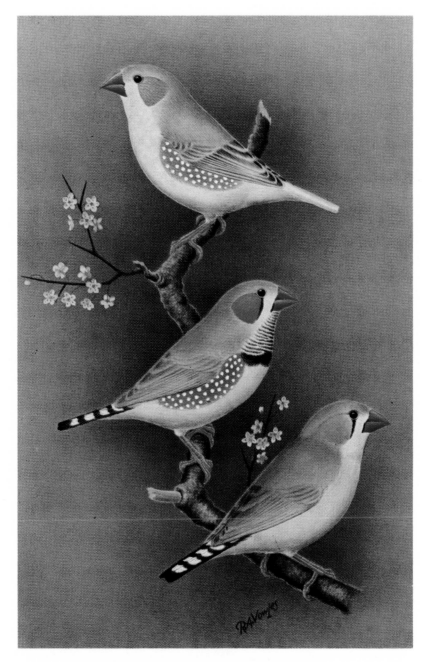

Plate 3. *Rare zebra finches. Top, Male normal penguin. Center, Male fawn. Lower, Recessive silver female. Rare mutations of zebra finches are being standardized by students of genetics and are bred in increasing numbers. (Courtesy of Bates and Busenbark: Finches and Soft-Billed Birds. Jersey City, N.J., T.F.H. Publications, Inc., 1963.)*

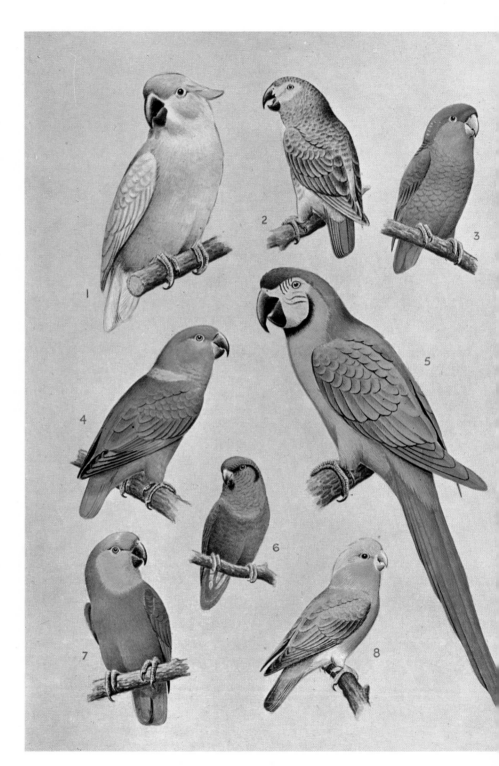

Plate 4. *1, Greater sulfur-crested cockatoo* (Kakatoe galerita). *2, African gre[y]
parrot* (Psittacus erithacus). *3, Finsch's amazon* (Amazona finschi). *4, Yellow-nape[d]
amazon* (Amazona auropalliata). *5, Blue and yellow macaw* (Ara ararauna). *6, Blu[e-]
headed parrot* (Pionus menstruus). *7, Blue-fronted amazon* (Amazona aestiva[).]
8, Roseate or rose-breasted cockatoo (Eolophus roseicapillus). *Scale: 1/6 actua[l]
size. (Courtesy of All-Pets Books, Inc., Copyright 1953.)*

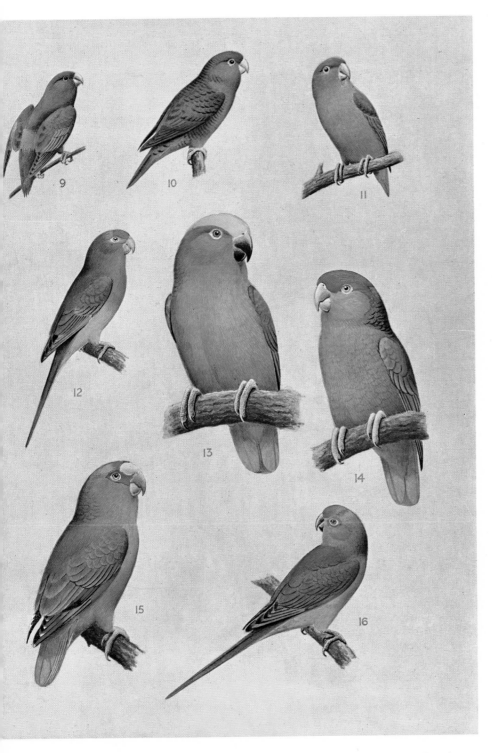

Plate 4 (cont.). *9, Blue-wing parrotlet* (Forpus vividus vividus). *10, Lineolated parakeet* (Bolborhyncus lineolatus). *11, Tovi parakeet* (Brotogerys jugularis). *12, Petz conure* (Eupsittula canicularis). *13, Yellow-fronted amazon* (Chrysotis ochrocephala). *14, Green-cheeked amazon* (Amazona viridigena). *15, Spectacled amazon* (Amazona albifrons). *16, Golden-crowned conure* (Eupsittula aurea). *Scale: 1/4 actual size. Courtesy of All-Pets Books, Inc., Copyright 1953.*)

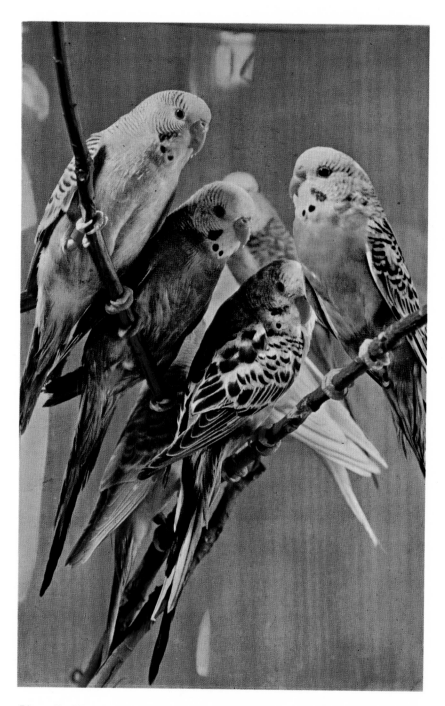

Plate 5. "Rare" parakeets. These budgerigars, showing various newer color combinations, were very expensive a few years ago. Now, through skilled handling by breeders, the so-called "rares" are as inexpensive as the older color varieties called "normals." (Courtesy of Bates and Busenbark: Parrots and Related Birds. Jersey City, N.J., T.F.H. Publications, Inc., 1959.)

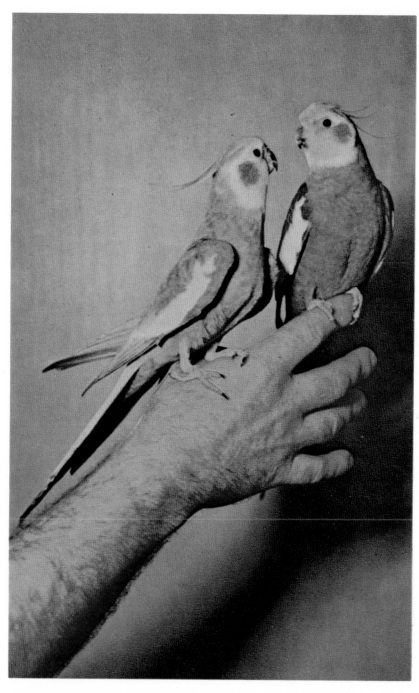

Plate 6. *Cockatiels. (Courtesy of Bates and Busenbark: Parrots and Related Birds. Jersey City, N.J., T.F.H. Publications, Inc., 1959.)*

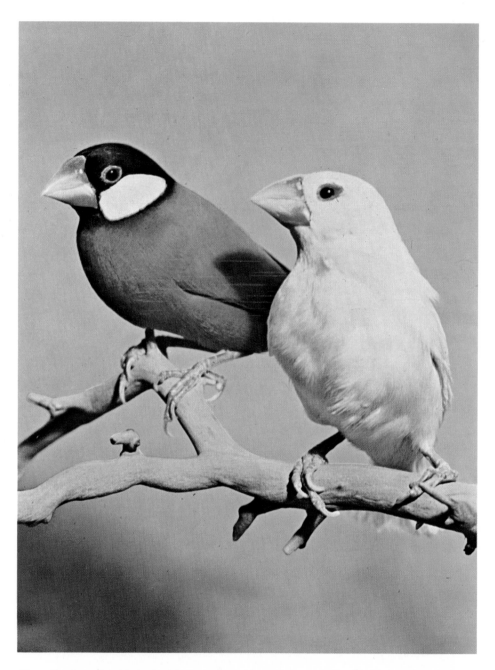

Plate 7. *Java rice birds, both in the white and grey varieties, are among the hardiest and most popular of the larger finches. These birds can be kept with parakeets with no fear of aggressiveness on the part of either species. (Courtesy of Bates and Busenbark: Finches and Soft-Billed Birds. Jersey City, N.J., T.F.H. Publications, Inc., 1963.)*

PART II

CLINICAL CONSIDERATIONS

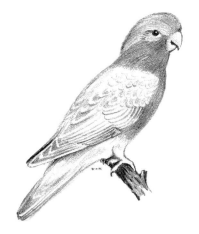

9

Clinical Examination and Methods of Treatment

Robert Millard Stone

It should be noted that, unless another bird is specifically mentioned, the discussion in this Chapter refers to the budgerigar (*Melopsittacus undulatus*), since birds of this species are the most numerous among those kept as pets.

PRELIMINARY PROCEDURES

Instructions to Client

The first contact with the client is usually made by telephone. It should be explained that diagnosis and subsequent treatment of illness is impossible without seeing the patient. The following instructions for transporting the bird to the veterinarian's office should be given and followed:

(1) Bring the patient in its own cage.
(2) Remove the water from the cage.
(3) Do not remove any of the droppings, or otherwise clean the cage.
(4) Cover the cage; and if the weather is cold and the trip is to be made by automobile, warm the car in advance.
(5) Bring all medication and feed used, past and present.

History of Patient

When the patient has been brought into the office, the answers to the following questions should be routinely recorded:

(1) What is the age, sex, color, and name of the patient?

(2) How long has the patient been in the present home, and is there any knowledge of previous ownership?

(3) Are there or were there any other pets in the home?

(4) Was there any previous illness, and what medication, if any, was used?

(5) What is the major complaint?

(6) How long has the condition persisted?

(7) How frequently do the symptoms occur?

Observation of Patient

Before an attempt is made to remove the patient from the cage, its actions and the contents of the cage should be closely noted.

THE ATTITUDE OF THE PATIENT:

(1) Does the patient ruffle its feathers and sit with its eyes closed and its head tucked under its wing?

(2) Is the patient alert to the strange surroundings, or is it completely uninterested?

(3) Does the patient stand on one or both legs, or does it sit on the floor in the corner of the cage?

(4) Does the patient open its mouth and gasp when breathing?

(5) Does the tail bob up and down when the patient breathes?

(6) Does the patient hold its wings away from its body and puff up?

THE CAGE AND CONTENTS:

(1) Are there any toys or mirrors present which might increase the tendency to regurgitate seeds?

(2) Is the cage painted, and, if so, is it a lead paint that can cause serious gastrointestinal difficulties?

(3) Are all of the perches of the same diameter or are they varied (such as a branch from a tree with the bark removed) to give the feet more exercise?

(4) Are there any small red mites on the perches or under the toys and other objects in the cage?

(5) Are there any sticky clusters of regurgitated seeds on the bottom of the cage or on the bird?

THE EVACUATIONS

Normal droppings are dark green or black and of a firm consistency, with a soft white center. The dark-colored is the fecal portion, and the white portion is the urinary excretion. The normal number of evacuations per day will vary between 25 and 50. Wet droppings are seen many times when the patient is a fruit-eating parrot or belongs to another nectar- or fruit-eating species. On many occasions there may be several fresh watery movements whereas the remainder of the evacuations appear normal. Since many of the birds have never been out of their current home since their acquisition, they become frightened by the strange surroundings, and this is reflected by a "nervous diarrhea."

Watery, pasty droppings are usually intermixed with white urine and surrounded by a water stain, indicating diarrhea and enteritis, a common finding in many conditions.

FEED

The normal consumption of seed by budgerigars is approximately 1–2 teaspoons daily, or 100 times the weight of the bird per year. The usual mixture is 40% canary seed, 50% millet seed, and 10% oats, but the proportions will vary with the individual, and will also depend to some extent on the activity of the bird. There is some evidence that the smaller yellow millet seed is nutritionally superior. It also should be kept in mind that commercial seed mixes are usually deficient in lysine and arginine and low in vitamins A, D, and B_{12}. The availability of cuttlefish bone, grit, greens, egg yolk, milk protein, vitamin-mineral mixtures, and such additions as sponge cake, oatmeal, and old bread should also be checked. All of these additions are beneficial.

WATER CONSUMPTION

If at all possible, effort should be made to determine how much water is being consumed. If the client can possibly do so, and the condition warrants it, effort should be made to determine the water intake by measurement at home. The normal intake will vary between 1 and 2 teaspoonfuls a day.

GENERAL PHYSICAL EXAMINATION

Precautions and Restraint

To remove a smaller patient, such as a canary or budgerigar, from the cage, it should be carefully approached, after first making sure that all entrances and exits of the room are secure against its escape. Taking care to cover the area surrounding the arm which is inserted into the cage, move the hand slowly toward the patient and, when contact is made, carefully pin the wings to the sides of the body and pick up the patient, holding the head between the thumb and index finger. After the bird is removed from the cage, if preferred, it can be handed to an assistant to hold (Fig. 9-1), but the examination can satisfactorily be completed when it is held by the clinician. Special care should be taken when handling the more fragile patients, such as canaries and other finches. Birds of this type can easily be injured and on occasion may be killed by rough handling.

The "medium-sized bird," such as a cockatiel or a half-moon conure (*Aratinga canicularis*), can be handled in the same manner as a smaller bird, with the one addition of a heavy leather glove, such as a driving glove (Fig. 9-2). A wool glove usually will not suffice as a protection against biting.

For the handling of larger birds, such as parrots or macaws, the best protection is provided by use of heavy but soft pliable leather gloves (Fig. 9-3).*

Covering the patient with a towel in an attempt to capture it can lead to injury or escape, since the clinician is blindly grasping whatever part of the bird happens to be accessible.

*Hand Guard Glove Co., 2599 N. Lexington Ave., St. Paul, Minn.

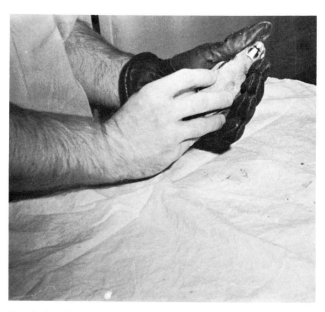

Fig. 9-2. *Position of handler and patient when medium-sized bird is being restrained.*

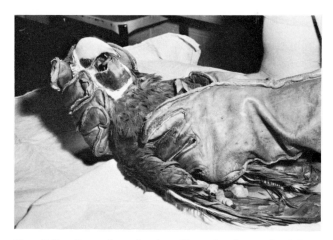

Fig. 9-3. *Procedure for handling the large-sized bird.*

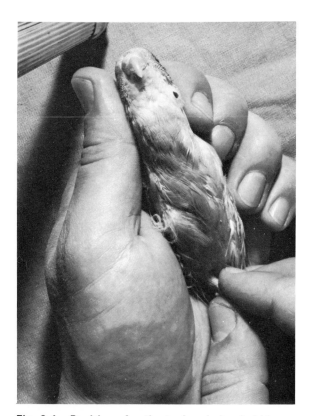

Fig. 9-1. *Position of patient when being held by an assistant for examination or other procedure.*

Examination of the Head

Start the examination by checking the head. Look for large atypical feathers, often found on the top of the head, abrasions or tears in the skin, and palpable fractures. Check for abnormal contour of the skull, such as was seen in one budgerigar which, on postmortem examination and microscopic examination of tissue sections, proved to have an ependymoma of the brain originating from the wall of the lateral ventricle.

One canary had what appeared to be a subcutaneous mass just above the eye; when this was removed and sections were examined under the microscope, it was identified as an epidermoid inclusion cyst.

THE EARS

The ears, which have no pinna, are below and behind the eyes. They should be examined closely for exudate, obstruction, foreign bodies, and wounds.

THE EYES

The eyes should be examined and notation made of swollen, edematous lids with subcutaneous hemorrhage, such as are seen in canaries with malaria. Examination should also be made for abrasions of the cornea, abscesses, and protrusion of the membrana nictitans as a result of infection. Both slow pupillary reflex and iritis are found in many canaries with *Paracolon* infections. Blepharitis in canaries is often associated with pox. A protruding orbital mass in one budgerigar proved to be a lipoma originating deep in the orbit; in another a fibrosarcoma was removed from the conjunctiva. One patient with a visibly enlarged orbit and a diffuse keratitis failed to respond to therapy. The eye was removed, and histological examination revealed suppurative panophthalmitis. The eye should be examined for cataracts, which are found occasionally in budgerigars but most often in cockatiels. When there is a history of nervousness, the bird should be checked carefully for blindness.

THE CERE

Normally the cere is blue in the male budgerigar and brown in the female, but in many instances the color varies anywhere between the two. This can make it very difficult at times to differentiate between the sexes. Hypertrophy of the cere is unimportant as far as the health of the bird is concerned. The cere should be checked for swellings due to abscesses which communicate with the sinuses. It should also be checked for proliferation of exuberant tissue which is honeycombed in appearance. This is found in infestations by the scaly-leg mite (*Cnemidocoptes* spp.)

THE NARES

Opening on the cere are the nares, or nostrils. These should be examined to see if they are occluded. An extension of sinusitis many times will result in a caseous exudate. The nasal sinuses open into the nostrils, and the presence of such an exudate causes difficulty in curing a sinusitis since the sinuses must drain in an upward direction.

THE BEAK

The beak should be inspected for fractures, overgrowth, wry beak, atrophy, tumors, scissor bill, excessive fragility, and flakiness. The lower mandible must also be examined because it too often shows abnormality of growth or shape. The honeycombed appearance of a thickened beak is again an indication of infestation by the scaly-leg mite. The commissures of the mouth should be inspected for granulation tissue or fibroepithelial polyps that ulcerate.

THE MOUTH

The mouth should be checked for stomatitis or the presence of growths. One budgerigar was found to have a squamous epithelial papilloma which was attached to the pharynx.

THE TONGUE

The tongue should be examined carefully for such things as a nylon thread or a strand from a woman's veil which may have wound around the base of the tongue. Check should also be made for lesions produced by caustic substances, tears caused by sharp objects, or burns resulting from eating hot food.

Examination of the Neck

CROP

The most prominent structure in the area of the neck is the crop. It lies to the right of the center line and extends down for a variable distance almost to the thoracic inlet, depending on the age and size of the bird. The crop is an expansion of the esophagus and contains circular muscle fibers. It is used as a storage depot, permitting the bird to digest food at a later time, and as a place to moisten the food. The structure is prominent in budgerigars and almost absent in canaries. The structure should be palpated for the presence or absence of contents, dilation and loss of tone of the muscle, and neoplastic masses inside the wall, which are usually accompanied by a fetid odor. Of five masses surgically removed from the area of the crop and neck one was a xanthoma and involved only the subcutaneous structures, one was an undifferentiated sarcoma, one a leiomyoma, and one a fibrosarcoma which involved the crop wall. The other was an epidermoid inclusion cyst in the area of the jugular vein. The cyst had ruptured, and the swelling gave the appearance of a distinct mass. By passing a blunt probe into the throat and down to the crop, the examiner can determine if there is a blockage or an impaction. A common cause of blockage in the budgerigar is thyroid dysplasia, which is occasionally complicated by cysts.

Examination of the Torso

PECTORAL AREA

By palpation with the fingers, the examiner can check for normal configuration over the pectoral area. The amount of muscle mass (as an indication of the degree of fleshing) and presence or absence of fat can be determined by digital palpation of the area. Fat canaries are rare, but obese budgerigars with fatty masses over the pectoral area and lower abdomen are found quite often. The pectoral area is also a common area for abnormal growths. Among 49 masses removed from the pectoral area and examined histologically there were 16 xanthomas, 27 lipomas, 1 neurofibroma, 1 fibroepithelial papilloma, 1 plasma cell tumor, and 1 neurosarcoma. On two occasions the apparent masses were composed of necrotic fat. In obese individuals fatty tissue over the pectoral area is often mistaken for a neoplasm and removed surgically. These deposits of fat are of a soft pliable consistency, bilaterally symmetrical, and an evenly shaded pale yellow in color.

Hemorrhage from a ruptured blood vessel can sometimes cause sudden death. Often the site is the pectoral vein, under the skin covering the thorax and under the skin of the abdomen.

The stethoscope can be used as on any other individual for listening to heart sounds (Fig. 9-4). The normal heart rate is 300–500 beats per minute. This rate is normally too rapid for the examiner to count. A bradycardia in which each individual beat can be easily counted usually portends impending circulatory collapse. Auscultation of the lungs is easily performed and the presence of respiratory distress is easily determined. Normally the respiratory rate is 85 per minute. The respiratory capacity is increased by a system of air sacs, air tubes, and air cavities in the principal bones. This helps in flight and eliminates heat. There are 11 air sacs: 2 each of cervical, axillary, anterior thoracic, posterior thoracic, and abdominal, and 1 interclavicular. The air ducts connect the bronchi and the air sacs and communicate further with air cavities in bones and throughout the body to the quills of the feathers. When chronic infection of the air sacs develops the patient may make an intermittent or at times a constant chirping sound.

A subcutaneous accumulation of air may sometimes develop as a result of rupture of an air sac.

ABDOMEN

Palpation of the abdomen is done best with the index finger (Fig. 9-5). Normally the examiner can feel the tip of the liver and the abdominal organs, which have a soft, resilient consistency.

In egg retention palpation reveals a firm oval mass in the area of the cloaca. Heavy egg producers often develop herniation of the ventral abdominal wall. Palpation of the area will reveal a surplus of flaccid skin, but by carefully rolling the tissue between the thumb and index finger, the examiner can palpate the viscera.

Abdominal distention may indicate internal tumor, cyst, or peritonitis from ruptured egg.

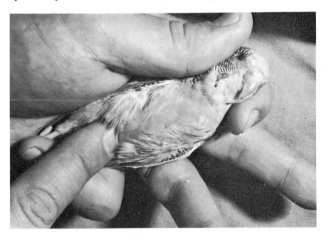

Fig. 9-5. *Position of patient and examiner's index finger when palpating for intra-abdominal mass.*

POSTERIOR PART

The base of the tail should be examined for possible involvement of the uropygial or preen gland with a tumorous mass. Growths surgically removed from this area included six squamous cell carcinomas, two leiomyosarcomas, two xanthomas, three epidermoid inclusion cysts, one lipoma, and one fibrosarcoma.

The preen gland, which is found in most birds except

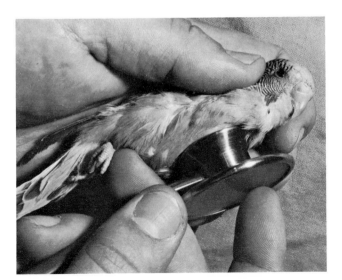

Fig. 9-4. *Position of patient and stethoscope for auscultation of heart and lungs.*

some parrots and doves, sometimes becomes impacted, resulting in a condition known as uropygitis or "pip."

The examiner should check for broken tail feathers which can be the cause of considerable hemorrhage; if any are found they should be pulled out.

Examination of the Wings

The wings should be carefully extended and checked for tears or abrasions in the integument. They should be examined for subcutaneous growths, which are most prominent in the areas of the joints. Of four masses removed from the wing, there was one xanthoma, two lipomas, and one undifferentiated sarcoma. Close examination should be made of the joints for the presence of chalklike deposits, or tophi, which accompany gout. Swollen wing joints in pigeons that show hard, yellowish, tumor-like masses are indicative of tuberculosis. At times the examiner may see swollen joints containing fluid varying from clear to grey in color, which often accompany *Salmonella* infections.

The wing feathers should be carefully checked because of the frequency with which infected shafts are found here. If the wing is abnormally carried by the bird, gentle manipulation by the examiner will reveal if fracture is present. The examiner should keep in mind, however, that the joints of the wing are very flexible and easily moved in all directions, and a fracture can easily be misdiagnosed in a wing that is merely bruised.

Examination of the Pelvic Limbs

After the patient is observed in the cage and it has been noted if the bird is using the limb to grasp the perch and to stand, the next step is careful manipulation of the limb to determine if fracture is present. An intra-abdominal mass or an aortic thrombus can at times so disrupt the blood supply to the limb or limbs that the patient is lame. Since the lips are more sensitive to temperature variation than the hand, the examiner can hold first the affected limb and then the normal limb to his lips to see if there is an appreciable difference in their temperature. The leg should also be examined for abnormal enlargement of the muscle mass. Of three patients with such abnormal enlargement one had a leiomyosarcoma which involved the whole limb and the two others had subcutaneous sarcomas.

The joints of the limbs should be examined for swellings which could be deposits of gout (tophi) as previously mentioned, or a condition known as "bumble-foot," or staphylococcal arthritis.

The toes should be carefully examined for overgrown

nails which can catch in the many crevices around the patient's home and haunts. Careful search should be made for fine thread or similar material which could cause impairment of circulation. Check should be made for deformity of the toes, usually the result of past injury, but on rare occasions caused by riboflavin deficiency, producing the condition in canaries known as "stiff claw," or "slipped toe."

Examination of the Skin and Feathers

Normal molting for the canary or parrot occurs in July and August, whereas in the budgerigar it occurs two or three times a year, at any time. New feathers come in as old ones fall out, and it usually takes from 6 to 8 weeks.

The integument of the bird is very thin, especially in the smaller individuals such as the canary or the budgerigar. When a wing is lifted, it can be seen that there are no feathers in the axillary region. Feathers grow in tracts over the body, and this area is void of tracts. By close observation it can be noted that muscles under the skin appear dark red in color, and fatty tissue appears yellow.

The examiner should check for malformed feathers, which are usually due to infected feather follicles, and broken feathers, which usually result from injuries.

METHODS OF TREATMENT

After the patient is examined and a diagnosis is made, the next step of the clinician is administration of the drug or drugs of choice. There are several routes of administration, each with advantages and disadvantages, and they should all be evaluated before a selection is made. With very few exceptions, the bird is best handled as an out-patient, for the following reasons:

(1) Pet birds are easily upset by a change in the environment.
(2) In most conditions close supervision and tender care are necessary, and the client is usually the best "veterinary nurse" one can find.
(3) The economics of hospital care for the pet bird are such that many clients are unable to financially accept the burden.

Medicated Water

If the client is unable or unwilling to handle the patient and if the bird must be treated as an out-

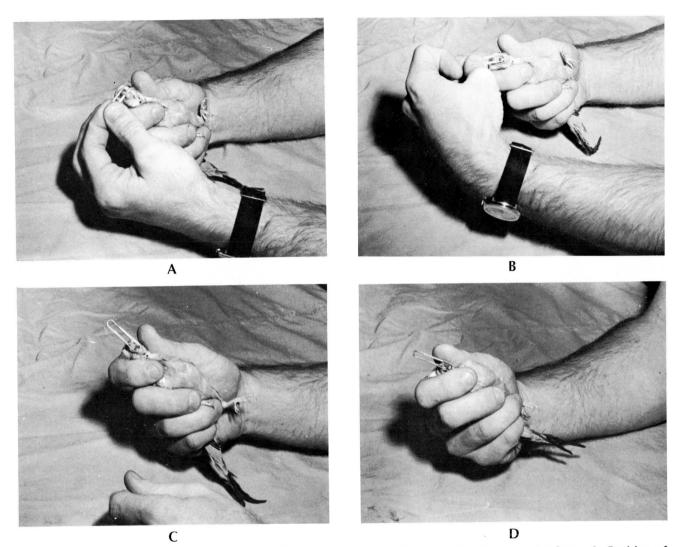

A

B

C

D

Fig. 9-8. *Use of paper clip as speculum to facilitate oral administration of medication to budgerigars. A. Position of handler and patient when inserting the paper clip speculum. B. Rotation of paper clip to open the beak. C. Paper clip in place, separating the upper and lower mandibles. D. Stabilization of paper clip and patient's head by thumb and index finger.*

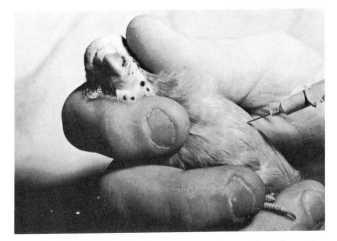

Fig. 9-9. *Position of handler, patient, and syringe for administration of medication intramuscularly.*

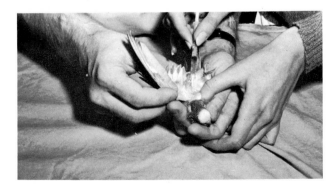

Fig. 9-10. *Position of patient, assistant, and handler for administration of fluids subcutaneously.*

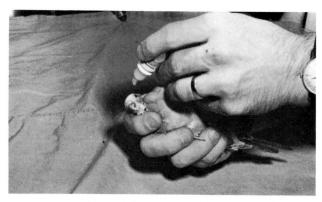

Fig. 9-11. *Position of handler and patient for intraocular administration of medication.*

use. In the case of respiratory conditions, steam inhalators or aerosol-dispersion of antitussive medications can be used to saturate the air in small enclosed rooms or areas holding the patient. There are also certain antimicrobial preparations in powder form which can be absorbed after the enclosed area is dusted with them.

Topical Administration

External lesions can easily be treated by topical application of medications. This can be handled as an out-patient or as a hospital procedure. The veterinarian

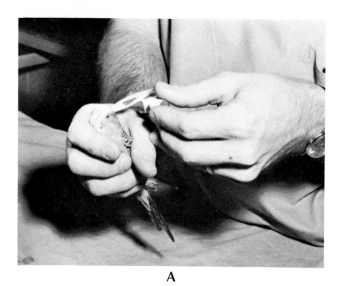

A

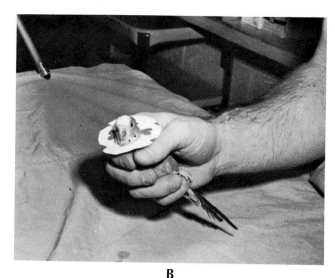

B

Fig. 9-12. *Use of playing card as Elizabethan collar. A. Reflecting the collar when applying it to the neck of the patient. B. Position of the collar after it is placed around the patient's neck, with Scotch tape used to hold edges of the card together.*

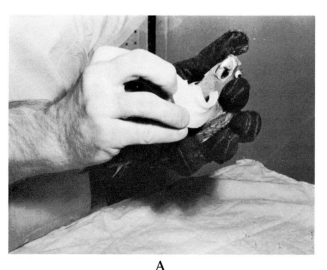

A

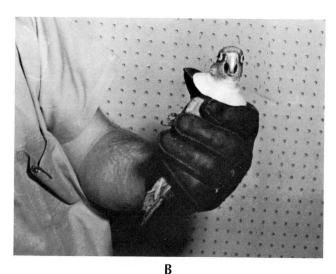

B

Fig. 9-13. *Use of top of plastic detergent bottle as collar for a larger-sized bird. A. Retracting edges of top of bottle when placing it on the neck of the half-moon conure. B. Bottle top in place about neck of the bird.*

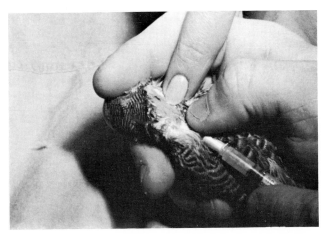

Fig. 9-14. *Position of patient and handler for administration of medication intravenously; an assistant is holding back the feathers in the area of the right jugular vein to facilitate its exposure.*

should keep in mind the fact that the patient can easily reach every area on the body, and may thus ingest any medication that might be applied. If the medication is innocuous orally, there is no problem, but if ingestion could cause trouble, a so-called "Elizabethan collar" can be placed about the neck to restrict movement of the head. A playing card with a 3-inch maximal measurement would be ideal for a budgerigar or similar-sized bird (Fig. 9-12 A and B). The center opening for the neck is slightly larger than the diameter of a pencil. In middle-sized patients, such as half-moon conures, the top of a plastic bottle, such as a detergent container, can be split and applied to the neck to prevent picking (Fig. 9-13 A and B).

Intravenous Administration

Intravenous administration can be used when the drug of choice must be given by this route. In smaller birds the right jugular vein can be used, since in most of the species the left jugular vein is absent (Fig. 9-14). Extreme caution should be taken in the very small fragile birds, because rough handling can cause death. In larger birds such as the parrot, the wing vein can be used.

Reference

1. BLACKMORE, D. K., and LUCAS, J. F.: A simple method for the accurate oral administration of drugs to budgerigars. J. small anim. Pract. 6:27–29, 1965.

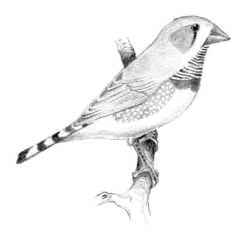

10

Clinical Laboratory Examinations

John Lynn Leonard

This Chapter presents some methods of clinical laboratory examination of cage birds the results of which will be useful in helping diagnose their diseases. The Chapter is based mainly on unpublished studies of the blood of the budgerigar (*Melopsittacus undulatus*) by Leonard and by Gallagher.[15]

BLOOD CONSTITUENTS AND METHODS OF STUDY

COLLECTION OF BLOOD SPECIMEN

In order to determine a red blood cell count, white blood cell count, differential count, and hematocrit value, only a few drops of blood are needed; that is, one drop for the blood film, a red cell pipette filled to the 0.5 ml. mark, and a filled capillary tube are sufficient for making all these studies. Obviously, there is no value in drawing enough blood to make a bird anemic and then finding that the number of blood cells in the sample is normal. Therefore, the primary consideration in choosing a method of blood collection should be to take as small a sample as possible. Of the various methods I have tried I consider clipping of the toenail to be the best. Blood was collected directly from the clipped nail into the pipettes and capillary tubes, so that no more blood was taken than was absolutely necessary. Bleeding from the jugular vein[20] seems to cause too much stress, especially if the collector is not very experienced, and more blood must be taken than is actually needed. Hardly any blood was obtained by clipping the shafts of mature or immature feathers.

Gallagher collected about 0.5 ml. of blood from each of his budgerigars by incising the wing vein. This method resulted in excessive blood loss, since it was difficult to stop bleeding from the vein. Puncture of the cere and of the heart were also tried by Gallagher and found unsatisfactory.

Murdock and Lewis[28] described a simple method of obtaining blood from the leg vein of ducks. After the scaly skin is washed with saline, the vein is visible on the medial side of the leg. A 20-gauge needle attached to a 10-ml. syringe is inserted in the vein in the region of the hallux. If blood is drawn slowly, 30–40 ml. may be taken without difficulty. Bleeding is easily stopped by applying pressure over the site for a few minutes. Murdock and Lewis reported taking several 30-ml. specimens at two-week intervals before a duck showed any signs of weakness.

I tried holding the budgerigar myself or having an assistant hold it. I found that if the person collecting the sample holds the bird, he is better able to anticipate the bird's movements and change its position as needed. The bird's back is placed against the palm, and the head steadied between the thumb and forefinger. If the left hand is used to hold the bird, the bird's left leg is held between the ring and middle fingers. The little finger is used to hold the tail against the palm of the hand, and the hand and fingers are bent to fit the contour of the bird's body. The chest is visible at all times, so the collector can be sure the bird is breathing normally and is not overly excited.

At the time of blood collection, all equipment should be conveniently placed so the collector can hold the bird in one hand and manage the equipment with the other. At least two red cell pipettes with mouthpieces attached should be available in case too much blood is drawn into one pipette. One must work quickly when collecting from a clipped nail, since the blood coagulates rapidly. Blood collected from the jugular vein coagulates more slowly.

The longer anterior toenail was found to be the most accessible. A fingernail clipper was used to clip the nail about midway between the base and the end of the vessel visible in the nail. The nail was clipped in an anteroposterior direction, since this tends to dilate the vessel. Clipping the nail sideways tends to compress it.[42] The toe was not held between the fingers since this would greatly decrease the blood supply to the nail. The leg was not grasped so firmly as to interfere with the blood supply to the distal portion. Blood flow was stopped almost immediately by application of firm pressure to the toe with the thumb and forefinger and cauterization of the surface of the nail with a silver nitrate applicator stick. Any blood present must be wiped off before the nail can be properly cauterized. If another blood sample is to be taken several weeks later, a different nail should be used, inasmuch as the blood supply to a nail is reduced after it has been clipped.

HEMOGLOBIN

Hemoglobin values were determined by the method of Denington and Lucas,[12] as cited in Lucas and Jamroz.[24] Whole blood, 0.02 ml., was collected directly from a clipped nail into a Sahli hemoglobin pipette, and mixed with 10 ml. of 0.4% solution of concentrated ammonium hydroxide in distilled water. After an hour,

Table 10-1. Normal Hemoglobin Values* for Budgerigars

	Leonard		Gallagher[15]		
	Age of Birds in Weeks		*Age of Birds in Weeks*		
Hemoglobin (Gm. per 100 ml.)	*8–28*	*48*	*3*	*13–26*	*52*
Mean	15.2	15.5	12.8	17.0	16.7
S.D.	1.1	0.83	1.3	1.0	0.9
Mean ± 3 S.D.	11.9–18.5	13.0–18.0	8.9–16.7	14.0–20.0	14.0–19.4
N	37	16	20	11	20

*S.D. = Standard deviation.
Mean ± 3 S.D. = Range within which 99 per cent of the values determined should occur.
N = Number of birds tested.

Table 10-2. Hemoglobin Values and Red Cell Counts of Young European Tree Sparrows and Black-headed Gulls, Showing an Increase from Birth to 30 Days of Age[19]

Bird	Hemoglobin (Gm./100 ml.)	Red Blood Cells (millions/cu. mm.)
European Tree Sparrow (*Passer montanus*)		
Age in days		
1–5	4.0	1.028
10–15	6.8	1.645
16–20	7.7	2.177
21–30	11.4	2.425
Black-headed Gull (*Larus ridibundus*)		
Age in days		
1		0.850
5–14	7.0	1.515
20–30	10.0	2.435

0.36 ml. of concentrated hydrochloric acid was added and the tube was inverted several times. The acid was added to rid the solution of cloudiness, which does not occur when mammalian blood is used. After 15 minutes, the optical density was read at a wavelength of 410 μ. The hemoglobin value (grams of hemoglobin per 100 ml.) was determined by comparison with a special graph. The graph was made by using an undiluted sample and one-half and one-quarter dilutions of human blood known to have 15.4 grams of hemoglobin per 100 ml.

Gallagher used a standard cyanmethemoglobin method and cleared the solutions by centrifugation.

Despite the different methods used, my results agree fairly closely with those of Gallagher. The ranges given for hemoglobin values are no greater than those given for dogs and cats by Schalm.[37] I did not find any significant differences in hemoglobin values due to age, sex, color, or weight. Gallagher's results indicate that hemoglobin values are lower in birds that are four weeks old or younger (Table 10-1). Sparrows and gulls younger than 30 days have lower hemoglobin values than older birds (Table 10-2). Hemoglobin values for birds of a variety of other species are shown in Table 10-3.

HEMATOCRIT

Blood was collected from a clipped nail directly into heparinized capillary tubes. The tubes were centrifuged in a microhematocrit centrifuge for three minutes. By use of the "t" test[22] with the level of significance set at 1 per cent, it was shown that results obtained when using column heights of 1.0–2.0 cm. were not significantly different from those obtained when using column heights of 2.1–5.8 cm. Therefore, results using columns only 2.0 cm. high should be as accurate as those obtained when higher columns are used. Gallagher also used a microhematocrit technique. After the hematocrit value is determined, the serum in the capillary tube can be drawn off with a micropipette and used for blood chemistry determinations.

I found no significant difference in hematocrit values related to age, sex, color, or weight. Gallagher's results indicate that hematocrit values are lower in birds that are four weeks old or younger (Table 10-4). Hematocrit values for birds of a variety of other species are shown in Table 10-5.

Bierer *et al.*[3] stated that the average hematocrit of eight parakeets with psittacosis was 41 and the range was 35 to 45. These values are definitely below normal according to my results and those of Gallagher.

RED CELL COUNT

For counting red cells blood was collected directly into a red cell pipette which had been rinsed in heparin solution (10 mg. heparin sodium/ml.) to prevent coagulation of the blood. After filling the pipette to the 0.5 ml. mark Natt and Herrick's solution* was added until the 101 mark was reached. Pipettes were then agitated for

(*continued on p. 201*)

*Natt and Herrick's Diluting Fluid[29]:

NaCl	3.88 Gm.
Na_2SO_4	2.50 Gm.
$Na_2HPO_4.12H_2O$	2.91 Gm.
KH_2PO_4	0.25 Gm.
Formalin (37%)	7.50 ml.
Methyl violet 2b	0.10 Gm.

Dissolve in distilled water and dilute to total volume of 1,000 ml. in a volumetric flask. Filter.

Table 10-3. Hemoglobin Values and Red Blood Cell Counts of Birds of Various Species

Bird	Hemoglobin (Gm./100 ml.)	Red Blood Cells (millions/cu. mm.)	Author
Ostrich (*Struthio camelus*)	14.6–17.2	1.653–2.266	De Villiers[13]
Canary (*Serinus canarius*)	7.08–12.04	3.5–5.7 4.5–5.0	Young[44] Ben-Harel[1]
Emperor Penguin (*Aptenoides forsteri*)	20.3	2.2	Schmitt and Righton[40]
King Penguin (*Aptenoides patagonicus*)	19.2	2.21	
Jackass Penguin (*Spheniscus demersus*)	18.2	2.23	
Rockhopper Penguin (*Eudyptes crestatus*)	17.5	2.91	
Humboldt Penguin (*Spheniscus humboldti*)	18.2	2.97	
White-throated Sparrow (*Zonotrichia albicollis*)	13.1–13.9	4.010–6.770	Nice *et al.*[32]
Junco (*Junco hyemalis*)	14.5–16.9	4.495–7.645	
Song Sparrow (*Melospiza melodia*)		4.460–5.225	
White-crowned Sparrow (*Zonotrichia leucophrys*)		4.640–5.690	
Tree Sparrow (*Spizella arborea*)		5.610	
Chipping Sparrow (*Spizella passerina*)		5.533	
Lincoln Sparrow (*Melospiza lincolni*)		5.230	
Cardinal (*Richmondena cardinalis*)	15.7–17.9	4.488–5.605	
Rufous-sided Towhee (*Pipilo erythrophthalmus*)		4.200	
House Sparrow (*Passer domesticus*)		4.231–5.769	
Tufted Titmouse (*Baeolophus bicolor*)	13.3–13.6	3.930–4.685	
Cowbird (*Molothrus ater*)		5.420–6.690	
Bronzed Grackle (*Quiscalus q. aeneus*)	16.5	5.405	
Brown Thrasher (*Toxostoma rufum*)	16.0	5.904	
Hermit Thrush (*Hylocichla guttata*)		4.810	
Bob-white (*Colinus virginianus*)		3.080–3.805	
Carrion Crow (*Corvus corone*)		2.490	Ponder[33]
Peregrine Falcon (*Falco peregrinus*)		2.547	
Grey Heron (*Ardea cinerea*)		2.478	
Spoonbill (*Platelea*)		3.400	
White Stork (*Cinconia alba*)		2.189	
Arabian Ostrich (*Struthio camelus*)		1.620	
Eagle Owl (Uhu) (*Bubo bubo*)	10.8	1.690	Christoph and Frank[5]
Long-eared Owl (Waldohreule) (*Asio otus*)	11.4	2.209	
Short-eared Owl (Sumpfohreule) (*Asio flammeus*)	14.9	2.720	

Table 10-3. (Continued)

Bird	Hemoglobin (Gm. / 100 ml.)	Red Blood Cells (millions / cu. mm.)	Author
Wood Owl (Waldkauz) (*Strix aluco*)	11.0	2.174	Christoph
Little Owl (Steinkauz) (*Athene noctua*)	11.5	2.267	and Frank[5]
Barn Owl (Schleiereule) (*Tyto alba*)	11.7	2.225	
Pheasant	13.7		Dukes and
Swan	13.4		Schwarte[14]
Brant	14.7		
Peafowl	12.0		
Goose	14.9		
Turkey	10.7		
Mallard Duck (*Anas platyrhynchos*)	12.9–18.2	2.51–3.67	Magath and Higgins[25]
Duck (mixed breeds—White Pekin, Mallards and hybrids)	7.5–16.5	2.23–3.75	Hewitt[16]
White Pekin Duck		1.84–3.32	
Dove			Riddle and
male	14.56	3.045	Braucher[34]
female	13.97	2.989	
Pigeon			
male	15.97	3.228	
female	14.72	3.096	
Pigeon		3.8	Scarborough[36]
Pigeon		2.84–3.9	Klineberger[21]
Pigeon			De Eds[11]
heart blood		2.625–4.325	
leg vein blood		2.275–4.475	

	Hemoglobin (Sahli°)	Red Blood Cells (millions / cu. mm.)	Author
Herring Gull (Silbermöven) (*Larus argentatus*)	90.25	2.14	Christoph and
Common Gull (Sturmmöven) (*Larus canus*)	92.10	2.55	Traue[7]
Laughing Gull (Lachmöven) (*Larus atricilla*)	86.50	2.67	

Table 10-3. (Continued)

Bird	Hemoglobin (Sahli°)	Red Blood Cells (millions/cu. mm.)	Author
Common Buzzard (Mäusebussarde) (*Buteo buteo*)	67–85	1.77–3.09	Christoph and Borowski[4]
Kestrel (Turmfalken) (*Falco tinnunculus*)	72–85	1.92–3.11	
Black Kite (Schwarze Milane) (*Milvus migrans*)	74–91	1.86–3.19	
Red Kite (Roter Milan) (*Milvus milvus*)	84	2.50	
Marsh Harrier (Rohrweihen) (*Circus aeruginosus*)	65–84	2.09–5.38	
Honey Buzzard (Wespenbussard) (*Pernis apivorus*)	76	1.97	
Gray Sea Eagle (Seeadler) (*Haliaetus albicilla*)	94	2.44	
Golden Eagle (Steinadler) (*Aquila chrysaetos*)	74	2.56	
Tawny Eagle (Steppenadler) (*Aquila rapax*)	76	2.20	
Imperial Eagle (Kaiseradler) (*Aquila heliaca*)	87	2.44	
Andean Condor (Kondor) (*Vultur gryphus*)	103	2.38	
Griffon Vulture (Gansegeier) (*Gyps fulvus*)	86–89	2.35–2.51	
Egyptian Vulture (Schmutzgeier) (*Neophron percnopterus*)	76	1.54	
Greater Sulfur-crested Cockatoo (Gelbhaubenkakadu) (*Kakatoe galerita*)	117	2.47	Christoph and Traue[8]
Bare-eyed Cockatoo (Nacktaugenkakadu) (*Kakatoe sanguinea*)	100	2.18	
Umbrella-crested Cockatoo (Weisshaubenkakadu) (*Kakatoe alba*)	92	2.54	
Rose-breasted Cockatoo (Rosakakadu) (*Kakatoe roseicapilla*)	106	2.79	
Leadbeater's Cockatoo (Inkakakadu) (*Kakatoe leadbeateri*)	100.5	2.04	
Blue and Gold Macaw (Gelbbl. Ararauna) (*Ara ararauna*)	100	2.45	
Mauge's Conure (Grunflugelara) (*Aratinga chloroptera*)	98	2.73	
Jenday Conure (Jendayasittich) (*Aratinga jendaya*)	112	3.22	
Nanday Conure (Nandasittich) (*Nandayus nenday*)	92	2.85	
Green Conure (Guyanasittich) (*Aratinga leucophthalmus*)	116	2.50	
Finsch's Amazon (Blaukappenamazone) (*Amazona finschi*)	109	2.53	
Festive Amazon (Blaubartamazone) (*Amazona festiva*)	105	2.55	
Yellow-fronted Amazon (Surinamamazone) (*Amazona ochrocephala*)	84	2.73	
Blue-fronted Amazon (Rotbugamazone) (*Amazona aestiva*)	108	2.63	

Table 10-3. (Continued)

Bird	Hemoglobin (Sahli°)	Red Blood Cells (millions/cu. mm.)	Author
Panama Amazon (Panamaamazone) (*Amazona panamensis*)	95	2.28	Christoph and Traue[8]
Vinaceous Amazon (Taubenhalsamazone) (*Amazona vinacea*)	86	2.53	
Versicolor Amazon (Blaustirnamazone) (*Amazona versicolor*)	94	2.66	
Bodin's Amazon (Rotstirnamazone) (*Amazona bodini*)	100	1.84	
Senegal Parrot (Mohrenkopfsittich) (*Poicephalus senegalus*)	91	2.73	
African Grey Parrot (Graupapagei) (*Psittacus erithacus*)	98	2.58	
African Ringneck (Halsbandsittich) (*Psittacula krameri*)	101	2.84	
Plum-head Parakeet (Pflaumenkopfsittich) (*Psittacula cyanocephala*)	89	3.77	
Red Rosella Parakeet (Rosellasittich) (*Platycercus eximius*)	104	3.44	
Redrump Parakeet (Singsittich) (*Psephotus haematonotus*)	113	3.78	
Cockatiel (Nymphensittich) (*Nymphicus hollandicus*)	110	3.23	
Hybrid—Red Rosella (male), Crimson Rosella (female) (Buschwaldsittich) (*Platycercus elegans*)	138	3.73	
Pelican	88.93	2.415	Christoph and Schube[6]
Domestic Chicken (*Gallus gallus domesticus*)	74	3.62	Yamamoto[43]
Silky Chicken (*Gallus gallus domesticus*)	82	3.505	
Grey-breasted Guineafowl (*Numida galeata*)	75.5	3.315	
King Quail (*Coturnix coturnix japonica*)	96	4.175	
Domestic Duck (*Anas platyrhynchos domestica*)	82.5	3.205	
Spotbill Duck (*Anas poecilorhyncho zonorhyncha*)	73.5	3.205	
Mandarin Duck (*Aix galericulata*)	83	3.33	
Budgerigar (*Melopsittacus undulatus*)	103.5	4.86	
Nyassaland Lovebird (*Agapornis lilianae*)	91	3.97	
Pigeon (*Columba lilianae domestica*)	99.5	3.98	
Eastern Turtle Dove (*Streptopelia orientalis*)	91.5	4.08	
Meadow Bunting (*Emberiza cioides ciopsis*)	92.5	4.41	

Table 10-3. (Continued)

Bird	Hemoglobin (Sahli°)	Red Blood Cells (millions/cu. mm.)	Author
Canary (*Serinus canarius*)	80.5	4.06	Yamamoto[43]
Tree Sparrow (*Passer montanus saturatus*)	78	4.29	
Skylark (*Alauda arvensis japonica*)	98	5.71	
Indian White-eye (*Zosterops palpebrosa japonica*)	83	4.31	
Brown-eared Bulbul (*Ixos [Microscelis] amaurotis amaurotis*)	97.5	4.38	
Bush Warbler (*Horeites cantans cantans*)	82.5	4.38	
Java Sparrow (*Padda oryzivora*)	84.5	4.11	
Zebra Finch (*Poephila castanotis*)	103	5.38	
Striated Mannikin (*Urolonchura [Lonchura] striata*)	101.5	4.65	
Black-billed Magpie (*Pica pica japonica*)	87	3.80	

Table 10-4. Normal Hematocrit Values* for Budgerigars

Hematocrit (per cent)	Leonard		Gallagher[15]		
	Age of Birds in Weeks		Age of Birds in Weeks		
	8–28	*48*	*3*	*13–26*	*52*
Mean	51	51	41.3	53.7	53.2
S.D.	2.5	2.7	3.2	2.7	4.0
Mean ± 3 S.D.	43.5–58.5	42.9–59.1	31.7–50.9	45.6–61.8	41.2–65.2
N	35	15	20	11	20

*S.D. = Standard deviation.
Mean ± 3 S.D. = Range within which 99 per cent of the values determined should occur.
N = Number of birds tested.

Table 10-5. Hematocrit Values and Red Blood Cell Counts of Birds of Various Families (Measurements are averaged, with ranges shown in parentheses) (From Bennett and Chisholm[2])

Bird	Number	Age*	Sex†	Hematocrit (per cent)	Erythrocytes (millions per cu. mm.)
TETRAONIDAE					
Ruffed Grouse					
(*Bonasa umbellus*)	2	A	M	37.4	—
LARIDAE					
Herring Gull					
(*Larus argentatus*)	10	I		33.9 (28–36)	—
ALCEDINIDAE					
Belted Kingfisher					
(*Megaceryle alcyon*)	1	A	F	54.8	—
PICIDAE					
Yellow-shafted Flicker					
(*Colaptes auratus*)	1	A	F	42.6	—
Yellow-bellied Sapsucker					
(*Sphyrapicus varius*)	3	A	M	48.5 (46–49)	3.95 (1‡)
Hairy Woodpecker	2	A	M	47.0	4.03
(*Dendrocopos villosus*)	1	A	F	47.4	—
Arctic Three-toed Woodpecker					
(*Picoides tridactylus*)	1	A	F	42.5	4.22
TYRANNIDAE					
Yellow-bellied Flycatcher§					
(*Empidonax flaviventris*)	5	A	MF	51.7 (47–55)	—
(*Empidonax* spp.)	21	AI	MF	49 (30–59)	6.62 (1‡)
Eastern Wood Pewee§					
(*Contopus virens*)	2	I		46.5	5.70 (1‡)
HIRUNDINIDAE					
Bank Swallow					
(*Riparia riparia*)	9	A	MF	53.8 (48–59)	—
Barn Swallow					
(*Hirundo rustica*)	2	A	MF	56.1	5.35
CORVIDAE					
Canada Jay	9	A	MF	46.6 (44–53)	4.66 (2‡)
(*Perisoreus canadensis*)	6	I	MF	46.9 (44–47.2)	4.88 (1‡)

*A, adult; I, immature.
†F, female; M, male.
‡Number of birds measured for the value cited.
§Birds examined from mid-August through mid-September.

Table 10-5. (Continued)

Bird	Number	Age*	Sex†	Hematocrit (per cent)	Erythrocytes (millions per cu. mm.)
CORVIDAE (Continued)					
Blue Jay					
(*Cyanocitta cristata*)	4	A	MF	47.1 (46–48.5)	4.51 (2‡)
PARIDAE					
Black-capped Chickadee	10	A	MF	48.1 (40–56)	5.62
(*Parus atricapillus*)				50.2 (45–52)	
Brown-capped Chickadee					
(*Parus hudsonicus*)	4	A	MF	47.3 (42–53)	
SITTIDAE					
Red-breasted Nuthatch					
(*Sitta canadensis*)	1	A		46.9	—
MIMIDAE					
Catbird					
(*Dumetella carolinensis*)	1	A		42.6	
TURDIDAE					
American Robin	2	A	M	46.6	—
(*Turdus migratorius*)	3	A	F	45.4 (40–47)	4.35 (1‡)
	3	I		37.3 (35–40.1)	4.08
Veery§					
(*Hylocichla fuscescens*)	10	A	MF	51.8 (47–59)	5.45 (5.08–6.0) (4‡)
Olive-back Thrush	8	A	MF	46.1 (44–56)	4.83
(*Hylocichla ustulata*)	1	I		43.8	4.66
SYLVIIDAE					
Golden-crowned Kinglet					
(*Regulus satrapa*)	1	A	M	41.8	—
BOMBYCILLIDAE					
Cedar Waxwing§					
(*Bombycilla cedrorum*)	1	A		53.6	—
STURNIDAE					
Starling§	5	A	F	49.8 (48.6–52.8)	11.3 (10.6–12.1)
(*Sturnus vulgaris*)	6	I		47.3 (45–49.4)	

*A, adult; I, immature.
†F, female; M, male.
‡Number of birds measured for the value cited.
§Birds examined from mid-August through mid-September.

Table 10-5. (Continued)

Bird	Number	Age*	Sex†	Hematocrit (per cent)	Erythrocytes (millions per cu. mm.)
VIREONIDAE					
Solitary vireo§	1	I		45.7	
(*Vireo solitarius*)					
Red-eyed Vireo	3	A	MF	48 (44–50)	5.03
(*Vireo olivaceus*)	4	I		47.9 (46–49)	
Philadelphia Vireo					
(*Vireo philadelphicus*)	1	A		55.0	—
PARULIDAE					
Black and White Warbler	3	A	F	46.4 (44–50)	4.76
(*Mniotilta varia*)§	5	I		42.1 (36–48)	5.60
Tennessee Warbler§					
(*Vermivora perigrina*)	1		F	50.9	
Orange-crowned Warbler					
(*Vermivora celata*)	1	A	F	49.5	
Nashville Warbler	8	A	MF	46.5 (40–56)	3.99 (1‡)
(*Vermivora ruficapilla*)	4	I		49.3 (46–52)	
Magnolia Warbler	2	A	M	49.6	—
(*Dendroica magnolia*)	4	A	F	48.1 (44–53)	
	13	I		42.4 (30–52)	3.79
Cape May Warbler§	1	A	F	44.9	—
(*Dendroica tigrina*)	1	I		38.9	
Myrtle Warbler	7	A	M	51.1 (45–54)	—
(*Dendroica coronata*)	6	A	F	50.1 (48–53)	
	5	I		44.1 (39–47)	
Chestnut-sided Warbler	6	A	M	55.7 (51–60)	5.4 (1‡)
(*Dendroica pensylvanica*)	2	A	F	50.	
	1	I		41.7	5.54
Bay-breasted Warbler§	2	A	M	50	
(*Dendroica castanea*)	—	A	F	48.8 (42–53)	
Blackpoll Warbler					
(*Dendroica striata*)	2	A	F	51.4	
Ovenbird	13	A	MF	47.2 (43–51)	—
(*Seiurus aurocapillus*)	7	I		42.4 (36–55)	4.6 (1‡)
Northern Waterthrush					
(*Seiurus noveboracensis*)	3	A		49.8 (47–53)	4.83
Mourning Warbler§					
(*Oporornis philadelphia*)	1	A	M	50.8	
Northern Yellowthroat	3	A	MF	51.1 (43–56)	—
(*Geothlypsis trichas*)	9	I		43.1	

*A, adult; I, immature.
†F, female; M, male.
‡Number of birds measured for the value cited.
§Birds examined from mid-August through mid-September.

Table 10-5. (Continued)

Bird	Number	Age*	Sex†	Hematocrit (per cent)	Erythrocytes (millions per cu. mm.)
PARULIDAE (Continued)					
Wilson's Warbler	2	A	M	57.4	
(*Wilsonia pusilla*)	1	I	F	44.0	
Canada Warbler	7	A	M	52.1 (47–57)	
(*Wilsonia canadensis*)	9	A	F	53.6 (48–64)	
	3	I		49.6 (49–50)	
American Redstart§					
(*Setophaga ruticilla*)	4	I		41.1 (34–45)	
PLOCEIDAE					
House Sparrow	2	A	M	50.5	
(*Passer domesticus*)	2	A	F	50.5	
ICTERIDAE					
Common Grackle	4	A	M	49.9 (46–53.5)	3.77 (1‡)
(*Quiscalus quiscula*)	6	A	F	46.5 (41.4–52)	4.81 (2‡)
FRINGILLIDAE					
Rose-breasted Grosbeak	2	A	M	53.3	—
(*Pheucticus ludovicianus*)	1	A	F	43	
Evening Grosbeak	10	A	M	54.9 (44–64)	5.03 (4.3–5.6) (6‡)
(*Hesperiphona vespertina*)	4	A	F	56.8 (54–62)	
Purple Finch	6	A	M	59.4 (51–71)	4.01 (2‡)
(*Carpodacus purpureus*)	9	A		54.0 (48–63)	5.45 (2‡)
	2	I		51.9 (2)	
Pine Siskin					
(*Spinus pinus*)	6	A	MF	48.7 (40–56)	6.24
Slate-colored Junco	6	A	MF	47.0 (44–52)	—
(*Junco hyemalis*)	1	I		42.6	
Chipping Sparrow	4	A	M	54.5 (50–61)	—
(*Spizella passerina*)	3	A	F	53.6 (51–58)	
White-crowned Sparrow					
(*Zonotrichia leucophrys*)	6	A	F	51.4 (45–57)	—
White-throated Sparrow	9	A	M	48.3 (40–58.6)	—
(*Zonotrichia albicollis*)	12	A	F	44.6 (39–55)	3.76 (1‡)
Lincoln's Sparrow	2	I		40.9 (38.4–43.4)§	
(*Melospiza lincolnii*)		A		48.1	
Swamp Sparrow	2	A	M	52.2	
(*Melospiza georgiana*)	2	A	F	57.6	
	2	I		49.4	
Song Sparrow	1	A	M	51.0	
(*Melospiza melodia*)	3	I		44.8	

*A, adult; I, immature.
†F, female; M, male.
‡Number of birds measured for the value cited.
§Birds examined from mid-August through mid-September.

(continued from p. 191)

30 seconds with a Yankee pipette shaker.* Five of the secondary squares of the central primary square of the counting chamber were counted, which is the usual method when examining mammalian blood.

Gallagher used a different blood diluent†; he used the same area I used in counting the cells, but used a 1:20 dilution. I found that in dilutions lower than 1:200 too many cells overlapped and they were too numerous in the area to be counted accurately.

Schlumberger[38] used the diluting fluid of Darcel‡ in counting red and white cells in the blood of budgerigars.

Despite the different methods used, my results agree fairly closely with those of Gallagher. The ranges given for numbers of red cells are no wider than those given for dogs and cats by Schalm.[37]

Schlumberger and Henschke[39] found that the number of red cells in blood specimens from 20 budgerigars ranged from 2.95 to 4.80 million per cu. mm. These

*Clay-Adams, Inc., New York, N.Y.

†Gallagher's Diluting Fluid:

Trisodium citrate	3 Gm.
Formalin	40%
New methylene blue	0.01 Gm.
Distilled water	100 ml.

‡Darcel's Diluting Fluid[10]:

Solution 1:
Sodium chloride	0.66 Gm.
Sodium citrate	1.11 Gm.
Neutral formalin	5 ml.
Distilled water	95 ml.

Solution 2: Giemsa solution (B.D.H.) 1 ml. solution to be added to 9 ml. of solution 1. Filter before use.

figures are lower than those obtained in my studies or by Gallagher.

I did not find any significant differences in red cell counts due to age, sex, color, or weight. Gallagher's results indicate that the red cell count is lower in birds that are four weeks old or younger (Table 10-6). As shown in Table 10-2, younger sparrows and gulls also have lower red cell counts than older birds. Red cell counts of various other species are shown in Table 10-3 and Table 10-5.

RETICULOCYTE COUNT. Gallagher diluted 1% brilliant cresyl blue in 0.85% sodium chloride 1:4, with blood. After mixing gently and allowing to stand for 10 minutes, blood films were made and stained by Leishman's method. The percentage of cells in which the nucleus was completely surrounded by reticular material was determined. Gallagher's values are given in Table 10-7.

Anemia and basophilic stippling of red cells occurs in ducks poisoned by ingested lead shot. Large numbers of erythroblasts and megaloblasts may be found in the blood. The proportion of reticulocytes may be as high as 70 per cent of the red cells.[17] According to Magath and Higgins,[25] the blood of the normal duck contains 13.2–35.8 per cent reticulocytes.

A trumpeter swan (*Cygnus buccinator*) with many red cells in different stages of granular degeneration has been reported.[35] The bird had been abused in a fight with a man and died of two fractured cervical vertebrae. The authors suggest that this condition might have been due to the release of red cells which had been previously removed from the circulation.

Table 10-6. Normal Red Cell Counts* for Budgerigars

Erythrocytes (millions per cu. mm.)	Leonard		Gallagher[15]		
	Age of Birds in Weeks		Age of Birds in Weeks		
	8–28	48	3	13–26	52
Mean	5.66	5.48	3.15	4.49	4.50
S.D.	0.54	0.68	0.29	0.35	0.30
Mean ± 3 S.D.	4.04–7.28	3.44–7.52	2.28–4.02	3.44–5.54	3.60–5.40
N	35	16	20	11	20

*S.D. = Standard deviation.
Mean ± 3 S.D. = Range within which 99 per cent of the values determined should occur.
N = Number of birds tested.

Table 10-7. Normal Reticulocyte Counts* for Budgerigars[15]

Reticulocytes (per cent)	Age of Birds in Weeks		
	3	13–26	52
Mean	12.3	6.7	6.7
S.D.	3.1	0.9	1.2
Mean ± 3 S.D.	3.0–21.6	4.0–9.4	3.1–10.3
N	20	11	20

*S.D. = Standard deviation.
Mean ± 3 S.D. = Range within which 99 per cent of the values determined should occur.
N = Number of birds tested.

Table 10-8. M.C.V., M.C.H., and M.C.H.C. Values* for Budgerigars Calculated from Hematocrit and Hemoglobin Values and Red Cell Counts Given in Tables 10-4, 10-1, and 10-6, Respectively

	Leonard		Gallagher[15]		
	Age of Birds in Weeks		Age of Birds in Weeks		
	8–28	48	3	13–26	52
M.C.V.					
Mean	90.0	93.1	130.4	120.1	115.6
S.D.	12.5	9.3	12.2	10.1	7.9
Mean ± 3 S.D.	52.5–127.5	65.2–121.0	93.8–167.0	89.8–150.4	91.9–139.3
N	34	15	20	11	20
M.C.H.					
Mean	26.5	28.6	40.7	38.2	36.6
S.D.	3.3	2.4	3.6	2.4	2.5
Mean ± 3 S.D.	16.6–36.4	21.4–35.8	29.9–51.5	31.0–45.4	29.1–44.1
N	36	16	20	11	20
M.C.H.C.					
Mean	29.8	30.6	31.0	31.6	31.3
S.D.	2.1	1.8	2.3	1.4	1.2
Mean ± 3 S.D.	23.5–36.1	25.2–36.0	24.1–37.9	27.4–35.8	27.7–34.9
N	35	15	20	11	20

*S.D. = Standard deviation.
Mean ± 3 S.D. = Range within which 99 per cent of the values determined should occur.
N = Number of birds tested.

MCV, MCH, AND MCHC

Mean corpuscular volume (MCV), mean corpuscular hemoglobin (MCH), and mean corpuscular hemoglobin concentration (MCHC) were calculated from hematocrit and hemoglobin values and the red cell counts. These values (Table 10-8) may be helpful in differentiating types of anemia present in birds.

WHITE CELL COUNT

With avian blood, it is impossible to selectively destroy the red cells and leave only the white cells, as can be done with mammals. This is mainly because avian red cells and thrombocytes are nucleated.

I have had completely unsatisfactory results with Rees-Ecker solution as modified by Lucas[24] and Natt and Herrick's solution which are used to study white cell counts in chickens, and Stroud's solution[42] which was used to study white cells in canaries. Only rarely could I find a leukocyte when using these solutions. A solution prepared by diluting five parts of Natt and Herrick's solution with four parts of distilled water was found satisfactory, however. Apparently the osmotic pressure or pH makes the undiluted solution unsuitable for use with budgerigar blood. Red cell pipettes were used with the diluted Natt and Herrick solution to make a 1:200 dilution. Heterophils, which are homologous with the neutrophils of mammalian blood, were the easiest white cells to recognize in the counting chamber. Their large dark granules make them unmistakable, but it is difficult to recognize the other white cells in the counting chamber and to distinguish them from some immature red cells and thrombocytes. I decided that the most accurate way to obtain total white counts was to determine the number of heterophils per cu. mm. by use of the hemocytometer, and then to find the percentage of heterophils from the blood film. From these two values, the total white count was determined. Heterophils were counted in all squares of one side of the counting chamber. The number of heterophils seen was multiplied by 222 to determine the number of heterophils per cu. mm. If eight heterophils were counted and the differential count showed that 40 per cent of the white cells were heterophils, then the total number of white cells per cu. mm. was $8 \times 222 \times 100/40$, or 4440 white cells per cu. mm. Pipettes were not rinsed in heparin first, as was done when counting the red cells, because it was thought heparin might destroy some of the white cells, as occurs in cats.[18] Undiluted Natt and Herrick solution was used to determine red cell counts, but the diluted solution could be used when both red and white cells were to be counted.

Gallagher used the same solution for total white cell counts as for red cell counts. He used a 1:20 dilution and counted all the white cells, rather than just the heterophils, in an area about half as large as the one I used.

The results of my studies and of the studies of Gallagher are shown in Table 10-9.

DIFFERENTIAL COUNT. Smears used for differential counts were made with a drop of blood obtained directly from a clipped nail and quickly air dried. Films of avian blood require a longer staining time than those of mammalian blood. Slides were stained for 5 minutes with Wright's stain, and distilled water was then applied for another 5 minutes. The distilled water had a pH of about 5. Buffered solutions used for mammalian blood films which have a pH of about 7 will not properly stain avian blood cells. I used Wright's stain so that I could more easily recognize budgerigar cells from the illustrations of chicken blood stained with Wright's stain in the *Atlas of Avian Hematology* by Lucas and Jamroz.[24] Gallagher believed that Leishman's stain was better than Wright's.

Differential counts were used to find the relative percentages of heterophils, lymphocytes, monocytes, and basophils. One-hundred white cells were counted in each blood film. Cells were counted by starting at one edge and moving the slide back and forth approaching the opposite edge with the completion of each row. This method is suitable for avian blood since it has been shown with chicken blood that white cells occur randomly throughout the blood film. This differs from mammalian blood, in which they are located mainly at the edges of the slide.[23] I found the making of differential counts of budgerigar blood a tedious procedure, since there are fewer white cells in the smears than in mammalian blood films. In some cases most of the slide was scanned before 100 cells were found.

The *Atlas of Avian Hematology*[24] by Lucas and Jamroz was very useful, especially since it shows the many variations of each cell type. Although it illustrates the cells of the chicken, budgerigar blood cells were found to be quite similar.

The large number of "smudge" or "smear" cells proved to be an important problem. Lymphocytes seemed to become smudged more commonly than other white cells. Therefore, true lymphocyte percentages and counts are probably higher than the values given in Table 10-9. Gallagher found fewer smudged cells in blood collected into a vial containing an anticoagulant.

Before distinguishing the different types of white cells, one must be able to recognize red cells and thrombocytes and be familiar with the wide variation that may occur in red cells.

Both the nucleus and the body of red cells are oval.

Table 10-9. Normal White Cell and Differential Counts* for Budgerigars

	Leonard		Gallagher		
	Age of Birds in Weeks		Age of Birds in Weeks		
	8–28	48	3	13–26	52
Total White Cells (per cu. mm.)					
Mean	6,530	3,803	6,450	4,000	4,000
S.D.	3,550	627	3,265	2,250	1,440
Mean ± 3 S.D.	0–17,180	1,922–5,684	0–16,245	0–10,750	0–8,320
N	25	18	20	11	20
Heterophils (per cent)					
Mean	52.4	61.3	55.3	59.0	64.4
S.D.	15.0	14.4	11.8	12.3	8.4
Mean ± 3 S.D.	7.4–97.4	18.1–104.5	19.9–90.7	22.1–95.9	39.2–89.6
N	25	18	20	11	20
Heterophils (per cu. mm.)					
Mean	3,090	2,000	–	–	–
S.D.	1,780	1,290			
Mean ± 3 S.D.	0–8,400	0–5,870			
N	25	18			
Lymphocytes (per cent)					
Mean	33.3	21.9	37.1	33.1	29.4
S.D.	14.0	12.0	11.5	13.5	8.6
Mean ± 3 S.D.	0–75.3	0–57.9	2.6–71.6	0–73.6	3.6–55.2
N	25	18	20	11	20
Lymphocytes (per cu. mm.)					
Mean	2,320	721	–	–	–
S.D.	2,170	424			
Mean ± 3 S.D.	0–6,510	0–1,993			
N	25	18			
Monocytes (per cent)					
Mean	5.5	3.4	3.2	4.1	3.0
S.D.	4.0	2.4	1.3	1.3	1.5
Mean ± 3 S.D.	0–17.5	0–10.6	0–7.1	0.2–8.0	0–7.5
N	25	18	20	11	20
Monocytes (per cu. mm.)					
Mean	323	124	–	–	–
S.D.	210	94			
Mean ± 3 S.D.	0–953	0–406			
N	25	18			
Basophils (per cent)					
Mean	8.9	13.3	4.1	3.8	3.2
S.D.	4.8	5.5	3.7	1.9	1.5
Mean ± 3 S.D.	0–23	0–30	0–14.8	0–9.5	0–7.7
N	25	18	20	11	20
Basophils (per cu. mm.)					
Mean	550	478	–	–	–
S.D.	466	247			
Mean ± 3 S.D.	0–1,860	0–1219			
N	25	18			

*S.D. = Standard deviation.
Mean ± 3 S.D. = Range within which 99 per cent of the values determined should occur.
N = Number of birds tested.

The cytoplasm becomes orange-pink with Wright's stain. Thrombocytes are smaller and are usually more rectangular than red cells. Their cytoplasm is usually very pale and almost transparent, and contains one to three red granules. Lymphocytes and monocytes resemble their counterparts in mammalian blood. I found that in many cases it was difficult to differentiate the two because of the variety of their size and shape. Some immature red cells could be confused with the lymphocytes. These immature red cells usually have a blue-green cytoplasm which is more dense than that of a lymphocyte. The elliptical and rarely distorted cell outline is more characteristic of a red than of a white cell. Nuclei of granulocytes are usually partially lobed, but are never as segmented as those of mammalian cells or of those of the domestic chicken. Basophils and heterophils are easily recognized by their granules. Basophils contain dark blue spherical granules; the granules of heterophils are dark red and spherical to spindle-shaped. The nuclei of basophils are usually obscured by the granules. Some workers in poultry hematology believe that eosinophils cannot be differentiated from heterophils because of staining artifacts.[29] Despite the use of differential staining techniques, I do not believe that it is possible to distinguish eosinophils from heterophils in budgerigar blood. Gallagher stated that eosinophils contain many round granules that are larger than any of those of heterophils. He found fewer than 0.3 per cent eosinophils in differential smears. The ranges for total white counts and the values of the various types of white cells shown in Table 10-9 are quite wide. Lucas and his co-workers, who did extensive work with chickens, found wide variations in these values to be characteristic of normal birds.[24] As well as different birds showing considerable variation, repeated blood samples from the same bird differed greatly. Since the ranges are wide, repeated blood samples are necessary and the values in blood of diseased birds must differ greatly from the normal to be of diagnostic and prognostic significance.

Schlumberger and Henschke[39] found that the total white cell count in 20 budgerigars ranged from 12,220 to 46,660 per cu. mm. These counts are at least twice as high as those found by me and by Gallagher. I assume that Schlumberger included thrombocytes in the counts whereas Gallagher and I did not. Schlumberger and Henschke[39] found that the red and white cell counts of these birds were markedly reduced after total body irradiation with 2,000 R. Table 10-10 lists total white cell counts and differential white cell values for various species. The sources should be consulted for information on the various techniques used in their determination before these values or those given in other tables are used as a basis for comparison in future studies.

THROMBOCYTE COUNT

Gallagher counted the thrombocytes in the central and in one other ruled area of a counting chamber. Each area equaled one sq. mm. He used the same blood diluent for thrombocyte counts as for red and white cell counts. His values are given in Table 10-11.

BLOOD GLUCOSE

Blood glucose levels were determined with 0.05 ml. of whole blood, using a micromethod based on the Somogyi-Nelson method.[26] Values determined with a reagent strip test* agreed fairly closely with the micromethod.

I found that the mean blood glucose level of 10 budgerigars which had been fasted for 18 to 24 hours was 153 mg./100 ml. The standard deviation was 25.2. Schlumberger[38] stated that the blood sugar levels of 30 normal, non-fasted budgerigars ranged from 144 to 306 mg. per 100 ml., with an average of 210 mg./100 ml. Fasting the birds for 24 hours caused a drop of 30–50 mg. per 100 ml. Schlumberger found that most budgerigars with pituitary tumor transplants had higher than normal blood glucose values. In six budgerigars with large tumor transplants, non-fasting blood glucose levels were above 1,000 mg. per 100 ml. In eight birds with primary pituitary tumors and no transplants, the average non-fasting glucose level was 232 mg./100 ml., with a range of 97 to 366 mg. per 100 ml. Three non-fasting budgerigars which had large actively growing fibrosarcoma transplants had blood glucose levels of 273, 219, and 302 mg. per 100 ml. In none of the normal hens that became obese did Schlumberger find blood glucose levels above normal.

According to Nelson *et al.*,[31] the blood glucose level of the normal great horned owl (*Bubo virginianus virginianus*) varies from 200 to 350 mg. per 100 ml. Pancreatectomy results in blood glucose levels as high as 1200 mg./100 ml. Pancreatectomy does not significantly alter the blood glucose level of ducks.[27]

BLOOD URIC ACID

Determination of uric acid levels would probably be of value in the diagnosis of renal diseases of cage birds. Schlumberger and Henschke[39] found that the blood uric acid level of nine budgerigars exposed to radiation ranged from 5.3 to 8.0 mg. per 100 ml. They stated that these values were within normal limits for the budgerigar, but did not give the normal range.

---

*Dextrostix, Ames Company, Inc., Elkhart, Ind.

Table 10-10. White Blood Cell Counts and Differential Values of Various Species of Birds

Bird	Total White Cells (thousands/ cu. mm.)	Lymphocytes (per cent)	Monocytes (per cent)	Heterophils (per cent)	Eosinophils (per cent)	Basophils (per cent)	Thrombocytes (thousands/ cu. mm.)	Author
Ostrich (Struthio camelus)	12.3-32.3	19.2-37.0	0.5-8.5	40.5-78.5	0-19.5	1.0-10.5	2.5-20.1	De Villiers[13]
Emperor Penguin (Kaiserpinguin) (Aptenoides forsteri)	10.9							Schmitt and Righton[40]
King Penguin (Königspinguin) (Aptenoides patagonicus)	16.0							
Jackass Penguin (Eselspinguin) (Spheniscus demersus)	16.3							
Rockhopper Penguin (Felsenpinguin) (Eudyptes crestatus)	13.1							
Humboldt Penguin (Humboldtpinguin) (Spheniscus humboldti)	14.6							
Average differential counts of 15 penguins of the five species listed above		35.0	2.5	57.3	3.0	2.2		
Herring Gull (Silbermöven) (Larus argentatus)	16.000	68.59	1.89	24.83	2.01	2.67	7.6	Christoph and Traue[7]
Common, Mew or Short-billed Gull (Sturmmöven) (Larus canus)	13.955	62.39	1.07	30.31	1.19	5.05	5.9	
Laughing Gull (Lachmöven) (Larus atricilla)	15.433						12.3	
Common Buzzard (Mäusebussarde) (Buteo buteo)	14.0-49.0	35-65.5	0.25-3.75	20.5-39.8	5.5-19	0.25-8	3.5-44	Christoph and Borowski[4]

Table 10-10. (Continued)

Bird	Total White Cells (thousands / cu. mm.)	Lymphocytes (per cent)	Monocytes (per cent)	Heterophils (per cent)	Eosinophils (per cent)	Basophils (per cent)	Thrombocytes (thousands / cu. mm.)	Author
Kestrel (Turmfalken) (*Falco tinnunculus*)	14.5–57.0	24–57.5	0.25–3.0	11.3–33	8.75–59.3	1.5–3.8	11.5–51.5	Christoph and Borowski[4]
Black Kite (Schwarze Milane) (*Milvus migrans*)	10.0–28.0	29.5–50.5	0–2	28.8–35.3	12.8–35.5	2.3–3.5	3.0–15.5	
Red Kite (Roter Milan) (*Milvus milvus*)	12.0	48.8	0.75	19.5	28.3	2.8	10.5	
Marsh Harrier (Rohrweihen) (*Circus aeruginosus*)	9.0–33.0	48–59.5	2.5–10.5	26.5–39.5	1.5–6.5	2.8–5.3	9.5–14.5	
Honey Buzzard (Wespenbussard) (*Pernis apivorus*)	10.5	55.3	1.25	29.8	9	4.8	14.5	
Gray Sea Eagle (Seeadler) (*Haliaetus albicilla*)	19.5	55	2	32.3	9.5	1.3	12.5	
Golden Eagle (Steinadler) (*Aquila chrysaetos*)	23.5	34	4.3	52.5	6	3.3	16.0	
Tawny Eagle (Steppenadler) (*Aquila rapax*)	42.5	30	0.8	57.3	10	2	17.5	
Imperial Eagle (Kaiseradler) (*Aquila heliaca*)	15.0	40.3	1.3	44	11.8	2.3	11.5	
Andean Condor (Kondor) (*Vultur gryphus*)	13.5	42	1.8	42.8	11	2.5	14.0	
Griffon Vulture (Gänsegeier) (*Gyps fulvus*)	22.0–41.0	20–22.3	0.8–2	61–61.8	10.3–11.8	5–5.3	9.5–12.5	
Egyptian Vulture (Schmutzgeier) (*Neophron percnopterus*)	29.5	37.5	4.8	43.8	5.5	8.5	8.5	
Cockatoo	14.4			80.2				Cullen[9]
Storm Petrel (*Hydrobates pelagicus*)		91–98						
Loon				71.0				
Chinese Goose				43.8	17.7			

Table 10-10. (Continued)

Bird	Total White Cells (thousands / cu. mm.)	Lymphocytes (per cent)	Monocytes (per cent)	Heterophils (per cent)	Eosinophils (per cent)	Basophils (per cent)	Thrombocytes (thousands / cu. mm.)	Author
English Jackdaw				42.3		13.8		Cullen[9]
Canary (*Serinus canarius*)				50.3				
Kingfisher				14.5		11.3		
Blackbird						23.8		
								Christoph and Trau[8]
Greater Sulfur-crested Cockatoo (Gelbhaubenkakadu) (*Kakatoe galerita*)	11.5	36.3	0.43	58.6	1.8	2.9	63.5	
Bare-eyed Cockatoo (Nacktaugenkakadu) (*Kakatoe sanguinea*)	9.0	31.8	1.0	56.8	2.0	8.5	10.0	
Umbrella-crested Cockatoo (Weisshaubenkakadu) (*Kakatoe alba*)	16.0	25.3	—	73.5	—	1.3	23.0	
Rose-breasted Cockatoo (Rosakakadu) (*Kakatoe roseicapilla*)	11.6	35.6	1.7	58.4	1.8	2.6	38.8	
Leadbeater's Cockatoo (Inkakakadu) (*Kakatoe leadbeateri*)	7.5	37.4	0.8	55.5	—	6.4	19.0	
Blue and Gold Macaw (Gelbbl. Ararauna) (*Ara ararauna*)	23.0	37.6	0.6	57.9	2.9	1.0	74.0	
Mauge's Conure (Grünflügelara) (*Aratinga chloroptera*)	23.7	48.4	0.4	47.1	2.3	1.8	52.2	
Jenday Conure (Jendayasittich) (*Aratinga jandaya*)	10.5	53.8	1.1	40.8	1.7	2.6	9.5	
Nanday Conure (Nandasittich) (*Nandayus nenday*)	17.0	56.8	0.8	38.1	2.4	2.0	6.5	
Green Conure (Guyanasittich) (*Aratinga leucophthalmus*)	14.5	39.5	0.8	55.8	2.5	1.5	40.5	

Table 10-10. (Continued)

Bird	Total White Cells (thousands/cu. mm.)	Lymphocytes (per cent)	Monocytes (per cent)	Heterophils (per cent)	Eosinophils (per cent)	Basophils (per cent)	Thrombocytes (thousands/cu. mm.)	Author
Finsch's Amazon (Blaukappenamazone) (*Amazona finschi*)	8.5	42.2	2.0	51.6	2.0	2.1	25.0	Christoph and Traue[8]
Festive Amazon (Blaubartamazone) (*Amazona festiva*)	14.0	39.6	0.4	56.6	2.4	1.0	50.0	
Yellow-fronted Amazon (Surinamamazone) (*Amazona ochrocephala*)	7.0	28.0	–	67.5	2.0	2.5	8.0	
Blue-fronted Amazon (Rotbugamazone) (*Amazona aestiva*)	13.6	37.7	0.6	56.4	3.2	2.2	35.5	
Panama Amazon (Panamaamazone) (*Amazona panamensis*)	7.5	42.6	1.0	50.0	4.3	2.1	46.5	
Vinaceous Amazon (Taubenhalsamazone) (*Amazona vinacea*)	10.0	47.5	–	48.5	2.5	1.5	29.0	
Versicolor Amazon (Blaustirnamazone) (*Amazona versicolor*)	8.0	50.0	–	46.3	2.5	1.5	31.0	
Bodin's Amazon (Rotstirnamazone) (*Amazona bodini*)	7.0	33.0	0.5	58.5	3.3	4.8	10.0	
Senegal Parrot (Mohrenkopfsittich) (*Poicephalus senegalus*)	34.7	29.4	–	64.7	2.3	3.5	54.0	
African Grey Parrot (Graupapagei) (*Psittacus erithacus*)	9.7	36.9	1.1	57.3	2.5	4.5	46.1	
African Ringneck (Halsbandsittich) (*Psittacula krameri*)	10.0	41.4	0.6	47.4	2.1	8.5	15.7	

Table 10-10. (Continued)

Bird	Total White Cells (thousands/cu. mm.)	Lymphocytes (per cent)	Monocytes (per cent)	Heterophils (per cent)	Eosinophils (per cent)	Basophils (per cent)	Thrombocytes (thousands/cu. mm.)	Author
Plum-head Parakeet (Pflaumenkopfsittich) (Psittacula cyanocephala)	10.0	33.5	—	61.0	2.0	3.5	6.0	Christoph and Traue[8]
Red Rosella Parakeet (Rosellasittich) (Platycercus eximius)	9.0	72.0	1.5	15.5	—	11.0	8.0	
Redrump Parakeet (Singsittich) (Psephotus haematonotus)	9.0	78.8	1.5	10.8	—	9.0	18.0	
Cockatiel (Nymphensittich) (Nymphicus hollandicus)	12.2	68.3	0.4	20.0	2.79	8.5	174.5	
Hybrid—Red Rosella (male), Crimson Rosella (female) (Buschwaldsittich) (Platycercus elegans)	8.5	67.0	7.1	18.5	1.3	6.1	64.0	
Pelican	19.7	27.2	0.8	67.3	3.4	1.4	11.1	Christoph and Schube[6]
Eagle Owl (Uhu) (Bubo bubo)	17.0	53.5		35.3	9.3	1.8	17.0	Christoph and Frank[5]
Long-eared Owl (Waldohreule) (Asio otus)	18.0						17.0	
Short-eared Owl (Sumpfohreule) (Asio flammeus)	22.0						13.0	
Wood Owl (Waldkauz) (Strix aluco)	19.0	62.0		25.4	8.6	3.9	18.0	
Little Owl (Steinkauz) (Athene noctua)	17.0	57.8		16.8	23.8	1.8	21.0	
Barn Owl (Schleiereule) (Tyto alba)	20.0	43.3		36.5	17.5	2.7	19.0	

Table 10-10. (Continued)

Bird	Total White Cells (thousands/ cu. mm.)	Lymphocytes (per cent)	Monocytes (per cent)	Heterophils (per cent)	Eosinophils (per cent)	Basophils (per cent)	Thrombocytes (thousands/ cu. mm.)	Author
Domestic Chicken (*Gallus gallus domesticus*)	23.7	56.8	10.3	26.0	4.7	2.2	43.1	Yamamoto[43]
Silky Chicken (*Gallus gallus domesticus*)	20.3	66.8	10.2	18.1	0.4	4.5	23.8	
Grey-breasted Guineafowl (*Numida galeata*)	15.5	36.2	8.4	43.5	7.4	4.5	43.6	
King Quail (*Coturnix coturnix japonica*)	16.2	56.4	5.1	33.8	4.0	0.8	32.8	
Domestic Duck (*Anas platyrhynchos domestica*)	24.5	22.4	3.8	66.8	4.9	2.2	35.4	
Spotbill Duck (*Anas poecilorhyncho zonorhyncha*)	10.6	30.1	7.4	51.0	5.1	6.4	28.6	
Mandarin Duck (*Aix galericulata*)	13.6	56.5	5.0	35.9	0	2.6	17.1	
Budgerigar (*Melopsittacus undulatus*)	7.7	57.2	12.0	25.8	0.1	4.9	34.4	
Nyassaland Lovebird (*Agapornis lilianae*)	16.9	12.1	3.4	82.4	1.0	1.1	14.9	
Pigeon (*Columba lilianae domestica*)	16.5	63.0	6.2	24.4	4.8	1.6	26.5	
Eastern Turtle Dove (*Streptopelia orientalis*)	11.1	70.8	4.9	17.9	2.6	3.8	19.1	
Meadow Bunting (*Emberiza cioides ciopsis*)	6.0	40.9	8.3	33.3	3.8	13.7	25.6	
Canary (*Serinus canarius*)	10.9	53.1	8.0	21.6	2.4	14.9	37.4	
Tree Sparrow (*Passer montanus saturatus*)	8.3	18.7	3.2	60.2	0.8	17.1	12.5	
Skylark (*Alauda arvensis japonica*)	14.2	51.6	11.6	26.4	3.5	6.9	31.8	
Indian White-eye (*Zosterops palpebrosa japonica*)	11.9	43.7	8.4	28.7	7.6	11.6	23.3	

Table 10-10. (Continued)

Bird	Total White Cells (thousands / cu. mm.)	Lymphocytes (per cent)	Monocytes (per cent)	Heterophils (per cent)	Eosinophils (per cent)	Basophils (per cent)	Thrombocytes (thousands / cu. mm.)	Author
Brown-eared Bulbul (Ixos [Microscelis] amaurotis amaurotis)	16.9	31.5	15.2	28.9	3.7	20.7	23.0	Yamamoto[43]
Bush Warbler (Horeites cantans cantans)	14.3	31.6	14.2	38.1	6.5	9.7	19.7	
Java Sparrow (Padda oryzivora)	20.6	48.1	12.8	31.9	1.7	5.5	23.5	
Zebra Finch (Poephila castanotis)	24.1	38.3	5.1	43.9	1.0	11.7	31.7	
Striated Mannikin (Urolonchura [Lonchura] striata)	13.2	28.9	11.5	35.5	1.9	22.2	24.2	
Black-billed Magpie (Pica pica japonica)	14.3	20.0	15.2	53.6	6.4	4.8	22.8	
Pigeon (heart blood)	7.6–16.6						8.0–89.0	De Eds[11]
Pigeon (leg vein blood)	3.6–8.6						8.0–84.0	
Pigeon	13–28.6	31.5–52.0	1–3	40–64.5	1–7	1–6	28–47.1	Klineberger[21]
Pigeon A.M.	13.0	43.6–79.6	3.7–10.4	11–39.2	0.4–6.2	0.6–6.0		Shaw[41]
Pigeon P.M.	18.5	32.4–74.0	1.8–10.2	16.4–55.6	0.2–6.8	0.4–9.8		
Duck (Anas platyrhynchos)	11.5–51.2	45.5–83.0	4.0–20.0	0–9.0	8.0–40.5	0–4.0	30.7	Magath and Higgins[25]
Duck (mixed breeds, White Pekin, Mallards and hybrids)	25.3	18.5–70.0	0–5.0	17.5–85.0		0–6.0		Hewitt[16]
White Pekin Duck		11.0–75.0	0.5–13.5	12.5–100		0–5.0		
Duck (Anas platyrhynchos)		32	8	48	7	5		Lucas and Jamroz[24]
Canada Goose (Branta canadensis)		46	6	39	7	2		
Ring-necked Pheasant (Phasianus colchicus)		34	8	48	1	10		

Table 10-11. Normal Thrombocyte Counts* for Budgerigars[15]

Thrombocytes (per cu. mm.)	Age in Weeks		
	3	13–26	52
Mean	47,100	33,800	29,450
S.D.	21,555	8,760	7,280
Mean ± 3 S.D.	0–111,765	7,520–60,080	7,610–51,290
N	20	11	20

*S.D. = Standard deviation.
Mean ± 3 S.D. = Range within which 99 per cent of the values determined should occur.
N = Number of birds tested.

References

1. BEN-HAREL, S.: Studies of bird malaria in relation to the mechanism of relapse. Am. J. Hyg. *3:*652–685, 1923.

2. BENNETT, G. F., and CHISHOLM, A. E.: Measurements on the blood cells of some wild birds of North America. Wildl. Dis. *38:*1–22, 1964.

3. BIERER, B. W., THOMAS, J. B., ROEBUCK, D. E., POWELL, H. S., and ELEAZER, T. H.: Hematocrit and sedimentation rate values as an aid in poultry disease diagnosis. J.A.V.M.A. *143:*1096–1098, 1963.

4. CHRISTOPH, H.-J., and BOROWSKI, G.: Beiträge zur Hämatologie der Zootiere. IV. Das Blutbild von Greifvögeln (Accipitres) unter besonderer Berücksichtigung einiger in Deutschland noch heimischer kleinerer Arten. Kleintier-Praxis *6:*71–76, 1961.

5. CHRISTOPH, H.-J., and FRANK, R.: Beiträge zur Hämatologie der Zootiere. IX. Das Blutbild von Eulen. Kleintier-Praxis *10:*121–126, 1965.

6. CHRISTOPH, H.-J., and SCHUBE, G.: Beiträge zur Hämatologie der Zootiere. VIII. Das Blutbild von Pelikanen. Kleintier-Praxis *9:*18–22, 1964.

7. CHRISTOPH, H.-J., and TRAUE, H.: Beiträge zur Hämatologie der Zootiere. III. Das Blutbild von Möven. Kleintier-Praxis *6:*66–70, 1961.

8. CHRISTOPH, H.-J., and TRAUE, H.: Beiträge zur Hämatologie der Zootiere. V. Das Blutbild von Papageien. Kleintier-Praxis *6:*76–80, 1961.

9. CULLEN, E. K.: A morphological study of the blood of certain fishes and birds with special reference to the leucocytes of birds. Johns Hopkins Hosp. Bull. *14:*352–356, 1903.

10. DARCEL, C. Le Q.: Counting erythrocytes and leucocytes in fowl blood. Stain Techn. *26:*57–59, 1951.

11. DE EDS, F.: Normal blood counts in pigeons. J. Lab. Clin. Med. *12:*437–438, 1927.

12. DENINGTON, E. M., and LUCAS, A. M.: Blood technics for chickens. Poultry Sci. *34:*360–368, 1955.

13. DE VILLIERS, O. T.: The blood of the ostrich. Onderstepoort J. Vet. Sci. *11:*419–504, 1938.

14. DUKES, H. H., and SCHWARTE, L. H.: The hemoglobin content of the blood of fowls. Am. J. Physiol. *96:*89–93, 1931.

15. GALLAGHER, L.: Personal communication, 1964.

16. HEWITT, R.: Studies on the host-parasite relationships of untreated infections with *Plasmodium lophurae* in ducks. Am. J. Hyg. *36:*6–42, 1942.

17. JOHNS, F. M.: A study of punctate stippling as found in the lead poisoning of wild ducks. J. Lab. Clin. Med. *19:*514–517, 1934.

18. JONES, T. C.: Personal communication, 1965.

19. KALABUKHOV, N., and RODIONOV, V.: Changes in the blood of animals according to age. Folia Haemat. (Leipzig) *52:*145–158, 1934.

20. KERLIN, R. E.: Venipuncture of small birds. J.A.V.M.A. *144:*870–874, 1964.

21. KLINEBERGER, C.: *Die Blutmorphologie der Laboratoriumstiere,* Leipzig, Barth, 1927, as cited by Jordan, H. E., in *Handbook of Hematology,* H. Downey, ed. New York, Paul B. Hoeber, Inc., 1938. Vol. II, p. 700.

22. LI, J. C. R.: *Introduction to Statistical Inference.* Ann Arbor, Mich., Edwards Brothers, Inc., 1957.

23. LUCAS, A. M., and DENINGTON, E. M.: The statistical reliability of differential counts of chicken blood. Poultry Sci. *37:*544–549, 1958.

24. LUCAS, A. M., and JAMROZ, C.: *Atlas of Avian Hematology,* Agr. Monograph 25. Washington, D.C., U.S. Department of Agriculture, 1961. 271 pp.

25. MAGATH, T. B., and HIGGINS, G. M.: The blood of the normal duck. Folia Haemat. (Leipzig) *51:*230–241, 1934.

26. MEITES, S., and FAULKNER, W. R.: *Manual of Practical Micro and General Procedures in Clinical Chemistry.* Springfield, Ill., Charles C Thomas, publisher, 1962. Pp. 153–155.

27. MIRSKY, I. A., NELSON, N., GRAYMAN, I., and KORENBERG, M.: Studies on normal and depancreatized domestic ducks. Am. J. Physiol. *135:*223–229, 1941.

28. MURDOCK, H. R., and LEWIS, J. O. D.: A simple method for obtaining blood from ducks. Proc. Soc. Exp. Biol. Med. *116:*51–52, 1964.

29. NATT, M. P., and HERRICK, C. A.: A new blood diluent for counting erythrocytes and leucocytes of the chicken. Poultry Sci. *31:*735–738, 1952.

30. NATT, M. P., and HERRICK, C. A.: Variations in the shape of the rod-like granule of the chicken heterophil leucocyte and its possible significance. Poultry Sci. *33:*828–830, 1954.

31. NELSON, N., ELGART, S., and MIRSKY, I. A.: Pancreatic diabetes in the owl. Endocrinology *31:*119–123, 1942.

32. NICE, L. B., NICE, M. M., and KRAFT, R. M.: Erythrocytes and hemoglobin in the blood of some American birds. Wilson Bull. *47:*120–124, 1935.

33. PONDER, E.: *Erythrocytes and the Action of Simple Haemolysis.* Edinburgh, Oliver and Boyd, 1924. 192 pp. Cited by Nice *et al.*[32]

34. RIDDLE, O., and BRAUCHER, P.-F.: Hemoglobin and erythrocyte differences according to sex and season in doves and pigeons. Am. J. Physiol. *108:*554–566, 1934.

35. SAVAGE, A., and ISA, J. M.: An unusual blood condition in a trumpeter swan. Canad. J. Zool. *40:*1314–1315, 1962.

36. SCARBOROUGH, R. A.: The blood picture of normal laboratory animals. Yale J. Biol. Med. *4:*323–344, 1931.

37. SCHALM, O. W.: *Veterinary Hematology.* Philadelphia, Lea & Febiger, 1961. Pp. 130–131.

38. SCHLUMBERGER, H. G.: Neoplasia in the parakeet. II. Transplantation of the pituitary tumor. Cancer Res. *16:*149–153, 1956.

39. SCHLUMBERGER, H. G., and HENSCHKE, U. K.: Effect of total body X-irradiation on the parakeet. Proc. Soc. Exp. Biol. Med. *92:*261–266, 1956.

40. SCHMITT, J., and RIGHTON, M.: Hematological findings in penguins. Nord. Veterinaermed. *14*(Suppl. 1): 305–313, 1962.

41. SHAW, A. F. B.: The leucocytes of the pigeon with special reference to a diurnal rhythm. J. Path. Bact. *37:*411–430, 1933.

42. STROUD, R.: *Stroud's Digest on the Diseases of Birds.* Jersey City, N.J., T. F. H. Publications, Inc., pp. 476, 375, 1964 (Reprinted from 1943).

43. YAMAMOTO, T.: Study on the blood cells of birds. Igaku Kenkyu (Acta Medica) *28:*1057–1059, 1959.

44. YOUNG, M. D.: Erythrocyte counts and hemoglobin concentration in normal female canaries. J. Parasit. *23:*424–426, 1937.

Suggested Reading

BARTSCH, P., BALL, W. H., ROSENZWEIG, W., and SALMAN, S.: Size of red blood corpuscles and their nucleus in fifty North American birds. Auk *54:*516–519, 1937.

CLELAND, J. B., and JOHNSTON, T. H.: Relative dimensions of the red cells of vertebrates, especially of birds. Emu *11:*188–197, 1912.

ELLIOTT, J. H.: A preliminary note on the occurrence of a filaria in the crow. Biol. Bull. of the Marine Biol. Lab., Woods Holl, Mass. *4:*64–65, 1903.

GULLIVER, G.: Observations on the sizes and shapes of the red corpuscles of the blood of vertebrates, with drawings of them to a uniform scale, and extended and revised tables of measurements. Proc. Zool. Soc. London, 1875, pp. 474–495.

HARTMAN, F. A., and LESSLER, M. A.: Erythrocyte measurements in birds. Auk *80:*467, 1963.

JOHNSON, E. P., and LANGE, C. J.: Blood alterations in typhlohepatitis of turkeys, with notes on the disease. J. Parasit. *25:*157–167, 1939.

JORDAN, H. E.: Comparative Hematology. In *Handbook of Hematology,* H. Downey, ed. New York, Paul B. Hoeber, Inc., 1938. Vol. II, pp. 699–862.

McGUIRE, W. C., and CAVETT, J. W.: Blood studies on histomoniasis in turkeys. Poultry Sci. *31:*610–617, 1952.

OLSON, C.: Variations in the cells and hemoglobin content in the blood of the normal domestic chicken. Cornell Vet. *27:*235–263, 1937.

OLSON, C.: Avian Hematology. In *Diseases of Poultry,* 5th ed., H. E. Biester and L. H. Schwarte, eds. Ames, Iowa State University Press, 1965. Pp. 100–119.

SALGUES, R.: Notulae tumorologiae. V. Les érythrocytes,

l'hémoglobine et la valeur globulaire au cours des affections cancereuses chez l'oiseau. L'Oiseau et la Revue Française d'Ornithologie *6:*308–312, 1936.

SPECTOR, W. S., ed.: *Handbook of Biological Data.* Philadelphia, W. B. Saunders Co., 1956. Pp. 164, 277, 344.

STEWART, P. A.: A preliminary list of bird weights. Auk *54:*324, 1937.

STURKIE, P. D.: *Avian Physiology,* 2nd ed. Ithaca, N.Y., Comstock Publishing Associates, 1965. 766 pp.

UDVARDY, M. D. F.: Contributions to the knowledge of the body temperatures of birds. Zool. Bidrag Uppsala *30:*25–42, 1953.

VENZLAFF, W.: Über Genesis und Morphologie der roten Blütkörperchen der Vögel. Arch. f. mikr. Anat. Abt. I *77:*377–432, 1911.

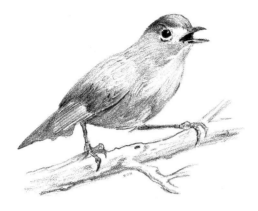

11

Surgical Techniques and Anesthesia

Charles P. Gandal

In the past many practitioners have avoided anesthetizing birds for fear of losing them. Once familiarity with avian species and techniques of anesthesia is gained it becomes apparent that the principles of mammalian anesthesia are quite applicable and form a sound basis for the safe and satisfactory anesthetizing of a wide variety of birds. Veterinary medicine and the pet bird industry have both progressed to the point where full medical and surgical coverage should be available for any and all of the avian species presented, and if this service is to be provided sound techniques in anesthesia must be developed.

GENERAL ANESTHESIA

Most of the smaller pet birds are quite delicate and extremely sensitive to rough handling, sudden changes in temperature, excitement, dietary changes, long car rides, and a new environment. Whenever possible, birds that are to be given a general anesthetic should be kept in a quiet part of the hospital overnight. Preferably they should be in their own cage and fed their accustomed diet. Rough handling is to be avoided. It is especially dangerous to physically examine a bird for several minutes, make a diagnosis, and immediately proceed to anesthetize the severely stressed patient.

Many avian patients are presented in advanced stages of disease and are poor risks for anesthesia and surgery. The guarded prognosis that is given in such cases need not be carried over to the relatively healthy birds that will be in the majority.

Familiarity with surgery of small birds reveals the

importance of hemorrhage control. It should be remembered that the weight of the average budgerigar is just over 1 ounce. This is about one-eightieth of the weight of a 5-pound poodle. Such a bird can ill afford to lose more than a few drops of blood. Many avian deaths following surgery are caused by excessive blood loss, shock, and circulatory collapse rather than anesthetic overdosage, to which they are customarily attributed.

Numerous agents have been reported as satisfactory general anesthetics for birds. Pentobarbital sodium,[23] chloral hydrate,[5] and tribromoethanol[24,29] have been used with success orally. Methoxyflurane,[22] fluothane,[18] ether,[3,9,13] and ethyl chloride[12,13,18] are the most reliable of the volatile anesthetics. Parenterally, sodium amytal,[7,11] pentobarbital sodium,[4,7,10,12,13,28] chloral hydrate,[7] and Equi-Thesin[14] have given good results when properly used.

Equi-Thesin* is the drug of choice for most procedures, although methoxyflurane† and ether are quite satisfactory if they are properly administered. The disadvantage of a volatile anesthetic is that it must be constantly monitored and supplemented, as opposed to a single injection of Equi-Thesin which leaves the surgeon relatively free of anesthetic problems for a reasonable period of time.

Arnall, on page 139 in the first of his series of articles on "Anaesthesia and Surgery in Cage and Aviary Birds,"[2] described "Criteria of Planes of Narcosis and Anaesthesia" as follows:

"Narcosis

· · · · · · · · · ·

"Medium narcosis. The feathers become ruffled. The head hangs progressively lower until it reaches the floor but the bird can be easily roused. Only a little struggling occurs when threatening movements are made near the bird's head or when it is picked up.

"Deep narcosis. There is little or no response to sound vibration but there may be some attempt at co-ordination when the bird is placed on its back. Purposeful voluntary movements (fluttering) are seen when painful stimuli are applied, and in some cases shrill cries are emitted after the stimulus is discontinued. The latter is more noticeable with barbiturate narcosis. Respiration is usually fairly rapid, regular and deep but, after stimulation, it may become irregular.

"Anaesthesia

"Light Anaesthesia. No response is provoked by vibration or postural changes but, although no voluntary purposeful movement is performed, all reflexes, palpebral, corneal, the cere and pedal are present and brisk. Pedal response may continue after stimulation ceases.

"Medium anaesthesia. The palpebral reflex is lost; corneal and pedal reflexes are sluggish, delayed and intermittent. Respiration is slow, deep and regular. Most operations can be performed at this level of anaesthesia.

"Deep anaesthesia. Corneal, digital, cloacal, buccal and cere reflexes are absent. Respirations are very slow but usually regular. If anaesthesia is further deepened the respirations become slower and shallower and finally cease."

And he goes on to state:

"In debilitated, toxic, obese or cardiovascular cases, Cheyne-Stokes type respiration may precede death in any plane of anaesthesia, or in a healthy bird when a highly toxic gas such as chloroform is used."

Anesthetic Agents

Volatile Anesthetics

Ether and more recently methoxyflurane have proved invaluable for procedures of short duration, with methoxyflurane being the inhalant anesthetic of choice from the standpoint both of safety and of duration of anesthesia.

As with mammals, inhalant anesthesia should not be used on birds that are suffering from respiratory distress. Birds that are in an obviously weakened condition should have the anesthetic dosage level adjusted accordingly.

Small birds may be satisfactorily anesthetized with ether by placing them in a 1-quart glass jar, spraying 1 ml. of ether into the jar through a 25-gauge needle, capping the jar, and waiting approximately 30 seconds. When the bird stops struggling it is immediately removed and, depending on the level reached, anesthesia may last 1 to 4 minutes. Further ether may be given intermittently by holding a cotton pledget moistened with ether close to the bird's nostrils, but great care must be exercised as a dangerous overconcentration may be rapidly attained.

A satisfactory ether cone for small birds may be fashioned from the cardboard cylinder on which bulk-packaged adhesive tape is stacked.[25] A 4-inch tube with a V-shaped notch cut out at one end allows the "cone" to fit snugly over the beak while cotton moistened with ether is placed at the other end.

---

*Equi-Thesin—produced by the Jensen-Salsbery Laboratories, Kansas City, Mo. Each 500 ml. contains 328 gr. of chloral hydrate, 75 gr. of pentobarbital, and 164 gr. of magnesium sulfate in aqueous solution of propylene glycol 35%; with 9.5 per cent alcohol.

†Metofane, Pitman-Moore Company, New York, N.Y.

Methoxyflurane may be administered in the same manner as ether but only 0.1–0.2 ml. is required in a 1-quart jar to achieve quick induction of surgical anesthesia. The bird will stop struggling within 30 to 60 seconds, and anesthesia will last from 4 to 10 minutes after its removal from the induction chamber, depending on the level reached initially. This may also be supplemented by the open drip method in the same way as ether. To date, in limited trials, methoxyflurane has been safer, more consistent in its action, and produced longer-lasting anesthesia than ether and it is considered well worth the difference in price.

Methoxyflurane may also be used on larger birds by holding the bird's head in a 1-quart jar into which 0.2–0.4 ml. of the drug has been sprayed and sealing the opening off with a towel. It may also be administered on a pledget of cotton held over the nostrils. Once a satisfactory stage of anesthesia has been reached an endotracheal tube may be inserted and attached to a gas anesthetic machine to facilitate long-term procedures.

Gas anesthetic machines may also be utilized for induction of anesthesia along with specially adapted face masks. Starting with the smallest available mask a thin sheet of rubber is stretched across the mask opening and secured to its borders. A small incision is made in this "rubber seal," sufficient to permit entry of the bird's head yet provide for a relatively air-tight fit. The bird's head is placed within the mask and his body gently restrained during induction. When a satisfactory plane of anesthesia is reached the flow is adjusted for continuation of that level. With this technique induction with controlled concentration may be rapidly achieved and oxygen may be efficiently administered if desired. This method may be advantageously used in small birds in which endotracheal intubation is impractical; in larger birds intubation may follow mask induction. The benefits of intubation for airway maintenance are well known, and this technique should be utilized whenever possible for long-term procedures.

Parenteral Anesthetics

Equi-Thesin is the drug of choice for most avian surgery and has the advantage of a single dose producing anesthesia lasting from 30 to 75 minutes. It is convenient to use (no dilution or preparation necessary), produces good surgical anesthesia, and is safe if certain precautions are observed.

SMALL BIRDS—INTRAMUSCULAR ADMINISTRATION

With the smaller birds Equi-Thesin is given intramuscularly on a weight basis, and the first and most important safety factor is accurate weighing of the patient

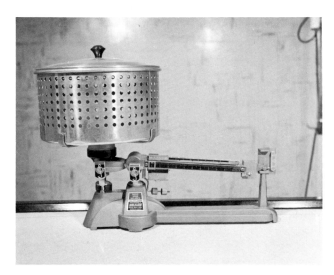

Fig. 11-1. *An accurate scale is a necessity for determining weight of a bird before inducing anesthesia by intramuscular injection of Equi-Thesin.*

(Fig. 11-1). The weight of budgerigars may vary from 25 to 55 grams and that of even "normal" appearing specimens may vary from 30 to 45 grams, a considerable range when one is utilizing weight to determine anesthetic dosage. The dose is 2.0–2.5 ml. per kilogram of body weight, or 0.20–0.25 ml. per 100 grams (see Table 11-1). The higher dosage level is safe for birds in good condition; the lower level should be used if the bird is weak, debilitated, or otherwise considered a poor risk.

The anesthetic is measured into a tuberculin syringe,

Table 11-1. Equi-Thesin Dosage for Small Birds (2.5 ml. per kilogram)

Reduce dosage by 10 to 20% for birds that are weak, debilitated, suffering from shock, have extremely large tumors, etc.	
Body Weight (grams)	**Amount of Equi-Thesin (ml.)**
23–26	0.06
27–30	0.07
31–34	0.08
35–38	0.09
39–42	0.10
43–46	0.11
47–50	0.12
51–54	0.13

utilizing a ½-inch 26- or 27-gauge needle, and is injected deep into the breast muscle. Following this the bird should be placed in a smooth-sided enclosure to avoid the possibility of its catching a leg or beak in the openings of a wire cage, drowning in the water dish, or otherwise damaging itself. It is interesting to note that only rarely does any gross swelling occur at the site of the injection.

Surgical anesthesia is usually attained in 7 to 10 minutes and may last for 30 to 75 minutes, depending on the dosage used and the individual bird. To prolong anesthesia a supplementary dose equivalent to 25% of the original amount of Equi-Thesin may be given intramuscularly 30 minutes after the initial injection. However, in general, it is preferable to use methoxyflurane for supplemental anesthesia, as it can be more readily and accurately controlled.

To avoid accidents, avian patients should be kept in a smooth-sided enclosure also during the recovery phase. A clear plastic box or upturned fish tank is ideal. Glass or plastic sides should be scratched, soaped, or taped so that the bird does not try to fly through them and incur serious injury.

Birds that are not back on their feet within one hour after surgery should be turned from side to side every 30 minutes, kept at a temperature of 80 to 85°F., and be given oxygen if indicated. A fish tank may be turned upside down and fitted with a valve to allow introduction of an oxygen hose and thus serve quite admirably as an avian "oxygen tent" (Fig. 11-2).

LARGE BIRDS—INTRAMUSCULAR ADMINISTRATION

Birds the size of a pigeon and larger may be readily anesthetized by injecting Equi-Thesin intramuscularly at the same dosage level as for small birds, substituting a 21-gauge needle for ease in injecting the larger quantity of anesthetic. Some of the larger birds have a longer induction period, and may stay anesthetized longer per unit dose, although individual variations are not much greater than those seen in mammals.

LARGE BIRDS—INTRAVENOUS ADMINISTRATION

The larger birds lend themselves more readily to intravenous administration of anesthetic agents, with the advantages of rapid induction, more accurate control of the plane of anesthesia, and ease and safety in supplementing an initial dose. The median vein as it crosses the ventral surface of the humero-radial joint is readily accessible for intravenous injection (Fig. 11-3). The bird is held gently, but securely, on its back with one wing folded against the body and the other extended. Equi-Thesin is administered to effect over a period of

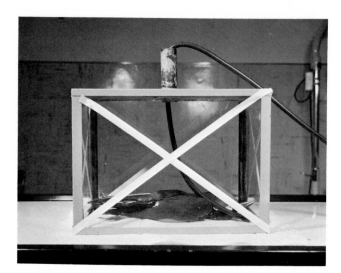

Fig. 11-2. *A makeshift "oxygen tent" for the smaller bird may be easily improvised, using a 2½-gallon fish tank. Also shown is taping of the walls to prevent the bird from making efforts to fly through them.*

3 to 5 minutes, utilizing a 25-gauge needle and a dose of 1.0 to 2.0 ml. of Equi-Thesin per kilogram of body weight (0.5–1.0 ml. per pound). At any time supplementary doses may be given intravenously to effect. The restraint required for this procedure makes it necessary to have semiskilled help and to exercise some care to avoid undue shock or possible damage to the bird's skeletal system. Sharp, small-gauge needles are also a necessity if one is to avoid the massive hematoma that results from tearing of thin-walled veins. Following withdrawal of the needle, pressure should be applied over the injection site for at least 1 minute as a precaution against hematoma formation.

Intravenous injection may also be accomplished satisfactorily in the smaller species by way of the jugular vein, although the problems of handling greatly favor intramuscular use of Equi-Thesin. It should be noted that in certain smaller birds, notably the budgerigar (*Melopsittacus undulatus*), only the right jugular vein is available for venipuncture.[20]

Problems of General Anesthesia

In cases of respiratory arrest from an overdose of inhalant anesthetic, artificial respiration should be initiated by *gentle* manual pressure on the breast. The mouth and trachea should be cleared of mucus to maintain an adequate airway, and further resuscitation should be attempted through use of oxygen by endotracheal intubation. Frequently, manual resuscitation along with free flow of oxygen from a tube leading directly into the mouth or held close to the external

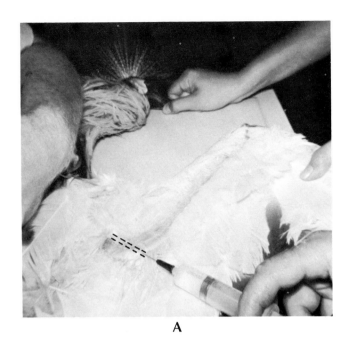

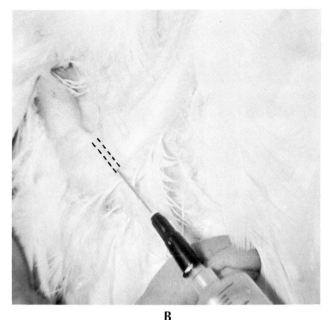

A   B

Fig. 11-3. *Technique for administration of intravenous anesthesia in a larger bird. A. Needle points to median vein as it crosses the ventral surface of the humero-radial joint. B. Position of needle as injection is made into the median vein.*

nares is all that is necessary. Regular endotracheal tubes may be used on larger birds, especially in the sizes commonly employed for cats and smaller breeds of dogs (French 12–26). On smaller species, a silver abscess cannula, filed-down 20-gauge needle, or metal mastitis injection tube on the end of a 10-ml. syringe will serve as an endotracheal tube. If the end of an oxygen tube is inserted into the syringe barrel (Fig. 11-4) and alternately placed against the opening in the hub end and withdrawn, respiration may be readily maintained, although one must be careful not to overinflate the lungs.

Equi-Thesin overdosage is not as readily counteracted. However, it must be remembered that signs of anesthetic overdosage show rather early in an operation, and as previously mentioned many "anesthetic deaths" are in reality the result of a combination of excessive blood loss, shock, and circulatory collapse. Recently we have had excellent results combating shock through the use of intravenous lactated Ringer's solution.

For combating Equi-Thesin overdosage, all of the above described procedures are of value, and intravenous or intramuscular administration of analeptics is also indicated. For larger birds they may be used on a weight basis as with cats and dogs, but such drugs must be diluted for use with smaller species. Friedburg[13] reported good results with methetharimide, using 0.2 ml. per 30 grams body weight of a mixture of 1 ml. of Mikedimide* and 8 ml. of sterile distilled water.

*Mikedimide—3% solution of methetharimide, Parlam Corp., Englewood, N.J.

LOCAL ANESTHESIA

To those unfamiliar with avian practice, the use of local anesthesia for minor surgical procedures might seem quite desirable. This does not always hold true, and, with the advent of methoxyflurane, a safe, easily administered, short-acting volatile anesthetic, there is much less need for local anesthetics.

In using local anesthetic agents, especially in the smaller pet birds, one must be aware of the potential hazard of shock inherent in restraining birds physically for undue periods of time. Budgerigars are relatively hardy, but finches, canaries, and other smaller species simply will not tolerate prolonged restraint under local anesthesia, even for minor procedures, and the resultant struggle can be fatal.

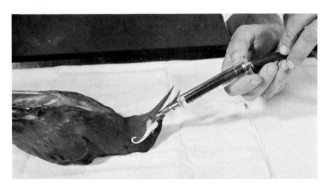

Fig. 11-4. *A simple apparatus for avian resuscitation may be improvised with a mastitis tube, 10-ml. syringe barrel, and oxygen hose (see text).*

With larger birds local anesthetics may be used to some advantage for very short procedures, but here again the use of methoxyflurane should be considered. Pigeons, ducks, geese, chickens, and swans seem to tolerate restraint much better than the more exotic species, and are better subjects for local anesthesia.

Anesthetic Agents

Procaine is well known for its fatal effects on certain birds and should never be used in the smaller species.[13] Doses as small as 0.1 ml. of 2% procaine hydrochloride may be fatal. When one considers the size of a budgerigar, canary, or finch, it becomes apparent that much further dilution of such agents is necessary, if they are to be used at all. In general, procaine should not be used in the smaller species, but with the larger birds moderate amounts of 2% procaine may be safely employed. We have utilized 2 to 4 ml. of 2% procaine in removing bumblefoot lesions from the feet of ducks and geese weighing from 3 to 8 pounds with no untoward symptoms.

Cetacaine,* applied topically, has been reported to be an effective local anesthetic agent.[13]

Ethyl chloride may also be utilized for local anesthesia, although its effects are of relatively short duration.

GENERAL CONSIDERATIONS OF AVIAN SURGERY

In general, avian surgery is no more difficult than the routine procedures most veterinary practitioners are accustomed to performing daily. A proper evaluation of each case is essential, as many avian patients are presented for surgery in an advanced stage of disease, and unsatisfactory results with such cases should not prejudice one against future attempts at surgery.

Much of the practitioner's bird surgery will involve small cage bird species, and the importance of adequate hemorrhage control and use of techniques to minimize blood loss cannot be given too much emphasis. The use of sterile cotton-tipped applicators for blunt dissection and sponging, use of small, finely made mosquito forceps, double ligation of vessels when indicated, and ready availability of sterile absorbable sponges will do much to ensure success. Ophthalmic instruments, such as fixation and dressing forceps and strabismus scissors, are of value in handling the delicate tissues of small birds.

Although birds are known to be quite resistant to infection, all avian surgery should be performed with

*Cetacaine, Haver-Lockhart Laboratories, Kansas City, Mo.

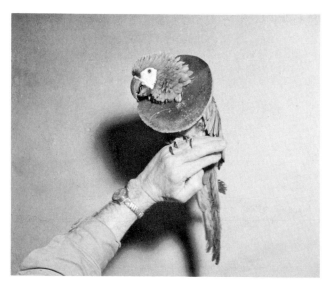

Fig. 11-5. *An Elizabethan collar may be fashioned of leather or plastic for larger birds, or of sturdy cardboard for smaller birds.*

aseptic technique. Feathers in the operative area should be plucked out (they will completely regrow in five or six weeks) and the area be prepared as for surgery in mammals. Small birds may be held in position on the operating table by adhesive tape once they are satisfactorily anesthetized, although it is generally preferable for an assistant to hold the bird gently. If, during the course of an operation, the bird seems in danger from respiratory failure or circulatory collapse, oxygen therapy should be instituted by holding the end of an oxygen tube at the bird's external nares and running the oxygen at a rate of 4 to 6 liters per minute. In the more serious cases intubation may be required, as described under the heading "Problems of General Anesthesia."

In birds, sutures are subject to continual inspection and to the ever-present possibility of "picking." Aseptic surgery will help to avoid some of the "picking" problems. In addition, all mirrors and shiny objects should be removed from the bird's cage to avoid its being constantly reminded of the operative area. The use of catgut swaged on an Atraumatic needle, along with a simple continuous stitch, is most important in avoiding irritation and attention-getting knots and suture ends. No problems have been encountered when using this suture material and technique for dermal closure, and it is far preferable to non-absorbable sutures and bulky interrupted or mattress sutures which have the added disadvantage of requiring further handling of the patient for their removal.

All birds should be closely observed for the first 3 to

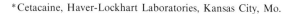

4 hours after surgery, as any serious tendency to pick at the sutures will occur during this time and may result in serious hemorrhage. After 4 or 5 days minor picking at the sutures is of little consequence. If birds show picking tendencies they should be fitted with a cardboard, plastic, aluminum, or leather Elizabethan collar (Fig. 11-5) large enough to protect the operative area but not to seriously incapacitate the bird. The average budgerigar collar should be 1¾ inches in diameter with a ½-inch hole in the middle.

SPECIFIC SURGICAL PROBLEMS

Head

EYES

Both enucleation and cataract removal have been satisfactorily accomplished in avian species. Such cases will only rarely be presented to the practitioner, and if surgery is indicated fair to good results may be obtained by following accepted mammalian techniques. Enucleation, even in budgerigars and canaries, may be successful provided the disease process does not contraindicate surgical intervention.

Cataract removal is rarely called for except in cases of bilateral affliction; although it may be successful in birds of pigeon size and larger, it is not recommended for the smaller species. In the cataract surgery that we have done no corneal sutures were used because of the small size of the eye. The lids were sutured together, for 3 to 5 days, with loosely placed nylon mattress sutures,[8] facilitating corneal healing.

SINUSES

Most pet birds are susceptible to recurrent attacks of sinusitis. Properly treated with broad-spectrum antibiotics many of these cases will not recur. In a certain percentage of cases the condition becomes chronic and ultimately a caseous mass may completely fill and markedly distend the facial area (Fig. 11-7). Removal of inspissated or caseous material may be readily accomplished. In larger birds and domestic fowl local anesthesia or simply manual restraint may be satisfactory. However, with smaller birds light general anesthesia is advisable. The area is plucked clean of feathers and thoroughly washed, and an incision is made over the swelling. The foreign material is readily removed, the area flushed with aqueous Zephiran, and the wound sutured. Broad-spectrum antibiotics should be administered for 3 or 4 days postoperatively to prevent a recurrence of the condition.

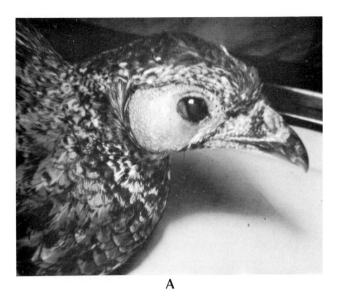

A

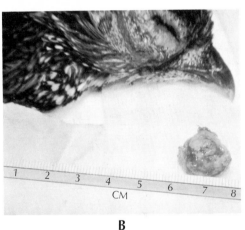

B

Fig. 11-6. *Post-ocular eosinophilic granuloma in scintillating copper pheasant. A. Photograph before surgery. B. Photograph after surgery, showing size of tumor removed.*

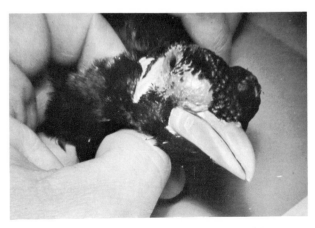

Fig. 11-7. *Chronic sinusitis in mynah bird, with caseous mass distending facial area. The mass was removed surgically, with successful results.*

CERE

Hypertrophy of the cere is not uncommon in budgerigars. A white flaky excess growth at the base of the beak, with concurrent feather loss, is associated with a *Cnemidocoptes* mite infestation. A true hypertrophy of the cere in which the overgrowth is a gray-brown color occurs almost exclusively in female budgerigars. If the external nares are seriously occluded by the growth, electrodesiccation or electrocautery may be used to remove the excess and restore an adequate nostril aperture, under general anesthesia produced by parenteral injection.

BEAK

Fractures may occur in birds with a thin, elongated beak. In smaller birds two or three layers of tape wrapped around the area will usually suffice to keep the area immobilized for the 2 or 3 weeks required for healing. In larger birds a flat aluminum sheet may be cut to size, shaped to fit, and taped to the fractured area to provide satisfactory immobilization. Small intramedullary pins may be used in some cases, although they may be difficult to anchor securely in the spongy bone.

In some fractures of the lower mandible circulation to the distal segment is so poor that necrosis will result. If, after a reasonable time, healing of the fracture has not occurred, surgical amputation of the distal fragment is advisable. Birds may get along quite well after such an operation if the upper bill is kept trimmed to allow for adequate prehension.

MOUTH

Small papillomatous masses may frequently be found at the base of the cere and at the corners of the mouth. Ligature and excision may be attempted under manual restraint, although the method of choice would involve use of light general anesthesia and removal by excision or electrofulguration.

Oral flukes (*Cathemasia* species) may sometimes be found in the posterior oral cavity and proximal portion of the esophagus. They may be readily removed with forceps, although their pathogenicity is not fully determined.

Miscellaneous tumors, both benign and malignant, are infrequently seen in the oro- and naso-pharynx (Fig. 11-8). These must be handled as individual cases, the prognosis being determined by their size, location, and the general condition of the bird.

A 10-year-old amazon parrot (*Amazona orchrocephala*) was presented with a history of inability to

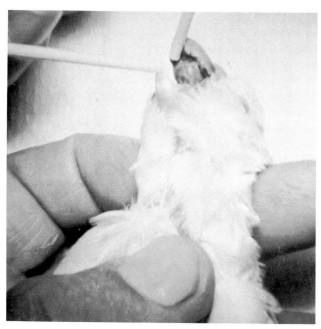

Fig. 11-8. *Leiomyosarcoma of soft palate in parakeet.*

swallow food. Examination revealed a soft, yellow, irregular, papillomatous mass approximately 1 cm. in maximum measurement on the left lateral fold of the larynx. The bird was anesthetized with Equi-Thesin, the growth curetted from the larynx, and the area cauterized with trichloroacetic acid. This was repeated three times at weekly intervals. The growth recurred in eight months and the initial series of treatments was repeated. Six months later the growth again recurred, and the treatment was again repeated. No further recurrence was noted in the five ensuing years.[26]

Crop

In most avian species the crop is subject to impaction, with secondary dilatation. The impaction may be of foreign material ingested by the bird, material normally ingested which has formed a dry mass that will not pass on through the digestive tract, or, uncommonly, a urate calculus,[6] all of which will ultimately necessitate surgery.

Good general anesthesia is essential. The area is prepared by plucking and thorough scrubbing with pHisoHex.* An incision is made through the skin, which is then bluntly dissected from the underlying tissues and crop. The crop is opened following much the same technique as in gastrotomy, the impacted mass is removed, and the walls are sutured with a Connell stitch using 000 to 00000 intestinal gut on an Atraumatic needle. The skin is sutured with gut, using

---

*pHisoHex, Winthrop Laboratories, New York.

a continuous suture. Food and water are withheld for 18 hours, after which the bird's normal routine is resumed. Careful closure of the crop wall will result in a high percentage of success, with few postoperative problems.

Chronic dilatation of the crop may occur and be refractory to medical treatment and drainage. By using delicate instruments, fine sutures, and careful technique 40 to 60 per cent of the hypertrophic organ may be successfully removed, with a fair to good chance of recovery. This depends, of course, on the bird's initial condition and the skill of the operator.

Body

NEOPLASMS

The most common neoplasms of pet birds, especially budgerigars, are lipomas and lipogranulomas (Fig. 11-9). Subcutaneous granulomas of the breast and abdomen are frequently mislabeled cysts or abscesses. The pathology and interrelationship of these two types of tumors have been well documented.[17] Papillomas are not uncommon, and fibromas have been recorded, especially in the larger species. Fibrosarcomas and adenocarcinomas are among the more commonly found malignant tumors.

In general, benign subcutaneous tumors may be successfully removed if the bird is in good physical condition. Malignant subcutaneous tumors may also be removed with good results if they have not become too invasive or have not metastasized. Benign subcutaneous tumors occur most frequently on the breast and abdomen (especially in budgerigars), and less frequently in the cervical area and on the leg and wing.

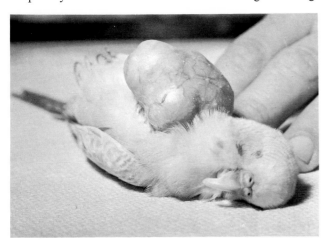

Fig. 11-9. *Massive lipogranuloma in a budgerigar. Such growths may be successfully removed if good technique is used, with adequate hemorrhage control.*

The malignant subcutaneous neoplasms are found more commonly in the cervical area and on the upper part of the leg and wing. They may be recognized by their firmer consistency and broad invasive base.

Tumor surgery, especially on a small bird, demands good surgical anesthesia. The feathers over the operative site and adjacent areas should be plucked and the area properly prepared. Adequate visualization is imperative for good hemorrhage control, and the incision should be of ample size.

The initial incision through the skin is made with a scalpel, with care not to cut into the underlying muscle which might result in hemorrhage that is difficult to control. The skin incision is lengthened using strabismus scissors in small birds or regular Mayo scissors in larger specimens; the lower blade is kept just under the skin, precluding the possibility of any muscle punctures. Blunt dissection is of value in most subcutaneous tumors and may be readily accomplished. Double clamping of vessels may be satisfactory for smaller vessels that must be cut, but in most cases it is worth the extra time it takes to ligate them. Hemorrhage prevention or control is one of the most important aspects of avian surgery. Electrocautery may be of value in controlling hemorrhage, but it must be carefully used, especially in the smaller birds, to prevent excessive tissue damage, or damage to adjacent structures. Oozing vessels that cannot be otherwise controlled, especially those in the breast muscle of smaller birds, may be compressed with Gelfoam* and the wound sutured.

In closing the incision in the skin an Atraumatic needle with the appropriate size gut is utilized, and a continuous stitch is employed as previously described.

Cervical surgery is apt to require special care to avoid the large, thin-walled crop and jugular and carotid vessels. Great care should be taken in dissecting subcutaneous tumors in the neck region if good results are to be achieved. Electrocautery is definitely contraindicated. Besides the tumors mentioned, colloid goiter may also be encountered and successfully removed.

Uropygial gland tumors are not uncommon, being chiefly adenocarcinomas (Fig. 11-10). In examination of a bird, the uropygial gland, or preen gland, should be palpated. If it is enlarged a close inspection should be made. Frequently plugging of the oil duct with inspissated material will cause swelling of the gland. In these cases, gentle manual pressure and injection of a softening agent into the duct (Sebumsol† has been found to do an excellent job) will facilitate breakdown of the occluding material. Gentle pressure on the gland will

* Gelfoam, Upjohn Company, Kalamazoo, Michigan.
† Sebumsol, Parlam Corp., Englewood, N.J.

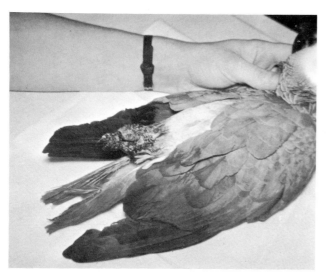

Fig. 11-10. *Epidermoid carcinoma of uropygial gland in African grey parrot. This is one of the more common neoplasms occurring in birds, especially in psittacines.*

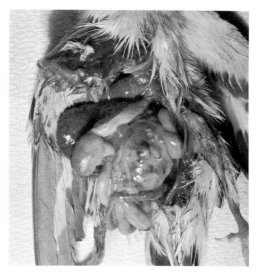

Fig. 11-11. *Carcinoma of gonadal origin as typically seen in parakeets. This lesion frequently involves the kidneys as well, and is not usually amenable to surgery.*

expel the remainder of the material and allow a return to normal function of the gland.

Malignant uropygial tumors are usually quite invasive; they are situated in close contact with the underlying bone, and present problems of hemorrhage control. The entire affected gland should be dissected out, but, if possible, adequate skin should be left for complete closure; the use of Gelfoam under the site of closure of the skin will help in controlling the oozing that is common in this area. Electrocautery or electrodesiccation may also be used for hemorrhage control when the growth is closely apposed to the bone.

Abdominal tumors are for the most part malignant, involving the reproductive system and/or kidneys (Fig. 11-11). Most of these patients are presented at such an advanced stage that surgery is impossible, owing to the large size of the tumor and the small working space. In birds of budgerigar size abdominal surgery for tumor removal has been uniformly disappointing. If it is attempted, an extensive cruciate incision should be employed to ensure adequate visualization. Oxygen should be given to the bird as soon as the body wall is opened. Extreme care should be used in dissection to prevent massive fatal hemorrhage.

In the larger birds some success with abdominal tumors may be expected, depending on the bird's condition and the size, type, and location of the tumor. The successful removal of a massive hemangioendothelioma from the abdomen of a pigeon (Fig. 11-12) has been described,[16] and Hasholt[19] has reported successful performance of laparotomy in budgerigars under local anesthesia.

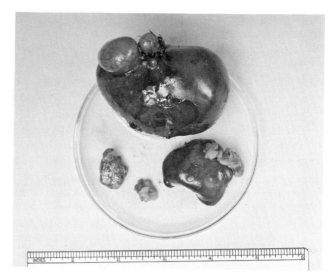

Fig. 11-12. *Intra-abdominal hemangioendothelioma successfully removed from a 495-gm. pigeon. The tumor weighed 113 gm.*

HERNIAS

Only female birds develop abdominal hernias (Fig. 11-13), seemingly a direct result of egg laying and pressure on the abdominal musculature. It is important to differentiate this lesion from the bulging of an abdominal neoplasm. Hernias may be repaired, using the same techniques as employed in mammals, with good results provided extensive adhesions have not occurred. A mid-line incision and suturing of the abdominal muscles in proper position, separately from the overlying skin, will usually suffice.

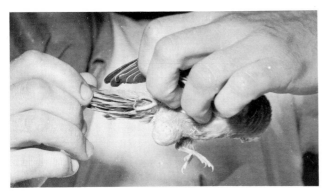

Fig. 11-13. *Hernia in a female budgerigar.*

DISORDERS OF THE OVIDUCT

The oviduct may be operated on by laparotomy if the patient is initially in good condition. Soft-shelled eggs may get lodged in the oviduct, the yolk material becoming inspissated and the shell leathery-walled. The oviduct may be opened and the mass removed, with repair just as for gastrotomy, using intestinal sutures, of suitable size. If removal of the oviduct is indicated, the vessels and oviduct should be carefully ligated prior to excision of the duct. This is a difficult surgical procedure; it should be attempted only if necessary, and then with a guarded prognosis.

At times the oviduct may prolapse, especially following egg laying. If simple replacement is not effective or cannot be readily accomplished, the bird should be anesthetized. The extruded portion is cleaned, sprayed with a local anesthetic, and replaced; if necessary a purse-string suture is placed about the vent.

Egg-bound birds may be "delivered" instrumentally if gentle manual pressure does not first produce results.[15] The bird should be anesthetized, methoxyflurane being quite satisfactory for this procedure. The vent is cleaned and dilated with a thumb forceps or nasal speculum. The oviduct is visualized, and a sterile probe is inserted to the egg shell. With a rotating motion the oviduct is dilated, while gentle pressure is placed on the egg to promote its passage. A small amount of sterile lubricant may be introduced to facilitate delivery. This method is quick and has the added advantage of not causing secondary problems as might be expected following long sessions of "steaming, shell rupture, etc.," which have been advocated in the past.

Wings

TUMORS

Tumors of the wing are not uncommon, the types most often seen being fibromas, fibrolipomas, fibro-myxomas, lipomas, fibrosarcomas, osteosarcomas, with an occasionally highly malignant sarcoma. The ratio of benign to malignant types is about 2 to 1.[1] Most frequently they are found on the dorsal surface of the wing at or near the humero-radial joint. If they are well localized, removal is indicated. However, many of them are diffuse and extremely difficult to dissect away completely. These are better handled by amputation, which gives satisfactory results provided the bird is in good condition and metastasis has not occurred.

The technique for amputation is very much the same as in mammals, and the procedure is actually easier in some respects, because of the paucity of tissue in the area and the ease with which hemorrhage may be controlled with a tourniquet. As in mammals, identification and ligation of the vessels and preparation of an adequate stump will enhance the cosmetic effects.

OTHER LESIONS

Tumors must be differentiated from feather cysts and the more fluid-appearing swellings seen most commonly in pigeons afflicted with paratyphoid infections. Feather cysts are easily recognizable. They involve one or more feather follicles and contain thick, grumous material and undeveloped feathers. They should be incised and thoroughly cleaned, and the lining cauterized with silver nitrate. If hemorrhage continues the follicle should be packed with Gelfoam, held in place with stay sutures.

Norwich, crest, and crest-bred varieties of canaries suffer from hereditary "feather cysts" (hypopteronosis cystica).[2,21] Heavily feathered birds seem most affected, and, although the cysts may be found on any part of the body that is feathered, they are most commonly seen on the wings and dorsal aspects of the body. Arnall[2] advocates utilization of a basal ligature along with incision and curettage, followed by cauterization. He notes that other cysts will frequently occur, and that affected birds should never be used for breeding.

FRACTURES—INTRAMEDULLARY PINNING

In small pet birds properly applied coaptation splintage and immobilization is so uniformly successful that there is little need for intramedullary pinning. If the use of intramedullary fixation is deemed necessary, a hypodermic needle stylet or a hypodermic needle itself may be utilized, much as a Steinmann pin would be applied in a dog. The ease of palpation of the bones in birds makes closed reduction relatively easy, and if one is careful to prepare the site properly and uses good aseptic technique, satisfactory results may be expected.

Simple coaptation and immobilization is not as effective in wing fracture in larger birds, in which the Jonas (sliding-sleeve) intramedullary pin is preferred.[27] This is inserted at the fracture site and provides an excellent method for achieving the best possible apposition. Following surgery the wing should be taped to the body in a normal folded position for two or three weeks, as the large medullary canal with its fine bony trabeculae may not adequately hold the pin in place if the wing is moved excessively.

Compound fractures of the humerus and of the radius and ulna may be ideally treated with the Jonas pin. Even after several days and occurrence of infection such fractures lend themselves to this type of fixation. Ideally, the wound should be cleansed and the bird treated with local and systemic antibiotics for several days prior to surgery. If this is not practical, thorough debridement is sufficient in most cases if antibiotics are administered systemically for 7 to 10 days postoperatively.

Old, partially or fully healed misaligned fractures may be repaired with the Jonas pin. With overlapping and extensive callus formation it may be difficult to bring the displaced segments into apposition. The removal of a small segment of the callus and bone will usually facilitate proper positioning, and any shortening that results will be readily compensated for. It is important in this type of surgery to preserve the large blood vessels as far as possible. They are not well protected by muscle and if they are inadvertently cut healing may be delayed or, in fact, necrosis of the distal portion of the wing may occur.

PINIONING

In rendering a bird flightless one must consider whether permanent or temporary results are desired.

For temporary effects all the primary feathers on one side may be cut close to their attachment to the wing. This leaves an undesirable row of quill stumps that ultimately may have to be removed manually to stimulate new feather growth, or at best will remain till the next normal molt. Alternatively 8 to 10 primary feathers may be pulled out on one side, unbalancing the bird sufficiently to prevent any real flight. Normally these feathers will regenerate in two or three months. It is well to remember that production of imbalance is the principle behind all pinioning, and if both wings are cut, plucked, or operated on, flight will not be completely lost. In addition, it should be pointed out that birds caged outdoors may in times of gusts of high wind be able to soar over fences in spite of proper pinioning.

Numerous methods have been advocated for permanent pinioning, including tenotomy and neurectomy,

but the only uniformly satisfactory method is amputation of the distal two-thirds of the fused second and third metacarpals, leaving the alula, or first digit, intact.

Ideally this is accomplished in birds under 7 days of age, and it may be done with a serrated scissors. Little or no hemorrhage results, and if some oozing occurs momentary clamping of the stump with a forceps is all that is necessary. When the operation is performed on an older bird, more extensive hemorrhage control precautions must be taken. After the bird is half grown, the use of an umbilical tape tourniquet just proximal to the site of amputation has proved to be extremely effective, although extra precautions must be taken in larger birds, as will be described.

The site of the operation is just distal to the point at which the alula (first digit, or spurious or bastard wing) joins the second and third metacarpals (Fig. 11-14). In birds the size of a duck the feathers at the site are plucked and a ligature or tourniquet is placed around the entire metacarpus, leaving out the alula, which to some extent camouflages the stump and gives a good cosmetic effect.

In larger birds, such as swans and geese, a doubled umbilical tape ligature is inserted in the interosseous space between the second and third metacarpals by means of a taper point needle. The needle is kept in close apposition to the posterior border of the second metacarpal (the anterior bone). The doubled end of the tape is then cut, and the two pieces are tied separately anteriorly and posteriorly, providing a separate tourniquet for each metacarpal and giving much better hemorrhage control than a single all-inclusive tourniquet. It is important to remove all feather quills from the

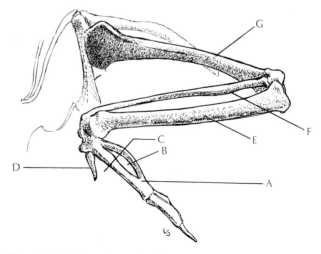

Fig. 11-14. *Drawing of wing skeleton, showing indicated line of amputation for pinioning: A, joined 2nd and 3rd metacarpals; B, interosseous space; C, line of amputation; D, alula, or first digit; E, ulna; F, radius; G. humerus.*

operative site, otherwise hemorrhage control will be impaired.

The portion to be amputated is removed with strong serrated scissors and bone cutters. A small skin flap may be left and sutured. However, in our experience a simple transverse cut, coated liberally with Smear 62* to repel flies, will heal quite satisfactorily.

Obviously, technical refinements of this procedure are possible, and yet simplicity and speed are important when handling unanesthetized birds and the procedure as outlined has proved very satisfactory in hundreds of cases and a wide variety of species.

Legs

TUMORS

Tumors of the legs are quite similar to those occurring on the wings and are handled in a similar manner. If they are extensive, malignant, or involve the bones, amputation is indicated. Most small pet birds, and all of the psittacine birds (which utilize their beak as an extra leg) get along quite well following amputation. However, the handicap of having only one leg should be given serious consideration and discussion both from the practical and from the esthetic standpoint.

The surgical procedure for amputation again varies with the subject and follows the basic principles utilized in such surgery in mammals. The use of a tourniquet to restrict blood flow, preparation of a flap to cover the stump, and strict attention to aseptic principles will help to ensure success.

OTHER LESIONS

Other swellings that occur on the legs and feet include the lesions of gout and of bumblefoot, the former occurring mostly at joints of the lower leg and foot, while the lesions of bumblefoot are seen on the plantar surface of the foot (Fig. 11-15). With gout, especially in small birds, urate deposits may completely occlude the circulation to one or more of the digits and auto-amputation occurs. If such occlusion is recognized at an early stage, surgical amputation of the affected digit will save the bird much prolonged discomfort.

Bumblefoot is especially common in waterfowl when they are kept on concrete covered with a thin layer of sand. It causes pronounced lameness and can be unsightly. Surgery for treatment of such a lesion is relatively easy, and several techniques yield good results.

Anesthesia for most waterfowl may be limited to

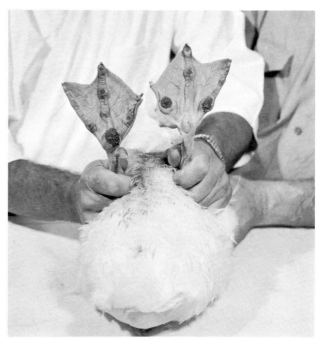

Fig. 11-15. *Multiple bumblefoot lesions on domestic duck. These can be successfully removed surgically, provided good aftercare is supplied.*

2 to 4 ml. of 2% procaine infiltrated about the lesion. In some of the more sensitive or delicate birds, light general anesthesia may be indicated in addition to procaine, to forestall any excessive struggling that might result in shock.

A tourniquet should be placed at the distal portion of the tarsometatarsus, and the operative site should be thoroughly cleansed and prepared. Electrocautery or electrodesiccation may be used with good success to effect complete removal of the lesion, and these methods have definite advantages in hemorrhage control. However, the resulting wound is somewhat slower to heal and must be kept well protected. Surgical excision with a scalpel is preferred for most bumblefoot lesions, followed by suturing with Vetafil* or nylon dermal suture. If well done, this procedure results in quicker healing of an area that at best is difficult to keep properly bandaged and free from bacterial contamination.

Local antibiotics, gauze packs, and thorough bandaging with elastic adhesive will do much to enhance healing of these lesions. If first intention healing has not taken place when the sutures are removed at 10 days, it is important to continue the bandaging for as long as necessary to effect complete closure. Following this, the bird should be kept in a clean enclosure, preferably on grass, with free access to clean water at all times.

---

*Smear 62, Diamond Laboratories, Des Moines, Iowa.

*Vetafil bengen, Dr. S. Jackson, 7801 Woodmont Ave., Washington, D.C.

FRACTURES

Most of what has been written about wing fractures applies also to leg fractures. The smaller birds are readily handled by a variety of coaptation splintage, with the "custom" intramedullary pins of needle stylets and hypodermic needles being used when indicated. Jonas-type intramedullary pins are preferred in most larger species and are very suitable for fixation of fractures in the femur, tibiotarsus, and tarsometatarsus. Some external support should be utilized for one or two weeks after pinning and may consist simply of two or three layers of tape, padded aluminum splintage, or any other appropriate device.

It should be pointed out that overly long and curled toenails are one of the chief causes of leg fractures in small birds. The bird may be scared while grasping the cage wire, and in its panic to suddenly get away the curled claw gets stuck and its violent efforts at release frequently result in a fracture. Large birds may sustain fractures in a similar manner, and zoo eagles have been known to receive bilateral tibial fractures when frightened in a violent thunderstorm.

Radiography

It is invaluable in all fracture work to have biplane radiographs of the affected area. The use of a paper cassette without intensifying screen is of great value in radiography of the bones of birds. It gives excellent definition and facilitates satisfactory exposures, even in the smaller species, which might require ultrashort exposure with regular cassettes and intensifying screens. Good-quality radiographs also define the pneumaticity of bones.

References

1. ARNALL, L.: Some common surgical entities of the budgerigar. Vet. Rec. *72:*888–890, 1960.
2. ARNALL, L.: Anaesthesia and surgery in cage and aviary birds. Vet. Rec. *73:*139–142 (Part I); 173–178 (Part II—A regional outline of surgical conditions); 188–192 (Part III—A systematic outline of surgical conditions); 237–241 (Part IV—A systemic outline of surgical conditions, concluded), 1961.
3. BACHRACH, A.: Strictly for the birds. Vet. Excerpts *14:*99, 1954.
4. BAILEY, R. E.: Surgery for sexing and observing gonad conditions in birds. Auk *70:*497–499, 1953.
5. BARGER, E. H., CARD, L. E., and POMEROY, B. S.: *Diseases and Parasites of Poultry,* 5th ed. Philadelphia, Lea & Febiger, 1958. Pp. 56–57.
6. BEACH, J. E., WILKINSON, J. S., and HARVEY, D. G.: Calculus in the crop of a budgerigar *Melopsittacus undulatus.* Vet. Rec. *72:*473, 1960.
7. BIESTER, H. E., and SCHWARTE, L. H., eds: *Diseases of Poultry,* 4th ed. Ames, Iowa State College Press, 1962. P. 931.
8. *Canine Surgery.* Santa Barbara, Calif., American Veterinary Publications, Inc., 1952. P. 313.
9. DONOVAN, E. W., and BOONE, M. A.: A method of anesthetizing the chicken with diethyl ether. Avian Dis. *9:*227–231, 1965.
10. DURANT, A. J.: Removing the vocal cords of fowl. J.A.V.M.A. *122:*14–17, 1953.
11. FRETZ, V. C.: Anesthetizing poultry. Vet. Med. *27:*109, 1932.
12. FRIEDBURG, K. M.: Problems encountered in pet bird practice. Vet. Med. *56:*157–162, 1961.
13. FRIEDBURG, K. M.: Anesthesia of parakeets and canaries. J.A.V.M.A. *141:*1157–1160, 1962.
14. GANDAL, C. P.: Satisfactory general anesthesia in birds. J.A.V.M.A. *128:*332–334, 1956.
15. GANDAL, C. P.: A practical technic for the relief of egg bound birds. Vet. Med. *55*(12):39, 65, November, 1960.
16. GANDAL, C. P.: Removal of an intra-abdominal tumor of a pigeon by radical incision. Avian Dis. *5:*250–252, 1961.
17. GANDAL, C. P., and SAUNDERS, L. Z.: The surgery of subcutaneous tumors in parakeets. J.A.V.M.A. *134:*212–218, 1959.
18. GRONO, L. R.: Anaesthesia of budgerigars. Australian Vet. J. *37:*463–464, 1961.
19. HASHOLT, J.: Current Diseases of Cage Birds. 31st report Veterinary Hospital, Copenhagen, Denmark, 1959. Pp. 1–20.
20. KERLIN, R. E.: Venipuncture of small birds. J.A.V.M.A. *144:*870–874, 1964.
21. KEYMER, I. F.: Cage and aviary bird surgery. Mod. Vet. Pract. *41*(11):28–31, June 1; (12):32–36, June 15, 1960.
22. LEININGER, F. G.: Clinical use of methoxyflurane anesthetic in small animal practice. Vet. Med. Small Anim. Clinician *60:*401–405, 1965.
23. LEONARD, R. H.: Parakeet and canary practice. J.A.V.M.A. *136:*378–380, 1960.
24. MOSBY, H. S., and CANTNER, D. E.: The use of Avertin in capturing wild turkeys and as an oral-basal anaesthetic for other wild animals. Southwest. Vet. *9:*132–136, 1955.

25. PETRAK, M. L.: Personal communication, 1965.

26. PETRAK, M. L.: Personal communication, 1965.

27. SECORD, A. C.: Fractures in birds repaired with the Jonas splint. Vet. Med. *53:*655–656, 1958.

28. WARREN, D. C., and SCOTT, H. M.: The time factor in egg formation. Poultry Sci. *14:*195–207, 1935.

29. WRIGHT, H. M.: A Suggested Method of Capturing Birds with a Narcosis Producing Drug, Mimeo. Missouri Conservation Comm. 1953.

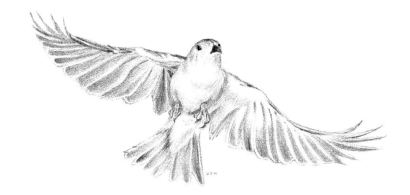

12

Nutritional Deficiencies

T. Geoffrey Taylor

Very few abnormal conditions associated with deficiencies of particular nutrients have been definitely characterized in pet birds. This is perhaps surprising, since many of the foods eaten by these birds, especially seed-eaters, are, by the standards commonly accepted for domestic poultry, very deficient in a number of important nutrients. The probable explanation of this paradox is that the requirements of mature, nonbreeding cage birds are substantially less than those of fast-growing chicks and laying hens.

SPECIFIC DEFICIENCIES

Deficiencies of proteins or of particular essential amino acids would not be expected in insectivorous species or in softbills generally, but it would not be surprising if seed-eaters suffered from such deficiencies, since many bird seeds are very low in total protein and in some essential amino acids (*e.g.,* lysine).[4] However, a protein deficiency has not been described in pet birds. Nor, indeed, have any vitamin-deficiency conditions been reported in the species commonly kept as pets, in spite of the fact that canary seed and millets are relatively low in a number of vitamins.[1]

The fact that all seeds are low in calcium is widely recognized, and most pet birds are supplied with cuttlefish bone or some other source of calcium, so that a deficiency of this mineral is unlikely to be encountered.

A deficiency of iodine has been shown to be widespread in budgerigars kept as pets in England.[2] Schlumberger[6] recorded the occurrence of goiter in budgerigars sent to him from New York, Pennsylvania, Ohio,

233

Indiana, Illinois, Wisconsin, Minnesota, Arkansas, Colorado, and Washington. These states are all considered to be in the goiter belt. Petrak[5] has seen many cases in budgerigars from the vicinity of Boston, Massachusetts, which is not in the goiter belt. Dysplasia of the thyroid was reported by Blackmore[2] in 85 per cent of the pet parakeets included in his survey. All of the usual seeds are very deficient in iodine, and the drinking water in many areas also has a low iodine content.

Lafeber[3] recommends placing one drop of a solution made up of 2 parts of Lugol's solution and 28 parts of distilled water in the drinking water twice weekly as a prophylactic and daily as a therapeutic measure.

REQUIREMENTS OF BREEDING BIRDS

The requirements of breeding birds for essential amino acids, total protein, vitamins, and minerals are far more exacting than those of nonbreeding birds kept as pets. Canaries and softbills are less likely to suffer from nutritional deficiencies than budgerigars, because their usual diet provides most of the nutrients which are essential to health. The diet of budgerigars, on the other hand, consists largely of seeds, which are notoriously deficient in a number of nutrients. Breeders recognize that some parents are better feeders than others; the effect of good and bad feeding on young budgerigars is shown in Figure 12-1.

In breeding budgerigars protein or amino-acid deficiencies express themselves in the form of reduced numbers of eggs and in high mortality of the chicks. These deficiencies are most likely to occur as a result of over-breeding, and they can be most easily prevented by including small amounts of high-quality animal protein in the diet, such as milk or egg proteins or fish meal. These may be incorporated in a supplementary food, or equal parts of milk and water may be provided in glass fountains instead of water.

Vitamin deficiencies are most likely to show themselves by poor hatchability of the eggs, and by weak young suffering a high incidence of mortality. Specific abnormalities in chicks "dead-in-shell" have not been reported. A deficiency of vitamin D_3 associated with rickets, leg weakness, and inability to fly is sometimes encountered in young budgerigars, but non-fatal deficiencies of other vitamins have not been identified with certainty. The administration of a multiple-vitamin prep-

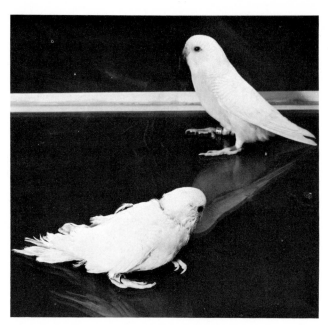

Fig. 12-1. *Young bird from "good-feeding parents" (upper right) and from "poor-feeding parents" (lower left). The well-fed bird weighed 32 gm. at 38 days of age, compared with 24 gm. at 55 days for the poorly fed bird. Birds were photographed on a glass sheet, which is difficult for birds to stand on; the well-fed chick would not normally be down on its hocks. (Courtesy of R. T. French Co., Rochester, N.Y.)*

aration in the drinking water is probably the most satisfactory way of preventing vitamin-deficiency troubles.

When breeding birds are fed a diet deficient in calcium, the eggs have thin shells and there is grave danger that egg binding will occur. A deficiency of vitamin D_3 produces similar symptoms and aggravates a calcium deficiency. Fortunately, the necessity for providing a calcium supplement is well known, so that conditions associated with a deficiency of calcium are rare.

The diet of most seed-eaters is liable to be low in a number of trace elements, in particular iron, copper, and manganese, but anemic conditions associated with a deficiency of either iron or copper or both have not been reported. Various unexplained leg deformities, similar to perosis in young chicks and turkeys, occur from time to time in young budgerigars, and it is possible that a manganese deficiency is implicated.

It would seem to be a wise precaution to offer a complete mineral supplement to all breeding birds as an insurance against mineral-deficiency conditions.

References

1. BISHOP, C., and TAYLOR, T. G.: Studies on the vitamin content of bird seeds. Vet. Rec. *75:*688–691, 1963.

2. BLACKMORE, D. K.: The incidence and aetiology of thyroid dysplasia in budgerigars (*Melopsittacus undulatus*). Vet. Rec. *75:*1068–1072, 1963.

3. LAFEBER, T. J.: Thyroid dysplasia in the Budgerigar. Animal Hospital *1:*208–218, 1965.

4. MASSEY, D. M., SELLWOOD, E. H. B., and WATERHOUSE, C. E.: The amino-acid composition of budgerigar diet, tissues and carcase. Vet. Rec. *72:*283–286, 1960.

5. PETRAK, M. L.: Personal communication, 1966.

6. SCHLUMBERGER, H. G.: Spontaneous goiter and cancer of the thyroid in animals. Ohio J. Sci. *55:*23–43, 1955.

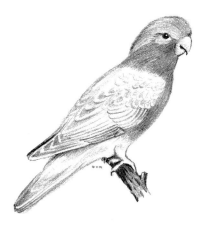

13

French
Molt

T. Geoffrey Taylor

French Molt is, primarily, a disease of young budgerigars, although it has also been reported in the young of lovebirds and other birds of the family Psittacidae. It is not fatal, but it is nevertheless extremely disfiguring, and affected birds are virtually useless. It has been known ever since the budgerigar first became domesticated and does, indeed, occur in the bird in the wild state. The incidence of French Molt is very widespread, and few experienced breeders are able to state that they have never bred a bird suffering from it. The cause of the disease has long baffled scientists and fanciers alike, and many theories have been put forward. No single theory, however, is wholly convincing and capable of explaining all occurrences.

DEFINITION AND SYMPTOMS

French Molt may be defined as a condition in which the flight and tail feathers of the young birds drop out or break off, at about the time the birds are ready to leave the nest box. Sometimes the feathers fall out after the birds have been flying several days. The symptoms of the disease vary considerably and depend a great deal on the severity of the attack. Although only the primaries and tail feathers are usually affected, in severe cases the secondaries may also be lost, and in the most extreme cases practically all the feathers of the body are shed, so that the birds are virtually naked. At the other extreme the attack may be so slight as to escape recognition. In very mild cases only the two longest tail feathers are shed, and the power of flight is in no way impaired.

One very interesting feature of the disease is that the flight feathers are usually shed symmetrically, that is, if a particular feather in one wing is lost, the corresponding feather in the other wing also falls out. The inner flight feathers tend to drop out first, and not infrequently all are lost except the two outer ones, which are the first to complete their growth. Fully grown feathers are not shed, only those which are still growing.

These variable symptoms have led some people to suggest that French Molt is not a single disease but that it includes several distinct, though related, feather diseases. It is not unusual to distinguish the condition in which the feathers drop out in their entirety from that in which they break off at the point where the web of the feather joins the quill. Bleeding may occur in both types. My own personal view is that these varying symptoms are of no fundamental significance and that there is no need to postulate the existence of separate diseases. It seems more reasonable to assume that the detailed symptoms in any particular case depend on the severity of the attack and the age at which the acute stage is reached, rather than that different diseases are involved.

OCCURRENCE

One of the most baffling aspects of this disease is its unpredictability. A particular breeder may never experience an outbreak of the disease for year after year and then, for no apparent reason, many of his pairs will produce a proportion of "runners," as birds suffering from the disease are called. Another puzzling feature of the disease is that some pairs continue to rear healthy young when fed and managed in exactly the same way as pairs that produce a high proportion of affected youngsters. It is a common experience that, once the disease has appeared in an aviary, it will continue throughout that season, becoming progressively worse with time. The only safe course, then, is to stop breeding and rest the birds for 6 months or more.

It is frequently observed that French Molt appears toward the end of a breeding season, often in third nests. It seldom develops in first-round youngsters, and in mild outbreaks healthy and diseased young occur in the same nest. Usually, the youngest chicks in a nest are more likely to suffer from French Molt than the oldest ones, but this is by no means an invariable rule.

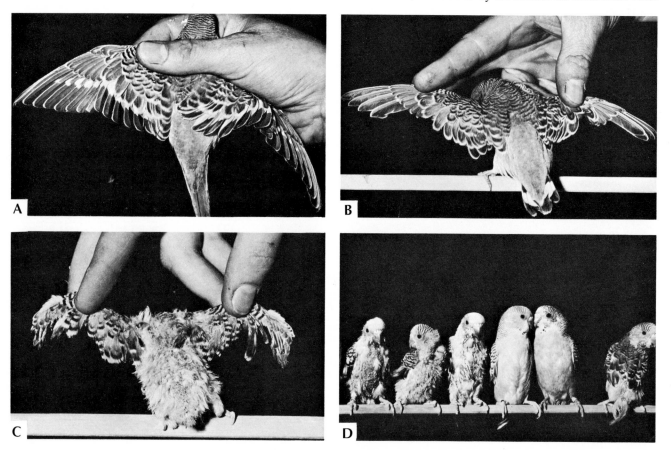

Fig. 13-1. A. *Healthy bird showing full complement of wing and tail feathers. B. Bird 5 weeks of age with French Molt of moderate severity. Note that the long tail feathers, the secondary wing feathers, and all except the last four primaries have been lost. C. Bird 5 weeks of age with very severe attack of French Molt. D. A row of "runners."*

Sometimes the disease appears to strike completely at random.

ETIOLOGY

Many theories have been put forward to account for the disease, and the most important of these are that it is due to:

(a) a bacterial or viral infection,
(b) a feather mite,
(c) the red mite,
(d) heredity,
(e) a nutritional deficiency.

Although systematic investigation has been carried out on all these possibilities, the true cause of the disease is still a matter for speculation.

The pathology of French Molt has been studied by Schofield,[1] who observed:

(a) no mites or other parasites,
(b) no evidence of dermatitis or other form of skin lesion,
(c) poor development of the keratin of the quill,
(d) extensive hemorrhage in the vascular pulp in the quill,
(e) a reduced rate of growth of the flight feathers.

Schofield concluded from his investigations that the etiology is complex and the disease cannot be attributed to a single cause. He recognized that a failure in the supply of nutrients to the growing feathers was the immediate cause of the trouble and suggested that genetic, nutritional, and environmental factors are all implicated.

EXPERIMENTAL INVESTIGATIONS

We have been carrying out research on French Molt at Reading for a decade or so, with most of our work being on the relationship between nutrition and the disease. We rejected the mite theory because the disease frequently occurs in the absence of mites and because healthy young are often reared in the presence of mites. After a few years we ruled out heredity as a primary factor, because we were able to induce the disease in birds bred from a wide variety of sources. The idea that toxic substances might be to blame occurred to us, but this possibility was not studied initially because it does not fit in with the observations which have been made on the circumstances under which French Molt occurs, in particular, with the progressive increase in the incidence of the disease with the increase in the number of rounds taken. We accepted Schofield's report that he could find no evidence for the involvement of microorganisms in the disease.

We had earlier shown[2] that the crop contents of chicks bred from pairs which had previously bred young suffering from French Molt contained less protein than those of chicks bred from pairs with no history of French Molt, and it was suggested that the cause of the disease might be a deficiency in the protein-rich secretion (known as "crop-milk"), on which the young are fed for the first 10 days or so after hatching. The theory we wished to test was that French Molt is caused by a shortage of an essential nutrient in which the normal diet is deficient and which is supplied from the tissue reserves of the parent birds in the "crop-milk." It was envisaged that French Molt might result when the reserves of the unknown nutrient were exhausted after a variable time, depending on the nutrient status of the adult birds at the start of breeding, the diet, and the number of young reared.

The general plan of our experiments at Reading was to deplete the tissue reserves of the parent birds by continuous breeding on a basal diet consisting of panicum millet (*Setaria italica*) only. Sea sand and oyster shell grit were also supplied. When a high incidence (over 50 per cent) of diseased young were being bred the pair was allocated to a particular experimental treatment for a further two nests and the number of diseased young was compared with the number bred by untreated control pairs. At least three pairs were placed on each experimental treatment.

Over the years, supplements of all the essential amino acids, vitamins, and minerals (including trace elements) were fed, but in no case was a significant reduction in the incidence of French Molt recorded. When deficiencies of amino acids and vitamins A and D had been eliminated, the seed fed to all birds was treated with 1 per cent cod liver oil and they were given sterilized milk, diluted with an equal amount of water, to drink. The birds bred freely on this diet and fertility and hatchability were good, but a high proportion of the young suffered from French Molt.

During the course of this research we investigated the origin of the so-called "crop-milk" on which budgerigars feed their young. The most likely source appeared to be the glandular stomach, or proventriculus, although the possibility that the glands of the lower esophagus also contribute to the secretion could not be ruled out. The evidence suggested that only the hen produces "crop-milk."

Another observation we made was that, in the majority of cases, eggs from birds with a long history of French Molt gave rise to diseased young when fostered by pairs whose own youngsters, reared in the same nest, developed into perfectly healthy birds. It appears that the disease may be "carried in the egg."

During investigation of the levels of certain minerals in the plasma of healthy budgerigars and birds with French Molt it was noted that the packed-cell volume was less in the blood from birds with French Molt than in that from the controls. The data obtained from six birds in each category, given in Table 13-1, show that the packed-cell volume is significantly less in the birds with French Molt than in healthy birds.

We then examined the bone marrow and found a striking difference between the smears obtained from birds with French Molt and from healthy birds. The marrow from the diseased birds was severely hyper-

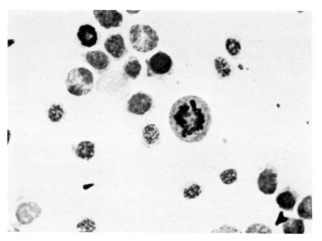

Fig. 13-2. *Bone-marrow smear from a bird having French Molt.*

plastic, with 50 mitotic figures being counted in 20 fields compared with only 4 in marrow from the control birds.

Hemoglobin levels were proportional to the packed-cell volume, and the anemia was thus a normocytic, normochromic type. Smears of the peripheral blood of diseased birds were indistinguishable from those of healthy birds. The red cells were abnormally fragile and it would appear therefore that, in birds suffering from French Molt, the life span of the erythrocytes is unusually short and that new cells are not produced fast enough to maintain a normal cell count, in spite of the hyperactivity of the hematopoietic tissues.

The possibility that the anemia was secondary to a severe hemorrhage appeared unlikely, since the feathers of the birds used in this investigation did not bleed.

ADDENDUM

A new sidelight on the etiology of French Molt was provided by subsequent research on another problem. During the course of an investigation into the biochemical effects of hypervitaminosis A on chicks of the domestic fowl it was observed that a low packed-cell volume was a consistent feature of this condition, and the possibility that excess vitamin A may be a factor involved in the development of French Molt was considered. This possibility was consistent with the fact that capillary hemorrhages are associated with hypervitaminosis A in some species and with the findings of a survey made in 1957 among 600 British breeders of

Table 13-1. Packed Cell Volume (PCV) of Blood from Healthy Budgerigars and from Ones Suffering from French Molt

	Healthy			French Molt	
Age (days)	Live Wt. (grams)	PCV (%)	Age (days)	Live Wt. (grams)	PCV (%)
28	47	55	30	37	43
52	35	56	75	31	51
75	33	50	77	28	47
76	33	50	77	36	41
81	34	58	79	40	48
83	36	53	80	37	45
	Mean 53.7			Mean 45.8*	
	Standard error ± 1.3			Standard error ± 1.5	

*Significantly less than mean for healthy birds $P < 0.01$ (t test).

budgerigars that the percentage of those who used cod liver oil was greater among breeders who had serious trouble with French Molt than among breeders whose birds were free from the disease. It could also explain the observations that French Molt is "carried in the egg" and that the disease seldom occurs in the first nest and becomes progressively worse as the number of nests increases.

We therefore carried out an experiment to test the theory that excess vitamin A may be a factor in the development of French Molt, when the vitamin is fed in the usual way, *i.e.*, by adding it to the seed in the form of an oily solution. Six pairs were fed on panicum millet treated with 1 per cent peanut oil containing 1,000 I.U. vitamin A and 1 mg. vitamin E per gm. of oil. Later, 100 I.U. vitamin D$_3$ was added per gm. of oil. This level of vitamin A is similar to that normally fed by breeders. As controls, six pairs were fed exactly the same except that the vitamin A was omitted from the feeding oil. After about 4 months a small amount of vitamin A (100 I.U. per gm.) was included in the oil given the controls to avoid the danger of a *deficiency* of vitamin A occurring in these pairs.

Several pairs on the control treatment refused to

breed to begin with, so that fewer nests were obtained from this group, but the number of young bred per nest was similar in both groups. The detailed results of this experiment are shown in Table 13-2. It will be seen that the incidence of French Molt was twice as great in the high-vitamin-A group as in the controls, 70 per cent compared with 35 per cent. One of the pairs fed the high level of vitamin A reared 16 young in 4 nests, and only 4 of these youngsters had French Molt. This pair was obviously very resistant to French Molt; with this pair omitted from consideration, the incidence of French Molt in the remaining five pairs was 90 per cent.

These results are consistent with the theory that high levels of vitamin A predispose budgerigars to French Molt, but the disturbingly high incidence of the disease in the control group, which certainly did not have excess vitamin A in their diet, suggests that the vitamin was exerting its influence indirectly.

Determinations of vitamin A were made on the liver and kidneys of a number of diseased and healthy birds on both treatments and the results are given in Table 13-3. In each group the birds suffering from French Molt stored greater amounts of vitamin A in both liver and kidney tissue than did the healthy birds,

Table 13-2. Effect of High Level of Vitamin A (10,000 I.U./Kg. Seed) on Incidence of French Molt

	High Vitamin A			Low Vitamin A (Control)		
	No. of Nests	No. of Young	Percentage of Young Affected	No. of Nests	No. of Young	Percentage of Young Affected
All pairs	15	58	70	9	34	35
Omitting one pair	11	42	90			

Table 13-3. Mean Concentrations of Vitamin A (I.U./Gm. Fresh Tissue ±S.D.) in Kidneys and Liver of Healthy Young and Young Affected with French Molt, on Diets High and Low in Vitamin A

High Vitamin A				Low Vitamin A			
French Molt		Healthy		French Molt		Healthy	
Kidney	Liver	Kidney	Liver	Kidney	Liver	Kidney	Liver
303.4 ±34.0	440.4 ±46.2	274.0 ±54.2	373.0 ±51.5	223.5 ±58.6	81.4 ±12.8	121.3 ±17.7	59.2 ±16.3

but these differences were not statistically significant. It is interesting to note that on the high-vitamin diet the livers contained a greater concentration of vitamin A than the kidneys, whereas on the low-vitamin diet the kidneys were the richer in both diseased and healthy birds.

The hypothesis that we now favor is that the primary cause of French Molt is a fragility of the capillaries in the pulp of the growing feather and that the factor or factors responsible also cause a weakening of the red cell membranes. An excess of vitamin A and a deficiency of vitamin E are among nutritional factors which alter the structure of biological membranes in such a way as to reduce their strength, and a third fat-soluble vitamin, vitamin K, appears to act on membranes in a manner similar to vitamin E. Capillary hemorrhages are a feature of a deficiency of both vitamin E and vitamin K in chicks.

It appears, however, that these dietary factors merely predispose young budgerigars to the disease and that the primary cause lies elsewhere. The possibility that French Molt may be due to a virus or virus-like agent has not been investigated experimentally and it is one which should now be taken seriously, since virtually all the other theories have been tested and found wanting.[1]

A viral infection is consistent with the observation that the disease appears to be transmitted in the egg and with the allegation frequently made by breeders that the disease often shows itself for the first time following the introduction of new stock. Furthermore, it is not inconsistent with any of the other observations which have been made. The increase in the incidence of the disease with the advance of the breeding season and, in individual pairs, with the number of nests bred, could be explained in terms of an increasing build-up in the virus population in the bird-room with the increase in the density of the bird population, so that, eventually, the virus reaches a level high enough to infect 100 per cent of the young birds. The ability of pairs formerly producing affected young to breed healthy young after a rest of 6 months or even less would be explicable, on this theory, in terms of a gradual reduction in virus particles in the blood and tissues to a low level while the birds were flying in an aviary where the population density was low.

The evidence in favor of a virus being responsible for French Molt is purely circumstantial, but my personal opinion is that it is sufficiently great to justify an investigation. Our nutrition experiments have now been wound up. In the final one chlortetracycline at a level of 400 p.p.m. was administered in the drinking fluid to eight breeding pairs, but no reduction in the incidence of the disease was observed over two rounds. We must now hand over the problem to workers in other disciplines.

References

1. SCHOFIELD, F.: A new look at an old problem: French Moult. All-Pets Mag., September, 1955.

2. TAYLOR, T. G.: *Feeding Exhibition Budgerigars,* 2nd ed. London, Iliffe Press, 1958. 52 pp.

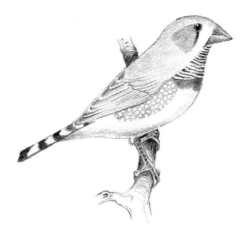

14

Conditions Involving the Integumentary System

Robert B. Altman

The avian integumentary system includes the skin, feathers, scales, claws, beak, and uropygial gland. Disorders involving these specialized structures occur commonly and present the practitioner with some of his more difficult diagnostic problems.

This Chapter endeavors to discuss the particular conditions, the cause, if it is known, and the treatment, if any is possible.

DEFORMITIES OF THE BEAK, FEATHERS, CLAWS, AND TOES

DEFORMITIES OF THE BEAK

In order to recognize beak deformities, one must know the normal conformation of the beak of the various species of cage birds. Basically, only two types of beak need be differentiated. The soft-billed birds and non-psittacine seed-eating species have a relatively straight bill of varying length, with the upper mandible slightly overlapping the lower. The second type is the hooked heavy bill seen in the seed-eating psittacines and carnivores such as the falcon, hawk, and owl.

The most common deformity is simple overgrowth (Fig. 14-1), resulting from malocclusion or insufficient normal wear. Various instruments suitable for its correction (Fig. 14-2) are easily obtainable. In the soft-billed and non-psittacine seed-eaters, overgrowth occurs at the tip and along the non-occluding edges of the upper mandible. This is easily trimmed with a pair of cuticle nippers. For trimming heavier bills, podiatrists' toenail nippers are excellent. By following the natural line of

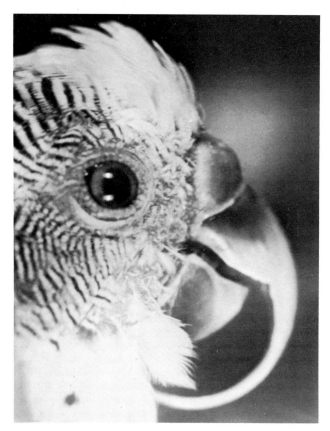

Fig. 14-1. *Overgrowth of upper mandible of a budgerigar.*

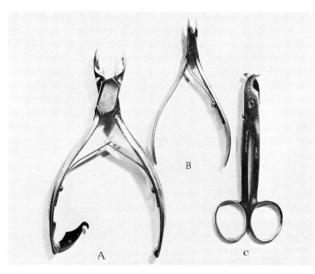

Fig. 14-2. *Instruments for trimming beaks and claws of birds. A. Podiatrists' toenail nippers for cutting a parrot's beak. Manufactured by H. E. Fragey, Germany; obtainable through most surgical supply houses. B. Cuticle nippers for cutting claws and beaks of smaller species. Manufactured by Revlon, Germany, No. 2023; obtainable in most drug stores. C. Canine toenail nippers for cutting claws and beaks of large psittacine birds. Manufactured by Amico, Germany; obtainable from most veterinary supply houses.*

the bill and removing only the overgrown edges, no blood vessels will be encountered.

Problems of malocclusion occur more frequently in the psittacine species. In the captive bird with the type of beak characteristic of these species, overgrowth of both the upper and the lower bill occurs. In parrots, macaws, and other larger psittacines, as well as in hawks and falcons, both the point of the bill and the lateral hooks must be trimmed if they are overgrown. Frequently the lower bill must be trimmed if it does not meet the upper bill evenly. In parrots and parakeets, if the bird is held up between the examiner's eye and a bright light source (transilluminated), the line of demarcation between the vascular and non-vascular part of the beak can be seen. Trimming should be done as frequently as is necessary.

Lafeber[8] suggests that the average rate of growth of the budgerigar's upper beak is about $\frac{1}{4}$ inch per month, or about 3 inches a year. I believe, however, that the growth can vary from $\frac{1}{4}$ inch to $\frac{1}{2}$ inch per month. Such growth is seen in many birds with malocclusion.

One of the most common causes of overgrown beaks, particularly in the budgerigar, is the parasitic infestation, "scaly face." The mite (*Cnemidocoptes* spp.) invades the matrix of the beak, destroying some of the germinal tissue. This results in a different rate of growth of the two sides of the beak, with consequent spooning and fissuring. The lower beak will also overgrow on non-occluding edges. Elimination of the mite will prevent further damage, but the already existing deformity is irreversible.

Overgrowth of the upper beak commonly occurs from a loss of contour and straightening (Fig. 14-3, *2*), often seen with advancing age. Beak deformity has also been observed in parrots with tuberculosis.[5]

Hereditary and congenital deformities are not often seen, because the young birds die or are euthanatized. Some less severely affected birds will live, and constant trimming of the beak is necessary. These deformities cause scissor bill (Fig. 14-3, *6*), epignathism, and prognathism.

Other causes of beak deformity in both psittacine and soft-billed birds, such as malnutrition, specific nutritional deficiencies, rickets, and osteodystrophy (often called "rubber beak" by the layman), are seen more often in captive wild birds. The tough chitinous consistency of the bill is lost, and a pliable rubbery bill which can easily be bent is evident. The bird is, of course, unable to eat, and usually starves to death. If force feeding is undertaken early enough, and calcium, in the form of dicalcium phosphate or Pervinal* powder or syrup, is

*Pervinal—concentrate of essential vitamins, minerals, lipotropics, and bioflavonoids (U.S. Vitamin & Pharmaceutical Corp., New York, N.Y.).

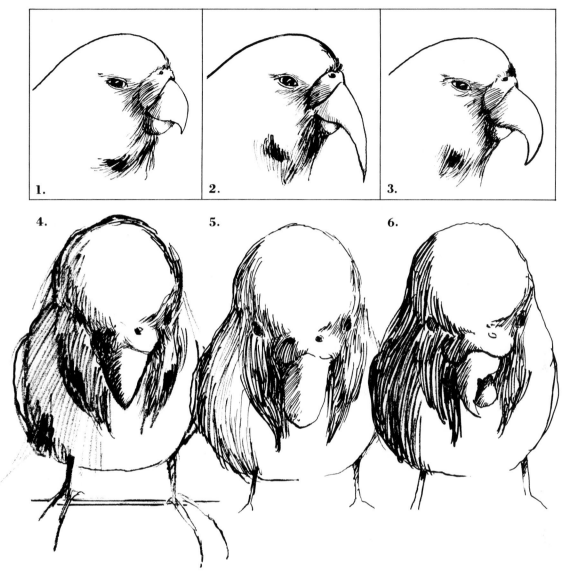

Fig. 14-3. *Normal beak, and variations occurring in the beak in budgerigars. 1. Normal beak (lateral view). 2. Straight beak showing loss of normal curvature. 3. Excessive curvature in upper beak. 4. Normal beak (anterior view). 5. Flattening with spooning. 6. Scissor bill.*

mixed with the food, the bill will often harden with relative rapidity. One of the most difficult problems encountered is the curling of the bill as it hardens. Splinting with adhesive tape and/or wire may correct the malocclusion while the beak returns to normal hardness. Feeding high-protein seeds and food rich in methionine is also helpful.

A deficiency of vitamins A and D, biotin, pantothenic acid, and folic acid causes abnormal beak formation.

According to Arnall,[2] food impacted on the hard palate in chicks which have not been cleaned by the parent hardens, and the pressure causes deformity of the upper beak.

A beak that has been split as a result of trauma will frequently grow out normally without any treatment. However, bleeding or inability to eat as a complication of the injury necessitates splinting. Wiring these beaks is a most efficient method of treatment. Drilling very small holes through the two halves of the beak and wiring with 00000 stainless steel will support the beak while it grows out. A bird with an avulsed upper or lower beak usually dies, since it is unable to eat. Hand feeding is extremely difficult, time consuming, and impractical, although it is not impossible.

Trauma can also cause hemorrhage between the layers (laminae) of the beak. Cage birds allowed freedom in a small enclosure, such as a room, may fly into objects and cause injury to their beak. Particularly with mirrors or windows, depth perception is lost and the bird often collides with the glass. Discoloration and deformity can result. The blood between the layers clots and dries; consequently, as the beak grows, flaking and fractures occur.

Tumors of the beak, seen occasionally in budgerigars (Fig. 14-4), cause severe deformity, and all have been found malignant. Euthanasia is the only recourse. A differential diagnosis must be made between invasive tumors of the upper beak and deformity or fractures of the beak due to intra-laminal hemorrhage. During the early stages the two conditions are similar, but since they differ so in prognosis the proper diagnosis is essential. In deformity and fractures from previous trauma and hemorrhage, there is usually little or no bleeding when the abnormal tissue is flaked away. With tumors, flaking or scarification of tissue results in hemorrhage and pain.

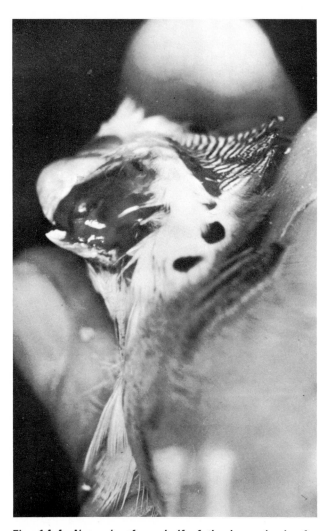

Fig. 14-4. *Necrosis of one-half of the lower beak of a budgerigar due to tumor formation.*

FEATHER DEFORMITIES

Deformity of the feathers may occur idiopathically, as the result of trauma, or from nutritional, parasitic, and probably metabolic causes.

Broken or split feathers should be extracted. The feather should be held firmly with the fingers or a hemostat, and the pull exerted perpendicularly to the follicle so that there is no tearing of the skin. Immature feathers are vascular and when broken will bleed profusely. Hemorrhage is easily controlled after removal of the feather by compressing the open follicle with a wet cotton pledget for a few moments.

Feathers that are incompletely developed or have defective barbules which cause imperfect interlocking and resultant fraying are the result of either genetic variations or abnormal feather development. It has been suggested by Kluver[7] that this condition is caused by a deficiency of the amino acids arginine and glycine.

In larger birds such as macaws or cockatoos, injury to the large tail feathers will produce fraying and breaking of the primary shaft. This may be caused by inadequate caging facilities, with resultant rubbing of the tail feathers on the sides or bottom of the cage.

DEFORMED CLAWS AND TOES

Deformities of the claws and toes (Fig. 14-5) are usually the result of injury. Such deformities or even absence of claws or of entire digits is noted frequently in canaries and finches. These deformities in no way handicap the bird. In many of the psittacines, claws are thick and straight and must be trimmed frequently. Cuticle or canine toenail nippers facilitate this. In parrots, care must be taken in trimming the claws. The claw of the short hind toe (hallux) bleeds easily, since the vessel extends close to the end. Electrocautery and chemical cautery (silver nitrate or copper sulfate) will control hemorrhage in the beak or claw that has been trimmed too close or broken.

When cauterizing the upper bill with silver nitrate, extreme caution must be taken to eliminate the possibility of ingestion of any of the chemical. Holding the lower and upper bills together with the fingers prevents this hazard. Legs severely infested with the scaly leg mite (*Cnemidocoptes* spp.) (Fig. 14-6) often have deformed toes and nails. The nails become thick and grow either straight or without the natural curve (Fig. 14-5, *2*), or curve excessively (Fig. 14-5, *3*) or abnormally, like a corkscrew (Fig. 14-5, *4*). In some cases toe nails will be completely missing and no regrowth will take place. Excessive length of the claws in large psittacines can be prevented by use of perches of larger diameter. This affords more surface for the normal wear of the nail.

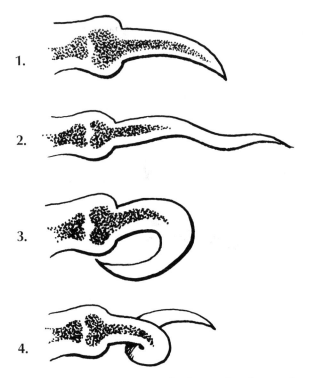

Fig. 14-5. *Normal claw, and claws showing various deformities.*
1. *Normal claw.*
2. *Spiral claw.*
3. *Excessive curvature of the claw.*
4. *Corkscrew nail.*

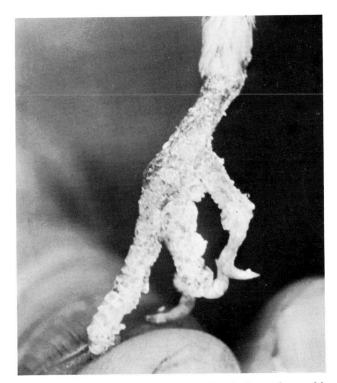

Fig. 14-6. *Foot of a budgerigar showing lesions of cnemidocoptic mange.*

Deformed and gnarled toes will be seen in cases of gout (articular). Diagnosis is based on the presence of yellow-white urate nodules at the interphalangeal joints.

FEATHER CYSTS (HYPOPTERONOSIS CYSTICA)

Feather cysts are subcutaneous swellings caused by growth of the feather shaft within the confines of the follicle. The feather, instead of protruding through the skin following its normal growing course, curls within the follicle. As the feather continues to grow, this cystic mass enlarges, with a cheesy exudate forming within the follicle and the wall becoming thickened. As the mass enlarges, the area surrounding the follicle may show an acute inflammatory reaction. This irritation causes the bird to pick at the area, which often causes ulceration of the cystic mass. Ulceration can also occur spontaneously. After the follicle has ulcerated, the feather then has a chance to escape through the open skin. The feather is generally engulfed in the cheesy exudate, which on contact with the air dries into a very hard, crustlike mass. Continual growth of the feather often raises this hard scablike mass well above the surface of the skin, and in the later stages it can appear very much like a tumor. One or many follicles can be involved. These cysts have been seen in many species, including canaries, parakeets, and parrots, with the highest incidence seen in canaries of the Norwich, crest, crest-bred, and plain head breeds. The wings are most frequently the site of this lesion.

Treatment depends on the number of cysts, their size, and the age of the bird. If only one or a few cysts are found, removal of the abnormal feather, wrapped in its exudate, and curettage of the lining of the follicle are of value in eliminating the cyst. Hemorrhage is often something of a problem, and hemostasis can be accomplished by cautery. If the lesion remaining after curettage is small, application of an antibiotic ointment will result in healing. Rarely will a new feather grow from this now destroyed follicle. If, however, the lesion is very large, it may be necessary to suture the edges of the skin to close the wound. This treatment is usually followed by systemic administration of antibiotics.

For cysts developing in other areas of the body, particularly over the back and around the pectoral area, the treatment of choice is excision of the entire cyst. This is easily accomplished without anesthesia, and by simple excision through the skin; closure of the wound by one or two sutures of 0000 medium chromic catgut eliminates necessity for later removal of the sutures. Recurrences of these cystic masses in areas on both the wings and the body are common, and there seems to be little effective means of inhibiting future cyst formation. This condition is thought to be hereditary. Arnall[1] quoted the statement of Crew and Mirskaia[4] that treatment of affected birds with injection of thyroid extract, in addition to initiating a fresh molt, stimulated appearance of a new plumage which did not carry fresh lesions, but was nevertheless partially depigmented.

MOLTING

Molting is the normal physiological means by which birds change their plumage. The various species generally molt at specific times. The true physiological nature of molting in birds is not completely understood. All birds molt in a fairly definite pattern, the old feathers being replaced by the growth of the new. In different species certain areas will grow new feathers before other areas.

Cage birds exist under various environmental conditions, and these factors have a tremendous influence on the molting cycle. Season, temperature, humidity, nutrition, egg laying, and sex are influencing factors. For example, female chicks usually feather more rapidly than the male chicks do; also, molting is more conspicuous in females. Most psittacine birds molt continually throughout the year. Molting is generally heavier in the spring and early summer than in the colder months. The passerines, such as canaries, start their molt in the spring, usually in May, and molt throughout the summer to late September. Most of the song birds will stop singing during the molt and start again in the fall. Egg laying ceases during this period.

During the molt, the bird loses feathers by either picking or shaking them out as they are shed from the follicle. New feathers appear as small shoots (pinfeathers), and the bird often scratches and picks at the skin and feathers. There apparently is some pruritus associated with a heavy molt. During the molt, birds are more susceptible to fracture due to the resorption of calcium in the Haversian systems of the long bones. It is therefore advisable to keep birds caged during this period.

ABNORMAL MOLTING

The differentiation between a normal heavy molt and a pathological molt is difficult. Both the previous molting habits of the bird and the current clinical signs must be evaluated. A canary losing many feathers in the spring can be undergoing a normal molt, yet the same feather loss in December could be pathological. Any bird losing feathers and not replacing them is undergoing an abnormal molt. This is demonstrated by the appearance of bare skin spots and the lack of any feather replacement.

A bird persistently losing feathers during a period when it should not normally lose them can also be considered to be in a pathological molt. Other signs of pathological molt are the replacement of normal feathers with abnormally formed feathers.

The etiology of an abnormal molt can vary, and determining it is difficult. Heavy to severe molts can occur from extremes in temperature or rapid temperature changes, and from severe shock or fright. Usually such a history can be extracted from the owner, and a molt resulting from such causes is temporary. Improper diet and avitaminosis can cause a heavy molt with subsequent poor feathering. Re-establishment of the proper diet and supplementation with a vitamin will bring the bird back to condition. A water-soluble multi-vitamin preparation placed in the drinking water daily is an adequate source of supplementary vitamins. The concentration will vary with the normal water consumption of the species. A soft-billed bird, such as a mynah bird, will consume far more water than a seed-eater. Therefore, lower concentration of the vitamin mixture is necessary. Approximately 10 to 30 drops per ounce of water is the standard dose of Vi-Aqua.* Direct oral administration of the concentrated vitamin mixture is also possible (1 to 3 drops), depending on the size of the bird.

External parasites will often cause feather loss, but such a condition is usually associated with pruritus and the organisms can be demonstrated.

Large bare spots not associated with feather loss frequently appear on the abdomen of a bird. Such areas can be caused simply by the wider separation of the feather tracts as the result of obesity or tumors, leaving large areas of skin uncovered.

One of the most common causes of feather loss with abnormal structure of the newly formed feathers is hypothyroidism. Thyroidectomy decreases the rate of feather growth, and the feathers become fringed and elongated, frequently with a loss of barbules.[9] Such feathers are uneven and appear like ostrich feathers. The addition of 5 to 10 grains of powdered thyroxin mixed thoroughly with 1 pound of seed, or 1 to 5 drops daily of a suspension of 10 grains of thyroxin in 1 ounce of water will alleviate this situation.

Unfortunately, the cause of a great majority of abnormal molts is undetermined. All treatment fails, and a partly feathered to completely featherless creature may result. Keeping such a featherless bird alive for a

---

*Vi-Aqua—A palatable water-soluble multi-vitamin preparation (U.S. Vitamin & Pharmaceutical Corp., New York, N.Y.).

long period of time is very difficult, since the bird has lost all of its insulation.

Some birds lose the tail and wing feathers very slowly, and these feathers, broken and frayed, remain in the follicles. If these feathers are pulled out, new feathers will grow to replace them in 6 to 8 weeks. According to Beach[3] feather loss causing a naked breast in one bird was thought to be hormonal in origin, resulting from an ovarian cyst.

FEATHER PICKING

Feather picking may be initiated by either a normal or an abnormal molt. Any dermatological condition which is accompanied by pruritus may result in feather picking. Boredom seems to be a major factor, although there is no scientific confirmation of this. Several species seem to be particular candidates for this condition. Although all species of parrots are affected, the African grey seems to be the worst offender. Cockatiels also show a high incidence. Of the larger birds, the cockatoos also are offenders.

The condition starts by just a few feathers being pulled. These can be old feathers ready to be pulled out, or new in-coming feathers which cause itching of varying intensity. The bird then continues to pick. The habit becomes a vice, and the bird picks itself bare. Frequently, chewing of the feathers breaks a feather shaft near the follicle, leaving only a badly split quill. These stubs then slow down the growth of the normal new feathers as they try to supplant the old. This occurs particularly with the flight feathers. The broken quills should be extracted by firm traction on the broken shaft, pulling perpendicularly to the follicle while the wing is held with the fingers, near the shaft being pulled. Occasionally some hemorrhage will result. Compression for 60 seconds with wet cotton will cause clotting.

If the bird chews through a newly formed feather, severe hemorrhage results. It may be difficult to find the feather since often the entire cage and bird are spattered with blood. Pulling the feather eliminates the problem. The only feathers that will hemorrhage to any extent are the large wing and tail feathers.

If the feather has broken below the surface of the follicle, it can be extremely difficult to pull the remaining shaft. However, this must be done, and it can be accomplished by use of a mosquito hemostat.

Treatment of feather pickers is difficult if the etiology cannot be determined. Elimination of the cause is the ideal course. If picking continues after the bird has been treated, the only means of hindering further picking is by placing a collar (the so-called Elizabethan collar) on the bird. These collars must be made to fit the individual, and their weight is important. For smaller birds such as finches, budgerigars, and canaries, oak tag is an excellent material for the purpose. A circle 3 inches in diameter is cut out of oak tag. A slit is made from the edge of the disk to the center, and a hole ½ inch in diameter is cut out of the center. The collar is placed around the bird's neck and the slit is closed with staples. For the first 30 to 60 minutes the bird will lose its balance and do "back flips," but it will then gradually become accustomed to the collar. The collar should be left on until the next molt has taken place and the new feathers have grown out. Birds have lived a life time wearing such collars with little ill effect. For the larger species of psittacine birds, a relatively strong material must be used, or the bird will chew its way through within hours. Various plys of acetate are excellent for this purpose. Frequent sprays or baths may help alleviate the picking habit.

BROWN HYPERTROPHY OF THE CERE

In psittacine birds, particularly budgerigars, hypertrophy of the cere is a common occurrence, the severity of the condition showing great variation. The cere, which is generally soft and blue (in males) or light brown to pink (in females), becomes cornified and keratinized. The cornified tissue proliferates, and the normally flat cere becomes elevated. In some cases pieces of the abnormal tissue will break off and only 1 or 2 mm. of thickness will remain. In other cases continuing development will produce a unicorn-like appearance (Fig. 14-7). Except for occluding the nares, this process does not affect the bird. The excess tissue may be removed by carefully

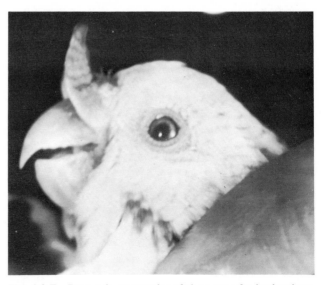

Fig. 14-7. *Brown hypertrophy of the cere of a budgerigar.*

separating or peeling the thickened, hard, keratinized tissue from the underlying normal layer. Softening for several days with a bland ointment such as boric acid ointment will facilitate removal and decrease the possibility of hemorrhage. Regrowth of the tissue can be expected. In the average case no treatment is required. Age increases the incidence of hypertrophy; although it develops in both sexes, it is more commonly seen in females. The etiology is unknown.

ABSCESSES

Because of the high body temperature of birds, abscesses are not commonly seen. The general appearance of the abscess differs from that typically seen in mammals. Inflammation and heat are usually absent. Most of the pus is a cheesy exudate rather than a liquid, and the abscesses are well walled-off and painless.

One of the most common sites of abscess formation in canaries and budgerigars is the periocular region (Fig. 14-8). Abscesses in this region may involve either or both the upper and the lower eyelid and the area below the lower lid. Their etiology is unknown; treatment is not always successful, and they frequently recur.

Treatment consists of plucking the feathers from the surrounding area. The skin is incised the length of the abscess, but care should be taken to avoid the larger blood vessels. The periocular area is usually very vascular. After incision the exudate should be removed and the abscess well curetted. If the lesion is not too extensive, cauterization with silver nitrate is indicated. An ophthalmic antibiotic ointment containing no steroids should be applied locally for 4 to 6 days; antibiotics should be administered in the food or drinking water for 7 days.

These abscesses are sometimes the result of inflam-

mation of the membranes lining the infraorbital sinuses, and must be differentiated from infectious sinusitis of turkeys, thought to be caused by a pleuropneumonia-like organism. The condition must also be differentiated from sinusitis associated with vitamin A deficiency, and from foreign body injury to the sinus. Periocular abscesses and foreign body sinusitis usually occur on only one side.

A small, hard pea-shaped mass of cheesy exudate may occur in mynah birds above the eye on the supraorbital crest and between the nostril and the eye. Excision is accomplished by making a small incision over the nodule and scooping out the cheesy material. Usually the mass comes out in one piece. One or two 0000 catgut sutures will close the incision. This procedure is simple and requires no anesthesia.

In parrots and budgerigars, an accumulation of exudate may distend and distort the cere. This exudate may be caseous or liquid. If it is liquid, there is usually a copious nasal discharge, with an accumulation of coagulated exudate on the beak. Sinusitis is the cause of this discharge. If the exudate clots in the cere, a very hard core will fill the nasal cavity. This core must be curetted out to re-establish free drainage. Infusion with Furacin* solution or use of Terramycin† ophthalmic ointment and antibiotics administered parenterally for 10 to 14 days is usually sufficient to eliminate the sinus discharge. Since this condition is chronic, its manifestations can be expected to reappear. Care must be taken during curettage of the nasal area, particularly in parrots, not to injure the vascular nasal septum in the cere.

Abscesses and necrotic foci are occasionally found in the hard palate of parrots. The symptoms usually displayed are anorexia and weight loss. When the mouth is explored during physical examination, a soft, white, cheesy exudate can be found in the cleft of the palate. Since tumors (sarcomas) are sometimes found in this location, differential diagnosis is necessary.

Treatment consists of curettage of the affected portion of the palate, local application of Furacin* solution, and systemic administration of antibiotics. Curettage several times a week for two weeks is generally necessary. Cauterization of the diphtheritic membrane with silver nitrate after curettage may be necessary.

Abscesses of the uropygial gland are seen in all species, but most commonly in budgerigars. As the result of either trauma or a blocked duct, one or both lobes of the gland enlarge and become abscessed. This area is very sensitive, and the bird displays signs of discomfort and pain, constantly flicking the tail and pick-

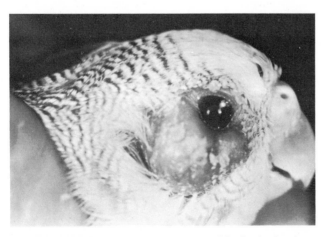

Fig. 14-8. *Abscess in region of lower lid of a budgerigar. Note the extensive subcutaneous vessels.*

*Furacin—nitrofurazone (Eaton Laboratories, Norwich, N.Y.).
†Terramycin—oxytetracycline hydrochloride (Pfizer Laboratories, New York, N.Y.).

ing at the area. An elevation with distortion of the feathers can be seen after the swelling has become extensive. Ulceration and bleeding may call the owner's attention to the condition.

Lancing and curettage should be performed after it is ascertained that an abscess and not a tumor exists. Neoplasms of varying types have been found in this area. Care should be taken to avoid damage to the ducts and the papilla.

Birds with chronic infection of the uropygial gland should be seen regularly, and the contents of the gland should be expressed. This is easily accomplished by compressing the lobes with blunt thumb forceps. Canaries should regularly have this gland expressed during physical examination.

Abscess of the footpads, particularly the large metatarsal footpad, is very common in parrots and budgerigars. This condition, similar to bumblefoot in chickens, is of unknown origin. On culture, staphylococcal organisms have been isolated, but by no means in the majority of cases. It is probable that these abscesses start with injury to the pads or are the result of unsanitary cage conditions. Treatment consists of curettage of the affected pad, followed by daily application of an antibiotic ointment or tincture of iodine. A chronic inflammation often persists, with resultant arthritic changes in the joint.

GRANULOMAS

Lipogranulomas are among the most commonly found tumors of budgerigars. Obesity is a constant hazard in cage birds, with the fat being distributed primarily over the pectoral and abdominal areas. Fatty degeneration occurs in the center of these fatty masses, and a small nodular granuloma develops. These granulomas enlarge very rapidly and are best removed surgically early in the course of their development, since the hazard of shock increases with the increasing age and size of the mass. Most of these birds are obese, and this too creates a problem relating to anesthesia. It is often advisable in the early stages of development of the tumor to place the bird on a diet in order to reduce both its weight and the risks of anesthesia. Many of these granulomas have a hollow, fluid-filled core caused by breakdown of necrotic fat. During excision care must be taken to remove the granuloma in its entirety and not to incise the mass. Most of these granulomas peel out with little difficulty, and careful blunt dissection of the surrounding connective tissue will decrease the amount of hemorrhage.

Granulomas can occur anywhere on the body, but rarely are seen on the extremities.

BURNS AND SCALDS

Burns and scalds are frequently seen in pets that are not caged, being found mostly in budgerigars. They frequently result from the birds flying over or falling on gas ranges or into pots of boiling water or hot soup.[6]

If the bird is in contact with a hot liquid for more than a few seconds there is little chance of saving its life. Burns of the feet, legs, and wing tips are the most common, because these non-feathered parts are more vulnerable to exposure. The limbs are the most likely parts to come in contact with flame or hot water. Birds that have been scalded or burned are usually in pain and stay on the bottom of the cage or in one spot on the perch and are reluctant to move. They are puffed up and have no appetite. Treatment consists of local application of Furacin* or a broad-spectrum antibiotic ointment for 4 to 6 days, followed by topical application of Aquasol A† until the lesions have healed. If the burns are extensive, 0.1 to 0.2 ml. of physiological saline solution injected intramuscularly daily and antibiotics administered parenterally are necessary. A guarded prognosis should always be given.

LACERATIONS

Both pet birds and wild birds are frequently seen with lacerations resulting from their falling prey to dogs or cats. Rarely will a bird impale itself or in any other way injure itself other than by being the unfortunate victim of a closed door or drawer.

Wounds caused by predators are either large superficial lacerations, which a cat's claw would cause, or small deep puncture wounds from the teeth of a dog or cat. Unless these wounds are complicated by internal injuries or have penetrated vital organs, recovery is usually uneventful and the prognosis excellent.

In deep wounds in which muscles are torn, the muscles are sutured with 0000 medium chromic catgut with a swaged-on needle. The skin is then sutured with the same material. Simple interrupted sutures are preferred, but if time is important a simple continuous stitch will suffice.

With lacerations in the area of the proximal end of the humerus, the wing should be immobilized by splinting close to the body to prevent further tearing of the friable skin after the wound is sutured.

Lacerations of the crop are a great problem; fistulas are a common sequel (Fig. 14-9), and very careful suturing is necessary. All seed should be removed from

---

Furacin—see footnote p. 250.

†Aquasol A—cream of vitamin A with panthenol (U.S. Vitamin & Pharmaceutical Corp., New York, N.Y.).

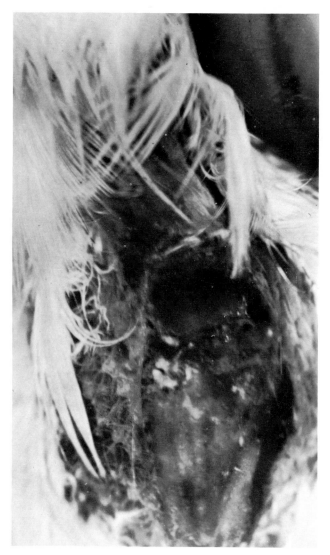

Fig. 14-9. *Fistula of the crop in a budgerigar.*

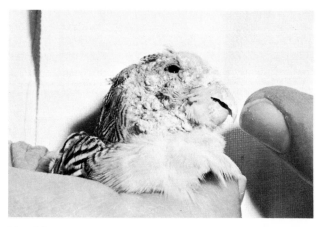

Fig. 14-10. *Extensive cnemidocoptic lesions of head of a budgerigar. (Courtesy of R. T. French Co.)*

the crop. If the laceration is of recent origin, separation of the very thin crop lining from the surrounding tissue is not too difficult. However, if more than 6 to 8 hours has elapsed, there is more difficulty in dissecting the lining mucous membrane. If possible, the crop should first be sutured with an inverting suture of 0000 stainless steel. Catgut of this strength absorbs too rapidly. The skin should then be sutured with stainless steel, using a simple interrupted stitch.

Fistulas will appear in 6 to 21 days. A guarded prognosis should always be given for the first two weeks after a laceration is sutured. A soft, seedless diet, such as one consisting of chopped hard-boiled eggs and fruit, should be offered for the first 24 to 48 hours.

DERMATITIS

Dermatitis is an uncommon occurrence in avian species. Most skin inflammations are secondary to trauma or parasitic infestations, such as scaly face (*Cnemidocoptes* spp.) (Fig. 14-10), and irritations caused by constant scratching because of presence of the red mite (*Dermanyssus*). The red mite is now infrequently seen in cage birds, and is more of a problem in a flock or aviary.

Occasionally, dry crusting of the skin under the wings and over the back occurs, leaving large raw lesions. Treatment with topical application of antibiotics or of steroid creams such as Panolog,* and oral administration of steroids such as Azium† solution, ½ to 2 drops twice daily, is often successful. The danger of self-inflicted trauma as a result of pruritus must be eliminated by constant observation or by use of an Elizabethan collar (discussed earlier in the section on Feather Picking; also discussed and illustrated in Chapter 9).

Attempts have been made to culture fungi and bacteria from many of these cases of dermatitis, but no specific pathogen has been incriminated.

The treatment of scaly face, the most common dermatitis, is discussed in Chapter 25.

Favus, a fungal disease caused by *Trichophyton megnini,* and fowl pox, a viral infection, both of which cause skin lesions, are discussed elsewhere.

ULCERS

Ulcers are commonly found as eroded skin lesions over tumors. The skin is stretched, and becomes thick-

---

*Panolog—a combination of triamcinolone acetonide, thiostrepton, neomycin sulfate, and nystatin (E. R. Squibb & Sons, New York, N.Y.).

†Azium—dexamethasone (Schering Corporation, Bloomfield, N.J.).

ened and friable. Trauma from picking by the bird or constant irritation from contact with the perch or bottom of the cage causes ulceration. Ulcerated areas frequently bleed profusely. In all cases, surgical removal of the primary lesion eliminates the cause. If surgery is not feasible because of location of the lesion, or the age or poor condition of the bird, topical application of Panolog,* Forte-Topical,† Furacin‡ ointment, or similar medications is useful in controlling, but rarely will it eliminate, the ulceration. Cauterization with 1% silver nitrate or by electrocautery will frequently by the only means of hemostasis.

Corneal ulcers rarely occur because the small area of cornea exposed in birds is well protected.

Occasionally, seed hulls or awns will become foreign bodies in the eye, and if they are caught under the nictitating membrane abrasion of the cornea can result. Topical application of ophthalmic ointment containing antibiotics and, after the first three days, steroids will usually lead to rapid, uneventful recovery.

CONTUSIONS AND HEMATOMAS

Contusions and hematomas occur frequently in cage birds allowed at times to fly freely or in birds whose cages are dropped. If they are uncomplicated by other structural or visceral injuries, the condition does not require any treatment and recovery is routine.

Hemorrhage is found most frequently around the sternum and over the parietal area of the head. A hematoma results occasionally from intramuscular injection into the pectoral muscles and practically always from venipuncture in the jugular or branches of the radial vein.

GANGRENE AND NECROSIS

Gangrene and necrosis occur primarily as the result of trauma. As one of the more common sequels to tight leg bands, necrosis occurs distal to the band. Pathological fractures under the tight band also result. Trauma to the banded leg results in swelling of the leg. In canaries, dry scaly legs will result in pressure under the band, with consequent necrosis. Fractures also can result in necrosis if there is vascular involvement.

The first sign of difficulty is lameness of the involved leg. The bird is reluctant to bear weight on it, and leans to the side. Swelling follows. The band becomes em-

bedded in the inflamed tissues. The grasping powers of the toes are reduced and the toes remain closed. The tissues become discolored; necrosis appears above the claws, and progresses up the leg. The dried-out toes then either fall off or are picked off (auto-amputation).

Removing leg bands can be very difficult, and great care must be taken not to produce fracture of the leg in which rarefaction of the bone may be occurring, and to injure as little tissue as possible. On the medial surface of the leg there is usually a fully engorged vessel, which should be avoided.

Use of curved dental crown scissors (Fig. 14-11) is of great value in removing these bands. One jaw of the scissors is worked under the band as gently as possible, and the band is severed with one cut if possible. Attempt should never be made at this point to spread the band to remove it. Although most of the bands are made of aluminum, much damage can be done to the leg by attempts to pry the band open.

The first cut generally results in loosening of the band; another cut is then made on the opposite side, and the band falls off easily. If there is any hemorrhage, compression of the leg for 1 to 5 minutes is usually sufficient to control it.

A guarded prognosis should always be given in cases of tight bands, and the owner of the bird should be made aware of the possibility of a pathological fracture, hemorrhage, or even of necrosis following removal of the band. If there is a fracture, the leg must be set.

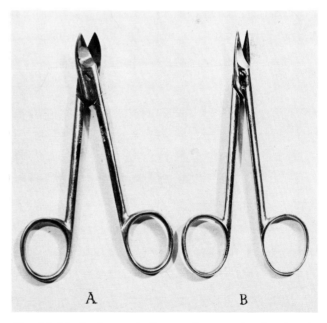

Fig. 14-11. *Instruments for use in removing leg bands. A, Wide-jaw dental crown scissors. Manufactured by Haslam, Pakistan; obtainable from surgical supply houses. B, Narrow-jaw dental crown scissors. Manufactured in Italy; obtainable from surgical supply houses.*

Panolog—see footnote p. 252.

†Forte-Topical—hydrocortisone, neomycin, penicillin, polymixin B (The Upjohn Co., Kalamazoo, Mich.).

‡Furacin—see footnote* p. 250.

An idiopathic condition prevalent in budgerigars results in dry gangrene of one or both legs. If advanced and extensive, the condition can spread to the skin directly over the sternum. Dry necrosis starts at the last phalanx of the digits and the claws fall off. Necrosis gradually progresses up the foot and usually terminates at the tibiotarso–tarsometatarsal joint. There is no pain associated with this condition, and it is sometimes self-limiting; only the toes are lost and the bird can live a functional life on the stumps. The majority of these cases, however, terminate fatally.

In 1959, Doctor John King at Cornell did some un-published work on feeding ergot in an attempt to pro-duce similar clinical responses, but was unsuccessful. Treatment of the condition is strictly empirical, and amputation proximal to the line of demarcation of necro-sis may be of value. Topical application of antibiotic and/or steroid preparations has been of little value.

References

1. ARNALL, L.: Anaesthesia and surgery in cage and aviary birds. III. A systematic outline of surgical conditions. Vet. Rec. *73:*188–192, 1961.

2. ARNALL, L.: Conditions of the beak and claw in the budg-erigar. J. small anim. Pract. *6:*135–144, 1965.

3. BEACH, J. E.: Diseases of budgerigars and other cage birds. A survey of *post-mortem* findings. Vet. Rec. *74:*134–140, 1962.

4. CREW, F. A. E., and MIRSKAIA, L.: Vet. Rec. *11:*541, 1931.

5. DURANT, A. J., and MCDOUGLE, H. C.: Diseases of the Digestive System. In *Diseases of Poultry,* 3rd ed., H. E. Biester and L. H. Schwarte, eds. Ames, Iowa State College Press, 1952. Pp. 1029–1041.

6. HASHOLT, J.: *Reprint from the Member Publication of the Danish Veterinary Association,* No. 12, June 15, 1960, pp. 6–8.

7. KLUVER, C. F.: Feather faults. All-Pets Mag. *30*(11):12, November, 1959.

8. LAFEBER, T. J.: Digestive System Disturbances of the Budg-erigar. In *Current Veterinary Therapy,* 1966–1967, R. W. Kirk, ed. Philadelphia, W. B. Saunders Co., 1966. Pp. 535–538.

9. STURKIE, P. D.: *Avian Physiology,* 2nd ed. Ithaca, N.Y., Comstock Publishing Associates, 1965. Pp. 624–625, 629.

Suggested Reading

ALTMAN, I. E.: Skin and Feather Problems. In *Current Veter-inary Therapy,* 1964–1965, R. W. Kirk, ed. Philadel-phia, W. B. Saunders Co., 1964. Pp. 424–426.

BACHRACH, A.: Skin and Feather Problems of Caged Birds. In *Current Veterinary Therapy,* 1966–1967, R. W. Kirk, ed. Philadelphia, W. B. Saunders Co., 1966. Pp. 549–553.

COFFIN, D. L.: *The Care, Feeding and Diseases of Psittacine Pets.* Angell Memorial Parakeet and Parrot Book, 1953, pp. 15–32, Boston, Mass.

EVANS, H. E.: *Guide to the Study and Dissection of the Chicken.* Ithaca, N.Y., Cornell University Press, 1952. P. 16.

Handbook on the Treatment of Exotic Pets. London, The British Veterinary Association, Part I, pp. 2–23, 27, 35–39, 71, 74.

STONE, R. M.: Pet bird practice. J.A.V.M.A. *137:*364–372, 1960.

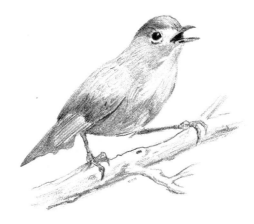

15

Disorders of the Skeletal System

Irving E. Altman

Disorders of the skeletal system of cage birds include primarily those conditions that are due to trauma, nutritional deficiences or imbalances, and infection. Congenital deformities are seldom encountered. Fractures of the wings and legs, a frequent consequence of caging, are a common problem to the veterinarian. Simple methods of external fixation of fractures are, therefore, dealt with extensively. The remaining conditions are discussed to the extent permitted by personal experience and access to the literature.

RICKETS

Rickets is seen in young birds just out of the nest. By the time the lesions are discovered, the pathologic process is usually irreversible. The pathogenesis is not wholly understood, but frequently some fledglings will be affected while others in the same brood remain normal. Nutrition of the young bird plays an important role in this condition. One theory is that the parent birds do not care for the nestlings properly, and that the stronger and larger birds take some of the food that should have gone to the weakened nest mates.

The birds show difficulty in standing and locomotion, swelling at the joints of the long bones, lack of appetite, softening of the beak, and, terminally, prostration and death.

Treatment consists of provision of supplementary calcium, phosphorus, and vitamin D_3. Vionate,* added

*Vionate—contains vitamins A, D_3, C, E, B-complex, and folic acid; also choline chloride, calcium, phosphorus, salt, iodine, iron, cobalt, copper, magnesium, and manganese (E. R. Squibb & Sons, New York, N.Y.).

to the seed or nestling food in the proportion of 1 ounce of powder mixed with 1 pound of seed or nestling food, can prove beneficial in the early stages.

OSTEOGENESIS IMPERFECTA

Arnall[2] reported on a suspected case of osteogenesis imperfecta in a newly imported young parrot. The case was typified by bending or folding fractures of one limb, together with thinness of the cortex of the long bones. Nutritional secondary hyperparathyroidism or nutritional osteoporosis is discussed in Chapter 22.

CONGENITAL DEFORMITIES

Congenital deformities of the skeletal system are not often seen by the practitioner because of the early death of the affected birds. The long bones of the legs are most commonly affected, and curling and twisting of the feet are the resultant anomalies. Frequently the parents will reject such deformed nestlings and they do not survive. For any that do, euthanasia is the best recourse.

Arnall[1] reported that congenital deformities of the shoulder, elbow, and carpus occasionally occur in the budgerigar. He further reported that congenital luxations involving the legs are more common, and dysplasia of the hip, splay legs, patellar luxation, and rotation luxation of the tibiotarsal joint due to slipped Achilles tendon are all seen occasionally. The more serious deformities affect the hip and cause a degree of permanent abduction of the limb, sometimes as much as 90 degrees. The knee is seldom deformed, but poorly developed trochleae and patellae have been observed. Single, displaced, twisted claws on one or both feet, and clubbed feet may be congenital.

Beach[3] recorded the occurrence of congenital deformities in 2 budgerigars out of 866 on which he performed necropsy. In one bird, both hips were affected, and in the other a tarsus.

Petrak[8] reported a congenital deformity of the knee joint in a cockatiel (*Nymphicus hollandicus*), resulting in a 90-degree lateral angulation of the leg from the knee down. The toes of the affected leg clutched normally. The bird was rejected by the parents at 2 days of age and was hand-raised after that.

LUXATIONS

Luxations are traumatic in origin and are infrequently seen. Because of the pneumatized structure of the bones and the well-developed ligaments and joints, fractures,

rather than dislocations, are produced by severe trauma. Occasionally luxations associated with fractures make it extremely difficult to accomplish reduction because of the size of the patient and the difficulty in manipulation. Manual reduction should be attempted and some means of coaptation splintage should be established in order to obtain stability of the injured part.

Hasholt[5] reported 77 cases of distortions and dislocations among 1592 cage birds brought to him for treatment. Of the 77 cases, 55% occurred in various toe joints, 20% occurred in the knee joint, 10% in the upper mandible, and 15% were equally distributed between the elbow and tibiotarsus.

The great majority resulted from catching of overgrown and deformed claws on various objects. Dislocation of the beak was due primarily to catching the beak in the slit of bells. Ankylosis usually occurred after healing. Hasholt considered that a dislocated toe was best treated by amputation.

ARTHRITIS

The causes of arthritic conditions include trauma, infectious diseases, and metabolic disturbances. In budgerigars and canaries, urate deposits at the joints of the long bones cause a very painful, acute inflammation of the joints. These urate deposits are the result of a metabolic disturbance, gout, for which there is no treatment or cure. Excision of the urate nodules with curettage will temporarily relieve the pain.

Arnall[1] reported that an acute arthritis similar to that found in young pheasants occasionally occurs in cage birds. Presence of a seropurulent material in the tarsal joints is accompanied by anorexia, rapid weight loss, and, commonly, death. Micrococci, staphylococci, streptococci, and the fungus *Aspergillus* have been isolated. He further reported that a chronic condition associated with swelling and frictional ulceration on the tibiotarsal joint may lead to ankylosis-in-flexion of the joint. This syndrome may follow a history of paresis, inability or disinclination to perch, or corns on the tibiotarsus. Recognizable pathogens are seldom cultured from these cases, but staphylococci, pasteurellae, a *Corynebacterium, Escherichia coli,* and some streptococci have been isolated.

Janovski[6] reported a crippling inflammation of the joints of the lower extremities associated with arthropathy and *Escherichia coli* septicemia in cage birds. The arthropathy was characterized by progressive polyarticular arthritis of serofibrinous or seropurulent type, with a granulomatous type of inflammatory response being observed occasionally. This led to gangrene of the phalanges, metatarsophalangeal joints, or the entire foot. The disease has been observed in canaries, parakeets, and finches. Gram-negative coliform organisms were found in affected limb tissues and *E. coli* in the viscera. The disorder was attributed to direct infection of the lower extremities by way of fecal contamination or to delayed hypersensitivity to *E. coli.*

Bumblefoot frequently is the cause of arthritic changes in the tarsometatarso-phalangeal joint. In pigeons, arthritis of the wings preventing flight can be caused by infectious diseases such as tuberculosis or paratyphoid.[7] Arthritic changes in the joints produce swelling, inflammation, and pain. The affected appendage is usually guarded. If the wing is involved, the affected wing droops, the bird is reluctant to run and unable to fly. If the leg is involved, the affected limb is held in flexed position, bearing no weight. Most arthritic changes are unilateral.

The parenteral administration of corticosteroids is helpful in relieving the inflammation. Intra-articular administration of Azium* or Predef 2×† with a ⅜-inch, 25-gauge tuberculin needle, at the dosage of 0.05 to 0.1 ml., should follow aspiration of synovial fluid. Much bleeding usually follows these injections, and compression after injection is necessary. Oral administration of Azium at a dose of ½ to 2 drops can follow intra-articular injection. It is advisable to administer antibiotics in conjunction with the steroids. Intra-articular injections should be repeated as necessary.

FRACTURES

Skull Fractures

The cranium of smaller birds is relatively thin and subject to fracture. Many birds are permitted to fly freely and they frequently collide with mirrors and windows, owing to a lack of depth perception. Fractures and concussions often result. Symptoms vary with the degree of cranial hemorrhage and pressure on the brain, ranging from unilateral paresis to convulsions or coma. Treatment is symptomatic. Birds should be kept in an environmental temperature of 85 to 90°F at complete rest. If convulsions occur, anesthesia may be induced with Equi-Thesin,‡ administered intramuscularly at a dose of 2.5 ml. per kg. of body weight.

---

*Azium–Dexamethasone (Schering Corporation, Bloomfield, N.J.).

†Predef 2× — 9-fluoroprednisolone acetate (2 mg./ml.) (The Upjohn Company, Kalamazoo, Mich.).

‡Equi-Thesin (Jensen-Salsbery Laboratories, Kansas City, Mo.) —each 500 ml. contains:

Chloral Hydrate	328 gr.
Pentobarbital	75 gr.
Magnesium Sulfate	164 gr.

in an aqueous solution of propylene glycol, 35%; with 9.5% alcohol.

Fractures of the Mandible

Fractures of the mandible are difficult to repair in the smaller species. Pinning with fine needle wires is sometimes possible. Cracks or fissures may be wired with 00000 monofilament stainless steel suture. Longitudinal fractures of the upper beak can be similarly wired. Avulsion of the upper or lower beak is impossible to repair.

Fractures of the Long Bones

The highest incidence of fractures in canaries is in the tarsometatarsus, whereas in the budgerigar it is in the tibiotarsus (Fig. 15-1). Fractures of the femur are encountered with less frequency in all species because of its being incorporated within the contour of the body. Birds that are molting are more susceptible to fracture, since during the molt cycle the Haversian systems of the long bones undergo enlargement by erosion and resorption of bone substance. This osteoporosis increases the fragility of the bones and makes them more susceptible to trauma.[4] The prognosis in most fractures depends on the age of the patient and the accompanying damage to the vascular and nervous supply of the part. If vascular interference is extensive, necrosis can be expected. The main vessel to the leg is the ischiatic artery.

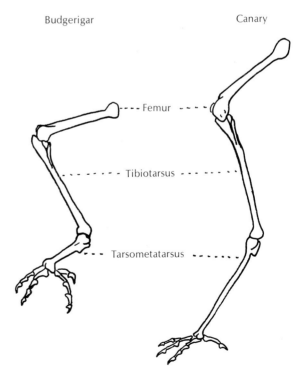

Fig. 15-1. *Bones of pelvic limb, showing differences in structure of tibiotarsus and tarsometatarsus of the budgerigar and the canary.*

TARSOMETATARSAL FRACTURES

My records of past cases indicate that 71 per cent of the fractures in birds have involved the tarsometatarsus. Of these, 70% involved the right leg and 30% the left. The tarsometatarsus, which is one of the longest and most prominent bones in the pelvic limb of birds, generally receives the brunt of trauma in accidents. There are many causes for these accidents:

(1) cage and stand being tipped over;
(2) cage falling from brackets;
(3) the bird's leg being caught between the bottom of the cage and the drawer pan, when the pan is carelessly replaced during cage cleaning;
(4) excessive pressure exerted by the fingers of the one holding the bird while the nails are being clipped;
(5) long toenails becoming hooked on the wire of the cage and the bird incurring injury while attempting to free itself;
(6) bird landing on a spring mouse-trap that is in the room for purposes other than catching birds;
(7) in combat, a large bird with a strong bill striking the tarsometatarsus of a smaller bird, a circumstance usually occurring in aviaries of wild birds.

Tarsometatarsal fractures may be divided into three categories:

(1) fractures of the upper third;
(2) fractures of the middle third;
(3) fractures of the lower third.

MIDDLE-THIRD FRACTURES. All fractures which can be splinted without involving the joints are considered middle-third fractures. This type of fracture of the tarsometatarsus can be set in a simple flap splint. A firm, easily adjusted splint is formed by rolling adhesive tape around the tarsometatarsal bone and leaving $\frac{1}{4}$-inch flaps as wings.

The bird is held by an assistant in such a position that the fractured leg is toward the operator. It is of prime importance, in holding a bird, to keep the wings closed and against the body at all times, to prevent embarrassing escapes. Should the bird escape, be certain all windows and doors are closed before an attempt is made to catch it. When the bird is within reach, one quick swoop of the arm is made from the shoulder, placing the hand over and around the bird to prevent it from spreading its wings.

Another method of holding the bird is to extend the wings up over the back and gently press them together with the thumb and forefinger. In the hands of amateurs this method may cause fracture of the wings unless extreme care is taken. Holding the bird by the wings

does not give complete control of the body as does keeping them against the body, but in certain cases the method is valuable. When the assistant holds the bird in his left hand, his right hand is free to grasp the middle toe and extend the leg upward in any position the surgeon directs. The fractured ends of bone are easily approximated by this means, and the surgeon is able to apply the cast.

A strip of adhesive tape, 3 or more inches long and about $\frac{3}{8}$ of an inch wide, is used. The width depends on the size of bird being treated. This strip of adhesive is laid against the posterior side of the leg to be set, and the leg is fixed in place by gentle pressure. There should be a $\frac{1}{8}$- to $\frac{1}{4}$-inch strip of adhesive extending beyond each side of the tarsometatarsal bone. The adhesive is then rolled or laid over the anterior face of the tarsometatarsal bone and the two adhesive surfaces are brought tightly together. Be sure that the fractured ends of the bone are in proper approximation. Continue rolling the adhesive until three layers have been applied around the leg. With a strong-jawed artery clamp, the $\frac{1}{4}$-inch flaps are clamped tightly together, forming a stiff non-flexible wing of the splint (Fig. 15-2). With good blood supply, fixation and callus formation are sufficiently advanced in two weeks to permit removal of the splint. Occasionally, three weeks may be required for complete healing.

This splint can be applied in two positions. The wings of the splint may be spread antero-posteriorly or laterally. The former position is the most readily accomplished, the tape being easily applied when the assistant holds the bird with its side toward the surgeon. The lateral application of the splint is a little more difficult because the tarsometatarsal bone is deeper antero-posteriorly than from side to side. For application in this position the assistant must hold the bird with its head or tail toward the surgeon, and the tape is applied as described above. It can easily be seen that when the

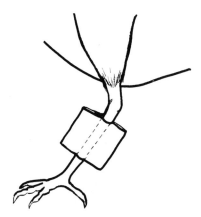

Fig. 15-2. *Tape splint for fixation of middle-third tarsometatarsal fractures.*

leg is flexed the wings of the splint lie flat against the body. I believe the bird is more comfortable in a splint applied in this manner.

UPPER-THIRD FRACTURES. In upper-third fractures, where the joint must be included in the splint, it is desirable to set the leg at as nearly normal an angle as possible. Normally, the angulation at the tibiotarso-tarsometatarsal joint is 45 to 75 degrees, depending on the type and stance of the bird. The assistant holds the bird in the manner described previously, but with its abdomen and legs toward the surgeon. The fractured leg is moved forward. A strip of adhesive, about 3 to 4 inches long and 1 inch wide, is used. The feathers covering the tibiotarsus should be removed. The posterior surface of the leg is now placed on the adhesive surface of the tape and the leg is adjusted to the normal angle with the fractured ends approximated. The adhesive is then laid over on itself, enclosing the leg, and the adhesive surfaces are fixed to each other. The distance from the posterior point of the flexed joint to the end of the splint will be ¾ to 1 inch. In this case three folds of tape are again required for proper strength. With a strong-jawed forceps, the splint folds are clamped together, conforming to the shape of the leg.

One of the pitfalls in treatment of this type of fracture is the tendency of the leg toward abduction, especially if the leg is too greatly extended in setting. When the bird rests on the bottom of the cage, the leg will be placed out sideways. This causes a great deal of pressure for long periods of time, with abduction resulting. Therefore, the setting of this fracture should be in as nearly normal a position as possible, with emphasis on flexion rather than extension.

The tibiotarso-tarsometatarsal joint must be fixed in complete extension when the fracture is close to the head of the tarsometatarsus. This gives rise to a straight, stiff leg. It is naturally impossible for the bird to place this leg under the body when resting on the bottom of the cage. Therefore, one must guard against bending of the fracture from abduction. The bird must be induced to stand on its perch with its good leg, while the extended fractured leg hangs down in back of the perch. Since it is easier for a bird to clutch its perch than to let go, this is not too difficult to do. Keep food and water in their usual cups. This will force the bird to its perch to obtain nourishment. As a matter of fact, this practice is suggested for all birds with fractures.

LOWER-THIRD FRACTURES. In fractures of the lower third of the tarsometatarsal bone the tarsometatarso-phalangeal joint must be included in the splint (Fig. 15-3). The assistant holds the bird on its back with the fractured extremity toward the surgeon. A strip of adhesive,

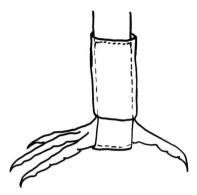

Fig. 15-3. *Tape splint for fixation of lower-third tarso-metatarsal fractures.*

1 to 1½ inches long and ¼ inch wide, is obtained and the width of the center portion is reduced to ⅛ inch for a length of ⅜ of an inch. This narrowed part is then placed underneath the foot (below the tarsometatarso-phalangeal joint) and the ends are brought up laterally along the side of the foot. The fractured ends must be in apposition before the adhesive is pressed firmly against the foot. These lateral strips are held firmly in place by rolling a ½-inch strip of adhesive around the lower half of the tarsometatarsal bone, as close to the joint as possible. In this case the splint is made without wings.

Within one week, if bone healing progresses nicely, the loop beneath the foot can be cut away; the splint is allowed to remain another week before it is removed.

FRACTURES OF THE TOES

Fractured foretoes are easily treated by the use of collodion. The toe next to the fractured one is used as a splint. The two toes are held together with the collodion, and healing occurs in about 10 days.

A fractured rear toe is somewhat more difficult to set. If there is no displacement of the fractured ends, some collodion or collodion and cotton is placed around the toe. Care should be taken not to make the splint too heavy. With displacement, and some difficulty in keeping the fractured ends together, a flap-winged splint of Scotch tape may be used. The wings of the splint are horizontal and will not interfere with clutching of the perch.

FRACTURES OF THE TIBIOTARSUS

With tibiotarsal fractures the method of splinting is similar to that described for upper-third tarsometatarsal fractures. The tibiotarso-tarsometatarsal joint is flexed so that the tarsometatarsal bone is held at a 90-degree angle. In this case, the bird rests on the tarsometatarsus or lower portion of the splint. The assistant holds the bird with the fractured leg directed cranially, its abdomen and legs toward the surgeon. The leg is placed on the adhesive, which encases the tibiotarsal and tarsometatarsal bones and extends about ⅛ inch below the tarsometatarsus. The long end of the adhesive that extends posteriorly is folded over the leg with a ¼-inch flap at the anterior edge. Because of the thickness of the musculature at the anterior edge, the flap will probably be ½ inch from the flexed tibiotarso-tarsometatarsal joint at the posterior edge. This adds strength and rigidity to the splint. The adhesive is laid over the leg with a niche cut into it about one-half to three-fourths of the length of the tarsometatarsal bone so that it may again be folded until three layers are applied. With a heavy-jawed artery forceps, the adhesive is clamped together to conform to the shape of the leg (Fig. 15-4). The adhesive posterior to the tarsometatarsal bone must be well clamped together to fix it at a 90-degree angle. Very often, after one week, this portion of the splint may be opened and cut away and the bird permitted to use the joint at will. After two weeks, the entire splint is removed.

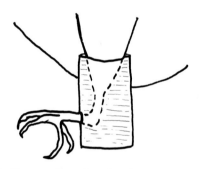

Fig. 15-4. *Tape splint for fixation of tibiotarsal and upper-third tarsometatarsal fractures. Note the 90-degree angulation of the joint.*

FRACTURES OF THE FEMUR

Fractures of the femur may present many and varied problems. The method of treatment that generally gives the best results is very simple. It produces complete flexion of the whole leg and thereby sets the femur in as nearly normal a position as possible. The femur in canaries is found under the skin of the body, so that no portion extends beyond the contour of the body itself.

The assistant holds the bird on its back with the fractured leg toward the surgeon. The leg is completely flexed and the feathers on either side of the leg are caught up and twisted and held together. This may be done by the assistant, or an artery clamp may be used to hold the feathers together as close to the flexed leg

as possible. These feathers are then tied tightly with thread. This forms a sling, keeping the leg firmly flexed. One must be careful at what position the feathers are tied together. If they are gathered too far forward or too far backward, the leg will slip out of its sling. Each bird is different, and the proper position is determined by the degree of firmness felt by the fingers when the leg is moved, before the feathers are tied. The leg is left in the sling for two or three weeks, and usually heals nicely.

PELVIC LIMB FRACTURES IN LARGER BIRDS

The fixation of tibiotarsal and tarsometatarsal fractures in birds weighing more than 100 grams is complicated by the need for stronger splinting material. Materials such as match sticks, tongue depressors, quills, aluminum sheeting, and fine-gauge wire have all been incorporated in softer dressings with varying degrees of success. Hasholt[5] recommends four to six layers of Porofix, which is a light, stiff, porous material. Parrots may dislodge any splint unless a device such as an Elizabethan collar is used. It may be helpful to place the bird in the dark for at least several hours immediately after application of the splint.

WING FRACTURES

Wing fractures in small birds, such as canaries, budgerigars, and finches, are fairly common. They are due to improper handling, catching of the wings in wires of the cage, and other accidents. The wing bones are very thin and some contain air spaces. A complete wing (see Fig. 5-13, p. 65) is made up of the scapula, coracoid, and clavicle in the shoulder region; the humerus in the arm; the radius and ulna in the forearm; two carpal bones (the radial carpal and the ulnar carpal); three metacarpal bones, and three digits.

In fractures of the humerus, the radius and ulna are usually involved also, and occasionally the metacarpus and digits (Phalanges) (Fig. 15-5).

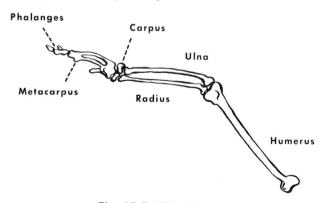

Fig. 15-5. *Wing bones.*

After examining a bird, and noticing how the wings are flexed and set against the body, it is easy to see how difficult it would be to place a splint on either the humerus or the radius and ulna. Therefore, I devised a plan to use the body as a splint (Fig. 15-6) and have had good results.

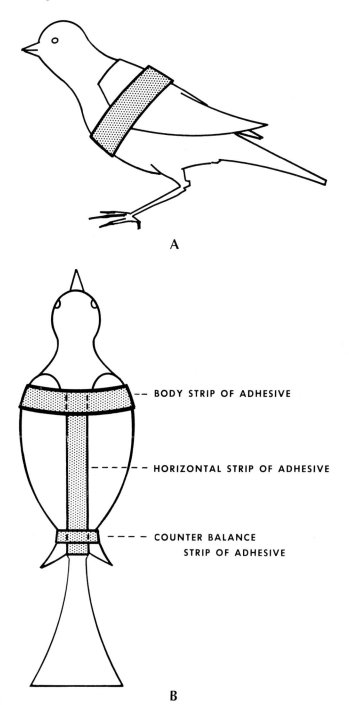

A

BODY STRIP OF ADHESIVE

HORIZONTAL STRIP OF ADHESIVE

COUNTER BALANCE
STRIP OF ADHESIVE

B

Fig. 15-6. *Use of the body as a splint for fixation of wing fracture. A. Placement of the first strip of adhesive tape around the body. B. View of the dorsal body surface of the bird, with all tapes in place.*

A fractured wing always droops, the degree depending on the severity of the fracture. In setting the injured part the wing is lifted to its normal position. Occasionally, this automatically reduces the fracture. Fractures with severe displacement are reduced by gentle manual manipulation. When the wing is set and in normal position, the tip of the fractured wing is placed on the tip of the normal wing.

The surgeon now hands the bird to the assistant, who grasps the caudal part of the bird between his fingers so that the wings are held as set, the legs are extended caudally, and the tail is included in his grasp. In fracture of the left wing the bird is held with the right hand; in fracture of the right wing it is held with the left, in each case so that the fractured wing is toward the surgeon. A 6-inch length of adhesive, $\frac{1}{2}$ inch wide, is placed around the body cranial to the legs, holding the wings to prevent extension (Fig. 15-6 A). This strip of adhesive is started on the ventral edge of the wing facing the surgeon, carried over the back and around to meet itself, the end being left to hang temporarily. Another length of $\frac{1}{2}$-inch-wide adhesive is placed longitudinally on the back of the bird. Starting at the anterior edge of the adhesive that goes around the body, it is carried back over the crossed wing tips and folded under for a distance of $\frac{1}{2}$ inch. The adhesive going around the body is then carried over the longitudinal strip to tie it down, going twice around the body.

The wing is now set, but if it were left this way the bird would be top-heavy and unable to stand. Therefore, a piece of $\frac{1}{2}$-inch-wide adhesive is placed around the wing tips (Fig. 15-6 B), tying them together and, of more importance, acting as a counterbalance for the bird. The splint remains on for two weeks. It is removed by cutting the anterior strip under the breast and the counterbalance strip on each side of the wing tips. The adhesive is gently pulled off, while pressure is being exerted against the base of the feathers. Ether may be used to loosen the adhesive.

Results will usually be good. In healed fractures of the humerus, the wing will often droop slightly but after exercise will correct itself and the bird will be able to fly.

PINNING OF FRACTURES

Pinning of fractures of long bones has great value in larger birds. In birds the size of canaries, budgerigars, and finches, it has less value. Using a 25-gauge hypodermic needle as a pin usually causes complete splintering of the bone. The technique used for pinning bones is presented in Chapter 11. Results of pinning compound fractures may be adversely affected by interruption of circulation to the fracture site.

References

1. ARNALL, L.: Anaesthesia and surgery in cage and aviary birds. II. A regional outline of surgical conditions. Vet. Rec. *73:*173-178, 1961.

2. ARNALL, L.: Further experiences with cagebirds. Vet. Rec. *73:*1146-1154, 1961.

3. BEACH, J. E.: Diseases of budgerigars and other cage birds. A survey of *post-mortem* findings. Vet. Rec. *74:*134-140, 1962.

4. BELLAIRS, A. D'A., and JENKIN, C. R.: The Skeleton of Birds. In *Biology and Comparative Physiology of Birds,* A. J. Marshall, ed. New York, Academic Press, 1960. Vol. I, pp. 241-300.

5. HASHOLT, J.: Current diseases of cage birds. J. small anim. Pract. *2:*97-108, 1961.

6. JANOVSKI, N. A.: Arthropathy associated with *Escherichia coli* septicemia in caged birds. J.A.V.M.A. *148:*1517-1522, 1966.

7. LEVI, W. M.: *The Pigeon.* Sumter, S.C., Levi Publishing Co., Inc., 1963 reprint. P. 385.

8. PETRAK, M. L.: Personal communication, 1966.

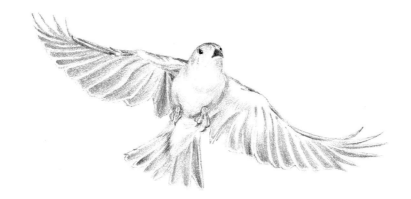

16

Diseases of the Respiratory System

Leslie Arnall

Evans, Farner, and Fiennes, in Chapters 5, 6, and 17, respectively, discuss the avian respiratory system, and its varied anatomy and physiology. In this Chapter, therefore, only brief reference will be made to its form and function.

Not only does the respiratory system in birds differ from that in mammals, but considerable variation in form and function exists between different species of birds, even between species that are outwardly quite similar. Additionally, beyond the quite apparent anatomical and associated physiological differences between species, appreciable differences in predisposition and resistance to certain pathological changes occur within species. Such different individual and strain susceptibilities to disease can be only partly accounted for by the interaction of a bird and its environment.

Some indication of relative susceptibilities can be given with regard only to the more common diseases and species (see Table 16-1). The range of species of birds is comparable to that of mammalian species, and the incidence of respiratory disease mirrors to a great extent the popularity and intensiveness of husbandry of the species, the scientific knowledge of the respective aviculturists, and the economics of investigating disease in the species concerned. Useful comparative knowledge is to be gained from the excellent work on avian disease and mortality carried out by researchers associated with wildlife trusts and other bodies concerned with nature conservation. This knowledge cannot, however, be applied *en bloc* to identical or closely related species kept in captivity.

Passeriformes and, in particular, gallinaceous and columbiform species reared for table purposes have of

Table 16-1. Comparative Incidence of Some Common Avian Disease Conditions Showing Respiratory Symptoms, and Relative Susceptibilities of the Species or Groups of Birds That Are More Commonly Affected

Disease Condition or Causative Agent*	Species, Group, or Type of Bird Affected†	Comments
IRRITANT AND TOXIC INHALANTS *e.g.,* Ammonia (wet, stale droppings) Coal tar (Kerosene) substances Paraffin Acaricides Disinfectant aerosols Sodium fluoride	Considerable species and individual variation (see next column), dependent to some extent on the numerous anatomical and physiological variations between species and other groups. The canary is traditionally used to detect noxious vapors in wells, mines, ship's holds, etc.	More rapid and serious effects in smaller, excitable, active, non-acclimatized, young and stressed birds
DISEASES OF INTEGUMENT Hyperkeratinization, or "hypertrophy," of cere	Essentially budgerigars + + + +	Rarely obstructs respiration
DISEASES OF CIRCULATORY SYSTEM CARDIOVASCULAR DEGENERATIONS Atheroma Thrombosis Ruptured aorta	Middle-aged and older birds, younger birds in zoological collections and as pets. Particularly large parrots + + + and other long-living species, especially psittacines + +; young turkeys + +	
DISORDER OF REPRODUCTIVE SYSTEM Egg peritonitis	Pet budgerigars + + +; aviary budgerigars +; many aviary bred species + or + +	Mainly in unbred, sporadically bred, or exploited birds, or birds with intercurrent (*e.g.,* *E. coli* or *Salmonella*) infection
DISEASES OF ENDOCRINE SYSTEM Thyroid dysplasia and "goiter"	Essentially budgerigars: pet—on low-iodine grain diet + + +; on iodine-fortified diet, rare; aviary budgerigars without special iodine +; other small and medium psittacines +; pigeons +	Tracheo-syringeal obstruction symptoms plus esophageal obstruction
INFECTIOUS DISEASES BACTERIAL Cocci: Diplococci and Streptococci	Passeriformes (canaries, finches—especially newly imported) + + +; Psittaciformes (budgerigars +; other members of Order + + +)	Septicemia-pneumonias; usually a powerful predisposing cause—excess heat, cold, exhaustion, starvation

Table 16-1. (Continued)

Disease Condition or Causative Agent*	Species, Group, or Type of Bird Affected†	Comments
INFECTIOUS DISEASES (Cont.)		
Staphylococci	Mynahs + + + (supraorbital or infraorbital granulomas or inspissated pus in sinuses); psittacines (parrots, budgerigars) + +; canaries + +; pigeons + +; in wounds, especially torn air sacs	Usually associated, in psittacines and some passerines, with arthritis or pyemic abscess in parenchymatous organs
Pasteurella septica and *P. pseudotuberculosis*	Ornamental and table members of Phasianidae + +; many finches + +; sparrows + +; canaries +; predatory birds + + and psittacines (+); *P. pseudotuberculosis* sporadic in finch-like granivorous and carrion species, from toucan to tit-mouse size	More in captive wild species Septicemic/Pyemic. Usually sporadic but epizootics in canaries and sparrows with both types causing septicemias
Salmonellae, especially *S. typhimurium*	Pigeons (especially squabs, squeakers) + + +; canaries, sparrows, and various finches + or + +; other passerines + +; water birds (*i.e.*, fish eaters) commonly infected, but low mortality and morbidity + + +	Sporadic and epizootic; enzootic, especially in pigeons and water birds. More omnivorous than solely granivorous birds involved
Escherichia coli	Budgerigars + +; other psittacines + or + +	Symptoms particularly if secondary to virus, egg peritonitis, or other predisposing factor
Erysipelothrix rhusiopathiae	Galliformes (turkey, pheasant, other table birds) + +; pigeons + +; greenfinch +; bullfinch +; zebra finch +; budgerigars (+); various waterbirds + +; predatory and carrion spp. +	Increasingly reported but epizootics rare except in domestic table birds
Listeria	Canaries +; reports rare	In one Canadian outbreak 5 out of 25 birds affected died
Mycobacterium tuberculosis	Wood pigeon + + +; canaries + +; sparrows + +; starlings + +; and carrion spp. + +; psittacines (especially parrots) +; water birds +; peacocks +	Ubiquitous. Less than 1% in aviary populations generally. Morbidity sometimes high but, except in parrots (human strain), mortality usually low
Mycoplasma (PPLO)	Galliformes (Phasianidae + + and Meleagrididae + + +); Columbiformes +; Psittaciformes (+); Passeriformes (+)	Usually associated with rhinitis or infraorbital sinusitis, but suspected of being contributory factor in other disease pictures

Table 16-1. (Continued)

Disease Condition or Causative Agent*	Species, Group, or Type of Bird Affected†	Comments
INFECTIOUS DISEASES (Cont.)		
VIRAL		
Pox	Canaries + + + +; sparrows + +; finches + + +; and other small passerines + + +; pigeons + + + +	Serous rhinitis and conjunctivitis *or* crusty facial exudates *or* fatal viremia
Newcastle disease	Galliformes + + + +; Anatidae + +; Columbidae + +; Corvidae (crows), Ploceidae (sparrows) +; rare in predatory birds, parakeets, including budgerigars +; canaries (+)	All species less or much less susceptible than the domestic fowl; most are isolated outbreaks only
Infectious laryngo-tracheitis (I.L.T.)	In addition to domestic fowl, only pheasants affected +	
Ornithosis—psittacosis	Wide range of species, including Anatidae +; Galliformes +; Columbiformes + + + +; Psittaciformes + + + +; Apodiformes (hummingbirds) +; Passeriformes (orioles, crows, magpies, titmice, starlings, sparrows, various finches, troupials, cardinals, canaries) + +	Strains from Psittaciformes more often reported because more often studied, and human pathogenicity often greater from parrot-like birds. Pigeons average 25% serologically positive; virus from 15–100% of these
PARASITIC DISEASES		
PROTOZOA		
Trichomonas spp.	Columbiformes + + + + + (canker); Falconiformes (hawks, falcons, owls) + + + (frounce); domestic fowl +; possibly others (*e.g.,* quail, sparrow, canary) (+); other flagellates affect waterfowl and domestic fowl, but effect on the respiratory system is very secondary	Especially pigeon squeakers and squabs; although essentially an alimentary infection, glottal, laryngeal, and tracheal involvement is common
HELMINTHS		
Gapeworms		
Syngamus trachea	Corvidae + + +; Sturnidae + + +; gamebirds + + +; other Galliformes + +	Especially in young orphaned birds and in those reared in captivity or bred or kept in zoological gardens
Cyathostoma bronchialis	Ornamental, wild, and table water birds + or + +	
Filarial Worms	Falcons (+)	Between serosal layers of air sacs
Flukes	Domestic and ornamental waterfowl +; coots (+)	

Table 16-1. (Continued)

Disease Condition or Causative Agent*	Species, Group, or Type of Bird Affected†	Comments
PARASITIC DISEASES (Cont.)		
ARTHROPODS		
Acarine Parasites		
Cnemidocoptes pilae	Budgerigars + + + + +; lovebirds; parakeets, and other small psittacines + or + +; pigeons (+) (rarely affecting respiration); occasional reports in small passerines	A small proportion only impair respiration directly, many lead to starvation inanition, some with terminal "chills," "asthma" syndromes, or secondary septicemic pneumonias
Cytodites nudus and *Sternostoma tracheacolum*	Canaries +; green and Gouldian finches (+); Madagascar lovebirds (+)	A few isolated reports only so far
MYCOSES		
FUNGI AND YEASTS		
Aspergillus	Penguins + + (in captivity + + + +); aquatic birds + + +; budgerigars + + +; other psittacines + + or + + +; scavenging species (*e.g.,* Corvidae) + +; canaries + +; mynahs + + +; domestic poultry +; other Phasianidae + +	Acute in most susceptible, chronic in Psittaciformes, especially, where survival for weeks or months is not uncommon. Probably all avian species can become affected, but rare in some groups. Higher morbidity where rotting food, bedding, or dusty food is present, and in airless, damp, and dark conditions of management
Candida (Monilia)	Phasianidae + +—especially gamebirds + + + +; Psittaciformes +; mynahs +; various finchlike passerines +; Corvidae (crows, rooks, magpies) + +; Sturnidae (starlings) + +	Especially found in aviary birds after prolonged antibiotic (tetracycline) therapy has greatly lowered the level of bacterial pathogens
NEOPLASMS		
Osteosarcoma of skull Carcinoma of beak Granulomas of orbit, nares, cere, *etc.*	Budgerigars + or + + (mainly malignant); mynahs + (mainly benign); pigeons and quail + (a few highly malignant)	Respiration usually affected only after gross facial distortion
Celomic: of gonads or kidney	Budgerigars + + + +; other species + or rare	Respiration greatly embarrassed— often first sign of illness; edema and congestion of lungs
Leukosis complex	Essentially Galliformes, especially domestic fowl + + + +; budgerigars (myeloid and lymphoid) +; other species + or rare	A few authenticated cases in pet, aviary, or zoo birds

Table 16-1. (Continued)

Disease Condition or Causative Agent*	Species, Group, or Type of Bird Affected†	Comments
DISEASES OF METABOLISM OBESITY	Pet budgerigars + + + + +; aviary budgerigars +; other cage birds + or rare, unless kept under abnormal conditions of management and diet	Direct respiratory embarrassment or secondary, via cardio-vascular degeneration
GOUT	Budgerigars + + +; other psittacines + + or +; other species + or rare	Air sacs, pleura directly affected with deposits; nephrosis favors secondary pneumonias
OTHER CONDITIONS ALLERGY AND ANAPHYLAXIS	Pigeons +; rare in other species, except poultry	Stings uncommon in temperate regions; anaphylaxis related to drugs and foods insufficiently studied in birds
ASCITES	Budgerigars + + +; other species uncommon or rare, except cachectic ascites	Pressure and cachectic effects on respiratory system. Sequel to neoplasia in most cases
INJURIES Torn air sacs Punctured lungs	Racing pigeons—flying injuries + + +; aviary birds due to predators (bird or mammal) + + as result of fighting in smaller or weaker species, and belligerent species	

*Arranged in order of their discussion in other chapters of this book.
†Incidence of condition and relative susceptibility of affected species are indicated by the symbols:

+ + + + +   Extremely common/highly susceptible.
+ + + +   Very common/very susceptible.
+ + +   Common/moderately susceptible.
+ +   Fairly common/mildly susceptible.
+   Uncommon/relatively resistant.
(+)   Occasional reports only/resistant.

course been most studied. Game birds and quail are significant in this group. Levi's book, *The Pigeon*,[32] is outstanding for an ornamental and sporting bird. The canary has been studied because of its susceptibility to viral and protozoal disease and its use in the detection of air pollution. The opportunity to examine disease and resistance to infections and toxins in carnivorous species has made the study of falcons, vultures, and other predatory and carrion-eating species of considerable comparative interest. In relation to these well-distributed studies of avian groups, it emerges that psittacines, and the budgerigar in particular, show a relative rarity of infectious disease, and it may reasonably be assumed that as a group they are somewhat resistant to infections.

EXAMINATION OF THE RESPIRATORY SYSTEM

Because of the small size of most of the birds under consideration, clinical examination is difficult, inexact, and often unrewarding. The relatively small size of the lungs, their insulation with respect to detection of sound by the pectoral approach, and the blurring effect of vibrations resulting from muscle tone when the bird is auscultated dorsally add to the difficulty of such examination.

Whenever a bird is to be examined, and not only when disease of the respiratory system is suspected, it should be observed for some time at long range, preferably in its own environment or after some 24 hours of hospitalization. A guide to the normal rate of respiration at rest for various species is given in Table 16-2. When a stranger enters an aviary the nervous response and apprehension of the birds can readily be sensed. Their respiratory rate and their activity are increased 20 to 50 per cent. Most healthy birds at rest and relaxed show negligible tail-dipping movements related to respiration. After a burst of energy expenditure, such as flight, tail-dipping is noticeable, and even marked. In healthy birds this feature disappears in 10 to 60 seconds, depending on the size of the bird, once activity ceases and composure is regained.

A bird with involvement of the respiratory tract at any level is liable to show tail-dipping on the slightest exertion or even at rest when the involvement is marked. In obstructive lesions of the upper parts of the respiratory tract other evidence of effortful breathing may be seen. These include heaving movements of the thorax, huddling, ruffling of feathers, and intermittent or continuous gaping. Even when consolidation of the air sacs is quite extensive, tail-dipping may be relatively gentle or barely perceptible when the bird is quietly at rest.

In true pneumonic conditions, despite the effort of breathing, the anoxia, hypercapnia, and systemic involvement of a septicemic disease, the main presenting symptoms are still likely to be those of a heavy-lidded bird which keeps nodding off to sleep. Such a bird cannot find the energy to perch and sits huddled on the floor, eyes closed, head drooping slightly when undisturbed, and rocking fore and aft with each respiratory movement. The tail-dipping cannot be seen so clearly, because the tail is supported on the floor. From time to time the bird staggers, nearly falls over, rights itself, opens a bleary eye, and nods off to sleep again. This syndrome may also be seen in any very sick bird but, apart from pneumonic and septicemic conditions, is most commonly observed in birds with conditions causing increased intracelomic pressure, such as neoplasms, ascites, retained eggs, or egg peritonitis.

The feature of tail-dipping is that, although it occurs in response to overheating, anxiety, handling, or effort, the cessation of such etiological factors allows rapid reversal to a eupneic state. When disease is present, even gentle handling will provoke a marked tail-dipping

and heaving respiration which take several minutes to abate. In severe disease conditions of the respiratory tract or in generalized disease states, the mere act of quietly picking up the bird and placing it on its back for examination of the ventral surface for a few moments may be sufficient to cause its death. For this reason, such affected birds should be handled for only very brief periods at a time, suspended by lateral pressure on the neck and held in a vertical plane for examination of the sternal and abdominal regions. Deep abdominal palpation should be avoided if at all possible, or should be only momentary in duration. With a very distressed bird, placing it on a piece of plate glass and viewing it from below is the only way one can examine its ventral surface with reasonable safety. Such a bird is unlikely to require more restraint than a cage of fingers arched over it as it stands or crouches on the glass.

As in mammals, the thoracic part of the respiratory tract is not the only portion worthy of auscultation. Examination of the frontal area of the head, the throat, and the clavicular zones is also pertinent. In all except the largest birds weighing over 0.5 kg., use of the unaided ear is preferable to use of insensitive aids such as the standard binaural stethoscope. If, however, sufficiently sensitive and compact free or contact microphones and matching amplifying circuits are available, their use can enhance the value of an aural examination. By the stockpiling of tape recordings of respiratory sounds, a library of records establishing standards for different avian species can be collected, and repeated comparisons can be made.

Little purpose would be served by attempting to describe in detail, with onomatopoeic terms, all the nuances of sound produced by a diseased respiratory system, but a general outline here will be useful.

Dry, partially obstructive lesions of the nasal passages, accompanied by visible external evidence of dried exudate, usually give hissing or whistling sounds. When obstruction is almost complete, or the material is movable, a click may be heard. Moist nasal exudate may be seen, as well as heard as a bubbling sound of varying pitch related broadly to the caliber of the affected airway.

The various obstructive lesions of the glottis and trachea produce bubbling, roaring, or rattling sounds, with or without sibilant overtones. In severe cases the well-recognized "gaping" is seen either only after slight exertion or continuously when death is to be expected. A sound between a cough and a sneeze is produced from time to time, often preceded or succeeded by gulping movements. Typical examples are seen in trichomoniasis, moniliasis (candidiasis), *Syngamus* infection, inspiration of crop contents or of irritant gases, solid

Table 16-2. Respiratory Rates Observed in Various Avian Species, with Heart Rate, Body Temperature, and Body Weight

Species*	Respiratory Rate†‡ (per minute)	Heart Rate† (per minute)	Body Temperature† °F.	°C.	Body Weight†
Ostrich					120 Kg.
Condor	6				
Turkey	28–49	93	105.4	40.7	6–10 Kg.
Goose	♂♂13–40 ♀♀20–40		105.1	40.5	4.4 Kg.
Duck	♂♂32–110 ♀♀42–110	210–220	106.0	41.1	1.7–2.4 Kg.
Chicken	♂♂12–21 ♀♀20–37	220–360	106.2	41.2	2.5–3.5 Kg.
Pheasant					1.2 Kg.
Pigeon	25–30	190–250	105.1	40.6	240–300 gm.
Eastern mourning dove			108.8	42.7	
Bobwhite quail			111.2	44.0	
Raven					1.2 Kg.
Crow		342	106.0	41.1	340 gm.
Glossy starling	64–72	200–220			80 gm.
Macaw	55–78 (fear ?)	120–220			710 gm.
Cockatoo					
Parrot (African grey)	36	140–200			360 gm.
Parakeet (ring-necked)	76	200			155 gm.
Conure (blue-crown)	44	240–260			92 gm.
Lovebird (Fisher's)	120	280			55–70 gm.
Lovebird (masked)	132	256			62 gm.
Budgerigar	80–100	250–600	107.5	42.4	35–60 gm.
Mynah (greater Indian hill)	22–50	110–192			180–260
Canary (various)	96–144	560–1,000			18–38 gm.
Robin (eastern)		570–900	109.6	43.6	
Goldfinch	116	320–480			
Sparrow (hedge)		460			27 gm.
Java sparrow		600 (–c. 950)			7–12 gm.
Zebra finch	132–192	(c. 600–1,000)			
Mannikin	120–220	360–880			5–11 gm.
Hummingbird	(c. 180–360)	(c. 800 +)	108–111.2	(42.2–44.0)	2.4–5 gm.

*The Table is arranged to facilitate comparison of the findings in birds of related types, origins, or similar habits, each group in a descending body-weight series, the largest species being at the head and the smallest at the foot of the table.

†These figures are based on personal observations and those made or quoted by Sturkie (Sturkie, P. D.: *Avian Physiology.* Ithaca, N.Y., Comstock Publishing Associates, 1954), or Marshall (Marshall, A. J., ed.: *Biology and Comparative Physiology of Birds.* New York, Academic Press, 1960. Vol. 1 [p. 353]). Figures in parentheses and preceded by *c.* (*circa*) are suggested ranges based on limited observation or on sources of doubtful authenticity. Some of the figures reflect degree of domestication, fear, ambient temperatures, and various degrees of acclimatization.

‡Females may show up to 100 per cent greater respiratory rates in some species, especially domestic chickens, ducks, and geese.

foreign bodies, and, less commonly, in some forms of gout, avitaminosis A, or aspergillosis.

Pressure on the syringeal region as a result of hypertrophied thyroid glands, local neoplasms, enlarged and fatty heart, or other displacement lesions may produce any of the above signs, but is evidenced particularly by a loss of voice or a change of vocal pitch, an explosive, chirping expiration, or merely dyspnea. The slightest exertion on handling is sufficient to provoke extreme distress, gaping, and sudden death.

Consolidation of the air sacs produces less spectacular symptoms. Respiration is deeper than normal, more effortful, and usually accelerated. Over the frontal region, the ventral surface of the neck, or in the clavicular zone, a low-pitched hiss or roar is often discernible on direct auscultation. This is undoubtedly due to the more rapid flow of air over the dry mucosa of the upper respiratory tract. A continuous or sporadic clicking sound is heard whenever loose flakes of exudate or fungal mycelia are raised by the rapid passage of air. This is most likely to occur in later stages when the body attempts to absorb and resolve the lesions.

Interpretation of lung sounds is more difficult. The sounds heard over the lungs have a wider range than those heard over the upper respiratory tract, and in many cases of severe lung involvement no adventitious sounds are heard. Auscultation of the lungs of a eupneic bird with no lesion related to the respiratory tract generally yields a faint, soft, smooth rushing sound which shows little change in character after exercise, although its volume and rate are increased. A softer "flip," or clicklike sound, is noted in many budgerigars and some other birds as a constant and, one must concede, normal feature, occurring with each expiratory movement. Although avian physiologists in general deny existence of any valve,[29,39,40] this may indicate a flaplike valve action between the afferent and efferent secondary bronchi. Alternatively, it may indicate the collapse and re-inflation of the air sacs, or of the thinner-walled parts of the bronchi or capillaries. Whatever the mechanism, this sound is readily observable in normal, healthy birds of certain species.

In congested and edematous lungs, and when serous or mucoid exudation is present in the lower airways, hissing, bubbling, wheezing, or muffled rattling sounds can be auscultated between the scapulae and between the clavicles, and heard more faintly over the sternum. Respiratory rate is increased, but usually the depth of respiration is reduced. The bird often huddles with ruffled feathers and withdrawn neck, and tends to close its eyes and rock gently on its perch. In mild cases, the only external sign is a dipping of the tail with each respiratory movement. Shivering and anorexia are frequent accompaniments.

SPECIFIC CONDITIONS OF THE AIRWAYS OF THE HEAD

Rhinitis

Under this heading will be described local inflammatory and obstructive lesions of the cere and operculum, and the posterior nares, or sagittal palatal cleft. Such changes *per se* are often more distressing to bird and owner than they are dangerous. In addition to these purely local lesions, brief reference will also be made to specific microbiological conditions in which changes in the upper respiratory tract produce prominent symptoms.

The specialized fleshy structures of the face—the cere of the budgerigar, operculum of the pigeon, and other modified or elevated areas around the nares—are more properly part of the outer integument. However, because certain dry, crusty, exudative lesions of these areas often spread into or have spread from the lining membranes of the nasal passages, discussion of these structures is included here.

ETIOLOGY

Cere hyperkeratosis; cnemidocoptic mange; erosive, necrotic, and ulcerative local infections; neoplasms; foreign bodies, including regurgitated material; avian pox; moniliasis; trichomoniasis, and arthropod bites are the most important lesions and causes of disorder in this portion of the respiratory tract. Recognizable pyogenic bacteria do not as a rule produce typical abscesses. Ulcers and granulomas are the usual responses. Conditions produced by specific organisms are discussed later in this Chapter, as well as elsewhere in the book. These etiological factors are all calculated to produce exudation. This exudation may be serous (pox and certain other viruses), hard and encrusted (*Cnemidocoptes*), catarrhal (*Trichomonas*), or ozenic (various ulcers). Its nature varies as much with species and age of the bird as with the causal agent. *Mycoplasma,* various poultry viruses, *Aspergillus,* and sometimes avitaminosis A can less commonly, or with less certainty, be incriminated as the primary cause of a discharge or encrustation around the external nares.

SYMPTOMS

The symptoms range from noisy friction sounds as the result of a narrowed orifice, to sneezing and bubbling sounds, or clicking sounds made when loosened dried exudate or other foreign material oscillates within the nasal chambers. In hyperkeratosis and *Cnemidocoptes* infestation the cumulative exudate rises around the external nares but seldom occludes them. Unilateral catarrhal, ozenic, and hemorrhagic lesions and neoplasms do cause obstructions quite frequently. Pox lesions may be dry and scabby in pigeons, and viscid or sero-catarrhal in canaries and sparrows. In moniliasis and trichomoniasis, the mucoid or tenacious exudate is more noticeable in the oropharynx than in and around the nostrils.

TREATMENT

Treatment of the specific viral, bacterial, fungal, and protozoal infections is discussed elsewhere in the appropriate chapters. Infected wounds, ulcers, granulomas, and small benign neoplasms within and around the nares are best treated by excision, curettage, or coagulating diathermy. The surgical procedure is followed by topical application of an antibiotic cream appropriate to the sensitivity of any significant organisms found in the lesion. Care must be taken not to fill the nares or occlude the nasal chambers.

Organisms seldom spread systemically from superficial pyogenic foci, apart from those caused by pasteurellae, *E. coli,* and certain staphylococci. Staphylococcal arthritis, however, is occasionally associated with a superficial staphylococcal granuloma. But it is not usually necessary to give any antibiotic orally or parenterally as supportive therapy, provided the general health of the bird remains good.

The etiology of "hypertrophic" or hyperkeratotic lesions of the cere of budgerigars is unknown. Vitamin A deficiency does not appear to be implicated. The only effective treatment—and this is a temporary one at best —is to scrape off the keratinous crusts until normally colored cere appears or abrasion results; a protective dressing of animal or vegetable oil is then applied.

For mosquito and other arthropod bites, and for facial swellings of suspected allergic origin, dexamethasone or an antihistamine may be administered systemically in carefully computed doses.

When a true rhinitis is present, unassociated with systemic disturbance, local treatment is unsatisfactory. With such local bacterial and possible *Mycoplasma* infection, some response may be expected to tetracycline or chloramphenicol therapy. For birds over 200 gm. body weight, oxytetracycline or chlortetracycline, a 50-mg. capsule or tablet daily, can readily be administered for up to a week with minimal risk of toxic side effects; for birds weighing more than 1 kg., even higher doses may be used. For birds weighing 200 gm. or less, these drugs are best given in solution or suspension, *e.g.,* chlortetracycline bisulfate* or chloramphenicol palmi-

* Aureomycin Soluble Powder—American Cyanamid Co., Princeton, N.J.

tate,† by the method described by Blackmore and Lucas.[10] (See discussion of Direct Oral Administration and Figure 9-7 in Chapter 9, Clinical Examination and Methods of Treatment.)

Conditions that respond poorly to treatment include avian pox, possibly other viral diseases, ulcerative and necrotic conditions extending into the nasal mucosa and vestigial turbinate bones, malignant or inaccessible neoplasms, some foreign bodies, and locally invasive conditions caused by drug-resistant organisms.

Necrosis of Turbinates and Nasal Septum

Necrosis of the simple turbinate ridges and nasal septum is likely to arise during or after severe and chronic infections of the nasal mucosa. Nasal discharges are then viscid, catarrhal, mucopurulent, or hemopurulent, and may be fetid. Such ozena, or nasal gleet, is encountered much less commonly in cage birds than in poultry but is likely to be very resistant or intractable to treatment. Erosion extends until the infected necrotic material is inspired and leads to lower respiratory tract infection. Because of their potential danger to other stock, affected birds should be euthanatized if no response to therapy is obtained within a week. The pathological process should be confirmed and the sensitivity of any organisms present should be determined within this period. Affected birds should preferably be isolated when necrotic nasal lesions first appear.

Disorders of Internal Nares, or Choana

The terminal part of the nasal chambers may be involved by edema, inflammation, erosion, neoplasm, and other obstructive lesions. As part of the roof of the pharynx it is probably best described with the alimentary canal. Even with an occluded nasal system a bird can exist and breathe quite readily except when eating certain foods. As true of lesions in the mouth, the most important exudative and obstructive lesions include those of trichomoniasis, candidiasis, and, less frequently, those of avitaminosis A and aspergillosis, and bacterial lesions.

Sinusitis

Infraorbital sinusitis, often associated with conjunctivitis and rhinitis, and sometimes with blepharitis, is

† Chloromycetin Palmitate—Parke, Davis & Co., Detroit, Mich.

relatively common in the large parrots and mynahs; it is less frequent in most other species of cage birds, in which it occurs sporadically as a chronic condition. The acute epidemic form is frequently associated with conjunctivitis in canaries, the smaller finches, and other passerines, and in various columbiform and galliform birds.[26]

ETIOLOGY

No doubt the list of causative agents could be much more comprehensive but staphylococci, other nominally pyogenic organisms, and *Aspergillus* are among the important pathogens. The role of *Mycoplasma* in the causation of sinusitis in cage birds is very doubtful, but it is probable, from the frequent failure to find pathogenic bacteria, that *Mycoplasma* in conjunction with unspecified viruses may represent another cause. Vitamin A–deficiency is a potent predisposing cause but adult cage birds are seldom deficient in this vitamin. Sinusitis is often a sequel to various upper respiratory tract and ocular infections, and is sometimes initiated by injury incurred in fighting or resulting from other causes. It can therefore be unilateral or bilateral.

SYMPTOMS

The commonest picture is that of a bird with a swelling below the eye on one side or both. The swelling is often firm and may be pebble-like. The eye or eyes tend to close, giving a drowsy or depressed appearance. In extreme cases the swelling distorts the bone of the orbit and pushes the eyeball dorsally, causing extrusion of the third eyelid in the process. Differing anatomically but presenting similar features and sometimes co-existing, is the collection of similar soaplike, lenticular deposits of exudates under the upper or lower eyelid or beneath the nictitating membrane. These deposits can be manipulated and removed by expression, leaving little except moderately inflamed conjunctiva. Topical application of an ophthalmic antibiotic cream will usually promote rapid resolution in these cases. In true infraorbital sinusitis of the cumulative type, such expression of exudate is not possible.

An apparent supraorbital sinusitis, but actually a supraorbital subcutaneous and retroconjunctival accumulation of inspissated puslike material, is seen in parrots and mynahs (Fig. 16-1). A booklet devoted to the care of mynahs[38] lists the condition among the first six of about one dozen common conditions. Necrotic-cored lipomas present similar features, and should always be considered in differential diagnosis. The reason for the frequent occurrence of such masses at this site is un-

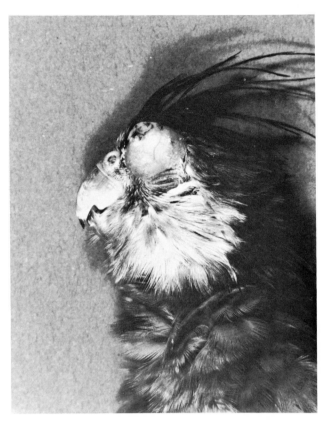

Fig. 16-1. *Supraorbital sinusitis in a cockatiel* (Nymphicus hollandicus). (*Courtesy of T. J. Lafeber.*)

known, for superficial abscesses are relatively rare among avian species. The lacrimal apparatus does not usually become involved. Treatment is similar to that described below for infraorbital sinusitis.

Acute sinusitis is not common as a discrete entity but may be expected in association with epizootic or enzootic conjunctivitis or other respiratory disease. Swelling and reddening of the face below the eye and a watery, catarrhal, or mucopurulent discharge from nostrils and eyes are the most prominent signs. Sneezing, head-shaking, head-hanging, closed eyes, and anorexia and other systemic signs may also be seen, singly or in combination.

TREATMENT

Apart from specific antibiotic therapy, given orally, parenterally, or by topical instillation, it is often necessary, in the more chronic cases, to remove the inspissated exudate surgically. The skin over the facial swelling is swiftly incised, generally without anesthetic, and the pebble of exudate is expressed or curetted away. The more fibrous the mass, the more likely is *Aspergillus* to be found. Irrigation with hypertonic (5%) saline solution, detergent antiseptic (*e.g.,* quaternary ammonium compound), phenylmercuric nitrate, or 4% aqueous silver nitrate, as for turkeys,[34] should then be carried out. Finally the sinus is filled with an aqueous intramammary suspension of the antibiotic of choice.

When the facial swelling is fluctuating, the more fluid mucoid contents can be aspirated by hypodermic syringe without prior incision, and irrigation as mentioned above be performed through the same needle.[21] In general, more permanently good results are obtained when incision is made. In the smaller passerine birds the exudate is usually catarrhal or serous, and systemic antibiotic therapy with or without trocharization of the sinuses themselves is usually effective. If deficiency of vitamin A is considered a probability, the vitamin can be supplied alone, or a multiple vitamin plus mineral food supplement can be used.

Disorders of the Glottis: Glottitis

Inflammations of the glottis are potent causes of dyspnea. Like the posterior nares, or choana, the glottal opening is a slit-shaped orifice which approximates to the choana (palatine cleft) during respiration. Any distortion of this part of the airway, or the presence of edema, congestion, exudate, or other foreign material, hampers the airflow. As the most distal part of the respiratory tract to have no alternative route, patency of the glottis is vitally important. The surface of the glottis is traversed by food materials and is exposed to both normal and abnormal oral and alimentary flora. It is to be expected that many conditions involve the glottis, and even mild involvement results in production of an audible or raucous respiratory sound. The glottis is rarely involved alone; consequently, the following comments apply also in some degree to similar changes further down the trachea and in the bronchi.

Any pathological changes in and around the glottis that interfere with airflow rapidly lead to superimposed changes such as congestion and edema, owing to alteration in the rate of the flow of air and the increase in physical effort involved. Panic aggravates this process. Neurological disturbances affecting movements of the tongue and glottis, although uncommon, can be extremely puzzling, with their production of snoring respiration and dysphagia in an otherwise obviously healthy bird. Sudden death is likely to be the result of starvation rather than of hypoxia.

SYMPTOMS

Symptoms have already been discussed under the heading, Examination of the Respiratory System.

ETIOLOGY

Trichomonas spp. are probably the most potent causes of upper respiratory tract disease in pigeons and doves. *Candida* (*Monilia*) affects a wider range of species, but has a somewhat lower morbidity rate. Candidiasis may follow intensive and prolonged therapy with antibiotics, especially tetracyclines or chloramphenicol. Mynahs, various finches, pigeons, and various members of the Corvidae (crows, magpies) and Sturnidae (starlings) are among those affected; *Aspergillus* only occasionally extends up to this level of the respiratory tract, but exudate and mycelia have been found in the trachea, glottis, and even the pharynx, mouth, and nasal chambers, especially in aquatic birds. Blackmore[7] has seen tuberculosis affecting the glottis in peacocks.

Occasionally gapeworms can be seen in the upper trachea through a dilated glottis, but generally congestion, edema, and froth with occasional streaks of blood are the only visible evidence of their presence. Wild birds found by the public and hand-reared, and specimens in zoological gardens are those mainly affected. Orphan nestlings of the Corvidae (crows, ravens, magpies), Sturnidae (starlings), and other soft-feeders and carrion-eaters are most commonly affected, and the incidence in galliform birds, especially game birds, is high. It is probable that the disease is a considerable hazard in many gregarious, intensively kept, or ground-feeding birds. This would be expected from the life history and ecology of the parasite.

The exudate or false membrane of avitaminosis A is not commonly seen, but deficiency of vitamin A should be considered when these findings are observed in debilitated individuals or birds on a poor or stale diet.

LESIONS AND DIAGNOSIS

When the conditions mentioned occur more typically in other portions of the respiratory tract, the lesions are described in the discussion of those regions. When laboratory examination of material from the nasal chamber, glottis, or oropharynx can be used to aid diagnosis, those methods are outlined here.

Trichomonads can readily be demonstrated in the viscid frothy exudates from infected young pigeons; with a sterile swab some of the exudate is smeared over a microscope slide on which a drop of isotonic saline solution has been placed. No staining is necessary, and with a high-power lens the flagellate can be seen readily in specimens less than 2 hours old, provided they have not been allowed to dry out before examination. The specimen may be stained with methylene blue if a permanent record is required for purposes of taxonomic identification.

Candida albicans can be readily seen as budding yeast cells in scrapings from diphtheritic membranes and necrotic debris. The yeast can be cultured on malt agar if living preparations are required.

Aspergillus species in creamy deposits appear under the microscope as moderately branching mycelia; in chronic cases in which the coloration of the deposit is a deeper yellow or greenish, the conidiophores bearing conidia may be recognized on microscopical examination of a teased specimen.

The paired Syngamus worms in the typical Y form may, with luck and some skill, be withdrawn from the glottis or upper trachea, but asphyxiation of the bird during examination and extraction is a very real hazard. Safer, more certain, but by no means guaranteed, is the identification of typical ova in the droppings of the bird. The gapeworm *Cyathostoma bronchialis* is found in waterbirds, the sexes separate, unlike *Syngamus* worms.[27]

The *tubercle bacillus* is unlikely to be found, in view of the relative rarity of tuberculosis in this portion of the respiratory tract, but it should be considered and the sample stained with Ziehl-Neelsen stain to aid in search for the organism. The complete absence, in a generous sample of caseous, necrotic material, of any of the pathogens mentioned above would lead one to suspect avitaminosis A. A similar material in parrots and the young of other species, lying mainly under the tongue but extending to the pharynx and glottis, may represent a collection of food debris.

TREATMENT

Description of the treatment and control of the specific infectious and deficiency diseases is to be found in discussion of the particular diseases. It is important to assess whether the condition is entirely a localized one or whether it is merely a prominent symptom of a general respiratory, alimentary, or other systemic disease. It is unlikely that the disorder is restricted to the glottis.

DISORDERS OF THE LARYNX, TRACHEA, SYRINX, AND BRONCHI

Etiology in General

Unlike the more protected glottis and larynx and the intrathoracic parts of the respiratory tract, the trachea is a long and relatively vulnerable organ. However, in some species part of the trachea is protected within the sternum or thorax; for example, the sigmoid convolution of the swan (*Cygnus* spp.), and the "quacker box" of ducks (Anatidae).

Wounds resulting from fighting, persecution, and panic, although quite common and sometimes serious in cage birds, seldom penetrate the trachea. Among free-flying birds such as racing or homing pigeons, and birds in large planted aviaries, exhaustion and panic injuries to the trachea result from flying into projecting objects. Contact with telephone wires and angular roofs or fencing causes extensive wounds, although the thinner cervical air sacs rather than the trachea are the respiratory structures most often damaged. Marauding cats, other carnivora, rats, stoats, and the usual native predators are more likely to cause deep punctures and lacerated wounds which *ab initio* are dangerously infected. Tracheitis, pneumonia, and septicemia rapidly follow in most such cases.

The changes described for the glottis in bacterial, fungal, protozoal, and helminth diseases and avitaminosis A occur equally or to an even greater extent in the trachea and larger bronchi.

Changes produced in these organs by viral conditions vary greatly among species. In general, changes such as are characteristically seen in poultry are milder or non-existent in cage and aviary birds and in those in zoological collections, with the exception of ornamental species closely related to the chicken, game birds, and waterfowl. Infectious viral laryngotracheitis (I.L.T.), for instance, from examination of available literature would appear to be confined to the chicken and pheasant, and their hybrids.[24] Most evidence for Newcastle disease in non-galliform birds has consisted of identification of the virus, or surveys of serological evidence in the commoner wild bird population. Although many of the specimens studied have been obtained because they were found sick or dead, Koch's postulates have not necessarily been fulfilled, and the birds in many cases may have been passive carriers of the virus.

Some strains of ornithosis-producing bedsoniae will produce overt signs of disease in parrots, pigeons, and numerous other species, whereas many strains produce little besides the build-up of measurable antibody level. Other strains cause illness and death only when an enzootic or superimposed bacterial or helminth challenge is added to the bedsonial infection.

Pox virus is one of the few viruses that regularly produce upper respiratory tract exudative lesions, for example, in canaries and finches (Fig. 16-2). It is highly probable that unidentified virus or virus combinations are responsible, alone or with other classes of organisms, for causing illness and death in cage birds that show only non-specific respiratory changes.

Foreign material within the airways and lesions impinging from without are discussed later in this Chapter.

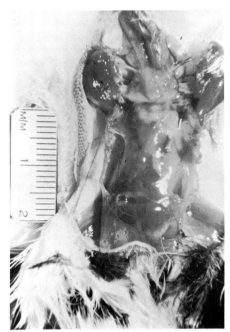

Fig. 16-2. *Visceral exudate at necropsy from a case of canary pox. (Courtesy of D. K. Blackmore.)*

Tracheobronchitis

Tracheobronchitis as a clinical entity is found in most avian species. The great predominance of the complex of upper respiratory tract disease in poultry is partly, at least, the product of intensive management and breeding for special qualities. In other avian species the incidence of tracheobronchitis is less prominent. Among other domestic and ornamental gallinaceous birds, similar infectious diseases are to be expected, although the epizootiology and etiology are often less certain. Conditions in such species will not be stressed here, and the reader is referred to standard textbooks and recent articles on poultry disease.

Other Non-specific Disorders

A greater hazard among the smaller, granivorous species commonly kept in aviaries is the inhalation of irritant materials. Exposure to ammonia, coal tar antiseptics, paraffin (kerosene) vapor, volatile-base aerosols, and lime is capable of causing effusive exudates, not only of the trachea and bronchi but of conjunctivae and lungs as well. Bubbling and rattling respirations and sneezing are to be expected. The susceptibility of birds to this form of assault is to be expected because

of the limited protection afforded by the nominal nasal chambers and turbinates, the specialized respiratory mechanism, and the high metabolic rate. Certain more drastic treatments, such as use of sodium fluoride powder in a "flutter box" for gapeworm, and use of an insecticide in a similar closed box, are other sources of danger. The ways of controlling such hazards are self-evident once their danger is realized.

LESIONS AND SYMPTOMS

The changes in the trachea and major bronchi in obstructive lesions range from a mechanical inflammatory edema with dry mucous membranes accompanied by harsh respiratory (snoring) sounds, to a severe catarrhal change characterized by bubbling sounds, a choking sneeze, gaping, severe distress, and at times attempts at regurgitation. The obstructive lesions include solid exudate, fungal mycelia, urate concretions, false membranes, *Syngamus* worms, and other foreign bodies. In the budgerigar, less commonly in other psittacines, and rarely in pigeons or other species, thyroid dysplasia,[2,6] goiter,[22] neoplasms at the entrance of the chest, focal infections, and cicatricial contractions have been found to produce a similar clinical picture. Hyperemic and congestive lung changes are to be expected, and, in long-standing cases, dilatation and even rupture of the heart chambers or great vessels are occasionally found in birds that have died suddenly. Movable or elevated flaps of solid exudate or of necrotic epithelium produce severe, paroxysmal, but often intermittent bouts of symptoms.

The congestive septicemic pox lesions seen in canaries and sparrows extend to the upper respiratory tract.[11] Greig and Beauregard[19] noted an adherent yellow or white material in the larynx, but did not specifically mention the trachea or bronchi.

Pigeons and falcons suffer distressing symptoms of asphyxiating tracheitis and even tracheobronchitis from the lesions of trichomoniasis.[35] Moniliasis usually is restricted to the upper alimentary tract of game birds[28] and only occasionally extends any distance below the larynx in the respiratory tract. The disease has been described in partridges[28] in which incoordination was the main symptom, in pheasants and ruffed grouse (*Bonasa umbellus*), and in capercaillie (*Tetrao urogallus*) by Kuprowski.[30]

It is difficult to be certain how many of the symptoms derive from deeper-seated lung and air-sac changes and systemic involvement generally, and how many derive solely from changes in the upper respiratory tract. A rapid, shallow or deep thoracic movement with little effort or adventitious noises suggests the lower respiratory tract as the main site of involvement.

TREATMENT

When bacteria or *Mycoplasma* is the suspected cause, a high dosage of a broad-spectrum antibiotic of low toxicity may be effective. With the smaller viruses, the appearance of severe symptoms in cage birds may often suggest an underlying or superimposed infection with *Escherichia coli* or other gram-negative organism. Tetracycline therapy often markedly alleviates symptoms. The over-all mortality may, however, remain at the same high level, although the deaths occur over a much longer period. It should be stressed, nevertheless, that prolonged administration of tetracyclines may allow a previously non-clinical enzootic disease, such as aspergillosis or candidiasis, to become overt and lethal.

The use of potassium iodide in the treatment of aspergillosis would appear to be of palliative rather than of curative value. Keymer and Austwick[28] and Blackmore[7] report nystatin* to be effective in the control of moniliasis in game birds. No effective dosages have been worked out for the disease in cage birds.

Although some appreciable response occurs to treatment of trichomoniasis in pigeons and falcons with such drugs as sulfamethazine (sulphadimidine), sulfaquinoxaline, 2-amino-5-nitrothiazole,† and various antimalarial and antibabesial drugs (such as quinacrine hydrochloride), the use of dimetridazole‡ has been found most effective. Aminonitrothiazole§ is effective, but is likely to prove somewhat toxic.[7]

DISORDERS OF THE AIR SACS AND PNEUMATIC BONES

The precise function of these spaces is not certain, and physiologists generally agree that the leavening influence is negligible in most avian species, rarely exceeding 4 per cent of body weight. It is, however, the largest flying species which have the most extensive bony air spaces. That birds can exist, breathe, and even fly some distance with opened abdominal or cervical air sacs is an observed fact.

The air sacs are serous-lined and undergo a marked inflammatory response to the direct entry of cold, unfiltered, and contaminated air. They form an admirable reservoir for the nourishment of pathogens and the retention of exudates. The entry of blood or ascitic, peritonitic, or other fluid into an air sac is followed in a matter of seconds by asphyxiation through "drowning,"

*Mycostatin—E. R. Squibb & Son, New York, N.Y.

†Enheptin—American Cyanamid Co., Princeton, N.J.

‡Emtryl—May & Baker (Pharmaceuticals), Dagenham, Essex, England.

§Entramin—May & Baker (Pharmaceuticals), Dagenham, Essex, England.

as the fluid pours into the tertiary bronchi and air capillaries of the lung.

Injuries and Infected Wounds

Infection of the superficially situated air sacs frequently follows injury. Free-flying pigeons, sick birds of gregarious species, and migrating wild birds suffer injuries of this type from misjudging their landings. Aviary birds attacked by more belligerent species, rodents, cats, or other predators frequently suffer torn cervical or interclavicular and, more rarely, thoracic or abdominal air sacs. Constant movement, combined with the poor elasticity of the skin, militates against rapid sealing of such wounds. Healing, if it occurs at all, is delayed, and the wound usually remains infected. When a flap valve occurs the picture is likely to become complicated by subcutaneous emphysema (see below).

Common contaminants and pathogens are *Aspergillus* species, possibly other fungi, staphylococci, and, less frequently, *Pasteurella multocida, P. pseudotuberculosis,* streptococci, *Klebsiella, Escherichia coli,* and anthracoids. The appearance with the more usual chronic response is that of a fibrous tumor-like protuberance showing within a thickened fleshy aril, somewhat like the dermal or feather cyst observed in hypopteronosis cystica.[1] These can be treated by curettage, freshening of the wound, application of antibiotic cream, and finally by suturing. Irrigation must never be employed because of the risk of aspiration. Freshly torn skin and air sacs may be sutured after a preliminary cleaning and debridement; use of 00 to 0000 catgut swaged on round-bodied malleable needles is excellent, as the risk of small tears is minimal, and the bird need not be handled again for removal of the sutures. Non-toxic antibiotics may be given orally or parenterally in support of surgical treatment, but are usually unnecessary. Acute infections usually extend rapidly to other air sacs, the lungs, and through the blood stream. Death from septicemic spread is a common sequel to wounds by predatory animals, but rarely follows flying injury or other accidental wounds.

Asphyxiation via the Air Sacs

Asphyxiation from the aspiration of fluids such as blood, exudate, or transudate through an internal or external tear or incision of the air sacs has already been referred to. Prevention of such a calamity in connection with surgical intervention can be reasonably assured by confining incisions to the mid-ventral line for abdominal operations and by performing mid-line trocharization for abdominal paracentesis. Saline irrigations during the repair of torn air sacs should be avoided, and access to ponds and waterbath should be withheld for aquatic birds and cage birds, respectively, until such wounds are healed.

Arthropod Infestation

Isolated reports of "air sac mites" have appeared. *Cytodites* spp., *Cytoleichus nudus,* and *Sternostoma tracheacolum* have been reported by Benbrook,[5] Keymer,[27] and Zwart[42] to have caused mild disease and some losses in cage and aquatic birds and in zoological collections. Keymer[27] refers to the condition in canaries, Gouldian finches (*Poephila gouldiae*), and Madagascar lovebirds (*Agapornis cana*). Murray[37] discussed the control of *Sternostoma tracheacolum* infestation in Gouldian finches by feeding carbaryl.*

Helminth Infection

The significance of gapeworms has already been discussed. Aquatic birds, in addition to infection by *Cyathostoma bronchialis,* the gapeworm of waterfowl, have

---

*Sevin-1-naphthyl-N-methyl-carbamate—Union Carbide Australia Ltd.

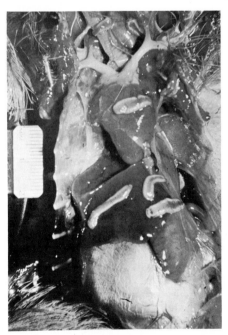

Fig. 16-3. *Flukes infecting the air sacs of a coot (water hen). (Courtesy of D. K. Blackmore.)*

occasionally been found to suffer clinical infections with flukes. To date, reports have been limited to free-living and domestic waterfowl[31] and coots (*Fulica atra*)[7] (Fig. 16-3). Filarial worms up to 4 inches long have been found in the air sacs of falcons.[12] The rarity of these infections and the known difficulty of their elimination make recommendations for therapy in such cases of doubtful use or value.

Consolidation and Occlusion of the Air Sacs and Pneumatic Spaces in Bones

ETIOLOGY

Apart from the filling of individual air sacs by exudate and necrotic debris as a sequel to external injury, several or all of these spaces may become involved in a number of generalized conditions.

One of the commonest infectious conditions seen in the budgerigar is aspergillosis. Marine and fresh-water birds, penguins,[15] and many aviary birds show sporadic outbreaks. The thoracic sacs are usually the first to be involved; the changes, however, spread and may involve all sacs, and even extend to the pneumatic bony spaces and to the lungs and other viscera. The lesions of the air sacs and other spaces commence as a plastic fibrinous response to mycelial growth. The walls of the sacs tend to adhere, and the lumen is at first occluded. Later, as the contents increase, the sacs are distended with creamy or cheesy lenticular masses. Air spaces in the bones may be similarly filled with a firm cheesy plug. Focal lesions involving only one wall of an air sac are also seen when the disease is less advanced. The lesions may be white, cream, yellow, or green in long-standing cases when many conidia are present. It is probable that infected birds are an appreciable hazard to other stock only when fruiting heads of the fungus are present in patent airways. Most infections come from the free-living forms of the fungus in decaying organic matter. For discussion of other lesions and therapy the reader is referred to Chapter 26.

Visceral gout is often accompanied by definite signs of nephrosis and lesions may spread over the visceral serosa. The visceral form appears to be less common than the articular in cage birds, but this impression may be the result of the more spectacular appearance of the symptoms presented by the articular form.

A viscid inflammatory change in the air sacs is to be found in affected birds of many species in association with Newcastle disease,[3] ornithosis,[13] avian pox (especially in small passerines[11]), and also other acute infections such as pasteurellosis, colibacillosis, and possibly mycoplasmosis.

The pathological changes produced in the air sacs as a result of inhalation of irritant chemical vapors are of minor importance compared with the changes produced in the lungs.

SYMPTOMS

The clinical signs of air-sac consolidation are not always spectacular. If the exudate is solid and firmly attached, the bird often appears normal at rest, even when the sacs are greatly dilated by the material. After a short flight, or a bout of struggling in one's hand, respiration becomes very labored and death of the bird from pulmonary edema or circulatory collapse may be expected. No adventitious sounds may be heard when the ear is placed near the head or throat, and very few may be heard on direct auscultation dorsally over the thorax, provided the bird is calm.

When the changes are of considerable duration, and especially when some shrinkage or absorption of the core of debris has occurred, the mass becomes a movable foreign body. It lifts and "ruttles" (oscillates) in the flow of air, and auscultation reveals a regular click, chirp, or hiss. If the exudate is more fluid, as in more acute or virulent infections, the sound is more like a gurgle, a squelch, or a bubbling.

Even after considerable experience with several avian species, one cannot always differentiate abnormal tracheobronchial, air-sac, and lung sounds on grounds of pitch, quality, and timing alone. Interpretation may still remain an inspired guess.

TREATMENT

Treatment of consolidated air sacs is and probably will remain ineffective, although in the case of aspergillosis some clinical response appears to follow oral potassium iodide therapy supported by antibiotics and multiple vitamin supplements by mouth. The bird may sometimes be kept alive and in moderate health for 3 to 6 months, but some respiratory difficulty remains throughout. Only in the case of an isolated pet, such as a talking mynah, parrot, or budgerigar, should the harboring of an affected bird be tolerated. Even so, talking usually ceases in affected birds. Communally kept affected birds should be destroyed because of their possible threat to the others.

There may be some hope of promoting absorption of air-sac exudates by use of such proteolytic agents as chymotrypsin or hyaluronidase, but to date I have found little evidence of response to these agents. Non-fungal exudates may be slowly resorbed once the causal agent

has disappeared. Gouty deposits tend to be relentlessly progressive unless they are purely dietary in origin and any renal changes are reversible.

Complications Involving the Pneumatic Bones

Bony air spaces do not appear to be essential to the Class Aves as a whole. Broadly, but by no means consistently, the more powerful or rapid flyers among the larger birds have more, larger, and more extensive systems of air-filled cavities in the bones. In some species (*e.g.,* eagles, albatrosses), the trabeculated spaces which pouch off bronchi directly, or by way of the air sacs, extend not only into the humerus and femur on either side but even into the sternum, some vertebrae, and the pelvic bones as well. The heavy ground-habitat and non-flying birds mainly have vestigial or no air spaces in bone (*e.g.,* penguins), but a well-pneumatized skeleton is found in such relative non-flyers as hornbills and the domestic fowl.[4] The obvious but by no means proved assumption is that the spaces make for lightness combined with strength.

The more extensively pneumatized bones are more prone to complications in the event of fracture or of infection of the air sacs. The splintering tendency of the brittle avian bone, coupled with the apparently high pain threshold, allowing vigorous movement of a badly damaged limb, readily leads to compounding of a fracture. Secondary fungal or bacterial infection and subcutaneous emphysema are sequels to be expected.[1] Osteomyelitis is uncommon in birds, but when established it may spread directly to the respiratory system.

Methods of fixation of such fractures are dealt with in Chapter 11. However, owing to the ready fragmentation of the porcelain-like bone, it is extremely difficult to maintain immobilization after the fracture has been reduced. With internal fixation, postoperative splintering of bone may lead to secondary compounding of the fracture with inflammatory involvement of the pneumatic spaces in the bone.

Subcutaneous Emphysema

Subcutaneous emphysema, a spectacular condition, is almost always caused by a flaplike skin wound, staggered over a tear in an air sac. Less often it is produced by air-sac rupture alone, which can occur when the bird is crushed or blunders in flight into a solid object while its glottis is closed. Erosive lesions of air sacs are a third, but uncommon, cause. Wounds of the skin of axilla or groin without air-sac involvement, fractures of

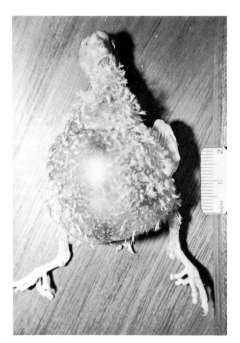

Fig. 16-4. *Extreme case of subcutaneous emphysema in a budgerigar. (Courtesy of D. K. Blackmore.)*

pneumatic bones, and clostridial infection are other possible causes.

The condition is characterized by a rapid blowing up of the contour of the body as a result of the presence of air or other gases in the subcutaneous or intermuscular connective tissue (Fig. 16-4). It is produced as a result of external injury by a trapping of air entering during a phase of lowered pressure (such as the expanding of a concavity "dead-space") followed by a positive-pressure phase when the dead-space is compressed while the two covering layers slide past one another, separating the wounds in the two layers and forming a sliding flap valve. The net result is a local, then a generalized, infiltration of gas until, in extreme cases, the contour of the bird becomes spherical. In emphysema resulting from internal rupture or injury the same process operates, but no escape of gas to the surface of the body is possible at all.

TREATMENT

Simple incision or trocharization often only temporarily alleviates the condition and may even aggravate it. When the condition results from internal rupture or injury, no treatment should be attempted unless very gross distention causes locomotor or other incapacity. When an obvious external injury is present, opening the skin wound and approximating and suturing the firmer tissues around the tear in the air sac should be

sufficient. If air is gaining entry only through the skin, complete closure of the skin wound will suffice. When it is impossible to reach and occlude the tear in an air sac, removal of some skin to leave a permanently gaping wound will allow granulation slowly to occlude the tear. Secondary pyogenic infection is a very uncommon sequel, but a little antibiotic cream may be applied if desired. Fungal contamination is unlikely if the treatment is instituted early and surgery is as aseptic as possible.

DISORDERS OF THE LUNGS AND PLEURA

Etiology and Pathology in General

The lungs of birds are small in comparison with those of mammals. They are slung, fitting tightly to the thoracic vertebrae and the dorsal parts of the thoracic ribs. Their expansion is possible, therefore, without the presence of a full, muscular diaphragm.

Although the lungs are superficially well protected from injury (deep puncture wounds are an exception), their situation leaves them vulnerable to the effects of pressure by neighboring organs. A dilated fatty heart, a fatty liver, very enlarged dysplastic thyroid glands, neoplasms at the entrance to the thorax, and gonadal, renal (Fig. 16-5), and hepatic neoplasms and cysts may

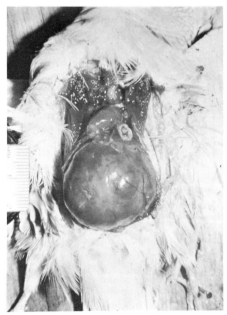

Fig. 16-5. *Cystic neoplastic kidney in a budgerigar causing increased intracelomic pressure and consequent respiratory distress. (Courtesy of D. K. Blackmore.)*

embarrass their function by exerting such pressure. The lungs respond to these mechanical factors with congestion, edema, and some evidence of collapse.

Ascitic fluid and sterile (egg) or infected peritoneal fluid may bathe the lungs, exerting pressure and shock effects; infected peritoneal fluid may also directly extend infection to any celomic organ, including the lungs. Hematogenous spread or direct extension to the lungs occurs frequently with *Pasteurella multocida, P. pseudo-tuberculosis, Salmonella typhimurium, Escherichia coli, Mycobacterium tuberculosis, Aspergillus,* viral, and other infections in susceptible species. Gouty deposits often encrust the lung, and infiltration of lymphoid foci, attributable to lymphatic leukosis, occurs in some species. Myeloid leukosis has occasionally been suspected with lesions occurring primarily in bone marrow and liver but secondarily in the lung. Surprisingly, the tendency of primary neoplasms elsewhere to metastasize to the lung is slight or delayed. Even osteosarcomas are well developed before a local spread to the neighboring thoracic wall occurs, and multiple metastases are rare.

Congestion of the Lungs

A frequent diagnosis of many antemortem respiratory involvements and even of conditions found at necropsy is "congestion of the lung." It is unlikely that active congestion of the lung, found with or without edema, can be said to constitute a disease. Rather, it is an agonal lesion. As a necropsy finding it is very common, especially in the frequently examined budgerigar. Chilling, exhaustion, starvation, or other stresses appear to be the only causes of the congestion in some cases.

PASSIVE VENOUS CONGESTION is a frequent terminal finding in species such as the budgerigar, when long-standing obesity has involved the liver and myocardium with subsequent dilation of the heart. In senile parrots and other long-lived birds, especially those in zoological collections, atheroma and atherosclerosis similarly lead to deficient heart action and congestive lung changes. Mechanical pressure effects of dysplastic thyroid glands acting directly on the heart and great vessels, impeding filling and emptying of the heart, and indirect pressure effects from space-occupying lesions located more posteriorly in the celomic cavity, kill by producing circulatory and pulmonary congestive changes.

ACTIVE VENOUS CONGESTION of the lung is also a frequent postmortem finding. The number of such cases in which potentially pathogenic bacteria are isolated from lung or liver or from heart blood is surprisingly small. Heat stroke, panicky over-exertion, serious fighting, crushing, and suffocation account for a varying proportion of deaths with active venous lung congestion as the main finding at necropsy. The condition occurs most frequently in small, gregarious, timid birds, or in birds that are in poor condition or that are badly housed.

In a large number of birds in which active congestion of the lungs occurs, with or without similar but probably milder changes in liver, kidneys, or elsewhere, the cause of death or of the lesions remains undiagnosed. These cases come from both pet owners and breeders of birds. There is a strong current of opinion which holds that a virus or virus complex is the cause. Unfortunately, to date there is no research devoted entirely or mainly to the solution of problems of virus disease in cage, aviary, and zoo birds. It is hoped that investigators in the field of comparative medicine will follow up this neglected branch of avian medicine.

CONGESTION WITH EDEMA, in some cases, can be related to the inhalation of irritant substances (such as disinfectants, sodium fluoride, insecticides, and certain volatile substances), but in a few cases an allergic response may be suspected. With the profuse output of papers on immunological responses in man and other mammals, and more rarely in poultry and other table birds, it is probable that allergic and anaphylactic reactions will be increasingly recognized in cage birds. At the present time, our knowledge of this subject is sketchy.

It must be emphasized that these changes are usually found after death with few, if any, antemortem signs of disease. The sole item of history is sudden death of a bird in apparently good condition. If premonitory signs are present, these include obesity, poor exercise tolerance, a small reduction in appetite, and sometimes alteration in the rate or depth of respiration. Auscultation at this stage may reveal moist or bubbling sounds dorsally over the thorax. If the lung changes are secondary to pathological changes in other systems or regions of the body, the range of symptoms is, of course, greatly widened. Treatment depends on the underlying causes and the pathologic changes suspected.

Asthma

The term "asthma" is frequently used by aviculturists to describe a vast range of diseases of many etiologies in their later stages. The lungs are congested and edematous, and have some exudation in the majority of serious diseases of cage birds. An active constriction of the tertiary bronchi and capillaries with superimposed edema of the epithelium probably occurs in birds only rarely; in the opinion of some it never occurs. With our present limited knowledge of allergic and anaphylactic responses in cage birds it is probably too early to say that asthma cannot occur, but certainly its presence can account for only a small number of the cases which are so diagnosed.

When presence of asthma is reasonably certain, the inhalation or parenteral administration of antihistamines, corticosteroids, or sympathicomimetic drugs may be judiciously tried.

Hypostasis

Hypostasis is uncommon and rarely occurs in birds to the same degree as in mammals. This is partly accounted for by the different structure, attachment, and shape, and relative size of avian compared with mammalian lungs. More important is the fact that long periods of recumbency are unknown in birds unless serious limb injury or paresis exists. In all other conditions the bird will stay on its feet until it is moribund.

Pneumonia or Pneumonitis

ETIOLOGY

True inflammatory changes in the lung are relatively uncommon apart from their occurrence as part of acute septicemias. Changes arising in or confined to the lung result mainly from inhalation or from direct implantation of infective material by way of a deep puncture wound. It is difficult to describe pneumonic changes *in vacuo*, that is, without reference to relevant features of the infections mentioned. However, clinical, pathological, and therapeutic aspects of specific infections and other conditions referred to here will be found discussed in greater detail in the appropriate chapters.

Acute Infectious Pneumonias

PASTEURELLA INFECTIONS

Pasteurella multocida and *P. pseudotuberculosis* are both capable of causing acute and often fatal illnesses in many species, especially game birds, ornamental fowl, many finches, sparrows, canaries, predatory birds, and psittacines. The acuteness of the condition varies with species, age, and individual, but, although *P. multocida* almost always produces an acute or peracute condition, *P. pseudotuberculosis* can, in older or resistant species, produce both acute and chronic changes, the latter with

caseous or tumor-like nodules throughout the body. Some of these chronically ill birds survive for considerable periods.

Infection may occur via the respiratory or alimentary system or by inoculation through a puncture wound. Lesions are either a diffuse deep congestion of the lung, or multiple petechiae or pinhead-sized necrotic foci of liver and lung. Symptoms include a heaving, silent or wheezing respiration, huddling, shivering, anorexia, depression, a closing of the eyes, and, at times, creamy, ochre, grey, or green diarrhea with or without streaks of blood in the droppings. The urine fraction may be watery, owing to renal involvement. In chickens, the face may be edematous and cyanotic. Catarrhal exudation of the oro-nasal and other mucous membranes is sometimes seen. Death occurs in 12–72 hours in many cases.[36] The chronic type of *P. pseudotuberculosis* infection is described later in this section.

INFECTION DUE TO ESCHERICHIA COLI AND OTHER GRAM-NEGATIVE ORGANISMS

Escherichia coli, Salmonella typhimurium, and other gram-negative organisms produce both sporadic and epizootic septicemia in which the organism may be isolated from the lungs, liver, and other organs, and from heart blood. These infections are seen much more frequently in fish-eating birds and omnivores than in granivorous species, indicating that an increased opportunity for infection is as important as any species susceptibility, in these cases. It is probable that an underlying or enzootic viral infection, especially ornithosis or Newcastle disease, only becomes overt when it is lit up by a superimposed bacterial infection. There is considerable evidence to indicate that this is true of ornithosis with *Escherichia coli* infection in budgerigars.

A high mortality from *Salmonella typhimurium* and other salmonellae alone occurs especially in some outbreaks of infection in pigeons (squabs and squeakers), canaries, and smaller finches. Infected adult pigeons may show little except green diarrhea, loss of condition or performance, and isolated limb joint swellings.[32] Budgerigars show considerable resistance to this group of organisms, as they do to most agents causing epizootic infectious diseases. Specific lung changes are secondary to the digestive and general septicemic changes.

Vermin in the loft, wild garden birds near the aviary, and foodstuffs contaminated by vermin are the major sources of infection. The public health hazard is self-evident.

Escherichia coli, Klebsiella, and other gram-negative organisms are not normal flora of the psittacine gut. Gram-positive lactobacilli are apparently the functional flora.[8] This is also true for some other avian species.[14]

Any coliform microorganisms are therefore of significance as potential pathogens in psittacines, no matter how few are present. This applies to organisms in the lung or other organs as well as to those in the alimentary canal.

Changes in the lung are usually limited to marked congestion, some edema, and little exudation. Birds seem incapable of producing copious amounts of purulent exudate in response to pyogenic organisms. Massive lobar-type consolidations are not to be expected with these acute infections. Miliary necrotic foci are seen whenever the bird survives long enough for these to develop, that is, for 2 or 3 days or longer. Similar changes are found in diseases of comparable duration, for example, in the more virulent forms of aspergillosis, tuberculosis, and pseudotuberculosis.

ERYSIPELAS

Erysipelothrix rhusiopathiae has been found occasionally in the bullfinch (*Pyrrhula pyrrhula*) and in zebra finches (*Poephila castanotis*), with accompanying septicemic signs. The greenfinch (*Chloris chloris*) is also believed to be susceptible.[25] Blackmore and Gallagher[9] reported erysipelas in various aquatic birds, house sparrows, and predatory, carrion-eating, and gallinaceous and columbiform birds. Lung changes were largely congestive and occurred in only some of the affected birds. The liver, spleen, and kidneys showed the main lesions.

STREPTOCOCCAL INFECTIONS

Streptococcal infections in canaries, thought to be spread by blood-sucking dermanyssid mites, were reported by Gray.[18] Symptoms were lethargy, diarrhea, and marked dyspnea, with exaggerated tail-dipping, gaping, and occasional wheezing sounds. Symptoms lasted 3 to 7 days before death. In my opinion, coccal infections invading the lung are uncommon and sporadic. A pneumococcus was isolated from two canaries which died suddenly after having respiratory symptoms for only 6 and 12 hours, respectively. A wide range of antibiotics are now available for use in such infections.

MYCOPLASMA INFECTIONS

Mycoplasma, which, like *Toxoplasma,* could be called an organism in search of a disease, has been isolated from a small proportion of fatal acute or chronic inflammatory lesions of the lungs of cage birds. Whether it is the primary pathogen or whether it is a secondary invader in viral or stress disease is still an open question. It may also kill or weaken embryos, producing caseous exudations of the tarsometatarsal and other joints.

VIRAL INFECTIONS

Infections by viruses, such as those causing ornithosis, Newcastle disease, and avian pox, produce diffuse changes in some species and with certain strains of virus. In many cases in which the virus can be isolated or in which serological examination reveals a current or recent infection, *Escherichia coli* or a salmonella is found in lesions or exudates. From a survey of feral pigeons in Liverpool, England, Hughes[23] concluded that in the adults of many species, *ornithosis alone* has a low morbidity with negligible mortality but the birds show a high incidence of serological evidence of having encountered the disease.

Ornithosis is essentially a hepatic disease. Nevertheless, usually secondary to more obvious hepatic, splenic, alimentary, or cardiac lesions, the following changes can be found in the respiratory tract:

(a) thickened serosa of lung, air sacs, and trachea;
(b) intense inflammatory response of the serosa with many large mononuclear cells and lymphocytes and few heterophils in a fibrinous exudate;
(c) proliferative changes of the "alveolar"/capillary epithelium in the lung; in other organs, necrotic lesions are the main finding.

Proliferative lesions in the epithelium of the lungs are a special feature of avian pox in house sparrows (*Passer domesticus*).[7] In many other instances a virus is suspected, but facilities for its identification are lacking. Death may not be due directly to a virus, but an added stress, such as 24 hours' starvation, lack of water, chilling, panic, exhaustion, overcrowding, or huddling, can be a sufficient triggering factor to cause illness and death. Necropsy is as unrewarding as consideration of the symptoms or serologic findings alone, with congestive changes or minute necrotic foci often the only abnormalities observed. In combination, however, these three approaches permit diagnosis of viral disease with some certainty.

Chronic Infections

Tuberculosis is a ubiquitous and cosmopolitan disease of birds.[41] In free-living and captive wild species the incidence of clinical disease and mortality is generally low, but Francis[17] quoted incidence of tuberculosis up to 4.8 and 4–8 per cent in samples of sick or shot sparrows and starlings, respectively. The actual incidence in avian populations at large is probably well below 1 per cent for most species. The incidence rises sharply in captive birds on a low level of nutrition and in crowded, wet, cold, poorly ventilated, and unhygienic aviaries. It is also higher in captive birds which have close contact with infected wild bird populations, poultry, or swine.

Among the species with a relatively high incidence, the wood pigeon (*Columba palumbus palumbus*) appears to be particularly susceptible. Carrion-eating species, omnivores, aquatic birds, and predatory species are somewhat less susceptible. Among the primarily aviary birds, as opposed to the more exotic zoological specimens, Psittaciformes, especially budgerigars, are resistant, whereas canaries are moderately susceptible. Francis[17] quotes Fröhner as reporting in 1893 a 25 per cent incidence of tuberculosis in 700 parrots treated for various complaints at the Berlin Veterinary School, but this figure probably does not reflect present-day experience with parrots. Fox[16] reported an incidence of 5.4 per cent in 698 necropsies in psittacines and also found 6.2 per cent in 3505 captive birds of all species.

SPECIFICITY

In most species of birds the causal agent of tuberculosis is the avian variant of *Mycobacterium tuberculosis*. The larger parrots are also affected by the bovine and human strains. There is some doubt whether mammalian strains of the organism can produce lesions in canaries.

SYMPTOMS AND LESIONS

Spread is by way of the lymphatics from the primary site. Because the alimentary tract is the main route of infection, liver lesions are observed in the vast majority of cases. In 17 birds examined by Blackmore the liver was involved in every instance.[7] The spleen, lung, and intestines showed important lesions in approximately half the number. The lung is therefore an important site of tubercle formation, and it is believed that lung lesions may occur after entry of the organism by either the alimentary or the respiratory tract (Fig. 16-6). In experimental studies, inhalation of mammalian strains of the organism was found to cause caseous lesions in the lungs of parrots.

In most birds a gradual loss of weight occurs, a "going-light" syndrome as described by aviculturists. Appetite remains good until the disease is well advanced, by which time, especially when the alimentary tract and liver are involved, diarrhea may be seen, often with droppings rather sparse in quantity and greenish in color. This, however, may be observed in cage birds whenever food intake or utilization is greatly reduced from any of a number of causes.

Respiratory signs are not spectacular and in many cases are negligible until the bird is moribund, but respiration is often slightly increased in rate or exagger-

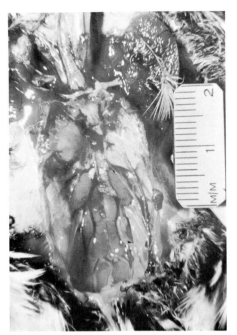

Fig. 16-6. *Tuberculosis lesions in the lung of a house sparrow. (Courtesy of D. K. Blackmore.)*

ated in depth, especially after the bird has been hustled. These symptoms, too, may appear in debility from several widely different causes.

In infected wood pigeons a darkening and dulling of the plumage, especially of the mantle, is so marked that it is claimed that affected birds can, with experience, be detected from a distance with binoculars or through the telescopic sight of a gun. McDiarmid[33] and Harrison and Harrison[20] describe integumental indications of tuberculosis in wood pigeons.

Atypical large lesions in the anterior parts of the body cavity may produce signs of impaired heart action with essentially circulatory effects. Blackmore[7] has noted tubercles of the trachea with partial obstruction of that organ.

Pasteurella Pseudotuberculosis Infection

Pasteurella pseudotuberculosis also affects a great number of species, and lesions have been reported in numerous finchlike small birds and various granivorous, omnivorous, and carrion-eating species from titmouse to toucan size. The disease is usually sporadic, but, with intensive husbandry, overcrowding, poor hygiene, or rodent-contamination of premises or food sources, a higher incidence—up to epizootic proportions—may be expected.

In breeding stock and the young, especially of canaries and sparrows, an acute outbreak of the disease may occur. The classic postmortem picture, however, is one of chronic productive nodules in any viscera, including lung, and in muscle and subcutaneous tissue.

Infection occurs mainly by ingestion and inhalation, but inoculation through puncture or laceration wounds accounts for some of the sporadic cases. The initial infection is generally followed by a bacteremia. In highly susceptible birds, this leads to death from a septicemia, with hepatomegaly and splenomegaly seen at necropsy. In many similar cases, in somewhat less susceptible hosts, these changes are accompanied by cream-colored miliary foci of necrosis in liver, spleen, kidneys, lungs, and pectoral muscles.

The pneumonic changes caused by *P. pseudotuberculosis* form part of a generalized disease picture in most cases. When the infection is the result of inhalation or thoracic inoculation of the organism by an infected claw, lesions occurring predominantly in the lung may be encountered.

Treatment is unwise except in the case of an isolated valuable or pet bird, but prophylactic use of an antibiotic selected on the basis of sensitivity tests for in-contact stock is advisable when necropsy has confirmed the presence of the disease in an aviary population.

Aspergillosis

INCIDENCE

Fiennes[15] discusses the alarming incidence of deaths from mycosis in 24 penguins at the London Zoological Gardens over a 3-year period—29 per cent, contrasted with only 4 per cent of deaths from the same cause among the 980 birds of all species dying during the same period. He lists some 14 general groups of species affected. To attempt to give a comprehensive list would invite comments on omissions. It is probably true that all birds are susceptible in some degree to aspergillosis and related mycoses.

The reported incidence in the various genera of birds is related to both the availability of fungal spores and conidia and interest in the susceptibility of the various species. The fungus is ubiquitous and grows readily on almost any rotting vegetable matter. Opportunities for infection are widespread.

EPIZOOTIOLOGY

Although primarily causing a respiratory disease in birds, with inhalation the route of infection, the fungus can gain access by way of the alimentary tract or through cutaneous wounds, and can infect the embryo by penetrating the shell of the egg. Granivorous birds (hard feeders), and aquatic and scavenging species are generally reported as showing the highest incidence. In most outbreaks the morbidity is low, with sporadic cases only. Epizootics of the "brooder pneumonia" type are rare in cage birds, but intensive husbandry and poor hygiene, or the introduction of "cured" sickly wild birds into or the mixing of different species in one aviary, at times lead to alarming outbreaks.

ETIOLOGY

The causal agent is usually *Aspergillus fumigatus,* but in favus-like lesions of the skin of the neck in mynahs the precise species of the fungus has not been determined. *Aspergillus glaucus* has been found in skin lesions of pigeons.

LESIONS AND SYMPTOMS

Lesions and, consequently, symptoms vary considerably among species. In parrots and parakeets, especially budgerigars, the disease is usually chronic, the bird remaining in indifferent health for weeks or even months before death occurs, often as the result of intercurrent disease. Lesions are dense, cheesy masses in any or all parts of the respiratory tract, including the lungs, with some spread via serous surfaces to other celomic organs (Figs. 16-7 to 16-11). In canaries and mynahs, and in the more acute cases in psittacines, lesions are noticeable in the mouth and pharynx as well as the respiratory tract, and more-fluid exudates are found. In long-standing infections in several species lesions have been found to involve kidneys, liver, brain, and even the great arteries, causing a mycotic arteritis. In such extensive

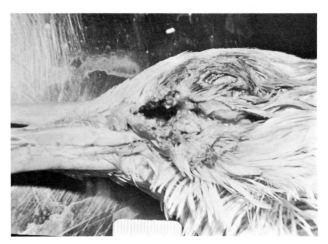

Fig. 16-7. Aspergillus *infection in the infraorbital sinus of a gull. (Courtesy of D. K. Blackmore.)*

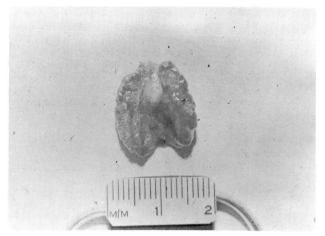

Fig. 16-8. Aspergillus *infection of the lung of a budgerigar. (Courtesy of D. K. Blackmore.)*

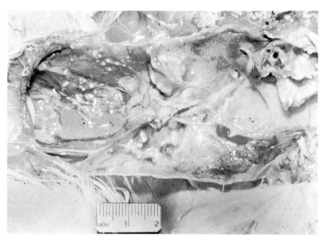

Fig. 16-10. *Multiple foci of* Aspergillus *throughout the serosa of a gull. (Courtesy of D. K. Blackmore.)*

infections there may be little evidence of respiratory disease, and aspergillosis may not be considered until necropsy evidence is available.

Symptoms are variable and, except in canaries, are seldom spectacular. Appetite is reduced, and loss of weight is considerable if the disease is of some duration. Anorexia is terminal unless the pharyngeal mucosa is affected, causing dysphagia. Under the fungal deposits the mucosa is eroded, and the condition undoubtedly is the cause of discomfort or pain.

Respiration, increased in depth and rate, is usually noiseless except in canaries, in which fluid tends to cause wheeze or rattle in the upper airways. When dry flakes of firm exudate lift in the air sacs or bronchi, clicking sounds or noises best represented by "pff, pff" occur with each respiratory movement. Condition is slowly lost and flying is curtailed in most affected birds, but climbing, hopping, or other light exercise is accomplished with minimal respiratory distress. A stage of

emaciation is seldom reached, in birds with mainly respiratory infection, before death supervenes. A mild malaise only may exist for months before the owner is convinced that the bird is really ill and seeks advice.

A provisional diagnosis can be made in life, but many conditions must be considered in differential diagnosis. Spores may be identified in sputum obtained by oral or tracheal swabs, or in the droppings, but this is possible only in the minority of cases in which the fungus is producing fruiting heads. If oropharyngeal plaques are seen, fungal mycelia may be identified in wet smears.

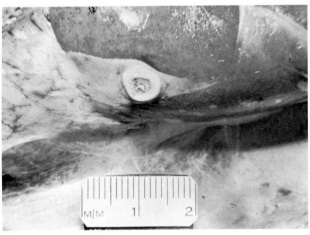

Fig. 16-9. Aspergillus *infection of serosa in a diver. (Courtesy of D. K. Blackmore.)*

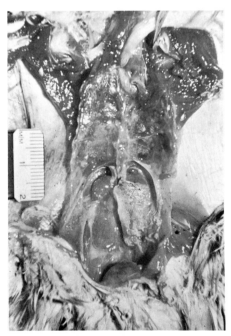

Fig. 16-11. Aspergillus *infection of the air sac in a parakeet. (Courtesy of D. K. Blackmore.)*

Infiltration of hyphae into the lung produces multiple small caseated, necrotic nodules in the lung tissue as well as on the pleural surfaces. The nodules are typical of chronic granulomas, and as such superficially resemble tubercles.

TREATMENT

When the presence of aspergillosis is suspected or confirmed, use of potassium iodide in water (0.1 to 0.2 per cent, or $\frac{1}{2}$ to 1 grain per pint) for drinking, or administered by stomach tube (2.5 ml./100 gm. body weight) has an ameliorating effect. Prognosis is very poor, even in treated cases. Intercurrent infections can be controlled with tetracycline or chloramphenicol. Prolonged use of such antibiotics (*i.e.,* for more than 10 days) should be avoided, as alterations in gut flora tend to lead to diarrhea and deficiencies of vitamin B_{12} (cyanocobalamin) and other vitamins. Additionally, in such bacteria-reduced birds, flare-ups of mycotic infections are likely to ensue. Toxic effects produced by the potassium iodide itself include a drooping of the head, temporary depression, and possible mucosal irritation and exudation.

CONDITIONS PRIMARILY INVOLVING THE PLEURA

Many of the disease conditions already described affect the pleural serosa secondarily or primarily. The lymphatics and serous surfaces generally allow transcelomic spread of infections such as tuberculosis and aspergillosis. Dissemination of the more acute infections, such as pasteurellosis and infections caused by gram-negative bacilli, is furthered by lymphatic as well as by hematogenous spread.

Gout

Another, eventually fatal, non-infectious condition of the pleura and other serosa is visceral gout. The exact renal or other excretory mechanism which is deranged is not usually established. Uric acid and urates accumulate in serous membranes and in periarticular connective tissue. Any celomic organs may be affected, and lesions at times superficially resemble those of tuberculosis or aspergillosis. At other times the deposit is a silvery-white, hoary film of varying thickness on serous surfaces.

The different connective tissue reaction, the gritty, crystalline nature of the lesions, and the positive reaction to the *murexide test* for urates readily differentiate the lesions of gout from other less common lesions, such

as calcified necrotic atheromas and secondary osteosarcomas. The depth within tissues, association with blood vessels, gross appearance, and histological and biochemical findings soon lead to differentiation. Direct microscopical examination of a crushed lesion is often sufficient to permit a fairly firm diagnosis to be made.

Symptoms do not generally include evidence of respiratory involvement until a late toxemic stage is reached, with concomitant anemia, weakness, and cachectic changes. (See also Chapter 28.)

OTHER CONDITIONS CAUSING RESPIRATORY TRACT SYMPTOMS

It cannot be stressed too often that, in the isolated pet bird or small closed private aviary, respiratory syndromes are unlikely to indicate viral, bacterial, protozoal, helminth, or arthropod infection or infestation of the respiratory tract. Mycosis is perhaps an exception to this statement, in that sporadic cases of fungal infection of the lungs can occur in isolation as well as in overcrowded conditions.

In pet birds, the following possibilities are worthy of the earliest consideration whenever respiratory action appears to be altered.

Neoplasms
    Local pressure effects (*e.g.,* on trachea or syrinx).
    General pressure effects (by large sublumbar mass, ascitic fluid)—important mainly in budgerigars.
    Invasion of lungs (rare).
    Cachexia.
Injuries
    Torn air sac or trachea, punctured lungs.
    Emphysema.
Hepatic and renal disease
    Fatty degeneration—obesity syndrome.
    Gout.
    Abdominal wall weakness, attenuation, and rupture.
Reproductive disturbance—"Egg peritonitis"
    Shock, toxemic syndrome.
Circulatory disturbance
    Atherosclerosis, aneurysm.
    Cerebral anoxia.
    Anemia (red mites, hemorrhage).
Central nervous system lesion
    Orbital or brain neoplasm.
    Depressed cranial fracture.
    Degenerative lesion of blood vessels of brain.
Endocrine and other metabolic disorders
    Largely unknown, probably uncommon in relation to respiratory disorders.

In large aviaries where morbidity ascends to a peak, peaks, or a plateau before slowly falling, followed by deaths giving a graph of similar but delayed form, an infectious disease is highly probable. The first birds to die must be examined post mortem in attempt to establish diagnosis of the disease. In smaller establishments with mixed species, mixed age groups, and small total numbers of birds, the epizootiology is severely blurred by a large number of variables. Three sporadic deaths from different causes and three deaths among 20 birds at the beginning of an epizootic may be identical in timing and follow illnesses with identical symptoms. For these reasons, an early narrowing of the possible diagnoses is essential to avoid unnecessary losses. A full clinical examination of all sick birds should be made, taking samples of any abnormal secretions, droppings, or deposits, as may be indicated, for subsequent examination.

Whenever there is reason to suspect infectious disease, immediate antibiotic or other appropriate provisional treatment should be given until sensitivity tests have been performed.

References

1. ARNALL, L.: Experiences with cage-birds. Vet. Rec. *70:*120–128, 1958.

2. ARNALL, L.: Further experiences with cagebirds. Vet. Rec. *73:*1146–1154, 1961.

3. BEAUDETTE, F. R.: A review of the literature on Newcastle disease. Proc. 47th Ann. Meeting U.S. Livestock San. A., 1943. Pp. 122–177.

4. BELLAIRS, A. D'A., and JENKIN, C. R.: The Skeleton of Birds. In *Biology and Comparative Physiology of Birds,* A. J. Marshall, ed. New York, Academic Press, 1960. Vol. I, pp. 241–300.

5. BENBROOK, E. A.: External Parasites of Poultry. In *Diseases of Poultry,* 5th ed., H. E. Biester and L. H. Schwarte, eds. Ames, Iowa State University Press, 1965. Pp. 925–964.

6. BLACKMORE, D. K.: The incidence and aetiology of thyroid dysplasia in budgerigars (*Melopsittacus undulatus*). Vet. Rec. *75:*1068–1072, 1963.

7. BLACKMORE, D. K.: Personal communication, 1965.

8. BLACKMORE, D. K.: The Pattern of Disease in Budgerigars: A Study in Comparative Pathology. Doctoral thesis, University of London, 1967.

9. BLACKMORE, D. K., and GALLAGHER, G. L.: An outbreak of erysipelas in captive wild birds and mammals. Vet. Rec. *76:*1161–1164, 1964.

10. BLACKMORE, D. K., and LUCAS, J. F.: A simple method for the accurate oral administration of drugs to budgerigars. J. small anim. Pract. *6:*27–29, 1965.

11. CAVILL, J. P.: Canary pox—Report of an outbreak in roller canaries (*Serinus canarius*). Vet. Rec. *76:*463–465, 1964.

12. CAVILL, J. P.: Personal communication, 1968.

13. DAVIS, D. E., and DELAPLANE, J. P.: Ornithosis in turkeys. Proc. Book A.V.M.A. 1955. Pp. 296–301.

14. FIENNES, R. N. T-W: Report of the Society's Pathologist for the Year 1957. Proc. zool. soc. Lond. *132:*129–146, 1959.

15. FIENNES, R. N. T-W: Report of the Society's Pathologist for the Year 1960. Proc. zool. soc. Lond. *137:*173–196, 1961.

16. FOX, H.: *Disease in Captive Wild Mammals and Birds.* Philadelphia, J. B. Lippincott, 1923. 665 pp.

17. FRANCIS, J.: *Tuberculosis in Animals and Man:—A Study in Comparative Pathology.* London, Cassell and Company Limited, 1958. 357 pp.

18. GRAY, H.: The diseases of cage and aviary birds, with some reference to those of furred and feathered game. Vet. Rec. *16:*343–352, 377–386, 417–425, 1936.

19. GREIG, A. S., and BEAUREGARD, M.: Laboratory studies of an outbreak of canary-pox. Canad. J. Comp. Med. *21:*407–414, 1957.

20. HARRISON, J. M., and HARRISON, J. G.: Plumage changes in wild tubercular wood-pigeons. Bull. Brit. Ornithologist's Club *77:*144–149, 1956.

21. HINSHAW, W. R.: *Diseases of Turkeys,* Calif. Agr. Exper. Sta., Bull. 613, 1937.

22. HOLLANDER, W. F., and RIDDLE, O.: Goiter in domestic pigeons. Poultry Sci. *25:*20–27, 1946.

23. HUGHES, D. L.: Personal communication, 1966.

24. JORDAN, F. T. W.: A review of the literature on infectious laryngotracheitis (ILT). Avian Dis. *10:*1–26, 1966.

25. KEYMER, I. F.: Some ailments of cage and aviary birds. Proc. B.S.A.V.A. First Annual Congress, London, 1958. Pp. 19–24.

26. KEYMER, I. F.: Infectious sinusitis of pheasants and partridges. Vet. Rec. *73:*1034–1038, 1961.

27. KEYMER, I. F.: Postmortem examinations of pet birds. Mod. Vet. Pract. *42*(23):35–38, December 1; *ibid. 42*(24):47–51, December 15, 1961.

28. KEYMER, I. F., and AUSTWICK, P. K. C.: Moniliasis in partridges (*Perdix perdix*). Sabouraudia *1:*22–29, 1961.

29. KING, A. S.: Structural and functional aspects of the avian lungs and air sacs. Int. Rev. Gen. Exper. Zool. *2:*171–267, 1966.

30. KUPROWSKI, M.: O moniliasie głuzców i o entero-hepatitis (Moniliasis in capercaillie in relation to blackhead). Méd. Vét. Varsovie *12:*201–204, 1956. In Polish, with German and Russian Summaries.

31. LAPAGE, G.: *Veterinary Parisitology.* London, Oliver and Boyd, 1956. 964 pp.

32. LEVI, W. M.: *The Pigeon.* Sumter, S.C., Levi Publishing Co., Inc., 1963. 667 pp.

33. McDIARMID, A.: The occurrence of tuberculosis in the wild wood-pigeon. J. Comp. Path. Therap. *58:*128–133, 1948.

34. MADSEN, D. E.: *Sinusitis of Turkeys.* Utah Agr. Exper. Sta., Bull. 280, 1938.

35. MESA, C. P., STABLER, R. M., and BERTHRONG, M.: Histopathological changes in the domestic pigeon infected with *Trichomonas gallinae.* Avian Dis. *5:*48–60, 1961.

36. MURRAY, C.: Fowl Cholera. In *Diseases of Poultry,* 2nd ed., H. E. Biester and L. H. Schwarte, eds. Ames, Iowa State College Press, 1948. Pp. 299–310.

37. MURRAY, M. D.: Control of respiratory acariasis of Gouldian finches caused by *Sternostoma tracheacolum* by feeding carbaryl. Austr. Vet. J. *42:*262–264, 1966.

38. Pet Mynah—T.F.H. Publications, Inc., 3rd ed. 1964, Jersey City, N.J.

39. SALT, G. W., and ZEUTHEN, E.: The Respiratory System. In *Biology and Comparative Physiology of Birds,* A. J. Marshall, ed. New York, Academic Press, 1960. Vol. I, pp. 363–409.

40. STURKIE, P. D.: *Avian Physiology.* Ithaca, N.Y., Comstock Publishing Associates, 1954. Pp. 96–100.

41. WILSON, J. E.: Avian tuberculosis: An account of the disease in poultry, captive birds and wild birds. Brit. Vet. J. *116:*380–393, 1960.

42. ZWART, P.: Acariasis in canaries. Nord. Vet. Med. *14* (Suppl.):292–296, 1962.

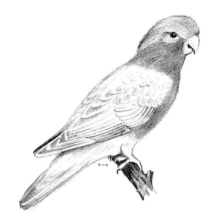

17

Diseases of the Cardiovascular System, Blood, and Lymphatic System

R. N. T-W-Fiennes

GENERAL PROBLEMS RELATED TO THE CIRCULATORY SYSTEM OF BIRDS

Birds as a Class are remarkable for their many adaptations to specialized ways of life. The specialized ways of life of most Orders include various types of aerial flight, at high or low altitudes, and of short duration or sustained over thousands of miles. In addition there are flightless birds, mostly plains-living creatures, remarkable for their ability to run at high speeds on two legs. Birds of other Orders are aquatic. Some can both dive in water and fly in the air; some, such as penguins, are adapted solely to a terrestrial and aquatic existence, and can dive to considerable depths in water.

The changes of physical environment to which birds are subjected as a result of these modes of life could not be sustained by any other group of animals. Birds may fly or soar from ground level to over 30,000 feet, and may sustain continuous flight during migrations of many thousands of miles without feeding. During their migrations they expend energy in a way impossible for any mammal except possibly sea-living creatures such as the Cetacea. Pressure changes at great depths in water are of such magnitude as to have made great modifications necessary in the venous system in aquatic mammals such as seals and whales.[8] How the physiological problems imposed by such conditions are overcome by birds has not been investigated, but evidently their anatomy is largely adapted to meet problems of rapid and extensive changes of pressure and oxygen tension in the surrounding environment. This is reflected in the anatomy of the circulatory, respiratory, and muscular systems. Avian pathology cannot be fully understood without a knowledge of the physiology of these systems. Unfortunately, they have been little studied, and knowledge concerning them is scanty.

The heart rate of birds is generally higher than that of mammals of comparable size, ranging between 100 and 1,000 beats per minute. The body temperature is higher, the normal temperature of many groups being as high as 106°F. (41°C.). Information regarding blood pressure is scanty. Although blood pressure may be high compared with that in mammals, the possible range undoubtedly must be very great to enable birds to overcome the physical changes of their environment.

The ratio of heart to body weight in birds, particularly in those capable of sustained flight such as the pigeon, is very high (13.8 gm./kg. is the figure given by Sturkie[15] for the pigeon). In addition to this, as much as one third of the body weight may be contributed by the muscular system.

In diving birds and birds capable of sustained flight, the muscles are very dark in color owing to the character and quantity of myoglobin that is present. Myoglobin is associated with the transfer of oxygen from the blood to the muscles and possibly with oxygen storage. The range of color seen in the musculature of birds is greater than that seen in other animal species. This variation in color is readily apparent from the white flesh of the breast muscles of poultry and the red flesh of their legs; the red pectoral muscles of game birds, such as partridges; and the very dark muscles of aquatic species, such as penguins, which in this respect resemble seals and aquatic mammals.

The most remarkable feature of the anatomical system of a bird, however, lies in the boxlike structure of the axial skeleton and the associated air-sac system. The skeleton is rigid but elastic; it is involved as a whole in the rhythmic movements of expansion and contraction associated with respiration. The whole body of birds is permeated by the nine air sacs, with their numerous diverticula which, in all but flightless species, pass into the cavities of many bones of the body. There are four paired air sacs—the cervical, anterior (cranial) thoracic, posterior (caudal) thoracic, and abdominal. In addition, there is one unpaired sac—the interclavicular, which gives off many diverticula. In all but flightless birds, many of the bones are pneumatic, including the femur, humerus, sternum, and the vertebrae.

The lungs of birds are relatively smaller than those of mammals, and the manner of their function, being related to the air-sac system, is different. The lungs contain no alveoli but consist of a honeycomb of tubes, which has been likened to the radiator of a car. The air traverses these tubes in its passage to and from the air sacs, and for this reason they are known as "air capillaries." It is believed that *during inspiration* air passes through the air capillaries on its way to the anterior air sacs. Air passing to the abdominal air sacs bypasses the lungs during inspiration, but passes through the air capillaries *during expiration*. This argues of course that there must be a system of valves and controls on the main bronchi, which directs the incoming and outgoing air along the correct channels.

Although the respiratory movements are periodic because of the air-sac system, the flow of air through the air capillaries is regular and smooth and not intermittent as in mammals. Furthermore, during both inspiration and expiration, oxygen-rich air is continuously passing through the lung capillaries, and for this reason the lungs can be of smaller relative volume than those of mammals. The air sacs provide birds with buoyancy; in addition they act as regulators of the air flow, ensuring a smooth and uniform passage to and fro, acting in this way as does the secondary bulb of a rubber hand inflator.

The effect of the air-sac system of respiration on the venous return of blood to the heart does not appear to have been studied, but must be of profound importance. It is difficult to imagine what can be responsible for maintaining the various pressures that will ensure blood return, other than the forces created by the acts of inspiration and expiration and the changes of volume and pressure exerted by the air sacs. The tremendous modifications of the venous system, described by Harrison and Tomlinson[8] in seals and whales, are evidence of the magnitude of the pressure systems involved in diving alone. Modifications involved in flight at high altitudes or sustained over long distances, or in diving to great depths in water, would require the utmost efficiency of the physical systems concerned. However, even the anatomy of the caudal vena cava (postcava) in different groups of birds is unknown. I have discovered, by means of Marco resin casts of the abdominal venous system, that in some families, especially the Anatidae (ducks, geese, swans), no caudal vena cava as such exists. In its place an enlarged sinus, into which the blood drains from the great veins of the posterior part of the body, is connected directly to the right atrium.

A knowledge of the mechanisms of blood return to the heart is crucial because of the frequency with which death may result from hemorrhage of different organs. These hemorrhages will be understood only in the light of knowledge, so far not available, of the various pressures which may affect the great veins of the body, organs such as the liver and heart, and the capillaries of the cranial region. In the next section the types of hemorrhage that occur in birds are described, and attempt is made to distinguish those which arise from injury or disease and those which may be the result of undue pressures in the vascular system.

Hemorrhage

Hemorrhage in birds may occur agonally or terminally or may be the result of shock, dietary deficiencies, injury, or disease of various organs. The various types are discussed in the following paragraphs.

AGONAL

When the skin is removed from the head of dead birds, hemorrhages are often noted between the compact layers of bone of the calvaria (Fig. 17-1). These are often misinterpreted as being due to some injury or to a blow on the head, or they may be thought to be hemorrhages of underlying meninges or cerebral tissue. Such an interpretation is usually incorrect; confirmation requires discovery of bruises of the overlying skin, injury of the underlying cerebral tissue, or further hemorrhages into the nasal cavities and sinuses, which would indicate that some injury had been sustained. The hemorrhages into the calvaria, which may be small and discrete or widely splashed, are in most cases agonal and arise from capillary rupture consequent to right heart failure.

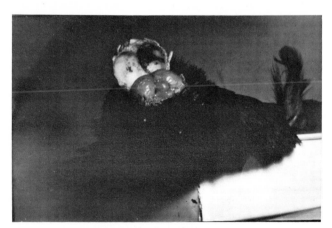

Fig. 17-1. *Agonal hemorrhage in the calvaria of a crow. Note the lack of hemorrhage in the brain.*

TERMINAL HEMORRHAGE

In septic or septicemic conditions, a dead bird may exhibit internal hemorrhages arising from rupture of the caudal vena cava or of the right atrium. Usually such a catastrophe represents merely a terminal event in some disease process. The mechanics of these cases will not be understood until more is known of the physiology of the venous return to the heart. Sick birds frequently conceal the fact that they are sick, possibly as an instinctive measure of protection, because sick birds are often killed by their companions. Many aviary owners are surprised when an apparently healthy bird suddenly falls dead while sitting on its perch or even while on the wing.

It would appear that the attempt to maintain normal activity when sick frequently results in failure of the right heart with consequent massive dilatation and rupture of a vein or of the right atrium. These same influences often result in congestion of the lungs and even hemorrhage into the lung substance, either of which may prove fatal. Lung conditions in birds, particularly congestion and hemorrhage, are often the result of passive congestion; if so, they are purely mechanical in origin and have no direct connection with the disease from which the bird has been suffering. A distinction between lung hemorrhage and active disease of the lung is obviously important, particularly when such a dangerous disease as ornithosis (psittacosis) might be involved. Terminal hemorrhages sometimes arise as the result of rupture of various organs, particularly of the liver and kidneys. This more commonly occurs in cases of disease of these organs; such hemorrhages are discussed under the heading, Hemorrhage Associated with Organic Disease.

HEMORRHAGE ASSOCIATED WITH SHOCK

Hemorrhage into the substance of the adrenal glands, arising from stress or shock, has been described less commonly in birds than in mammals. This is probably because the adrenals are less accessible than in mammals and consequently are less frequently examined. Stress or shock in birds is, however, commonly accompanied by hemorrhage into the lumen of the bowel, in which event the condition is frequently mistaken for hemorrhagic enteritis of infectious origin. Failure to understand this mechanism has led to many misdiagnoses, and the frequency with which enteritis is diagnosed as a cause of death in birds is almost certainly to be attributed to inexperience in this respect. Many species of birds, like other wild animals, including snakes, are sensitive psychologically and become readily stressed or shocked. This can arise from a simple change of cage or ownership; within a day or two, the bird may be found dead with hemorrhages, usually of the small intestine. Alternatively, the stress may trigger the activity of some latent pathogen of the bowel and cause death from infection as a secondary effect. Bowel hemorrhages associated with shock and stress are probably most commonly due to the hypotensive state usually present, and are probably caused by some impediment to the return of blood to the heart. Such hemorrhages in human subjects and dogs have been described by Marston.[11]

HEMORRHAGE ASSOCIATED WITH DIETARY DEFICIENCIES

Most investigators will, from time to time, be puzzled by unexplained hemorrhages found in various parts of birds' bodies, either internal or external. If they are observed frequently in a particular collection or aviary, the prevalent dietary methods should be investigated, since the hemorrhages may well be due to deficiency of vitamin K. This vitamin is known to be synthesized by bacteria in the bowel of some birds, but a supplementary supply is sometimes required. Vitamin K is present in the leafy parts of plants, carrot tops, alfalfa meal, kale, soy bean oil, and in young vegetable shoots. In vitamin K deficiency, the blood fails to clot, owing to lack of prothrombin. The affected bird may become anemic as the result of the loss of small quantities of blood, or hemorrhages of greater extent may lead to death. The condition is quickly and successfully treated by the addition of vitamin K to the diet.

HEMORRHAGE ASSOCIATED WITH INJURY

In any case in which injury is suspected as a cause of fatal hemorrhage, the body of the bird should be skinned and the inner surface of the skin should be examined for puncture wounds or bruises. Injury is often caused to birds, especially cage birds, as a result of flying into inanimate objects, with consequent hemorrhage into the nasal cavities, sinuses, or brain. Occurrence of such injury is easily determined by making the appropriate dissections of the head. Apparent injury of the brain may, in fact, be due to some infectious process which has extended into the cranial cavity from the respiratory passages. Hemorrhages from organs such as the liver more easily result from injury if the organ is diseased (see following section).

HEMORRHAGE ASSOCIATED WITH ORGANIC DISEASE

Death from rupture of the liver (Fig. 17-2) commonly occurs in all species of birds, particularly, it seems, in highly pigmented species, in which the metabolic strain on the liver is greater and in which there is a greater tendency for the organ to become fatty. However, fatty liver is a common disease in most species of birds, and this is the commonest cause of rupture. Rupture of the liver can also occur directly as a result of injury, as

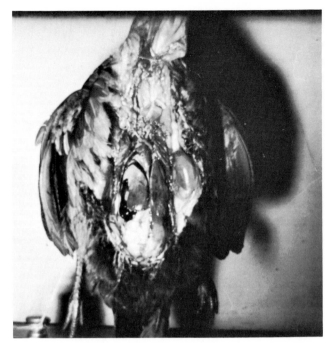

Fig. 17-2. *Rupture of the liver causing death in a jungle fowl.*

noted in the preceding section, or when the organ is diseased, as in tuberculosis. Fatty livers may be the result of faulty nutrition, poisoning, or bacterial toxins; the condition probably results also from a variety of unknown causes. The other organ commonly involved with hemorrhages is the kidney, usually, as in the case of the liver, occurring as the result of disease. Fatty degeneration of the kidney is often secondary to fatty degeneration of the liver, but rupture of a kidney is a less common cause of death than is rupture of the liver.

DISEASES OF THE HEART

PERICARDITIS

Occasionally, but rarely, a typical infectious pericarditis of a serofibrinous nature is encountered in birds. More commonly, either hemopericardium or hydropericardium is seen. Although serofibrinous pericarditis is a direct result of infection, hemopericardium or hydropericardium is a secondary effect consequent upon primary disease of the heart, disease of the lungs, or generalized passive congestion from some other cause. The pericardium is commonly found filled with clear serous fluid in such birds as parrots that have died of heart failure during the convalescent period following an attack of pneumonia. Indeed, in my experience, parrots rarely recover from true pneumonia; in spite of apparent recovery, death usually occurs from heart failure with pericarditis in the convalescent period.

The pericardium is often the site of extensive deposition of uric acid salts in the condition known as "visceral gout." These salts give the membranes a glistening, translucent appearance (see Chapter 28).

MYOCARDITIS

Myocarditis in birds is usually a chronic condition and is frequently the result of bacterial toxemia. It may also be idiopathic and accompany fatty degeneration of the liver; in such cases the heart, like the liver, is obviously fatty even to the naked eye. Myocarditis may thus be traumatic or degenerative, and death may occur either from cardiac rupture or from syncope. Cardiac degeneration has been stated to be especially common in ostriches, storks, and cassowaries,[5] but this statement, repeated from textbook to textbook, may well be inaccurate. It is obvious that an animal such as a bird, which often remains active in spite of serious disease, will commonly succumb to syncope if the heart is affected by infection or toxemia.

Heart failure (see above) frequently causes passive congestion of the abdominal organs and of the lungs, which may lead to hemorrhages of the bowel or lungs, or rupture of the right atrium. As in other animals, hypertrophy of the heart may occur after severe illness or strain; this is particularly common in predatory birds and all birds which habitually fly to great heights or over long distances. During the course of septicemic conditions, or as the result of poisons such as arsenic or phosphorus, some epicardial or endocardial hemorrhages frequently occur.

PARASITISM OF THE HEART

Adult filariae, although common in birds, are not found in the cavities of the heart. The only parasites which commonly affect the heart in birds are Sarcosporidia, which can be seen as nodules or spots on the muscle. These parasites are supposed to be non-pathogenic, but may cause local necrosis of the myocardium.

NEOPLASIA

In addition to being caused by Sarcosporidia, white nodules in the heart may be due to leukosis, and may be a manifestation of the lymphomatosis/leukemia/osteopetrosis syndrome which is described later. Such nodules may also be present in the pericardium. Very occasionally birds' hearts contain malignant tumors, usually lymphosarcoma or sarcoma.

TOXIC HEART DEGENERATION (ROUND HEART DISEASE)

The condition known as toxic heart degeneration, or round heart disease, has not been described in birds other than poultry, apparently occurring in pullets kept on built-up litter. It is probably of infectious origin, although this has not yet been proved.[16] The disease has been described in New Zealand, in the United Kingdom,[1] in the United States, and in India.[12]

Death occurs suddenly after a flapping of the wings, although occasionally the fowl may be lethargic for a few days, and the comb blue and shriveled at the tips. At necropsy, appearances are those of acute heart failure. The liver and kidneys show acute passive hyperemia, and the lungs are often edematous. The spleen, however, is usually normal in size and color. The volume and weight of the heart are generally increased, owing to thickening of the myocardium. The muscle has a parboiled appearance, and the apex of the organ is rounded, with an indentation at its point. In less advanced cases there is a more patchy degeneration of the myocardium, chiefly in the left ventricle, the effect being destruction of the symmetry of the organ.

Microscopically the heart muscle shows acute degenerative changes, ranging from cloudy swelling, fatty degeneration and sometimes infiltration, to necrosis. The general picture is one of acute diffuse myocarditis.

CONGENITAL DEFECTS OF THE HEART

Siller[14] described the presence of defects of the ventricular septum in poultry. These were generally unaccompanied by clinical symptoms, and Siller believed that they were due to genetic causes. There was evidence of anatomical communication between the ventricles in a high proportion of cases, but functional valves had developed in many defects and prevented any significant shunt. He considered that it is almost certain that septal defects in birds often close later in life.

DISEASES OF ARTERIES

ARTERITIS

Inflammation of arteries may be due to trauma, infectious conditions including those caused by viruses, bacteria, and fungi, and parasitic conditions, usually caused by migrating helminth larvae.

Traumatic arteritis in birds may, of course, be due to accidental wounding, but the commonest cause is frostbite of the feet which affects many tropical species during the winter months if they have access to outside flights. The result is gangrene of the feet and frequently loss of one or more toes. Apart from this, true arteritis of inflammatory origin appears to be rare in birds, although cases of arterial mycosis in budgerigars, caused by invasion of the arterial wall from outside by *Aspergillus fumigatus,* have occurred.

Arteritis and phlebitis are common sequelae of injury to the legs or feet (*e.g.,* bumblefoot) of long-legged birds such as storks or flamingos. The length of the arteries and veins in such birds makes them particularly vulnerable, and it is often impossible to save them if they should sustain an infected leg wound, a fracture, or sepsis of the foot.

Apart from these instances, arteritis does not appear to be commonly encountered in birds, and their arteries are usually free from parasitic infection.

DEGENERATIVE CONDITIONS OF ARTERIES

Idiopathic sclerotic conditions of the medial coat of the arteries are frequently found in pigeons, but are rare in other genera. A condition which conforms to accepted definitions of atherosclerosis, as seen in man or other animals, is commonly found among captive birds of certain species[4] (Tables 17-1 and 17-2). In general, seed-eating species of birds do not naturally suffer from this condition, whereas it is commonly found in captive specimens of fruit- and meat-eating species.

So-called dissecting aneurysms are common in arteries of turkeys and lead to rupture of the vessel and death in a significant proportion of young birds. Gresham and Howard[6] have summarized their own views on dissecting aneurysm and presented evidence for their theory that it is due to a true atheroma, which is an initial lesion of the abdominal aorta. In this condition, a sudden change of structure occurs at the origin of the anterior mesenteric artery. The wall of the aorta becomes thin, and consists largely of smooth muscle fibers separated by thin elastic strands. At this point, the aneurysm develops, and rupture and hemorrhage may occur.

Physiological fatty streaking* is present in young chicks and in the young of other birds at the time of hatching. In the case of chicks, and probably other birds too, it disappears at the age of 6 weeks.

Atheromatous lesions of varying extent, usually quite harmless, can frequently be found in the brachiocephalic trunks and abdominal aorta of susceptible species. A typical site of small plaques is at the junction of smaller tributaries, such as intercostal arteries. Lesions of increasing degrees of severity may be found in older birds, until the vessels appear to be completely occluded by the atheroma. In many cases there are calcium de-

*For definitions of fatty streaking and atheroma see *Classification of Atherosclerotic Lesions.*[17]

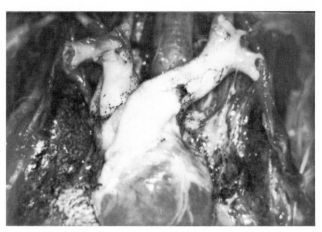
Fig. 17-3. *Heart and great vessels of elderly cockatoo with atherosclerosis and anthracosis.*

posits in the arterial wall and the elasticity of the vessel is lost. It should, however, be remembered that arteries are very elastic, and when an artery is distended with blood the atheromatous plaque is usually depressed into the arterial wall unless the vessel is calcified. In the absence of thrombus and calcification, therefore, plaques which appear to occlude the vessel may not in reality be of great significance (Fig. 17-3).

Nevertheless, in old birds, uncomplicated atheromatosis causes death as a result of interruption of the circulation. Plaques of lethal size and extent have been described in the aorta, and in the brachial, axillary, coronary, and renal arteries. They are somewhat uncommon in the coronary arteries, and have not been described in the arteries of the brain. They are virtually never found in the pulmonary arteries.

THROMBOSIS AND EMBOLISM

Atheroma of arteries is a condition which progresses through life, usually causing fatal hindrance to the blood flow only in old age. Associated thrombosis, which is so serious in the human, is very rare in birds. A few such cases have been described by Hamerton[7] and others, one such case being a ball thrombus in the heart of a trumpeter swan that apparently caused its death. Thrombosis does, therefore, occasionally occur, but is of little importance in the pathology of the circulation in birds.

DISEASES OF THE BLOOD

Anemia

Anemia may be due to constitutional, traumatic, dietetic, or parasitic causes. The anemias of poultry have not been studied, and nothing worth while can be said about them except that those most generally recog-

Table 17-1. Reported Cases of Arterial Disease among the Orders of Aves*

1. **Struthioniformes, Rheiformes, Casuariiformes, Apterygiformes, Tinamiformes**
   (a) Fatty streaking   Nil
   (b) Atheroma   8 ostriches

2. **Sphenisciformes**
   (a) Fatty streaking   Nil
   (b) Atheroma   1 Humboldt's penguin

3. **Gaviiformes, Podicipediformes, Procellariiformes**

4. **Pelecaniformes**
   (a) Fatty streaking   Nil
   (b) Atheroma   pelican
        gannet
        3 cormorants

5. **Ciconiiformes**
   (a) Fatty streaking   Nil
   (b) Atheroma   2 flamingos
        white ibis
        shoebill
        3 herons
        2 goliath herons
        2 storks
        1 cattle egret
   (c) Arteritis   Nil
   (d) Aneurysms   1 flamingo

6. **Anseriformes**
   (a) Fatty streaking   Nil
   (b) Atheroma   31 varied ducks and geese
        1 swan
   (c) Medial sclerosis   Nil
   (d) Arteritis   Nil

7. **Falconiformes**
   (a) Fatty streaking   Nil
   (b) Atheroma   14 vultures
        1 falcon
        2 bateleur eagles
   (c) Other lesions   Nil

8. **Galliformes**
   (a) Fatty streaking   fowl
   (b) Atheroma   1 peafowl
        14 pheasants
        turkeys
        fowl

*Adapted from Fiennes,[1] with references omitted.

Table 17-1. (Continued)

9. Gruiformes	
(a) Fatty streaking	Nil
(b) Atheroma	9 cranes
(c) Medial sclerosis	Nil
(d) Arteritis	Nil
10. Charadriiformes	
(a) Fatty streaking	Nil
(b) Atheroma	1 lapwing
	1 sheathbill
11. Columbiformes	
(a) Fatty streaking	Nil
(b) Atheroma	pigeons
(c) Aneurysms	pigeon
12. Psittaciformes	
(a) Fatty streaking	Nil
(b) Atheroma	1 parakeet
	conures
	lories
	parrots
	2 macaws
	1 cockatoo
(c) Other conditions	Nil
13. Cuculiformes	
(a) Fatty streaking	Nil
(b) Atheroma	1 Guira cuckoo
(c) Arteritis	Nil
14. Strigiformes	
(a) Fatty streaking	Nil
(b) Atheroma	owls
(c) Other lesions	Nil
15. Caprimulgiformes, Apodiformes, Coliiformes, Trogoniformes	
(a) Fatty streaking	Nil
(b) Atheroma	aged hummingbird
16. Passeriformes	
(a) Fatty streaking	Nil
(b) Atheroma	1 jay
	4 birds of paradise
	2 rooks
	1 Indian crow
	2 starlings
(c) Arteritis	1 Indian silverbill
(d) Aneurysms	1 sparrow

Table 17-1. (Continued)

17.	Coraciiformes	
	(a) Fatty streaking	Nil
	(b) Atheroma	hornbills and motmots 1 kingfisher
	(c) Other lesions	Nil
18.	Piciformes	
	(a) Fatty streaking	Nil
	(b) Atheroma	7 toucans
	(c) Arteritis (parasitic)	Nil

nized are due to parasites. The parasites responsible may be blood-sucking ectoparasites, helminth parasites of the bowel, or blood parasites, the last being either filariae or protozoa. Diseases of the bone marrow are discussed under Leukemia, under Diseases of the Lymphatic System.

Almost nothing is known about the constitutional and dietary anemias of poultry. Anemia arising from bone marrow damage is not uncommon in birds and arises usually from traumatic causes. Because of the connection of the air sacs with the pneumatic spaces of many bones—the humerus, femur, sternum, and vertebrae—any volatile or noxious drugs or fumes inhaled by birds can damage or destroy the bone marrow. Birds can

thus be given volatile anesthetics such as chloroform and ether only at some risk, and volatile drugs in a room where birds are kept can have harmful results. Often bird cages are placed in kitchens during winter nights, to keep the birds warm. Coke fumes escaping from a faulty stove in an unventilated room can prove fatal to birds that have been left there.

ANEMIAS CAUSED BY PARASITES

The ectoparasites of birds belong to two classes, the Insecta and the Arachnida. The nests or holes in which birds build them often harbor numbers of fleas and lice which are parasitic on the birds. If numerous, the para-

Table 17-2. Susceptibility to Atheroma of the Orders of Aves

	Fatty Streaking	Atherosclerosis	Other lesions
Aves*			
Groups 1–4, 14, 15, 16	+	+	−
Groups 5, 7–11, 13, 17, 18	+ + to + + +	+ + to + + +	+
Group 12 (parakeets, etc.)	+ + +	±	−
Group 12 (parrots, etc.) and Group 6	+ + + +	+ + + +	−

*Key to Orders composing the various groups:

1. Struthioniformes, Rheiformes, Casuariiformes, Apterygiformes, Tinamiformes
2. Sphenisciformes
3. Gaviiformes, Podicipediformes, Procellariiformes
4. Pelecaniformes
5. Ciconiiformes
6. Anseriformes
7. Falconiformes
8. Galliformes
9. Gruiformes
10. Charadriiformes
11. Columbiformes
12. Psittaciformes
13. Cuculiformes
14. Strigiformes
15. Caprimulgiformes, Apodiformes, Coliiformes, Trogoniformes
16. Passeriformes
17. Coraciiformes
18. Piciformes

sites may contribute to anemic conditions, both by the actual deprivation of blood and by the continual irritation they cause. Parasites such as red mites will not usually be seen on birds, since they emerge from cracks or holes in the trees only when the birds are roosting.

It may therefore be difficult at times to discover what ectoparasites are the cause of anemic conditions. It is also often difficult to locate internal parasites in an avian cadaver because they may be present in sites that are easily overlooked. At necropsy, therefore, smears of bowel contents should be examined under the microscope for helminth ova, the discovery of which may lead a worker to find a parasitic infection that he would otherwise overlook. This is particularly true of many of the trematodes which affect water birds, and which may be present in the bursa of Fabricius or other obscure sites. Trematodes may be the cause of anemic conditions in water birds, especially exotic ducks kept for ornamental purposes in crowded conditions on water.

A common cause of anemia in avian species is filariasis, especially among South American, and to a lesser extent among tropical Asian and African, species. The adult worms may be found in the peritoneal cavity, and the blood may contain large numbers of microfilariae. Filariasis may also be associated with lesions of the skin, and when diagnosis is difficult in living birds skin scrapings should be examined for microfilariae under the microscope. Filariasis is one of the commonest causes of parasitic anemia in birds.

There is a large amount of literature on the blood parasites of birds, which is reviewed in Chapter 25, on Parasitic Diseases. When anemia is suspected, blood films should be prepared and examined for the presence of parasites. The finding of a few blood parasites does not, however, necessarily indicate that these are the cause of the anemia, and discretion in making a diagnosis is necessary.

The main infecting blood parasites of birds include:

(1) *Trypanosoma* spp., most commonly *T. avium;*
(2) *Haemoproteus* spp., the best known of which is that of pigeons and doves, *H. columbae*[10];
(3) *Leucocytozoon* spp.;
(4) *Plasmodium* spp., of which there are a number that infect many different species of birds;
(5) *microfilariae*, being the larvae of numerous species of Filaroidea, the adults of which are to be found in the body cavity;
(6) *Aegyptianella* sp., a parasite of poultry almost entirely confined to Egypt, although Coles[3] described an outbreak in Pekin ducks in South Africa.

Many birds reveal the presence of *Haemoproteus* or *Plasmodium* in the blood, and filariasis is a common infection of tropical birds, especially those from South America. In birds in their natural habitats, these parasites probably do little harm, but they may become dangerous under conditions of captivity, when the birds are exposed to stressing circumstances. Furthermore, blood parasites can be dangerous in an unnatural host. The classic example of such a situation is seen in penguins in temperate zones infected by malarial parasites transmitted by mosquitoes from the common sparrows.[13] Again, malaria can be dangerous in many species of birds, including canaries.

For detailed descriptions of parasitic diseases, see Chapter 25.

DISEASES OF THE LYMPHATIC SYSTEM

The lymphatic system of birds is essentially similar to that of mammals in its physiology, but differs in the distribution of the lymphatic tissue because of the absence of lymph nodes. Aggregations of lymph follicles (Peyer's patches) are present in the bowel, and aggregations of lymphoblastic tissue occur in the bone marrow. There are no true lymph nodes along the course of the lymphatic vessels, although there are small aggregations of lymphoid tissue at intervals along their course. These, however, have not the structure of a lymph node as understood in mammalian anatomy. There is a pre-pubertal thymus, which extends in a thin strip, ventrally situated, along the greater part of the length of the neck. In addition, similar tissue is present in the bursa of Fabricius, or cloacal bursa, an epithelial diverticulum opening on the dorsal wall of the proctodeum. This, like the thymus, contains lymphatic-type tissue and is supposed to be associated with the development of immunity in young birds. Like the thymus, it involutes about the time of development of sexual maturity.

The number of lymphocytes in the circulating blood of fowl may be 13,000 to 15,000 per cu. mm., but varies greatly. Little is known of the number present in the blood of other groups of birds.

The avian spleen varies in size and shape from group to group and even among birds of one species. The splenic capsule is thin and does not contain muscle fibers; the organ, therefore, can hardly be an important reservoir of red blood cells. Splenomegaly is found in a great many infectious diseases, particularly fowl typhoid, and the spleen, together with the thymus and bursa of Fabricius, probably plays a role in immunity and defense against infection.

There is no reason to suppose that the lymphatic vessels of birds could not become infected and so give rise to lymphangitis, particularly in large running birds like ostriches. However, no such diseases are described in the literature on avian pathology, and they therefore can be ignored. Consequently, the only group of diseases which must be described is that of the avian leukemias or lymphomatoses.

Leukemia

This group of diseases is well known in poultry but there are very few references to it in other groups of birds. The chapter on the avian leukosis complex in *Diseases of Poultry*[9] also includes a very full bibliography. There is, however, little knowledge of this condition except in domestic birds, and even in pheasants it is known only from experimental attempts to transmit the disease in the wild and from cases occurring naturally in birds raised in captivity. For this reason the subject is somewhat academic for the pathologist interested in the diseases of cage and aviary birds; therefore only the general principles are described here.

The lymphomatosis complex of diseases is caused by a relatively large number of related viruses, which give rise to a number of different conditions, characterized by various levels of cellular disorders. The disorders constituting the main group are as follows:

(1) lymphoblastosis, associated with proliferation of lymphoblastic tissues;
(2) erythroblastosis, associated with proliferation of immature erythroblastic cells;
(3) myeloblastosis, being proliferation of the parent cells of the granular white cell elements of the blood;
(4) *osteopetrosis gallinarum,* being a viral infection of the skeleton, particularly of the long bones, which gives rise to bony thickening, a coarse and rarefied structure of the bones, and eventual obliteration of the marrow cavity. This condition is accompanied by widespread lymphomatous deposits in the soft organs.[2]
(5) The Rous sarcoma group of diseases, which are caused by a number of related viruses.

Those diseases that involve the blood and the blood-forming organs may be either leukemic or aleukemic. They are, however, all characterized by neoplastic invasion of various tissues throughout the body by those cells that are attacked by the virus. The best known of these conditions are probably the lymphomatoses, which may occur in several forms, being nervous, ocular, or visceral, or affecting the skeleton, as in osteopetrosis. Characteristically, the affected organs are invaded by neoplastic elements of the cell groups affected, producing the lesions characteristic of the particular type of disease.

The probability exists that many of the tumors found in cage and aviary birds, described in Chapter 27, may be associated with Rous sarcoma virus. For further discussion of Leukemia, see the section on virus diseases in Chapter 24.

References

1. BLAXLAND, J. D., and MARKSON, L. M.: Toxic heart degeneration, or "round heart disease" of poultry. Vet. J. *103:*401–405, 1947.

2. CAMPBELL, J. G.: A proposed classification of the leucosis complex and fowl paralysis. Brit. vet. J. *117:*316–325, 1961.

3. COLES, J. D. W. A.: An outbreak of aegyptianellosis in Pekin ducks. J. S. Afr. v. m. a. *5:*131, 1934.

4. FIENNES, R. N. T-W-: Atherosclerosis in Wild Animals. In *Comparative Atherosclerosis,* J. C. Roberts, Jr., and R. Straus, eds. New York, Hoeber Medical Division, Harper & Row, 1965. pp. 113–126.

5. FOX, H.: *Disease in Captive Wild Mammals and Birds.* Philadelphia, J. B. Lippincott & Co., 1923. Pp. 50–52.

6. GRESHAM, G. A., and HOWARD, A. N.: Aortic rupture in the turkey. J. Atherosclerosis Res. *1:*75–80, 1961.

7. HAMERTON, A. E.: Report on the deaths occurring in the Society's gardens during 1937. Proc. zool. Soc. Lond. *108:*489, 1938.

8. HARRISON, R. J., and TOMLINSON, J. D. W.: Observations on the venous system in certain Pinnipedia and Cetacea. Proc. zool. Soc. Lond. *126:*205–233, 1956.

9. JUNGHERR, E., and HUGHES, W. F.: The Avian Leukosis Complex, in *Diseases of Poultry,* ed. 5, H. E. Biester and L. H. Schwarte, eds. Ames, Iowa State University Press, 1965. Pp. 512–567.

10. LEVINE, N. D., and KATOR, S.: Check list of blood parasites of birds of the Order Columbiformes. Wildlife dis. No. 1. Jan. 59.

11. MARSTON, A.: The bowel in shock. The role of mesenteric arterial disease as a cause of death in the elderly. Lancet *2:*365–370, 1962.

12. RAMACHANDRA, P. K., PATHAK, R. C., and SINGH, A.: Observations on round heart disease in fowls. Indian vet. J. *36:*1–5, 1959.

13. RODHAIN, J.: Une infection à Plasmodium chez *Spheniscus demersus* (manchot du Cap). Ann. Parasit. *15:*253–258, 1937.

14. SILLER, W. G.: Ventricular septal defects in the fowl. J. Path. Bact. *76:*431–440, 1958.

15. STURKIE, P. D.: *Avian Physiology,* 2nd ed. Ithaca, N. Y., Comstock Publishing Associates, 1965. P. 119.

16. WILSON, J. E.: Round heart disease in poultry. J. Comp. Path. Therap. *67:*239–250, 1957.

17. WORLD HEALTH ORGANIZATION: *Classification of Atherosclerotic Lesions. Report of Study Group.* Technical Report Series No. 143, 1958. P. 4.

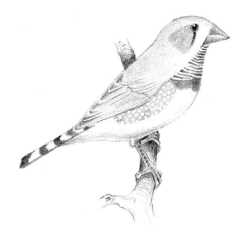

18

Diseases
of the
Digestive System

*Lawrence Minsky and
Margaret L. Petrak*

Despite differences existing in the digestive tracts of the pet birds generally encountered in veterinary practice (see Chapter 6), these differences have not proved a significant factor in diagnosis and treatment of disturbances of the digestive tract. Unless otherwise indicated, most of the remarks which follow in this Chapter relate primarily to the budgerigar.

FOREIGN BODIES

Contrary to what one might expect in small pet birds, the ingestion of foreign bodies does not appear to be a common problem. This is true in spite of the fact that budgerigars are very inquisitive little birds that frequently have the freedom of the house, in which they can and do pick at almost everything that catches their fancy. The rarity of the problem does not, however, indicate that foreign body ingestion or even impaction in the mouth is not possible. In hundreds of necropsies of budgerigars and canaries which included examination of the mouth, esophagus, crop, proventriculus, and gizzard, Minsky does not recall seeing a foreign body problem in the digestive tract. He once recovered by surgery a 2½-inch corsage pin from the gizzard of a pet peacock, which had suddenly become very listless and inappetent. Fortunately, in the process of examining the bird, a radiograph was taken which revealed the presence of the pin in the gizzard. Within five days after surgery, the peacock appeared well and ate normally.

Arnall[2] reported that wire, beads, string, and fine chains may lodge anywhere in the digestive tract, from the crop to the gizzard. Associated symptoms may be mild or remain unnoted for some time, and they may simulate those of indigestion or a dietary deficiency.

Beach *et al.*[6] recorded the occurrence of a urate calculus in the crop of a 2½-year-old opaline skyblue hen. The bird was in apparently good health when it fell off the perch dead. The authors theorized that the bird might have died in the process of trying to regurgitate the calculus. The calculus was $1.0 \times 0.8 \times 0.6$ cm., grey, smooth, and slightly nodular. The external layer was brittle and laminated; the core, which composed 80 per cent of the total, was amorphous and white, with pale yellow areas, and included what appeared to be seed husks. In a subsequent case the crop was found to contain a mass of material that was positive for urates. This was in one of several budgerigars that died when their seed supply failed. The crop contained other material which was obviously excreta picked up from the floor, and the authors speculated that this could provide a clue to the origin of the calculus.

Radiography, combined with the use of barium if indicated, should be utilized in the diagnosis of foreign bodies. Lafeber[15] recommends placing 0.25 to 0.5 ml. of liquid barium in the crop of the budgerigar. Normally this should be in the large intestine within 3 hours.

BURNS

In trimming birds' beaks, it sometimes happens that trimming is done a little too deeply, resulting in varying degrees of hemorrhage. This problem is mentioned here because on one occasion, which came to Minsky's attention, a cockatiel's beak had been trimmed a little too short, resulting in bleeding. The beak was then cauterized with a silver nitrate stick, a fairly common practice. Unfortunately, the bird took hold of the silver nitrate tip and chewed it sufficiently to cauterize the inside of the mouth, and some of the material apparently found its way into the crop. The bird became very ill, and after a period of five or six days of treatment it died. Much irritation and damage in the mouth and crop were noted on necropsy. The use of high frequency current is a safer procedure, although a little more involved, to stop such bleeding. However, silver nitrate sticks are commonly used for this purpose and, if used judiciously, should cause no harm. Birds may also exhibit a transient inability to eat hard foods after burning their mouth with hot mashed potatoes. Treatment in such cases consists primarily of feeding soft foods until healing takes place. Foods such as hard-boiled egg, sponge cake, or pablum may be tried. A sugar solution may be utilized if the bird refuses all foods. Tube-feeding of sugar solution or milk is employed as a last resort.

OTHER DISORDERS OF THE MOUTH

Arnall[2] has reported lodgment under the tongue of whole peas, corn, or other material, occurring in birds with deformed or fragile beaks. If neglected, the foreign matter may cause ulceration and may migrate under the epithelium. Soft material tends to cake and often becomes complicated with fungus. Prominent symptoms are dysphagia and halitosis. Treatment consists of curettage, determination of the suitability of the food supplied, and trimming of the beak if necessary.

Gerlach[10] reported that carnivorous birds sometimes experience granulomas (at times ulcerated) of the mouth cavity. *Escherichia coli* or *E. coli* and fungi (*Aspergillus* or *Mucor*) can be isolated in pure culture. The microscopical appearance is typical of *E. coli* granuloma. Treatment consists of surgical removal of the granuloma if possible. Sometimes subcutaneous invasion occurs. Postsurgical treatment consists of local application of iodine for its fungicidal properties, and the parenteral administration of an effective antibiotic.

DISORDERS OF THE CROP

INFLAMMATION

It is not uncommon to observe budgerigars regurgitating seed and mucoid fluid. Sometimes it is a transient condition lasting only a few minutes or a few hours. Sometimes the condition assumes more serious proportions, and the regurgitating persists and may become chronic. In such cases the wall of the crop often seemingly loses muscle tone and becomes filled to varying degrees with a mucoid fluid. When this condition is present, the bird frequently regurgitates and may flip some of the material on top of his head and upper neck. This material then dries and causes the feathers to assume a "pasted-together" appearance. The bird may then rub or scratch at the feathers in an effort to fluff them up into a more nearly normal state.

This condition of the crop can prove to be a formidable problem. The etiological factors are not clear. One might speculate about chemical irritants, infectious agents, nutritional imbalances or deficiencies, or possibly some physiological breakdown in the digestive process. At any rate, the resultant condition is an abnormal crop, as previously described. Prognosis is directly related to the extent of crop involvement and the length of time the condition has been present. In Minsky's experience the most effective approach has been to empty the crop two or three times daily by *holding the bird head down* and "milking" out the fluid with gentle steady pressure on the crop until it has been evacuated. Oral medication is then administered immediately. We have relied mainly on an oxytetracycline hydrochloride solution,* and liquid multiple vitamin preparations. These drugs are given in doses measured by the drop for convenience of administration. The oxytetracycline is administered orally at the rate of 2 drops 3 times daily. This delivers approximately 8 mg. per day. The dosage is empiric and was arrived at by trial and observation over a period of years. The multiple vitamin preparation is administered orally at a rate of 1 or 2 drops daily or given in the drinking water at a rate of 5 drops per ounce.

Placing medicines in drinking water is not a very satisfactory method of administration, because changes in color or taste usually discourage water consumption which at best is quite limited (2–5 ml. daily) even in the normal bird. It cannot be denied that there are some problems in trying to administer medicine with a dropper directly into the oral cavity of a budgerigar, parrot, or canary, but it is a method which assures a reasonable degree of accuracy and constancy of dosage (see description in Chapter 9). Moreover, it can be done and has been done for many years by bird owners with the guidance of the veterinarian and the aid of a demonstration. It has been suggested that ophthalmic ointments carrying antibiotics can be administered orally; however, the problems of accurate dosage plus the characteristics of the vehicle seem to make this method of drug administration impractical.

Arnall[1] mentioned the regurgitation of brown fluid in budgerigars. He treated the condition successfully with oral administration of sulfadimidine 5% (sulfamethazine) with kaolin and precipitated calcium carbonate—3 drops three times daily. The birds were then given softer foods, powdered dried yeast (heat-killed), a little fruit and green food, milk, soaked seed, and vitamin B complex.

A common cause of regurgitation of seed and mucoid secretion in budgerigars is compression of the lower esophagus by hyperplastic thyroid glands. Dyspnea and various wheezing, clicking, or crying sounds may or may not precede or accompany the alimentary symptoms. For further discussion and treatment of this condition, see Chapter 22, on Diseases of the Endocrine System.

Beach[4] described an idiopathic necrotic inflammation of the crop observed in 55 budgerigars. Clinical signs included a green slimy froth exuding from the beak and almost always the presence of a green diarrhea. In one aviary in which 21 cases occurred, 18 birds were found dead. With the exception of these cases, the majority of birds died after 2 days of illness. Almost

*Liquamycin Injectable—Pfizer Laboratories, New York, N.Y.

all were aviary or recently purchased birds. The condition has not been found in pet birds kept indoors. Diets have consisted of canary and millet seed. In addition, some birds had green food and some had cod liver oil.

Necropsy findings revealed the epithelial surface covered with yellow caseous material with papilliform projections, giving it a terry-cloth appearance. This lesion sometimes extended over the whole crop and up the esophagus as far as the buccal cavity, or over a more limited part of this area. Varying amounts of caseous material occupied the lumen.

Histologic examination revealed congestion of the submucosa, some mucoid degeneration of the epithelial cells when these were still present, and areas where the whole depth of the epithelium had disappeared. The surface consisted of a thick layer of amorphous eosinophilic material, representing the caseous material seen macroscopically, in which occasional fragments of nuclear debris and clumps of bacteria could be seen. A layer of bacteria was sometimes seen on the surface.

Beach could not transmit the disease and did not recall seeing it before 1954. He claimed satisfactory results following the use of several antibiotics. The condition is not usually epizootic and does not appear to be transmitted directly from bird to bird. Keymer[14] reported that a similar condition was seen once in a violet-eared waxbill (*Granatina granatina*) and once in a star finch (*Bathilda ruficauda*).

IMITATION "COURTSHIP FEEDING"

Regurgitation of moist seed by an apparently healthy budgerigar is probably a neurosis. Male birds, primarily, will feed a mirror image, a favorite toy, or any shiny object. This is imitation "courtship feeding." Removal of the object of attempted feeding will usually cure the condition for the time being. Petrak saw one very stubborn case involving regurgitation of large quantities of seed by a budgerigar even to dull objects, if all shiny objects were removed. The bird became weak and depressed from semi-starvation. The only treatment that has been of any avail involves frequent environmental changes. Placing the bird in a different cage every two weeks keeps the condition under control. A hen as a companion has not helped. Parrots have been known to regurgitate to sweet-talking owners.

CANDIDIASIS

Keymer[14] reported that parrots, pigeons, pheasants, and partridges may develop monilial infection (candidiasis) of the crop. This usually takes the form of whitish flocculent mucus loosely adherent to the crop epithelium.

IMPACTION OF THE CROP

Impaction of the crop is rare in pet birds. Arnall[2] reported that a dry impaction of the crop may be encountered in most species. When the content is normal food, the cause may be neuromuscular stasis, greedy feeding in laying birds, obstructive foreign bodies, or inflammation of the lower alimentary tract. Caged wild insectivores may have an impaction caused by hair mixed with food or by overly fibrous foods. Beach[5] reported that crop impaction is not uncommon in young male budgerigars, and is usually attributed to overeating. Occasionally, a bird that has been denied grit for some time will gorge grit when it is newly available, and its crop will become impacted.[15] This should be kept in mind when grit has been withheld as a therapeutic measure.

The administration of a few drops of mineral oil, followed by gentle manipulation, should help to break up the impacting mass. If the mass fails to yield to such treatment, surgical intervention is indicated. (See Chapter 11 for a description of the surgical technique.)

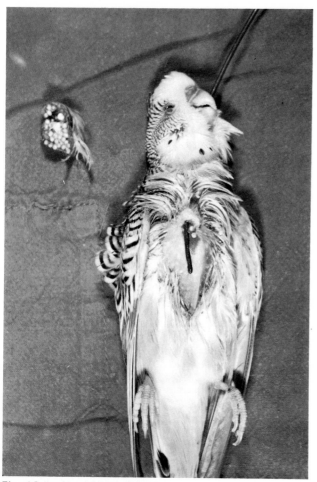

Fig. 18-1. *Impaction of the crop, with subsequent necrosis of the crop and overlying skin.*

INJURY TO THE CROP

Injury to the crop is not uncommon and is usually the result of a cat having clawed or bitten the bird, producing laceration of the crop. Repairing the crop is a rather delicate procedure. Standard surgical techniques are used, care being taken to completely close the crop wall. If the wound is not large, a purse-string suture works well. Occasionally, a wound or resulting infection may cause necrosis of such a large area of the crop that repair is impossible (Fig. 18-1).

DISORDERS OF PROVENTRICULUS AND GIZZARD

Proventriculitis and inflammation of the gizzard (ventriculus) are usually associated with a generalized condition rather than constituting specific problems in themselves.

Keymer[12] stated that catarrhal inflammation of the proventriculus and erosion or ulceration of the gizzard lining both cause regurgitation. This condition is commonest in debilitated, aged parrots and is rarely seen in budgerigars. Treatment consists of giving easily digestible and nourishing food such as bread and milk, cooked oatmeal with glucose and milk, banana, peanut butter on bread, and a paste made from crushed, hulled sunflower seeds. Antibiotics such as oxytetracycline* or chloramphenicol† should be administered orally. In waterfowl, the gizzard worm, *Amidostomum anseris*, is a common cause of erosion of the horny lining of the gizzard.

Keymer[14] reported that in debilitated waterfowl the proventriculus and gizzard are commonly the site of impaction with vegetation and mud or fine grit. The gizzard is most commonly impacted in gallinaceous birds, and lesions of the proventriculus are uncommon.

Beach[4] reported the occurrence of an intussusception of the proventriculus into the gizzard in a 2-year-old female budgerigar. The intussusception created a large bulge in the upper soft-walled part of the gizzard. The bird had shown symptoms of being cold and out of sorts for five months, during which time it had eaten only soaked canary seed, which presumably it could digest. A similar lesion was also seen in a 10-year-old parrot that collapsed 12 hours before death. The bird was thin, with an empty crop and gizzard. There was some erosion of epithelium at the site of the intussusception.

*Terramycin—Pfizer Laboratories, New York, N.Y.
†Chloromycetin palmitate—Parke, Davis & Co., Detroit, Mich.

Atrophy of the gizzard musculature was once observed by Petrak in an aged parrot. When presented for treatment the bird was cachectic. Hulled sunflower seeds were observed in the droppings. At necropsy the gizzard was found to be a thin-walled sac, with no musculature remaining. The cause was unknown. The same clinical picture occurred in a 4-year-old cockatiel, but this bird did not come to necropsy. The owner was advised to feed soft nutritious foods that would not require maceration by the gizzard.

DISORDERS OF THE INTESTINES

CONSTIPATION

Constipation as a separate entity is rather rare. Conditions such as abdominal tumors or cysts which may interfere with normal bowel activity may mechanically induce constipation. Usually there is a reduced frequency of elimination in such cases, with periodic large evacuations due to forceful efforts by the bird to defecate. Arnall[2] recorded the causes of constipation as:

(1) astringent substances;
(2) excess fibrous material or grit;
(3) poor muscle tone due to inactivity or obesity;
(4) pressure on rectum due to retained egg;
(5) neoplasm;
(6) hernia;
(7) pseudocoprostasis.

Treatment, if deemed advisable, consists of removal of the cause if possible, followed by soapy water enemas administered with a medicine dropper of appropriate size or soft plastic tubing, and gentle manipulation. The enema should be repeated in several hours if no results are obtained. Mineral oil may be administered orally with a medicine dropper. Fruit or green foods should be added to the diet. Grit should be removed temporarily if this is a factor in causation.

ENTERITIS

Enteritis is by far the most common condition noted in pet birds. It may be a primary condition or it may be part of the picture of a generalized disease. The complaint that the bird suffers from diarrhea with or without other symptoms is very frequent. Chilling may be a factor. The history usually reveals a sudden onset combined with some disturbance in ordinary routine or conditions, such as not covering the bird at night, an open window, a windy day with excessive drafts, or a rapid overnight fall in temperature. There may also be a history of a different seed being used, and the possibility of the presence of dirt or infected material

should be considered. Fright from a marauding cat or physical injury may be the exciting cause. Abdominal tumors affecting the kidneys or causing pressure on the intestine may also induce diarrhea.[11]

Clinical signs and symptoms are fluffing-up, malaise, diarrhea, soiling of feathers around the vent, increased grit consumption, polydipsia, and perching on both feet. Anorexia may follow, with the bird husking seeds but refusing to eat them.[23]

Stone[23] further reported that parrots and mynahs are prone to develop hemorrhagic enteritis. The ingestion of table food, spoiled food, and, at times, excessive liquor or beer may be the exciting cause. He suggests no food for 24 hours followed by seed and no other food. Various other treatments suggested are 25 mg. tetracycline dissolved in 1 oz. of water daily for 4 to 7 days, 3 drops of buttermilk by mouth to change the intestinal flora, and 5 drops of paregoric in 1 oz. of drinking water for 3 or 4 days.[23]

Keymer[13] reported that newly imported birds, deprived of grit for a long time, may eat it excessively when it is first supplied. He advises feeding small quantities until the appetite is normal.

Probably the most common cause of enteritis is bacterial infection. Vallée and Guillon,[24] as reported by Gerlach,[10] stated that *Escherichia coli* plays an important role in causing enteritis in canary flocks, particularly during the nestling period. Diarrhea occurs from the fifth day after hatching. Granulomas are seen not only in the abdomen, but also in the skin of the head and neck between the 10th and the 15th day of life. Sometimes the auditory canal is involved, which may result in symptoms of central nervous system disorder. Parents are considered to be carriers, because the nestlings are sick before they start eating by themselves. Infections with *E. coli* should be treated with antibiotics indicated by the results of sensitivity testing.

Beach[4] recorded 38 deaths from enteritis among 866 budgerigars examined post mortem. Of the 38, 12 birds were pets, 13 were from one breeder, and 13 were from seven other breeders; 18 were less than 1 year old. Cultures on ox-blood agar at 37°C. of material from 29 of the birds resulted in 5 with no growth and 15 with scanty mixed growths of unlikely significance; 3 yielded pure cultures of *E. coli,* which was considered significant, since gram-negative organisms are not usually present in the intestines of normal budgerigars. Other organisms which appeared to be significant were *Chromobacterium* (1 case) and *Staphylococcus* (2 cases).

Bacterial infection as a cause of enteritis is dealt with further in the first section of Chapter 24. The use of appropriate antibiotics, chemotherapeutic agents, and various supportive medications by oral and parenteral administration is helpful.

It is not uncommon to find birds eating an unusual amount of gravel during periods of digestive disturbances. Prevention of excessive consumption of gravel during such periods is advisable since the gravel may further contribute to the irritation of the digestive tract. Laxative foods such as greens and fruit should be avoided until the diarrhea has stopped.

The availability of clean fresh seed and fresh water, supplemented with multiple vitamin drops, is helpful in good nursing care of a sick bird. Increasing the environmental temperature until the fluffed-up appearance is gone should be standard procedure in any illness.

PROLAPSE OF THE CLOACA

If diarrhea persists, it may lead to prolapse of the cloaca, which may also result from efforts to pass a retained egg. This condition can prove quite serious and should be dealt with as soon as possible. The bird should be anesthetized and the cloacal mucous membrane coated with an ointment or oily medication containing either a local anesthetic or corticosteroid, or both, and an antibiotic, preferably neomycin sulfate. The prolapse is then reduced manually, and the cloaca can be further reoriented by introducing a thermometer and moving it about gently. A purse-string suture of light-weight non-absorbable material is then placed around the margin of the vent and tied; the opening should be just large enough to permit the entrance of the thermometer but with very little space to spare. This will permit evacuation but at the same time prevent recurrence of the prolapse. Treatment of the condition causing the diarrhea must follow. Usually the purse-string suture can be removed in one week unless the bird still has an obvious, persistent diarrhea.

PERITONITIS

In our experience, peritonitis has usually occurred as part of an air-sac infection or in conjunction with tumors or cystic conditions. "Egg peritonitis" is discussed in Chapter 20.

COCCIDIOSIS

Gerlach[10] reported that coccidiosis, as a rule, is not a problem in cage birds. In Passeriformes, species of the genus *Isospora* are seen. In Falconiformes, besides *Isospora, Caryospora* species are found. Neither genus has the strict host-specificity of *Eimeria* or the complete self-sterilizing effect, provided there is no reinfection (Schwalbach,[22] as reported by Gerlach[10]). Pathogenicity of these coccidia seems to be low and to depend on unsanitary conditions or stresses. *Isospora* oocysts are shed only in the late afternoon. This knowledge may be helpful when planning sanitary measures. Gerlach[10] knows of no reports of the effectiveness of coccidiostats against species other than *Eimeria* in birds. Lühmann,[19] as reported by Gerlach,[10] stated that many of the coccidiostats are more toxic to pet birds than to chickens and turkeys. Obviously, these drugs should not be used on a new species until they have been tested experimentally and favorable results reported. For further discussion of intestinal parasitism see Chapter 25.

LIVER DISEASE

According to Gerlach,[10] the liver parenchyma is involved in many pathological processes of infectious or non-infectious nature. Conditions of the liver and of the intestine may influence each other. Any disturbance of the liver may cause a diarrhea which is clinically indistinguishable from that resulting from enteritis. Specific clinical symptoms of liver diseases, such as jaundice, are rare. Gerlach stated further that greyish or yellowish foci and variously sized or confluent areas of degenerated cells, with or without hemorrhages or fibrinous exudate at the capsule surface, are generally indications of an infectious process. A congested and swollen dark-red liver may be due to cardiac failure or may be agonal.

Keymer[14] stated that congestion of the liver may be caused by an infectious disease, but if the liver of a dead psittacine is also swollen with rounded edges, psittacosis should be suspected. This is especially true if splenomegaly is also observed. He further stated that small pin-point, yellowish necrotic lesions may be seen in psittacosis, salmonellosis, or pseudotuberculosis. In tuberculosis the lesions are caseous and may be several millimeters in diameter. Histomoniasis is particularly common in peafowl and also occurs in pheasants, quail, and partridges. For a discussion of specific infections see the appropriate chapters.

ACUTE HEPATITIS

Beach[4] reported 20 cases of acute hepatitis among 866 budgerigars examined after death; two thirds of the cases were from aviaries, and all but 3 were in hens. Petrak encountered three cases of hepatitis in pet budgerigars, two in males and one in a female. Beach stated that the liver was enlarged or of abnormal color in some cases, but in many instances lesions were seen only microscopically. The birds seen by Petrak had enlarged, yellow-brown livers.

Several of the birds examined by Beach had died

without showing symptoms, but one or two had been ill for up to a month. In two of Petrak's cases there were signs of lethargy and diarrhea. One of these birds also exhibited polydipsia, and the other was thin and dyspneic before death.

Beach described the prominent lesions as discrete dense foci of round cells often associated with necrotic areas. In six cases the necrosis was very widespread and the cellular infiltration scanty. The predominant cells were usually lymphocytes, but in some cases with more obvious necrosis neutrophils were present, and in others most of the cells were histiocytes. Petrak's cases all showed fatty change and infiltration with heterophils. In addition, two birds had duplication of bile ducts and one of these also showed a fibrinous capsular exudate.

In three of Beach's cases an associated pneumonia occurred, and, in one, a focal nephritis. There were no consistent bacteriological findings; in about half the cases cultures from the liver showed no growth. In four other birds reported on by Beach, a more diffuse round cell infiltration was seen. The sinusoids were packed with lymphocytes in one. In another there were only occasional groups of round cells, but large areas of pink hyaline material were seen, leaving only small islands of liver cells. The etiology in all the cases was unknown.

CHRONIC HEPATITIS

Beach[4] reported five cases of hepatitis in budgerigars with lesions suggesting chronic inflammation. They were characterized by fibrosis. Petrak had four cases in budgerigars with lesions suggestive of chronic liver disease. Signs and symptoms in Petrak's cases included intermittent bouts of lethargy and reduced food intake for 6 months; not "seeming himself" for 2 years, with terminal diarrhea and lethargy for several weeks; and dermatitis in the cervical region. Petrak observed moist dermatitis in the axillary region in several budgerigars with liver disease; it is not known if there is a relationship between the two conditions.

In three of Beach's cases there was round cell infiltration, and in two there were proliferative changes in the bile ducts. One bird had a large, fibrous swelling $2.5 \times 2.0 \times 1.0$ cm., replacing almost the entire liver. Petrak's cases were characterized by cirrhosis, redundancy of bile ducts, bile retention, and in one case a heterophilic pericholangitis. In all cases, the stimulating cause or causes were unknown.

VIRUS HEPATITIS

Ratcliffe[20] first recognized virus hepatitis as a cause of death of birds in the Philadelphia Zoological Garden during 1946. For a discussion of the disease, see Chapter 24.

Burtscher,[8] as cited by Gerlach,[10] described a specific virus hepatitis in European owls. Miliary foci were seen in the liver and spleen. Reticulum cells in the liver and spleen showed intranuclear inclusion bodies. Intestines, larynx, lungs, and bone marrow may be involved in the pathological process. This condition is a frequent cause of death in owls in Europe.

Rosen *et al.*[21] have published a preliminary study of a specific virus hepatitis of pheasants in California. Inclusion bodies were seen in liver cells. Quail are considered to be carriers of the disease.

Levine and Fabricant[18] and Asplin and McLauchlan[3] reported the isolation of a specific virus from ducks with hepatitis in the United States and Great Britain, respectively.

FATTY CHANGE

Fatty change is a non-specific condition that occurs not infrequently in the livers of psittacine birds. It is noted most often in budgerigars, but this may be due only to the fact that they so outnumber all other psittacines in pet bird practice. Coffin[9] noted its occurrence in parrots; Arnall,[2] its occurrence in parrots and cockatoos; Beach[4] and Lafeber,[17] its occurrence in budgerigars; Buckley,[7] its occurrence in lovebirds. Petrak has seen it in budgerigars, cockatiels, parrots, and cockatoos.

The etiology is unknown. It may be postulated that there are genetic factors predisposing to its occurrence when certain nutritional, toxic, infectious, allergic, or environmental conditions act as triggering devices. Disturbances in carbohydrate and lipid metabolism may prove to be rewarding fields for future study.

Beach[4] recorded 37 cases in budgerigars in which fatty change in the liver was the main lesion. This was from his group of 866 necropsies in budgerigars, giving a frequency of occurrence of 4.3 per cent. The affected birds ranged in age from 6 months to 9 years, and twice as many males as females were affected. In 13 similar cases in budgerigars studied by Petrak, ages ranged from 1 year to 7 years, with an average of 4 years, and males outnumbered females 5 to 1. No statistical significance can be given to the age or sex distribution, since population studies have not been done.

Twenty-five of Beach's cases occurred in pet birds and the remainder in aviary birds. All of Petrak's cases involved pet birds. Symptoms and signs noted by Beach (and the numbers of cases in which they occurred) were:

(1) obesity (25);
(2) abdominal swelling due to enlarged liver (7);

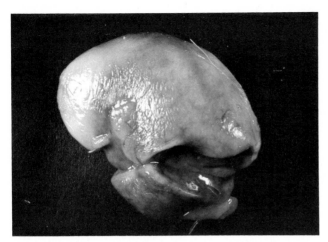

Fig. 18-2. *The liver of a 4-year-old male budgerigar, showing enlargement from extensive fat infiltration.*

(3) convulsions (2);
(4) blindness (2);
(5) inability to fly (2);
(6) "wheezing" respiration (2);
(7) sternal fat deposits (2);
(8) "off-color" one day (1);
(9) died following surgery (1).

Fifteen of the birds were found dead, without having shown premonitory symptoms.

Petrak noted the following signs and symptoms, with the number of cases indicated in parentheses:

(1) some degree of abdominal bulging (13);
(2) "off-color" (10—3 for 2 days, 1 for 3 days, 1 for 1 week, 2 for 1 month, 1 for 3 months, 1 for 8 months, 1 for 1 year);
(3) loose droppings (9)—white, green, black;

(4) obesity (7);
(5) subcutaneous lipomatosis (4);
(6) polydipsia (4)—all with loose droppings;
(7) regurgitation (2);
(8) thin (2);
(9) died after awakening from anesthesia (2);
(10) convulsive seizures (2), followed by blindness (1);
(11) Mild epistaxis (1)—evidenced by brown discoloration of the feathers adjacent to the cere.

In the majority of cases the liver is grossly enlarged (Fig. 18-2), and its color may range from varying shades of yellow or light brown to cream or light pink. Histological examination reveals replacement of liver cells with fat.

Diagnosis may be made by abdominal palpation and radiography if necessary. Treatment as described by Lafeber[17] consists of daily injections of a lipotropic substance* and vitamin B complex. This is followed by home treatment with the lipotropic substance and a multiple vitamin given in the drinking water daily and brewer's yeast or other nutritive powder added to the seed. Possible medication and dosages for budgerigars are listed by Lafeber[16] as follows:

Methischol*—0.01 ml. per 30-gm. budgerigar.
Bejectal Improved with vitamin C†—0.005 ml. per 30-gm. budgerigar.

The prognosis is good unless the condition is extreme. Success of treatment is evidenced by an increase in vigor and a decrease in size of the liver.[17]

---

*Methischol—U.S. Vitamin & Pharmaceutical Corp., New York, N.Y.

†Bejectal Improved with vitamin C—Abbott Laboratories, Chicago, Ill.'

References

1. ARNALL, L.: Experiences with cage-birds. Vet. Rec. *70:* 120–128, 1958.

2. ARNALL, L.: Anaesthesia and surgery in cage and aviary birds. III. A systematic outline of surgical conditions. Vet. Rec. *73:*188–192, 1961.

3. ASPLIN, F. D., and McLAUCHLAN, J. D.: Duck virus hepatitis. Vet. Rec. *66:*456–458, 1954.

4. BEACH, J. E.: Diseases of budgerigars and other cage birds. A survey of *post-mortem* findings. Vet. Rec. *74:*10–15, 1962.

5. BEACH, J. E.: Some of the major problems of budgerigar pathology. J. small anim. Pract. *6:*15–20, 1965.

6. BEACH, J. E., WILKINSON, J. S., and HARVEY, D. G.: Calculus in the crop of a budgerigar *Melopsittacus undulatus.* Vet. Rec. *72:*473, 1960.

7. BUCKLEY, P. A.: Personal communication, 1966.

8. BURTSCHER, —: Über eine virusbedingte Einschlusskörperchen-Hepatitis und -Lienitis bei Eulenvögeln. Allg. Path. *107:*96, 1965.

9. COFFIN, D. L.: *The Care, Feeding and Diseases of Psittacine Pets.* Angell Memorial Parakeet and Parrot Book, Boston, Mass., 1953. 32 pp.

10. GERLACH, H.: Lectures on Pet Birds, Mimeographed notes, U. of C., Davis, Calif., 1966.

11. JONES, O. G.: Common diseases of cage birds and other less usual pets. Vet. Rec. *68:*918–933, 1956.

12. KEYMER, I. F.: The diagnosis and treatment of common psittacine diseases. Mod. Vet. Pract. *39*(21):22–30, December 15, 1958.

13. KEYMER, I. F.: The diagnosis and treatment of some diseases of seed-eating passerine birds. Mod. Vet. Pract. *40*(7):30–34, April 1, 1959.

14. KEYMER, I. F.: Postmortem examinations of pet birds. Mod. Vet. Pract. *42*(23):35–38, December 1, 1961.

15. LAFEBER, T. J.: Personal communication, 1966.

16. LAFEBER, T. J.: The Medication of Budgerigars (Common Parakeets). In *Current Veterinary Therapy, 1966–1967,* R. W. Kirk, ed. Philadelphia, W. B. Saunders Company, 1966. Pp. 520–521.

17. LAFEBER, T. J.: Digestive System Disturbances of the Budgerigar. In *Current Veterinary Therapy, 1966–1967,* R. W. Kirk, ed. Philadelphia, W. B. Saunders Company, 1966. Pp. 535–538.

18. LEVINE, P. P., and FABRICANT, J.: A hitherto-undescribed virus disease of ducks in North America. Cornell Vet. *40:*71–86, 1950.

19. LÜHMANN, M.: Untersuchungen über die Verträglichkeit einiger Coccidiostatica im Aufzuchtfutter für Gänse. Arch. f. Geflügelk. *28:*368–377, 1964.

20. RATCLIFFE, H. L.: Hepatitis, cirrhosis, and hepatoma in birds. Cancer Res. *21:*26–30, 1961.

21. ROSEN, M. N., HUNTER, B. F., and BRUNETTI, O. A.: Preliminary study of an infectious hepatitis in pheasants. Avian Dis. *9:*382–393, 1965.

22. SCHWALBACH, G.: Die Coccidiose der Singvögel. I. Der Ausscheidungsrhythmus der Isospora-Oocysten beim Haussperling (Passer domesticus). Zbl. f. Bakt. I Orig. *178:*263–276, 1960. II. Beobachtungen an Isospora-Oocysten aus einem Weichfresser (Parus major) mit besonderer Berücksichtigung des Ausscheidungsrhythmus. Zbl. f. Bakt. I Orig. *181:*264–279, 1961.

23. STONE, R. M.: Prevalent problems and treatment of pet birds. Vet. Med./Small Anim. Clinician *62:*142–151, 1967.

24. VALLÉE, A., and GUILLON, J. C.: Coligranulomatose dans un élevage de canaris. Bull. Acad. Vet. France *37:*35–36, 1964.

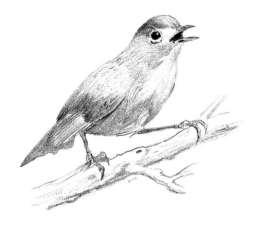

19

Diseases
of the
Urinary System

Jens Hasholt

Diseases of the urinary system are commonly diagnosed in birds, at necropsy. They have been demonstrated in practically every species of birds,[15] the rare exceptions being species of which only a few specimens, if any, have been kept in zoological gardens. The diseases are, of course, best known within the group of commercial poultry—fowls, ducks, geese, and turkeys—and in pigeons. Among cage and aviary birds, it must be admitted that, although within recent years a certain knowledge of the morbid anatomy relating to diseases of the urinary system has been acquired, little is known regarding the clinical manifestations of these diseases.

Care must be taken not to apply to birds the knowledge and experience gained regarding diseases of the urinary system of mammals; these two animal species differ too much anatomically, and even more physiologically. There is, for instance, no urinary bladder in birds. The ureters of birds, like those of reptiles, empty into the urodeum, and the urine is discharged together with the feces.

That the fluid balance must be different is evident from, among other things, the fact that the urine of birds normally varies in consistency from pasty to dry. Finally, the protein metabolism in birds proceeds in a different way. The difference in this respect is, perhaps, the most important one. The chief metabolic breakdown or waste product is not urea, as in mammals, but uric acid.

It would seem reasonable to compare the various species of birds, especially commercial poultry and cage birds. However, even the results of such a comparison must be accepted with great reservation, in the first place because of the great difference in the food consumed (as between seed-eaters, fruit-eaters, insect-eaters, nectar-eaters, birds of prey, and other types). Differences may even prevail within an apparently uniform group. Within the group of seed-eaters, for instance, it makes a difference whether birds of the species concerned husk the seed before eating it or not. Such a difference in habit will result in an appreciable difference in the amount and composition of proteins derived from the same kind of seed, and the birds that consume both husk and kernel will have a need for sand, gravel, or pebbles (so-called grit).

INCIDENCE OF URINARY SYSTEM DISEASE

To judge from the literature, there is little agreement concerning the incidence of diseases of the urinary system in birds, the characterization ranging from exceedingly frequent, relatively common and not infrequent, to rare. Exact figures are few. Fiennes[8] gives 17 per cent, Beach,[3] 9.7 per cent, Appleby,[1] 7 per cent in psittacine birds and only 3 per cent in passerines, and Lindt,[14] no more than 0.97 per cent.

This disagreement is doubtless due to differences in the evaluations on which the statements are based. Based on pure renal diseases alone (*i.e.,* diseases explainable solely or primarily by the renal changes) the figures are low. On the other hand, inclusion of all the cases in which a general debility or systemic disease is responsible for the renal changes (*e.g.,* organ degeneration in infectious diseases or intoxications) results in high but also somewhat varying figures. The few figures stated for clinically diagnosed diseases of the urinary system in cage birds are so low (0.88 per cent[10]) as to be of practically no value. It is, in fact, generally agreed that diseases of the urinary system are unrecognizable clinically.

All of the quoted statements include gout, which constitutes up to 50 per cent of the cases reported. This fact is pointed out because it is highly doubtful whether gout is referable at all to the diseases of the urinary system.

DIAGNOSIS OF DISEASES OF THE URINARY SYSTEM

TYPES OF DISEASES

ACUTE: Infectious nephritis occurs in fowl, and renal changes due to poisoning have been produced experimentally. In cage birds, necropsy has revealed acute renal changes, which could not be diagnosed clinically. Accidental injury to the kidneys resulting from bites or crushing has been seen in rare instances.

CHRONIC: Such lesions can be diagnosed with reasonable certainty in a number of cases.

NEOPLASMS: Deforming neoplasms in the abdomen are difficult to recognize in the early stages but are more easily diagnosed in advanced stages. However, the site of origin of the neoplasm can be established with certainty only by exploratory laparotomy or at necropsy.

NECROPSY DIAGNOSIS

Gross (Inspection)	*Microscopic (Histological)*
acute	nephrosis
	degeneration
	nephritis
	hemorrhage
	congestion (nephrosis)
chronic	degeneration (necrosis, fat)
	nephritis (glomerul. indurat.)
	infection (tuberculosis, lymphomatosis)
deforming	parasitic
	cyst
	tumor
	calculus
deposit	uric acid (tubules, ureter) concretions

DIFFICULTY IN ESTABLISHING DIAGNOSIS

Although the findings at necropsy, combined with those obtained by bacteriological and histological tests, are exceedingly interesting and instructive, it must be admitted that the owner and consequently the veterinarian are primarily concerned with the living bird. The signs and symptoms leading to the correct diagnosis and thus to proper treatment deserve the greatest attention.

A review of the literature on this subject was rather depressing. Only a few workers have concentrated on this question,[4,5,7,10,12,13,16] and Coffin's statement that "no symptoms are diagnostic and no treatment is worthwhile,"[4] is very much to the point as regards the results they have achieved.

Neither does the abundant literature on diseases of poultry give any criteria for establishing the diagnosis—not even Cumming's description[6] of infectious nephritis. The literature on experimental renal damage[18,19,21] is equally deficient in this respect. However, Selye[18,19] and Søndergaard *et al.*[21] stress the importance of extending the observations to include circulatory and nervous disorders as well, and, last but not least, they emphasize the appropriateness of laboratory analysis of the urine.

Acute Diseases

In an individual case it is impossible to make a diagnosis of acute renal disease on the basis of the clinical examination alone. It is similarly impossible to differentiate between the various acute renal diseases known from a single necropsy. However, if one is confronted with a relatively large series of birds, of which many are ill and some die, correlation of the results of clinical and postmortem examinations can provide a reasonable basis for a suspicion of acute renal disease. These diseases may be caused by infection (bacteria, viruses), parasitic invasion (coccidia, malaria), poisoning (chemical, vegetable, organic, enterogenous), and allergy.

In the great majority of cases the renal changes, ranging from reversible cytoplasmic changes (nephrosis) to severe degenerative lesions with disintegration of cell nuclei, from mild hyperemia and congestion to regular inflammatory states, are to be regarded as secondary. In such cases the renal changes are a consequence of or constitute part of a general disease, involving, for instance, the alimentary tract, liver, spleen, or circulatory system. This probably explains why so little interest has been shown thus far in the renal diseases. It is, admittedly, far more important to concentrate on combating the primary cause of illness, the more so because it is known, from the experimentally provoked renal diseases, that the nephroses, for instance, will subside spontaneously if the inciting cause is removed. The fact that the kidney condition is secondary to another disease doubtless accounts also for the nonspecific signs and symptoms. The quality of the urine cannot be evaluated on the basis of short-term observations. Accordingly, in acute cases even analysis of the urine will be of no aid in diagnosis.

The following uncommon diseases of the urinary system may be worth mentioning:

Acute purulent nephritis and ureteritis due to an ascending infection from an inflamed urodeum are occasional findings at necropsy, but these inflammatory processes usually are not diagnosed clinically, because death generally occurs at an early stage of the disease.

It is commonly believed that birds may die from shock (apoplexy) as a result merely of being held in the hand and examined. Personally I have never experienced this, but I have seen birds asphyxiated because the owner or assistant failed to hold them correctly. In the reported cases of shock, cerebral and spinal hemorrhages are mentioned as the causes of death. In various other cases, in which death occurred shortly after treatment (injection of penicillin), necropsy revealed pronounced renal hemorrhages and changes due to congestion. Such cases have been observed by Aronson *et al.*[2] among fowl, and by Hauser[11] among parrots. They all believe death was due to allergic shock.

In the case of a pet bird in which diarrhea suddenly develops, sodium chloride poisoning should be suspected. It is—at least in Denmark—a commonly held view among bird owners that cage birds need salt, and even a lot of it. There is, however, every reason to be on one's guard against provision of too great an amount. Selye[19] has shown that physiological saline solution used as drinking water causes severe damage to the urinary system, and Shaw[20] demonstrated that many migrating birds are killed every year by drinking brackish water. Selye[18] further called attention to the fact that desoxycorticosterone acetate (DOCA) may cause renal changes.

Acute, common-salt poisoning was diagnosed in a blue-fronted amazon (*Amazona aestiva*) after intake of some salted meat. The bird died in a short time from severe enteritis with blood-stained droppings. Necropsy revealed a hemorrhagic enteritis as well as moderately swollen, pale kidneys. Unwashed beach- or sea-sand scattered heavily on cage floors must be suspected as the cause of several deaths among canaries. The birds died without preceding signs or symptoms or after a short period of discharging liquid droppings. Necropsy either showed nothing abnormal—either histologically or bacteriologically—or revealed swollen kidneys, occasionally with marked deposits of uric acid. Such fatalities ceased immediately after removal of the sand.

If the kidneys, which lie thoroughly protected in recesses of the synsacrum, are injured by external violence the damage done is so excessive that it is always a greater act of mercy to kill the bird immediately and examine the kidneys afterward.

Chronic Diseases

Within this group of diseases, the making of anything like an exact diagnosis requires that the patient be kept under careful observation in the hospital. The data available from the owner are rarely of any aid. The bird is most often stated to have been ailing for some time; its mood is reported to have been changing, as has its appetite. Its drinking habits are hardly ever known. The droppings are stated to vary in consistency, but are most often liquid. To make a positive diagnosis the veterinarian must collect all the details available, compare them with his previous observations, and evaluate them on the basis of his earlier experience.

As stated previously, the general condition is rather poor, as, in fact, it is in the case of practically any disease. Only by observing the bird for a fairly long time will the slight differences become conspicuous and the bird's behavior become of importance. Its mood is changing, but the bird is most often dispirited and quiet. It rests with both feet on the perch; the body is kept in a more oblique position than usual, with head and neck bent slightly backward, so that it seems to be somewhat sway-backed. (This is unlike the posture in proventriculitis, when the bird is perched in a more upright position with head bowed and back hunched.)

The feathers over the synsacrum, and to some extent over the abdomen, are more or less bristly. The eyes are generally open and of normal size, but dull and uninterested. (In proventriculitis-affected birds the eyes are half-closed and sunken, giving evidence of pain.) The respiration is usually normal, but slight tail-dipping may be seen in some instances. The legs and cere vary from being slightly discolored to dark blue in color, and may be fairly dry (dehydration).

The appetite varies, but is most often subnormal, causing the bird to lose weight. The bird seems to have no desire for special kinds of seeds, nor does it seem to care particularly for vegetables and fruit. (Normally the bird gets a large proportion of its fluid requirement from the food.) Regurgitation, which is very common in association with diseases of the upper part of the alimentary tract, has not been noticed in these cases. Excessive thirst, as manifested in chronic nephritis in mammals, has been seen only in relation to certain infectious diseases (Newcastle disease, salmonellosis) and intoxications (ergot or sodium chloride). An excessive thirst may also be a symptom of a pituitary tumor in budgerigars.[17]

In advanced cases of nephritis the abdomen is seen to be distended (ascites); the abdominal wall is slightly bulging, with fluctuating tenseness. A similar abdominal bulge may be seen in cases of neoplasm in the abdominal cavity, but such a tumor is palpable deep in the cavity at an early stage. If kidney disease has been present for some time, general weakness with a consequent unsteadiness on the perch will be noticed, but central nervous system disorders (such as convulsions) have not been observed.

The urine, which normally constitutes a thin, pure-white to yellow-white layer or streak round the feces, is changed in character. When diarrhea is present it is extremely difficult to judge the quality of the urine. Possible soiling of the feathers around the vent is not diagnostically significant. Discharge of abundant "white excrements" is not a sign of increased excretion of uric acid, but is a relatively frequent phenomenon in diseases of the alimentary tract.

To judge the quality of the excrements it is necessary to cover the floor of the cage with paper—preferably white paper. In cases of diarrhea a large, wet dropping is seen, with no sharp distinction between feces and urine. Occasionally, however, the urine is distinguishable as thin white threads in the liquid discharge. Presence of small lumps surrounded by a moist zone of varying size will arouse suspicion of urinary tract disease. Close examination of the excrements in such cases will reveal fairly solid fecal matter centrally, surrounded by a ring of gruel-like to watery material, clouded by deposits of uric acid. If the bird is nervous, it may discharge almost clear water, but this seems to have nothing to do with the urine. A pungent, although not acrid, smell may occasionally be noticed.

In the cases of dogs and cats a veterinarian would hardly venture to make a diagnosis of nephritis without performing laboratory analyses of blood and urine. Why then should one do so where birds are concerned? The answer to this question is simply that no practical methods are available yet for making such analyses feasible in practice. With small cage birds, for instance, it has been thought difficult to obtain sufficient blood for quantitative analysis. Such analyses have been carried out on blood from ducks, in which a blood uric-acid level of 6.7 mg./100 ml. has been found.[9] Further, ligation of the ureters has been observed to cause a considerable rise of the uric-acid concentration (blood-40 times, muscles-15 times, kidneys and liver-5 times), resulting in death within 12 hours.[9] It is doubtless possible to collect the required amount of excrement, dry it, and analyze it for uric acid, but the result achieved would depend on so many external and internal factors that it would simply be of no value. Excrements from fowl have been subjected to such analyses, with findings of 50–90 mg. uric acid per gm. of air-dried excrement.[22] Experiments have even been conducted with urine and feces being collected separately (by colostomy). Such methods are, however, definitely unsuitable in practice.

Neoplasms, Lymphomatosis, and Other Disorders

These disorders may cause very considerable deformities of the kidneys. Common to these conditions is the fact that they must be developed to a certain degree before any signs are manifested at all, or before they can be diagnosed. The disorder may be localized in the kidneys alone, or involve other organs as well, for example, the liver. The veterinarian rarely sees the patient until the abdomen is bulging. However, in these cases, as well as in cases in which no more than a slight infiltration is palpable, in some instances covered by accumulated fluid, exploratory laparotomy is required to establish the diagnosis. Patients seen at a very early stage, having been admitted on account of changing moods and varying consistencies of droppings, are characterized by an upright position on the perch. The abdomen seems to be distended, but it is only the feathers that bristle, thereby concealing the feet (the bird "warms its toes"). This picture is characteristic of birds with tumors of the testes. Another sign very commonly seen in birds with tumors of the testes or the kidneys is unilateral and sometimes bilateral paresis or paralysis resulting from circulatory disturbances or compression of the large nerve trunks. The tumors are most often carcinomas, but sarcomas and adenomas may also be seen.

Cystic changes in the kidneys, which are rare, may occur either as a single large cyst (Fig. 19-1) or as a conglomeration of smaller ones. Such changes cannot be distinguished clinically from tumors, a fact which makes no difference, the treatment, or perhaps rather the impossibility of treatment, being the same.

Mineral deposits are not demonstrable clinically. Calcium deposits have been seen only as accidental necropsy findings. Deposition of uric acid may be suspected in relation to gout, but is in many cases not attended by clinical signs or symptoms. There is even a possibility that some deposition may occur after death.

PROGNOSIS OF DISEASES OF THE URINARY SYSTEM

The nephroses may have a chance of spontaneous cure when the causes are removed. For all other diseases of the urinary system the prospects of recovery are poor. In some cases, by appropriate feeding the disease can be kept quiescent and the bird be given tolerable conditions of life for months.

TREATMENT OF DISEASES OF THE URINARY SYSTEM

Preventive measures, such as prevention of spread of infection by means of isolation or euthanasia of affected birds, along with the necessary appropriate sanitary measures, must, of course, be adopted immediately. Likewise, nutritional disturbances (due to poisoning, deficiency, or an inappropriate diet) must be promptly corrected.

The treatment of the renal disease itself comprises various general measures, mainly of a dietetic nature, and drug therapy. The latter, however, is of doubtful value.

The patient must not be exposed to cold, drafts, or dampness, but should be placed in a dry and warm room with an unrestricted opportunity for exercise and free access to boiled water (a mixture of equal parts of water and claret is said to have a good effect). The food must be altered so as to contain the smallest amount possible of protein (mainly different sorts of millet seed with a little thistle seed added). Concentrates and, in particular, supplementary food of animal origin, should be avoided. A supplement of grape sugar should be given to birds that are particularly weakened. Unrestricted access to vegetables and fruits of different kinds is important. No matter what the food is composed of, a vitamin A supplement is recommended. The amount of this vitamin required has not been investigated in cage birds, but in poultry it is of the order of 6,000 to 9,000 I.U. per kilogram of feed.

The drug treatment definitely gives the impression of being based on the pharmacologic facts relating to domestic animals and humans, and to be directed against gout, the only disease involving the urinary system recognized clinically in birds. The drugs used will be briefly commented on. As stated earlier, none of them

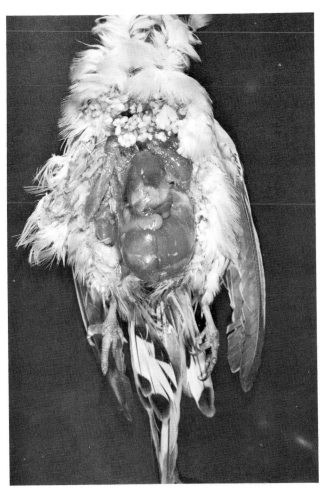

Fig. 19-1. *A large kidney cyst in a 5-year-old male budgerigar.*

can be claimed to have had any unquestionable clinical effect. We must look to other therapeutic possibilities for cure.

Colchicine, used in human medicine in cases of acute gouty arthritis, has been tried on birds in the form of a tincture, but without response. In this connection it should be borne in mind that the drug may have a highly irritating effect on the kidneys.

Salicylic acid and its salts, with their specific antirheumatic action, must also be reckoned among the proper gout-controlling drugs, and they also have a certain disinfecting effect on the urinary system. Salicylic acid has been given in doses of 0.05 to 0.2 gm., with no response.

Hexamine (hexamethylene tetramine) may be mentioned as a proper urinary tract disinfectant. (As is well known, the urinary tract is a very small organ in the bird.) Hexamine is said to be particularly active against *Escherichia coli* and to exert its effect by liberation of formaldehyde. However, as this liberation does not occur in alkaline or neutral solution, its action in birds, in whose urodeum the pH is 6.0–7.5, is undoubtedly questionable. Furthermore, the drug is stated to be highly irritating and to have caused hematuria.

Sulfonamides have also been claimed to be indicated, but no response to their use has been observed.

In cases of renal disease complicated by ascites use of a diuretic (*e.g.*, mersalyl) might be considered. In human medicine mersalyl is said to have a favorable effect on nephroses. However, since the drug is contraindicated in cases of nephritis and nephrosclerosis, it is hardly advisable to treat cage birds with it.

The most commonly employed therapeutic measure is addition of sodium bicarbonate to the drinking water (0.5–2%). However, the indication for this is not obvious, and clinical response to its use has been questionable as observed at the Veterinary Hospital in Copenhagen.

The veterinarian must realize and explain to his client that treatment of urinary tract diseases in cage birds at the present time has not gone beyond the experimental stage.

NECROPSY FINDINGS

It is extremely important for the veterinarian to supplement his clinical observations with postmortem examinations whenever possible. Permission for this, however, is often difficult to obtain. Aversion to necropsy, a desire for burial or—though more rarely—stuffing, and difficulties of transportation of the body, especially in the warm season, are among the most frequent problems arising in this connection.

At necropsy the organs should preferably be examined with a magnifying glass, because many changes cannot be seen with the naked eye. As stated previously, it is important to determine if the renal disease present is primary or secondary. When the condition has been acute, the kidneys are swollen, rounded, smooth, and moist in appearance. The color may vary somewhat; it is most often light yellow, but in cases of congestion and hemorrhage it is more or less red. Occasionally a distinct tubular marking is visible, and the ureters may be seen as thickened, slightly lobate cords filled with uric acid.

In case of chronic disease the lower surface of the kidneys is flattened or even concave and somewhat nodular or granular in appearance. The tissue is of a firmer consistency and is less likely to go to pieces during attempts to remove the organ. The color is dark brown, with a faint whitish marbling in some cases.

Differentiation of neoplasms, and histological examinations generally, should be referred to special laboratories.

References

1. APPLEBY, E. C.: Some observations on the diseases of finches and parrot-like birds kept in aviaries. Proc. B.S.A.V.A. Congress vol. I, p. 19, 1958.

2. ARONSON, F. R., BILSTAD, N. M., and WOLFE, H. R.: The pathology of anaphylactic shock in chickens. Poultry Sci. *40:*319, 1961.

3. BEACH, J. E.: Diseases of budgerigars and other cage birds. A survey of *post-mortem* findings. Vet. Rec. *74:*10, 63, 134, 1962.

4. COFFIN, D. L.: *The Care, Feeding and Diseases of Psittacine Pets.* Angell Memorial Parakeet and Parrot Book. Boston, Mass., 1953. 32 pp.

5. COFFIN, D. L.: Diseases of Parrots, in *Parrots and Parrot-like Birds,* by Duke of Bedford. Fond du Lac, Wis., All-Pets Books, Inc., 1954.

6. CUMMING, R. B.: Infectious avian nephrosis (uraemia) in Australia. Australian Vet. J. *39:*145, 1963.

7. DALBORG-JOHANSEN, J.: *Stuefuglenes Sygdomme og deres behandling.* København, J. Clausens Forlag, 1958.

8. FIENNES, R. N. T-W-: Report of the society's pathologist for the year 1961. Proc. Zool. Soc. Lond., *140:* 25–46, 1963.

9. FOLIN, O., BERGLUND, H., and DERICK, C.: The uric acid problem. An experimental study on animals

and man, including gouty subjects. J. Biol. Chem. *60:*361, 1924.

10. Hasholt, J.: *Fuglesygdomme.* Aa. Poulsen:Prydfjerkræ, Skibby bogtrykkeri, 1959.

11. Hauser, H.: Tödlicher Streptopenicillinschock bei Papageien mit Lungenmykose. Monatsschr. f. Vet. Med. *15:*632, 1960.

12. Keymer, I. F.: The diagnosis and treatment of common psittacine diseases. Mod. Vet. Pract. *39*(21):22, December 15, 1958.

13. Keymer, I. F.: The diagnosis and treatment of some diseases of seed-eating passerine birds. Mod. Vet. Pract. *40*(7):30, April 1, 1959.

14. Lindt, S.: Beitrag zur Pathologie und Klinik der Stubenvögel (Volièrehaltung). Kleintier-Praxis *9:*4, 1964.

15. O'Connor Halloran, P.: A Bibliography of References to Diseases of Wild Mammals and Birds. Am. J. Vet. Res., vol. 16, October, 1955, Part 2.

16. Plazikowski, U.: *Boken om Burfåglar.* London/Stockholm/New York, S. E. Berghs Förlag, 1959.

17. Schlumberger, H. G.: Neoplasia in the parakeet. I. Spontaneous chromophobe pituitary tumors. Cancer Res. *14:*237, 1954.

18. Selye, H.: Production of nephrosclerosis by overdosage with desoxycorticosterone acetate. Canad. M. A. J. *47:*515, 1942.

19. Selye, H.: Production of nephrosclerosis in the fowl by sodium chloride. J.A.V.M.A. *103:*140, 1943.

20. Shaw, P. A.: Duck disease studies. I. Blood analysis in diseased birds. Proc. Soc. Exp. Biol. Med. *27:*6, 1929; II. Feeding of single and mixed salts. *ibid.* p. 120.

21. Søndergaard, E., Prange, I., Dam, H., and Christensen, E.: Uricemia and kidney damage in galactose-poisoned chicks. Acta path. et microbiol. scandinav. *40:*303, 1957.

22. Sturkie, P. D.: *Avian Physiology,* 2nd ed. Ithaca, N. Y., Comstock Publishing Associates, 1965. Pp. 372–405.

Suggested Reading

Beach, J. E.: Some of the major problems of budgerigar pathology. J. small anim. Pract. *6:*15, 1965.

Berndt, R., and Meise, W.: *Naturgeschichte der Vögel.* Stuttgart, Franckh'sche Verlagshandlung, 1959.

Biester, H. E., and Schwarte, L. H., eds: *Diseases of Poultry,* 5th ed. Ames, Iowa, Iowa State University Press, 1965.

Blount, W. P.: *Diseases of Poultry.* London, Bailliere, Tindall & Cox, 1949.

Cosgrove, A. S.: An apparently new disease of chickens—avian nephrosis. Avian Dis. *6:*385, 1962.

Creek, R. R., and Vasaitis, V.: Uric acid excretion in the chick as related to the intake of its precursors and nitrogen. Poultry Sci. *40:*283, 1961.

Fritzsche, K., and Gerriets, E.: *Geflügelkrankheiten.* Berlin/Hamburg, Verlag Paul Parey, 1959.

Gray, E.: *Diseases of Poultry.* London, Crosby Lockwood and Son Ltd., 1955.

Gray, H.: The diseases of cage and aviary birds, with some reference to those of furred and feathered game. Vet. Rec. *16:*343, 1936.

Grzimek, B.: *Krankes Geflügel.* Stuttgart/Berlin, Fritz Pfenningstorff, 1950.

Hasholt, J.: Current diseases of cage birds. J. small anim. Pract. *2:*97, 1961.

Heinz and Haas: Ueber Kochsalzvergiftung. Münch. med. Wchschr. *70:*565, 1923.

Herpol, C., van Grembergen: Le pH dans le tube digestif des Oiseaux. Ann. Biol. anim. Biochem. Biophys. *1:*317, 1961.

Hilbrich, P.: *Krankheiten des Geflügels.* Schwenningen am Neckar, Verlag Hermann Kuhn, 1963.

Kemna, A.: *Krankheiten der Stubenvögel.* Minden, Philler Verlag, 1959.

Lesbouyries, G.: *Pathologie des oiseaux de basse-cour.* Paris, Vigot Frères, 1965.

Levine, R., Wolfson, W. Q., and Lenel, R.: Concentration and transport of true urate in the plasma of the azotemic chicken. Am. J. Physiol. *151:*186, 1947.

Marthedal, H. E.: *Fjerkræsygdomme I.* København, De studerendes raad, 1957.

Mercado, T. I., and von Brand, T.: Metastatic calcification induced by Hytakerol in chickens infected with Plasmodium gallinaceum. Poultry Sci. *43:*222, 1964.

Newton, L. G., and Simmons, G. C.: Avian nephritis and uraemia. Austral. Vet. J. *39:*135, 1963.

Parkhurst, R. T.: Avian nephrosis (Gumboro disease) in U.S.A. broilers. Treatment. World's Poultry Sci. J. *20:*208, 1964.

Pun, C. F.: Hereditary kidney hypoplasia in the domestic fowl. Poultry Sci. *40:*842, 1961.

Reinhardt, R.: *Lehrbuch der Geflügelkrankheiten.* Hannover, M & H. Schaper, 1950. 384 pp.

Sassenhoff, I.: Vergiftungen bei Hühnern and Wildgeflügel mit Metallphosphidgetreide. Arch. f. wissensch. u. prakt. Tierhlk. *74:*513, 1939.

Sturkie, P. D.: The effects of age and reproductive state on plasma uric acid levels in chickens. Poultry Sci. *40:*1650, 1961.

Wailly, P. de: *L'amateur des oiseaux de cage et de volière.* Paris, J. B. Bailliere et fils, 1964.

West, E. S., and Todd, W. R.: *Textbook of Biochemistry,* 3rd ed. New York, Macmillan Company, 1961. 1423 pp.

Wight, P. A. L.: Lymphoid leucosis and fowl paralysis in the quail. Vet. Rec. *75:*685, 1963.

Worden, A. N.: *Functional Anatomy of Birds.* Cage Birds. London, Dorset House, 1956. 136 pp.

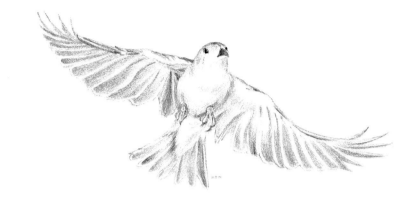

20

Diseases of the Reproductive System

David K. Blackmore

INTRODUCTION

Diseases of the female reproductive tract are relatively common in all species of cage and aviary birds, particularly in breeding birds, although they are by no means uncommon in nonbreeding pet birds. With the exception of neoplasms, diseases of the female reproductive tract have no particular species incidence.

The types of disease affecting the male genital system are far less numerous, and most of the information available concerns neoplastic diseases of the testes. Most references to such disease are concerned with psittacine birds, in particular with the budgerigar. The budgerigar, with its unique susceptibility to neoplasia, shows a high incidence of neoplasms of both the ovary and testes and a lower incidence of involvement of the oviduct.

None of the disorders described in this Chapter are contagious, so there is seldom a typical flock history to aid diagnosis. However, many of the more common conditions of the female reproductive tract are linked to a history of previous egg production or attempted breeding, and affected birds exhibit fairly characteristic signs and symptoms. Diagnosis of disease in individual birds always creates more difficulties than the management of a definite flock problem, and the treatment of reproductive disease is usually the treatment of the individual. Fortunately, some of the more common conditions, including impaction and prolapse of the oviduct, frequently respond to physical or surgical techniques.

Primary endocrine disturbances of the gonads will not be discussed in this Chapter, owing to a general lack of information on the subject. A brief mention of such conditions is made in Chapter 22, on Diseases of the Endocrine System.

The physiology of avian reproduction and the normal function of the reproductive tract are well described by Marshall[15] and Sturkie.[21]

Normal Anatomy

FEMALE REPRODUCTIVE TRACT

The gross anatomy of the avian female reproductive tract is relatively simple. In most species only the left ovary is functional, the right usually being vestigial except in birds of prey, in which both ovaries are often present although usually only the left is fully functional. The ovary is closely applied to the ventral surface of the anterior pole of the left kidney, and is supported by the mesovarium through which it receives its blood supply via the ovarian artery, a branch of the left renal artery.

The size and appearance of the ovary vary considerably, depending on the physiological state of the bird. The inactive ovary is a miniature white botryoid organ, the cortex consisting of a mass of small white developing follicles and the medulla of highly vascular connective tissue. The active ovary contains numerous much larger follicles, containing varying amounts of obvious yolk material. Apart from producing ova, the ovary has an important endocrine function.

The left and right oviducts (salpinges) develop from the Müllerian ducts, but the right oviduct is usually vestigial. Anatomically the oviduct can be divided into five parts: the infundibulum, the magnum (pars albuginea), the isthmus, the shell gland (pars calcigera), and the vagina (pars terminalis). Its size is subject to considerable variation, depending on the physiological state of the bird.

The infundibulum is funnel-shaped and is closely applied to the ovary; it receives extruded ova, and it is here that fertilization takes place. Communicating with the infundibulum is the magnum, which is the longest portion of the oviduct. The mucosa is highly glandular; it secretes mucin and a large proportion of the albumen which is applied to the ovum. The short non-glandular isthmus connects the magnum and the shell gland, or uterus. The shell gland is a comparatively short and dilated portion of the oviduct, with a glandular mucosa. Albumen is secreted here also, and the shell and shell pigments, if the latter are present, are applied to the ovum. The terminal portion of the oviduct, the vagina, is a muscular portion which communicates with the cloaca.

The whole oviduct is suspended by a cranial and a caudal ligament, through which it receives its well-developed blood supply.

MALE REPRODUCTIVE TRACT

The anatomy of the avian male genital tract is also relatively simple. It consists of paired testes, epididymides, deferent ducts, and in some species a penile organ.

The testes are ovoid encapsulated structures which are subject to considerable variation in size, depending on the physiological condition of the bird. In some species a 360-fold increase in size of the testes in the breeding season has been recorded (Marshall,[15] p. 183). The testes are usually white, yellow, or brown, but in some species the small testes of the nonbreeding birds are black, owing to large deposits of melanin. The major part of the organ consists of a mass of anastomosing coiled seminiferous tubules in which the spermatozoa develop. The two testes when fully active are of similar size, but it has been noted in the budgerigar that the right testis is usually slightly larger than the left. The testes are closely applied to the ventral surface of the anterior pole of the respective kidneys. The epididymides are small compared with those of mammals; they connect with the deferent ducts, which are in close apposition to the ureters and open into the cloaca. In the majority of birds no functional penis is present, although ducks and geese possess a muscular penile organ.

Apart from their function in the production of spermatozoa, the testes also have an important endocrine function.

DISEASES OF THE FEMALE REPRODUCTIVE SYSTEM

NEOPLASIA OF THE OVARY

Although Fox[8] records a sarcoma of the ovary of a king parakeet and Ratcliffe[17] an adenocarcinoma in a greater sulfur-crested cockatoo (*Kakatoe galerita*) and a fibrosarcoma in a crimson-winged parakeet (*Aprosmictus scapularis*), neoplasia of the ovary in cage birds appears to be confined mainly to budgerigars, in which species it is not uncommon. A relatively high incidence of the disease in budgerigars has been noted by several workers, including Gray,[9] Arnall,[4] Beach,[5] and Blackmore.[7]

There is apparently some confusion regarding the classification of these ovarian tumors. Ratcliffe[17] described an adenocarcinoma; Beach[5] recorded nine granulosa cell tumors, one spindle cell sarcoma, and one adenocarcinoma; and Arnall[4] used the terms adenoma, adenocarcinoma, dysgerminoma, and arrhenoblastoma.

In my experience these tumors are not clearly differentiated histologically. Of 24 budgerigar tumors examined in detail, 13 appeared to be granulosa cell tumors and 7 adenocarcinomas; 4 were atypical adenocarcinomas in which neoplastic smooth muscle predominated over the epithelial elements as described by Moulton[16] in the fowl.

In spite of the histological variations in the ovarian tumors, the gross morphology and effects on the bird are essentially similar. The tumors often become very large, and weights of over 10 gm. are not uncommon; one cystic ovarian tumor I removed from a budgerigar weighed 24 gm. and accounted for one third of the total body weight of the bird.

The tumors are white and pedunculated, with a smooth or slightly lobular surface (Fig. 20-1). The general shape is globular or ovoid, and occasionally the tumor may be bilobed. The whole neoplastic mass often measures more than 2.5 cm. in diameter. Cyst formation frequently occurs, and individual cysts containing a clear fluid may measure up to 1.5 cm. in diameter. Metastasis rarely occurs.[7]

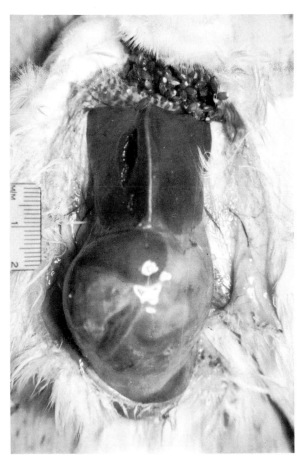

Fig. 20-2. *Budgerigar with distended abdomen due to ovarian tumor.*

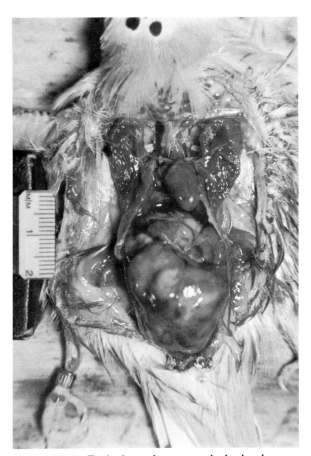

Fig. 20-1. *Typical ovarian tumor in budgerigar.*

Neoplasia of the ovary is essentially a disease of the older bird, although cases have been recorded in birds of only 2 years of age.[7] The signs manifested by affected birds are essentially similar to those seen with other forms of abdominal neoplasia. As the condition develops, the bird's abdomen becomes enlarged because of the size of the neoplastic ovary, and secondary ascites often develops (Fig. 20-2). The increase in volume of the abdominal contents may result in abdominal rupture or herniation, and, associated with the increased abdominal pressure, respiratory symptoms may develop.

A unilateral paresis or paralysis of the leg is frequently associated with neoplasia of the ovary (as with that of the testes in the male), presumably due to pressure on the sciatic nerve or plexus, although this symptom is more frequently seen in cases of kidney neoplasia. In a small proportion of cases there may be a change in secondary sex characteristics, such as a change in color of the cere from brown to blue. Palpation of the abdomen should reveal the neoplastic mass.

Surgical treatment of affected birds is often impossible, but if an early diagnosis is made tumor removal is indicated, as metastasis is unlikely to have occurred, and the tumors are usually well pedunculated. Hasholt[10] surgically removed ovarian tumors from 10 budgerigars and 1 amazon parrot; 7 birds recovered and 4 died.

CYSTIC OVARIES

Primary cystic change of the ovaries is rather infrequently recorded in cage birds, although cystic change secondary to neoplasia of the ovary is comparatively common in budgerigars. (See preceding section on Neoplasia of the Ovary.)

Beach,[5] in his survey of 866 budgerigar necropsies, recorded five cases of primary cystic change of the ovary in pet budgerigars between the ages of 2 and 8 years. Hasholt[10] recorded primary ovarian cysts in 9 budgerigars and 2 canaries among 140 pet birds with diseases involving the female reproductive organs. The mean age was 6 years. I have also seen six cases of the condition in pet budgerigars of a similar age group in my own series of over 900 budgerigar necropsies. Four of these birds also showed concurrent cystic change of the oviduct.

The cause of the condition is unknown, but Beach's observation[5] that two affected birds were suffering from a concurrent hyperostosis, together with Schlumberger's work[19] on the induction of hyperostosis with estrogen therapy, suggests the possibility of some primary endocrine disturbance.

The affected ovaries are usually grossly enlarged and consist of a mass of thin-walled cysts (Fig. 20-3) 0.4–1.5 cm. in diameter, containing a pale yellow fluid. The bird has a history of a slowly developing abdominal enlargement, together with the respiratory symptoms associated with increased abdominal pressure. Palpation of the abdomen reveals a poorly defined, soft fluctuating mass. Abdominal paracentesis with a small-gauge hypodermic needle will reveal the characteristic cystic fluid. Although removal of some of this fluid may cause a temporary improvement in the symptoms, it is unlikely to have any long-term effect. Complete ovariectomy is very difficult to perform by the time an affected bird is presented for examination. Of the 11 birds operated on by Hasholt,[10] 6 recovered and 5 died.

NEOPLASIA OF THE OVIDUCT

Although Gray[9] describes the oviduct as one of the five organs of the budgerigar most susceptible to tumor formation, specific references to the condition are few, and it apparently has not occurred in other than budgerigars.

Ratcliffe[17] recorded one case of an adenocarcinoma, Beach[5] described two cases of cystadenoma, and Blackmore,[7] an adenoma and an adenocarcinoma. One of the cases described by Beach was associated with concurrent multiple cyst formation in the oviduct and a change in color of the cere. The two birds reported by Blackmore[7] were 4 and 5 years old, and showed marked abdominal distention due to the neoplastic enlargement of the oviduct. In the case of the adenocarcinoma, the wall of the oviduct contained a white neoplastic mass 1 cm. in diameter, and there were two smaller metastatic lesions in the wall of the intestine, together with excessive ascitic fluid. In the second case the whole oviduct was distended, with a pedunculated tumor approximately 1.5 cm. in diameter within its lumen.

The definite clinical diagnosis of neoplasia of the oviduct depends finally on laparotomy, and in certain cases surgery may prove successful.

CYSTIC HYPERPLASIA OF THE OVIDUCT

Cystic hyperplasia of the oviduct, with subsequent dilatation of the whole organ, is a condition recorded mainly in budgerigars. Beach[5] described two cases of cystic hyperplasia of the oviduct of budgerigars; Arnall recorded two cases of cystic dilatation of the oviduct in one paper[2] and seven further cases in another.[4] The condition has also been recorded in Japanese quail (*Coturnix coturnix japonica*).[6] I have also seen seven other cases of the condition in budgerigars. The oviducts of these birds were considerably dilated and contained a white or brown mucoid fluid; in two cases the wall of the oviduct contained secondary cysts. Four cases were associated with concurrent cystic change of the ovary. This association may indicate some endocrine disturbance as a primary cause of the condition (see section on Cystic Ovaries).

Although Arnall[2,4] gave no information as to the histological appearance of the oviduct, it was suggested that the excessive fluid in the lumen was a direct result

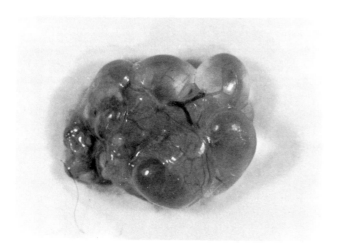

Fig. 20-3. *Cystic ovary in budgerigar.*

of cystic hyperplasia of the mucosa. Arnall also stated[3] that the fluid in the dilated oviduct may contain white or creamy masses.

Affected birds exhibit a progressive abdominal swelling, and often show respiratory embarrassment due to increased pressure on the respiratory tract. Palpation of the abdomen should reveal the distended oviduct, and abdominal paracentesis with a fairly wide bore hypodermic needle should reveal the cystic fluid. A conclusive diagnosis is obtained by laparotomy.

Arnall[2] described the surgical removal of the cystic portion of affected oviducts in four budgerigars, two of which showed some recurrence of the condition. It is suggested that complete removal of the oviduct is indicated in such cases. This surgical approach to the treatment of cystic hyperplasia of the oviduct would appear to be the only logical method of treatment for pet birds or for birds no longer required for breeding purposes.

OBSTRUCTION OF THE OVIDUCT

Obstruction of the oviduct is one of the most common diseases of the female reproductive tract encountered in cage birds. The obstruction may be caused by developing or fully formed eggs, concretions of egg material, calculi, or excessive secretions from the mucosa of the oviduct itself, the last condition being described in the preceding section on Cystic Hyperplasia of the Oviduct.

OBSTRUCTION DUE TO A DEVELOPING EGG (EGG BINDING).

Obstruction of the oviduct by a developing egg has been recorded in many different species of cage birds and is frequently seen in budgerigars and canaries.[4,9,13] I have noted the condition in nine different species of birds.

Hasholt[10] stated that the disease is always acute in passerine birds, death often occurring within a few hours. Psittacine birds, on the other hand, may survive for one to several days. When the egg is caught in the pelvic area, large blood vessels are compressed and severe circulatory disorders result. At the same time, intestinal and ureteral blockage may ensue.

Hasholt[10] described the occasional observation of an egg-bound bird ". . . sitting unsteadily on the perch with ruffled plumage and half-closed eyes. It makes frequent wagging and straining movements with the tail, and now and then moves over to the nest. The condition deteriorates quickly however and the bird takes refuge on the floor of the cage— . . . Egg-bound Canaries have hanging wings and tail, making them look as if they had a swelling over the root of the tail, whereas Budgerigars often sit on the tail with legs far apart, and with the wings and body erect, like penguins."

The obstruction usually occurs in the distal portion of the oviduct (pars calcigera or pars terminalis). On postmortem examination, apart from the obvious distention of the oviduct, there is often an associated egg peritonitis, due to escape of yolk material into the peritoneal cavity (see section on Egg Peritonitis). In only a very small proportion of cases is the obstruction caused by an abnormally large egg. In examination of 21 eggs removed from the impacted oviducts of budgerigars only 1 was found to be abnormally large, 6 appeared to be normal, and the other 14 were thin-shelled and soft. Similar findings were noted in other species of birds. Gray[9] recorded that in many cases the egg was not fully developed and was thin-shelled.

The exact cause of this stasis of eggs in the oviduct has not yet been determined. Keymer[13] thought the condition occurred most frequently in birds that had been overbred, or encouraged to breed at the incorrect season. Gray[9] suggested that the oviduct goes into a state of spasm or cramp, whereas Schwarte[20] stated that the retention of eggs is not uncommon in fowls during heavy production, and may be caused by a temporary suspension of normal physiological activity. This latter statement presumably implies a decrease in muscular activity. Hasholt[10] stated that this condition decreased tremendously in breeders' birds following improvement in feeding and management.

It is suggested that these facts and hypotheses indicate that cases of impaction are due to absence or decrease of peristalsis of the oviduct, and it is further tentatively suggested that this lack of peristalsis may be due to a drop in the level of blood calcium. Although there is no experimental evidence to support this theory, association of the condition with over-production of eggs, noted by Keymer,[13] together with the known incidence of soft-shelled eggs in affected birds, indicates an excessive drain on the calcium reserves. These arguments apply particularly to grain-eating birds which receive an essentially low-calcium diet. In my experience calcium borogluconate given by the intravenous or intraperitoneal route resulted in increased peristalsis of the intestine, and caused rapid expulsion of eggs in the few egg-bound budgerigars that were treated by this method.

There are several methods of treatment for egg-bound birds, and most authors agree that increasing the temperature of the bird's environment is often sufficient to effect a cure. Gray[9] considered that this form of treatment would result in 100 per cent recovery if the impaction was of recent occurrence. Jones[12] suggested a temperature of approximately 90°F., and both he and Keymer[13] recommended the use of infrared irradiation. Heated hospital cages would seem to be ideally suited for this form of treatment.

When there is no response to heat alone, the vent may be lubricated, and expulsion of the egg promoted by gentle manipulation of the bird's abdomen.[12] If the egg is in the pars terminalis or the cloaca, it may be punctured with a hypodermic needle and removed piecemeal.[12] This should be done only as a last resort. If the impaction is in the pars calcigera, laparotomy may have to be performed and the egg removed by means of a salpingotomy.[2] I have used this technique with reasonable success, and found that usually only one Lembert suture of 0000 chromic catgut is required to close the incision in the oviduct. Hoge[11] described a surgical technique whereby, under anesthesia, the egg is gently pushed backward until the membrane covering the egg is slightly everted through the vent. Retention sutures are placed over the egg, an incision made, the egg removed, and the incision closed by means of the retention sutures. An antibiotic powder is applied and the membrane is inverted back through the cloaca.

Gandal describes a method of "instrumental delivery" under "Disorders of the Oviduct," in Chapter 11, on Surgical Techniques and Anesthesia.

CHRONIC IMPACTIONS OF THE OVIDUCT.   The oviduct may become impacted and distended with material other than developing eggs. One cause of such distention is excess secretion of mucin and albumen associated with cystic hyperplasia of the mucosa of the oviduct, which is described elsewhere. Chronic impaction of the oviduct is often caused by inspissated egg material in the magnum, as opposed to obstruction with developing eggs, which usually occurs in the more distal portions of the oviduct. Keymer[13] referred to necrotic egg material in the oviduct of canaries, and Beach[5] recorded concretions of egg material in the oviduct of two budgerigars. I have seen impaction of the magnum with yellow inspissated, apparent yolk material in four budgerigars and in birds of two other species. The condition is due to stasis of eggs in the magnum of the oviduct. Impairment of normal oviduct function, as discussed in relation to more typical cases of egg binding, may be involved in production of this more chronic condition.

Hasholt[10] recorded 42 cases that would fall into this general category: 40 involving budgerigars, and 1 each in a cockatiel and a canary. The oviducts contained grey or yellow purulent matter, normal eggs, malformed eggs, calcareous deposits, and albumen. Five birds had a diffuse peritonitis with adhesions.

Affected birds are likely to show less obvious signs of impaction than typical egg-bound birds, owing to the smaller bulk of the impacting material. Unless there is a concurrent egg peritonitis or salpingitis, the birds will show no evidence of general malaise. Breeding birds will be unable to produce eggs, and careful abdominal palpation may reveal the enlarged portion of the oviduct. Alternating constipation and diarrhea may

occur. It is likely that the condition will often be undiagnosed until laparotomy or postmortem examination is performed.

One of the concretions Beach removed from the oviduct of a budgerigar consisted almost entirely of calcium carbonate.[5] I had a similar case in which the oviduct contained three small calculi, approximately 3 mm. in diameter, consisting of calcium carbonate. These calculi presumably originated in the pars calcigera.

Salpingotomy in treatment of chronic impaction of the oviduct was described by Arnall.[4] Hasholt[10] performed salpingectomy on 41 birds, and 35 lived. He described the surgical procedure.

PROLAPSE OF THE OVIDUCT

Prolapse of the oviduct can apparently occur in all species of birds, although most records refer to the budgerigar[4,5] or canary.[13] Gray[9] stated that the condition most frequently occurs in canaries, pigeons, and parrots.

The distal portion of the oviduct is prolapsed through the vent, often together with the cloaca and, in certain cases, the rectum. The condition is always associated with egg production and physiological hyperplasia of the oviduct. The prolapsed portion often contains a fully formed egg.

It is considered that the prolapse is due to excessive straining in an attempt to pass a partially impacted egg,[13,14] or to continued straining after the egg has been passed. These eggs are seldom abnormally large (see Obstruction of the Oviduct), and Gray[9] stated that the oviduct lacks muscular tone. It is therefore assumed that prolapse of the oviduct is due only to excessive contractions of the abdominal muscles and not to excessive activity of the musculature of the oviduct itself.

Hasholt[10] believes that prolapse is due to intense straining associated with flaccidity of cloacal muscles. He found that the egg and oviduct are usually prolapsed together. Out of 38 cases, different shell abnormalities existed in 28; in 5 the eggs were soft-shelled.

Hasholt stated further that the prognosis is good for birds treated early. However, most birds are not presented until the mucous membrane is soiled, abraded, and dehydrated. Of the 38 birds seen by Hasholt, 18 were treated successfully, 18 died, and 2 were euthanatized. These numbers point up the gravity of the condition.

Before the prolapsed portion is replaced, any egg contained within it must be removed. Arnall[4] recommends removal of the egg piece-meal, using a rolling movement with a pair of forceps to decrease the diameter of the egg. The prolapse can then be replaced by means of a lubricated thermometer and held in position by means of a purse-string suture about the vent until any signs of straining have ceased.[14] If the egg cannot be removed, or the oviduct held in position, salpingectomy may be performed. The prognosis is poor in such cases.

MISCELLANEOUS CONDITIONS OF THE OVIDUCT

Apparently very little information is available on other conditions of the oviduct. Although Keymer[13] recorded salpingitis associated with impaction of the oviduct and egg peritonitis in passerine birds, there are no detailed accounts of the condition. There also appears to be some confusion between cystic hyperplasia of the oviduct and a primary infectious salpingitis. As Keymer[13] suggested, one would expect to find a salpingitis as a complicating factor in cases of impaction of the oviduct and generalized egg peritonitis, and *Escherichia coli* would probably be associated with cases of salpingitis in budgerigars (see Egg Peritonitis).

Arnall[4] referred to rupture of the oviduct caused by abnormal eggs, resulting in an egg peritonitis, and Beach[5] recorded a similar case. Considering the relative frequency with which egg peritonitis occurs in cage birds, it is suggested that rupture of the oviduct may be secondary to a peritonitis and not the actual cause.

EGG PERITONITIS

Peritonitis due to escape of yolk material into the peritoneal cavity is a comparatively common condition in all species of cage birds and has been recorded by many workers.[1,2,5,14] Although most records refer to the budgerigar, I have seen the condition in other psittacine and in passerine birds; Keymer[13] recorded the condition in seed-eating passerine birds, and Bigland *et al.*[6] recorded a high incidence in Japanese quail.

Egg peritonitis apparently occurs as a direct result of the failure of ova extruded from the ovary to enter the infundibulum of the oviduct, or as the result of rupture of the oviduct. Arnall[2] suggested that rupture of the oviduct may occur as a result of stasis of normal or abnormal eggs. The condition is commonly associated with obstruction of the oviduct (see Obstruction Due to a Developing Egg, under Obstruction of the Oviduct). Arnall[3] also suggested that the condition may be due to reverse peristalsis of the oviduct.

The peritoneal cavity of affected birds is found to contain yolk material which varies in color from yellow to green or brown. There is an associated generalized peritonitis with adhesions between the various organs, especially between the loops of the intestine. The abdominal and thoracic air sacs are often involved (Fig. 20-4). As the condition always occurs in birds that are

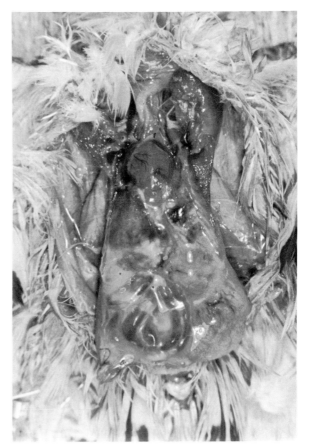

Fig. 20-4. *Egg peritonitis in budgerigar.*

attempting to produce eggs, the ovary is active and the oviduct hypertrophied.

Although the peritoneal cavity often appears to be bacteriologically sterile, in 50 cases I examined 18 showed evidence of secondary bacterial infection, 13 apparently due to coliform bacteria, 4 to enterococci, and 1 to a mixed infection by the two types of organisms. On primary culture, nine of the coliform bacteria exhibited marked beta hemolysis, and seven subjected to detailed biochemical investigation were confirmed to be *Escherichia coli*. Three of the enterococci isolated were shown to belong to Lancefield's Group D. Arnall[4] also recorded the isolation of *E. coli* from a budgerigar with egg peritonitis.

Although the condition can occur in single pet birds as well as in breeders' birds, all those affected have a history of active egg production. The abdomen is swollen and soft, and often the wall is erythematous. There is frequently some respiratory embarrassment due to either increased abdominal pressure or direct involvement of the respiratory tract. In acute forms of the disease, few symptoms may be noted and there may be no indication of the condition before the bird is found dead on the nest. In more chronic forms of the disease, progressive swelling of the abdomen, respiratory embarrassment, diarrhea, and possibly stasis of an egg in the oviduct may be noted. Keymer[13] suggested that radiography is an important diagnostic aid.

In the majority of cases, treatment is not possible, but Arnall[2] described exploratory laparotomy and irrigation of the peritoneal cavity as a method of treatment. Obviously the success of such surgical intervention depends on early diagnosis of the condition before extensive adhesions or secondary bacterial infection has occurred.

DISEASES OF THE MALE REPRODUCTIVE SYSTEM

TESTICULAR TUMORS

Apparently the only references to diseases of the male reproductive tract in cage and aviary birds concern neoplasia of the testes, which occurs frequently in budgerigars but far less commonly in other birds. The larger psittacines are sometimes affected,[7,8,17] and Rewell[18] recorded a seminoma in a collared turtle dove (*Streptopelia risoria*).

In budgerigars, older birds are most frequently affected. There is usually a period of general malaise varying from a few days to several weeks. The abdomen becomes progressively distended, and frequently there are signs of paresis of one leg, presumably due to pressure on the sciatic nerve or plexus. In a small proportion of cases, there is an apparent reversal of the secondary sex characteristics, indicated by a change in color of the cere from blue to brown. I have noted this change in birds affected by seminoma and by tumors considered to be interstitial cell tumors.

Tumors of the budgerigar testes have been described by a variety of terms according to their histological structure, and Beach[5] used the terms seminoma, Sertoli cell tumor, and interstitial cell tumor. Although this classification would appear to be the most logical, it is often extremely difficult to classify these tumors so precisely. On gross examination these tumors all appear somewhat similar. One or both testes may be affected, usually showing gross enlargement, and often weighing more than 5 grams. They are white in color with a smooth surface and uniform texture. Metastasis is not uncommon, with the liver appearing to be the organ most frequently affected.

The diagnosis of neoplasia of the testes is based on the signs already described, together with findings on abdominal palpation. It is doubtful whether the condition can normally be diagnosed in time for surgery to be attempted, and even if surgery appears to be successful, a guarded prognosis should be given because of the possibility of metastasis.

References

1. APPLEBY, E. C.: Some observations on the diseases of finches and parrot-like birds kept in aviaries. Proc. B.S.A.V.A. Congress, vol. I, p. 25, 1958.

2. ARNALL, L.: Experiences with cage-birds. Vet. Rec. *70:* 120–128, 1958.

3. ARNALL, L.: Some common surgical entities of the budgerigar. Vet. Rec. *72:*888–890, 1960.

4. ARNALL, L.: Further experiences with cagebirds. Vet. Rec. *73:*1146–1154, 1961.

5. BEACH, J. E.: Diseases of budgerigars and other cage birds. A summary of *post-mortem* findings. Vet. Rec. *74:*63–68, 1962.

6. BIGLAND, C. H., DaMASSA, A. J., and WOODARD, A. E.: Diseases of Japanese quail (*Coturnix coturnix japonica*)—A flock survey and experimental transmission of selected avian pathogens. Avian Dis. *9:*212–219, 1965.

7. BLACKMORE, D. K.: The pathology and incidence of neoplasia in cage birds. J. small anim. Pract. *6:*217–223, 1965.

8. FOX, H.: *Disease in Captive Wild Mammals and Birds. Incidence, Description, Comparison.* Philadelphia, J. B. Lippincott Company, 1923. 665 pp.

9. GRAY, H.: The diseases of cage and aviary birds, with some reference to those of furred and feathered game. Vet. Rec. *16:*343–352, 377–386, 417–425, 1936.

10. HASHOLT, J.: Diseases of the female reproductive organs of pet birds. J. small anim. Pract. *7:*313–320, 1966.

11. HOGE, R. S.: Anesthesia and surgery for egg bound parakeets. Animal Hospital *2:*46–47, 1966.

12. JONES, O. G.: Common diseases of cage birds and other less usual pets. Vet. Rec. *68:*918–933, 1956.

13. KEYMER, I. F.: The diagnosis and treatment of some diseases of seed-eating passerine birds. Mod. Vet. Pract. *40(7):*30–34, April 1; *40(8):*34–37, April 15, 1959.

14. KEYMER, I. F.: Cage and aviary bird surgery. Mod. Vet. Pract. *41(11):*28–31, June 1; *41(12):*32–36, June 15, 1960.

15. MARSHALL, A. J.: Reproduction. In *Biology and Comparative Physiology of Birds,* A. J. Marshall, ed. New York, Academic Press, 1961. Vol. II, pp. 169–213.

16. MOULTON, J. E.: *Tumors in Domestic Animals.* Berkeley, University of California Press, 1961. 279 pp.

17. RATCLIFFE, H. L.: Incidence and nature of tumors in captive wild mammals and birds. Am. J. Cancer *17:*116–135, 1933.

18. REWELL, R. E.: Seminoma of the testis in a collared turtle dove (*Streptopelia risoria*). J. Path. Bact. *60:* 155, 1948.

19. SCHLUMBERGER, H. G.: Polyostotic hyperostosis in the female parakeet. Am. J. Path. *35:*1–23, 1959.

20. SCHWARTE, L. H.: Poultry Surgery. In *Diseases of Poultry,* 5th ed. H. E. Biester and L. H. Schwarte, eds. Ames, Iowa State University Press, 1965. Pp. 1149–1161.

21. STURKIE, P. D.: Avian Physiology, 2nd ed. Ithaca, N.Y., Comstock Publishing Associates., 1965. Pp. 447–533.

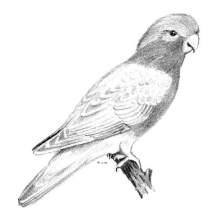

21

Diseases
of the
Nervous System

Jens Hasholt

The behavior of a bird, like that of any other living creature, depends on the proper integration of receptive impulses traveling through the communication lines (the nerves) to and from the coordination center (the brain). The behavioral patterns and reactions of birds appear to be less complex and more stereotyped than those of mammals, seeming to depend more on innate reflexes and instincts. Accordingly, the avian brain is less complex than the mammalian brain, and certain parts of the spinal cord, namely the cervico-thoracic and lumbosacral enlargements (intumescentia), reach a higher degree of development. This permits coordination of flight and walking movements in these two intumescentia rather than in the brain. This simplification appears to follow the principles of cybernetics, and it has been substantiated experimentally[6] by use of radio wave stimulation to map the pathways of the brain in the chicken.

Changes in the nervous system, particularly in the brain, are reflected in abnormal behavior. In order to diagnose these changes it is imperative that the normal behavioral pattern of each species of bird is known. This, however, is almost an impossibility when one considers the long list of species kept in captivity. Furthermore, birds that are kept as companions for people, so-called "pet birds," have an additional set of reactions related to the sleeping, eating, and social habits of their owners. It must be remembered that certain changes in the behavior of a bird are considered to be the results of short circuits between neural pathways. A bird has only a limited number of reflexes to handle ordinary situations; thus unusual stimuli provoke a whole chain reaction which may produce peculiar manifestations. These can be considered pathological only when they are repeated over and over outside the conflict situation which is usually responsible for their production.

Sleepiness, dullness, uneasiness, nervousness, anxiety, aggressiveness, dizziness, ataxia, circling movements, spasms (tonic, clonic, or epileptiform), paresis, and paralysis are all indications of disease somewhere in the nervous system, but none of the signs indicates the nature of the lesion, or the etiological agent.

As a result of this, the vague and unsatisfactory diagnosis of central nervous system lesion is frequently made, and one is not helped by the use of such terms as torticollis, vertigo, or ataxia to describe the symptom-complex. Unfortunately, neither laboratory examinations nor necropsy can assure the correct diagnosis in many of the diseases of the nervous system.

INCIDENCE AND CATEGORIES OF DISEASES OF THE NERVOUS SYSTEM

There is some disagreement regarding the frequency of nervous system lesions in birds, and published figures vary from 0.7 per cent[1] to 10 per cent.[7] However, it is difficult to ascertain how many diseases of the nervous system have been included under infections, poisonings, or deficiency diseases. It seems clear that lesions in the brain occur much more frequently and are more varied than those observed in the spinal cord and in the peripheral nerves. In the interest of convenience, the diseases of the brain can be divided into three main categories:

1. *Encephalitis*—inflammatory changes in the brain caused by either infection or trauma.
2. *Nutritional and toxic encephalomalacia*—primary degenerative lesions of both individual neurons and tracts, with possible secondary inflammatory reaction.
3. *Functional encephalopathy*—in which no morphological changes can be demonstrated and in which the clinical signs apparently are caused by chemical and electrical changes in the brain.

As neurological signs often are sequelae of various systemic infections, poisonings, and deficiency diseases, those are briefly summarized in the following paragraphs. More detailed descriptions of the diseases can be found elsewhere in the book; only the functional encephalopathies and some forms of neurosis are discussed in detail in this Chapter.

Encephalitis

Specific Infections

VIRAL INFECTIONS

AVIAN ENCEPHALOMYELITIS may affect galliform, columbiform, and anseriform species. It is manifested by ataxia, partial or total paralysis, and severe tremors in head and neck muscles, with less involvement of other muscle groups.

EQUINE ENCEPHALOMYELITIS can affect almost all species of birds, but galliform, passeriform, and anseriform species are most frequently involved. The clinical signs are paralysis and staggering.

AVIAN PNEUMOENCEPHALITIS (Newcastle disease) affects most frequently galliform and passeriform species, rarely anseriform species, and only exceptionally psittacine birds. The signs are tremors, rhythmic clonic spasms, torticollis, circling, and partial or complete paralysis. Guillon[4] observed an allergic encephalitis after vaccination against Newcastle disease.

POLIOMYELITIS has been reported to affect budgerigars.[9] However, attempts to transmit the disease were unsuccessful.[5]

BACTERIAL INFECTIONS

SALMONELLOSIS occurs in pigeons, canaries, and budgerigars.

TUBERCULOSIS of avian type occurs in poultry and small cage birds; the human type of infection occurs in parrots. If paralysis occurs it is due to tubercles in bone rather than in the brain.

STREPTOCOCCAL MENINGITIS occurs in sporadic cases only.

FUNGAL DISEASES

ASPERGILLOSIS occurs in penguins, waterfowl, turkeys, and baby chicks (brooder pneumonia).

PARASITIC INFECTIONS

TOXOPLASMOSIS may occur in chickens, pigeons, canaries, and budgerigars. The signs are tilted head, ataxia, and circling.

TRICHOMONIASIS may be observed in pigeons.

Conditions Resulting from Injury

ACUTE, from recent fractures of the skull.

CHRONIC, from formation of scar tissue following trauma.

Tumors

Gliomas, schwannomas, and hemangiomas.

Nutritional and Toxic Encephalomalacia

Such degenerative changes affecting the nervous system are usually the result of vitamin deficiencies or of poisoning with chemicals or with plant or animal substances.

Nutritional Deficiency Diseases

Only those nutritional deficiency diseases that affect the nervous system *per se* will be discussed, and not the deficiencies that result in muscular weakness, or in poor growth or skeletal development.

The most important deficiency diseases belong to the avitaminoses, and birds often suffer from varying degrees of suboptimal intake rather than a complete absence of any vitamin. The deficiency can be primary, due to lack of available vitamin in the feed, or secondary, due to poor resorption or deficient utilization in the body of available vitamins.

The vitamins whose deficiency may be detrimental and the manifestations of the conditions are listed below.

B-AVITAMINOSIS

The lack of various components of the B complex is manifested by various symptoms related to the nervous system.

Vitamin B$_1$ (Thiamine; Aneurin)—ataxia, paralysis, opisthotonos.
Vitamin B$_2$ (Lactoflavin, Riboflavin)—curling of toes.
Nicotinamide—tremor, paresis.
Vitamin B$_6$ (Pyridoxine)—spasmodic clonic or tonic movements.
Folic acid—paralysis with extended neck and tremors of drooping wings.
Vitamin B$_{12}$ (Cyanocobalamin)—clinically no significant nervous disturbances, but histological examination reveals neuronal degeneration with accumulations of fat.

E-AVITAMINOSIS

Deficiency of vitamin E may cause such symptoms as tilted head, ataxia, circling, and occasionally spasms.

The avitaminoses are naturally best known in poultry, in which clinical findings have been supplemented with numerous experimental observations. Among the cage birds it is predominantly the budgerigar, and especially the newly hatched young, that shows signs of deficiency with paralysis.

Poisoning

The toxic effect of any poison will depend on the amount, the chemical and physical properties of the substance, the rate of absorption, and individual characteristics of the poisoned bird (age, idiosyncrasy, and the like). The reaction can be acute, subacute, or chronic, and the clinical signs depend on whether the poison has local or systemic effect. Most systemic poisons cause marked alimentary, circulatory, or nervous signs (motor or cerebral). It is usually not possible from the clinical signs to tell what poison is responsible. A chemical analysis of the gastrointestinal contents will often provide the answer; however, it is usually a costly and time-consuming procedure. By carefully ascertaining what the bird has eaten or has been in contact with, it is often possible to establish a tentative diagnosis, sufficient for taking the necessary prophylactic measures, as therapy instituted after symptoms are evident is almost without value.

CHEMICAL POISONS

Such agents include lead, herbicides, insecticides, fertilizers, and wrongly administered medications.

VEGETABLE POISONS

Several house plants kept in pots in living rooms and even in aviaries are toxic. It must be remembered that the stones of prunes and cherries may contain toxic quantities of cyanide.

ANIMAL POISONS

Poisoning with material of animal origin is rare in cage birds; however, bird seeds contaminated with mites may be harmful. Earthworms have been reported to be toxic, particularly when the clitellum is well developed.

Bites by wasps and spiders may have serious clinical effects.

TOXINS PRODUCED BY BACTERIA AND PARASITES

Intoxications by certain enterotoxins of *Escherichia coli* and parasites may be harmful, but the mode of their action is not understood.

Functional Encephalopathies

Common to these diseases is the fact that they all manifest themselves by motor disturbance without demonstrable macroscopic or microscopic changes in the nervous tissue. The diseases can be categorized under two different headings: concussion, and increased intracranial pressure.

Concussion

Concussion is well recognized in cage birds; it is most often seen in free-flying budgerigars and more rarely in the larger parrots. Such injury occurs when the bird crashes into a window or mirror with great force, but it has also occurred when highly nervous birds are transferred into smaller cages, or when quail are kept in cages with low ceilings.

Birds that are kept in large cages or aviaries can also succumb to concussion; in this case it most frequently occurs during the night when the birds have been frightened by either sudden light, noise, or a predatory animal. In their panic they cannot find a new resting place and will invariably crash into walls or branches, only to be found unconscious the next morning where they have fallen. Drowning also has occurred under similar circumstances. A few cases of concussion have been attributed to rough handling by inexperienced owners who have attempted to catch and treat cage birds.

In the uncomplicated case of concussion the necropsy usually reveals nothing. However, hemorrhages are often present in severe concussions and contribute to aggravation of the condition by producing compression of the brain. Clinically it is often impossible to determine if this complication is present. Most of the contact that veterinarians have with cases of concussion in birds consists either of performing necropsy on a bird that has been found dead without previous signs of illness, or of being consulted because a bird suddenly behaves in an abnormal manner after a history of having flown into some object. The bird will often fall to the ground immediately and remain unconscious for a short time, after which it will appear confused. After a period of excitement the bird will often quiet down and go to sleep either on its perch or on the bottom of the cage. It will show no interest in food or water, and if disturbed it moves around in an ataxic fashion. It may manifest head-tilt, circling movements, or increasing paresis in either a leg or a wing. Increased excitation and nervousness are occasionally seen, as are clonic and tonic spasms. If all these signs increase in severity when the bird is disturbed or when attempts are made to catch it, a poor prognosis should be given.

External lesions are conspicuous by their absence, and rarely can one discern hemorrhages from the beak. Only in the most serious lesions of the skull will one find lesions in the skin covering the head. The red discoloration that occasionally can be seen after the feathers have been removed from the head region generally is the result of hemorrhages in the meninges, with blood penetrating the thin skull bones and skin. Hemorrhage will usually be seen in the leptomeninges rather than in the substance of the brain itself.

Subdural hemorrhages are not seen, whereas hemorrhages within the skull bones are not infrequent. The significance of these latter hemorrhages is not known. Appleby[1] has seen such hemorrhages at postmortem examination; Gray[3] and Beach[2] have seen them in birds that have been euthanatized and in which trauma and acute infection could be excluded. Occasionally, hypostatic congestion of the skull bones results in a greyish red, diffuse discoloration, often resembling a geographic map. When the skin is removed this maplike pattern becomes more evident, and when the skull is opened the inside of the calvaria appears smooth. After removal of the dura one can easily demonstrate that the extraneous blood is located in the bones of the calvaria, which consist of a thin compact layer on the outside and pneumatic spaces in the center.

When one removes the skin of the head of a normal, freshly killed bird, a change in color will often be observed in the bones. As air penetrates into the porous and pneumatic skull bones, a mother-of-pearl color will appear, and if one ruptures the blood vessels by either twisting or cutting the neck, many of the pneumatic chambers in the bones will fill up with blood, and the above-mentioned geographic map pattern will appear. Although these hemorrhages of the skull bones cannot be taken as proof of a severe concussion, they are probably of some importance as they may reflect changes of intracranial pressure.

The prognosis of concussion is always uncertain. If spasms occur, the chances of recovery are very small and euthanasia should be recommended. If effort is made to save the bird it should be placed as quietly as possible in a place where it is protected from sudden and loud noises, and from any sudden changes in light; unlike the recommendation in most other diseases in birds, the room should be rather cool. No drugs have proved to be of value, and force-feeding with various concentrates cannot be recommended as the excitement involved in catching and restraining the bird will be harmful.

Increased Intracranial Pressure

Under this heading will be included changes which directly or indirectly result in pressure upon parts of the brain without lesions appearing in the nervous tissue itself. The following conditions will be considered: tumors of the orbit, frontal bone, and pituitary; inflammation of the frontal bone; hemorrhages of the meninges; pigmentation of the calvaria; jugular stasis; and arteriosclerosis.

It is not currently known if some of the motor disturbances caused by these conditions are the result of changes in the brain or in the labyrinth. We know that the labyrinth is concerned not only with equilibrium but also with muscular coordination in general.

TUMORS

Although tumors of the orbit and frontal bone are extremely rare, tumors of the pituitary are fairly common in the budgerigar. According to Schlumberger,[8] tumors of the pituitary are so specific in effects that the clinical signs alone should lead to the correct diagnosis. Unfortunately, there is no known therapy for these tumors. Schlumberger's description of an affected bird is so vivid that it is quoted here:

"Cerebral involvement is indicated by somnolence and the occurrence of convulsive seizures. Although a terminal convulsion is often seen in birds dying of various causes, the convulsions observed in birds with a pituitary tumor have their onset several days before death. The seizures are accompanied by an incoordinated beating of the wings on the floor of the cage associated with clonic twitching of the legs and occasional piercing cries. The convulsion lasts for about 30 seconds followed by a 2–3-minute period of unconsciousness during which the bird appears to be dead. Recovery is usually abrupt, and the bird may subsequently climb back on its perch. Five or six seizures may occur before death."

In Denmark, where the entity even in budgerigars appears to be rare, we have seen the exact clinical signs that Schlumberger describes. One bird, however, presented a slightly different clinical picture. Over a course of six months the color of the head changed from egg-yolk yellow to a uniform green, and only during the last week before death was there any change in personality. The bird became quiet and showed complete apathy.

INFLAMMATION OF THE FRONTAL BONE

One case of a canary will be presented as representative of this entity. The bird, which was never out of its cage, began to sit quietly and sleep, with intermittent episodes of violent spasms. Palpation of the skull caused irregular severe spasms, which terminated in complete opisthotonos, with the bird lying on the bottom of the cage. On necropsy, the frontal bone was found to be greatly thickened, and the dura was grey but smooth in appearance.

HEMORRHAGES OF THE MENINGES

Hemorrhages of the meninges can vary in size from hardly visible petechiae to large hematomas. They can occur either as part of a systemic infection or as a result of accidental injury to the skull. The brain is usually damaged, but not always. One owner unintentionally caused a depression of the occipital bone with meningeal hemorrhage in two birds when attempting to restrain them. One bird survived with no ill effects, whereas the second bird died suddenly a few minutes later. Such sudden death makes one think of a state of apoplexy, a diagnosis that is not uncommonly used in passerine birds, especially canaries, that die suddenly while attempts are being made to capture or restrain them, or to administer treatment. However, not all such fatalities are due to cerebral apoplexy; some are caused by cardiac arrest and suffocation.

PIGMENTATION OF THE CALVARIA

This peculiar syndrome has been seen in budgerigars exhibiting apathy with intermittent periods of circling, often of such severity that the bird will tumble off the perch. On necropsy a yellow discoloration of hemosiderin was present in the skull bones only, particularly in pneumatic cavities of the temporal bone. A clutch of Bourke's parakeets (*Neophema bourkii*) were affected, spending almost the entire day at the bottom of the cage doing left and right pirouettes at varying intervals. It is not possible at this time even to state what the correlation is between the pigmentation and the clinical condition. The pigmentation may be merely a physiological phenomenon akin to the melanin pigmentation of the dura of the Japanese silk fowl, and thus be of no significance; on the other hand, if the pneumatic spaces of the skull take part in the regulation of the cerebrospinal fluid pressure, the pigmentation may be significant.

JUGULAR STASIS

Jugular stasis, caused by enlarged thyroid glands, has been seen to result in congestion of the brain with violent generalized spasms in budgerigars.

ARTERIOSCLEROSIS

Arteriosclerosis has been seen in three old amazon parrots which had carotid arteries that looked like calcified tubes. All three parrots had been euthanatized because they repeatedly fell off their perches and remained unconscious on the floor for several minutes after each fall. The clinical findings can probably be explained by cerebral ischemia and possible hypertension as a result of the sclerosis of the vessels.

Neuroses

Another group of functional disorders appropriately discussed in this Chapter are various neuroses.

The neuroses are psychic disturbances which can be of either hereditary or environmental origin. A neurosis will characteristically appear without any demonstrable specific cause. It is thought that for birds being forced to live in a cage in close contact with human beings is a stress of considerable magnitude. Caging is particularly stressful to a bird that normally lives in a flock with hundreds of its own kind. In addition to this, a pet bird has to adjust to idiosyncrasies of its owner and to new feeding and sleeping patterns and often to a completely strange diet. The bird which suffers least from captivity would seem to be the budgerigar. One of the reasons that it adapts so well is that it is usually extremely young when it is acquired; during its development it adjusts so well to its owner that it possibly considers itself the playmate of a human being rather than of any other bird. Another factor which has probably contributed to the uniquely successful domestication of budgerigars is their cheerful, lively, and sociable nature, together with their ability to mimic the human voice. These features tend to make the owners spend more time with the birds and thus occupy the birds' interest.

FEATHER-PICKING

Feather-picking, one of the most annoying of the neuroses, may result from lack of activity. The bird picks either its own feathers or those of others, particularly nestlings. There is no effective therapy; mineral and vitamin supplements are without effect, as are various collars and protective bandages. It seems that once a bird becomes a feather-picker it will always remain one. Transfer of the bird into an outside aviary in the spring will usually result in growth during the summer of a normal plumage which suddenly disappears during a night of feather-picking. Similar to this habit are those of chewing everything in sight to shreds and pieces, often encountered in budgerigars, and the various forms of to-and-fro movements. Gould's amadins and leafbirds

(Chloropseidae) invariably, when kept in too small cages, begin constantly repeated head and neck movements with the beak pointed toward the ceiling as if they were looking for an escape hole. The truly neurotic aspect of this behavior is emphasized by the fact that the movements are continued after the birds have been transferred to large aviaries. A slightly different manifestation was seen in two vasa parrots (*Coracopsis* spp.) that continuously tried to force their way out between the bars of the cage. The birds eventually had to be euthanatized, despite a change to different cages and the adoption of various protective measures, because of injuries to their skin.

SUDDEN CHANGES IN PERSONALITY

Sudden changes in personality have been seen, particularly in the larger parrots but also in budgerigars. Birds that have been friendly and playful have suddenly become hostile and aggressive, often without any detectable reason. Occasionally it may happen in conjunction with being boarded during the owner's vacation, and thus it could be interpreted as an expression of revenge or jealousy. Uneasiness in birds has been attributed to lack of peace during the birds' rest periods at night, because of radio or television.

SEXUAL ABERRATIONS

Sexual aberrations are not infrequent in budgerigars. In the male, copulating movements on the finger or in the hair of the owner may possibly be an expression of affection. If the bird utilizes the bars of the cage and it happens repeatedly even when daily free flight outside the cage is permitted, it is a neurosis. No changes have been found in the gonads on histological examination of tissue obtained at necropsy in many such birds. Also, testicular tumors of birds do not seem to be associated with such behavior disturbances. Certain of the larger parrots seem to prefer either men or women to members of the other sex, but this should not be interpreted as an expression of sexual attraction. It probably represents an adaptation to the sex of the person who raised them.

IMITATION "COURTSHIP FEEDING"

Another peculiar neurosis is the tendency of certain birds to feed either their owner or their own mirror image. The bird may spend most of the day filling its crop with seeds, only to regurgitate them later either on its owner or at the mirror. Such neurotic birds will often lose weight and deteriorate because of starvation. Treatment consists of removing all mirrors and providing the bird with a mate.

DISORDERS OF EGG LAYING

Female birds may show a disturbance of their normal egg-laying habits by depositing eggs in coat pockets, vases, or on the bottom of the cage. Another deviation consists of prolonged egg laying and nesting periods, possibly due to removal of eggs from the nest by the owner.

References

1. APPLEBY, E. C.: Some observations on the diseases of finches and parrot-like birds kept in aviaries. Proc. B.S.A.V.A. Congress vol. I, p. 19, 1958.

2. BEACH, J. E.: Diseases of budgerigars and other cage birds. A survey of *post-mortem* findings. Vet. Rec. *74:*10, 63, 134, 1962.

3. GRAY, H.: The diseases of cage and aviary birds, with some reference to those of furred and feathered game. Vet. Rec. *16:*343, 1936.

4. GUILLON, J. C.: Aspects histopathologies des maladies nerveuses des volailles. World vet. poultry assoc. III Congres internat. 1965, p. 93.

5. HICKEY, F.: Budgerigars and poliomyelitis. New Zealand Vet. J. *8:*15, 1960.

6. HOLST, E. v., and SAINT PAUL, U. v.: Vom Wirkungsgefüge der Triebe. Naturwissenschaften *47:*409, 1960.

7. LINDT, S.: Beitrag zur Pathologie und Klinik der Stubenvögel (Volièrehaltung). Kleintier-Praxis *9:*4, 1964.

8. SCHLUMBERGER, H. G.: Neoplasia in the parakeet. I. Spontaneous chromophobe pituitary tumors. Cancer Res. *14:*237, 1954.

9. SOMMERVILLE, R. G., MONRO, I. C., and CUTHBERT, C. C.: Poliovirus type 1 isolated from a budgerigar. Lancet *1:*512, 1958.

Suggested Reading

ARNALL, L.: Experiences with cage-birds. Vet. Rec. *70:*120, 1958.

ASCHENBORN, C.: *Krankheiten der Stubenvögel und ihre Behandlung.* Minden/Westf., A. Philler Verlag, 1953.

BERNDT, R., and MEISE, W.: *Naturgeschichte der Vögel.* Stuttgart, Franckh'sche Verlagshandlung, 1959.

BIERING-SØRENSEN, U.: Fjerkrætoxoplasmose. Nord. Vet.-Med. *8:*140, 1956.

BIESTER, H. E., and SCHWARTE, L. H., eds.: *Diseases of Poultry,* 5th ed. Ames, Iowa State University Press, 1965.

BLACKMORE, D. K.: The incidence and aetiology of thyroid dysplasia in budgerigars (*Melopsittacus undulatus*). Vet. Rec. *75:*1068, 1963.

BLOUNT, W. P.: *Diseases of Poultry.* London, Bailliere, Tindall & Cox, 1949.

COFFIN, D. L.: *The Care, Feeding and Diseases of Psittacine Pets.* Angell Memorial Parakeet and Parrot Book. Boston, Mass., 1953. 32 pp.

COFFIN, D. L.: Diseases of Parrots. In *Parrots and Parrot-like Birds,* by Duke of Bedford. Fond du Lac, Wis., All-Pets Books, Inc., 1954.

DALBORG-JOHANSEN, J.: *Stuefuglenes Sygdomme og deres Behandling.* København, J. F. Clausens Forlag, 1958.

DATHE, H.: Einige Worte über die Schreckmauser. Gefiederte Welt 1959—85.

DURANT, A. J., and McDOUGLE, H. C.: Apoplexy in a canary. J.A.V.M.A. *87:*265, 1940.

FEYERABEND, C.: Diseases of budgerigars. All-Pets Magazine 1951.

FEYERABEND, C.: *Your Budgie's Health Book.* Fond du Lac, Wis., All-Pets Books, Inc., 1957.

FRITZSCHE, K., and GERRIETS, E.: *Geflügelkrankheiten.* Berlin/Hamburg, Verlag Paul Parey, 1959.

FROST, C.: Experiences with pet budgerigars. Vet. Rec. *73:*621, 1961.

GALLI-VALERIO, B.: Sur une toxoplasmiase du Melopsittacus undulatus. Schweiz. Arch. Tierhlk. *81:*458, 1931.

GEISSLER, H.: *Die wichtigsten Küken- und Aufzuchtkrankheiten.* Frankfurt, Verlag Neue Presse, 1951.

GRAY, E.: *Diseases of Poultry.* London, Crosby Lockwood and Son Ltd., 1955.

GROTH, W.: Zur histologischen Diagnostik einiger Erkrankungen des Nervensystems der Hühner (Newcastle Krankheit, Mareksche Geflügellähmung, infektiöse Encephalomyelitis, Encephalomalacie). Berl. Münch. tierärztl. Wschr. *75:*24, 1962.

GRZIMEK, B.: *Krankes Geflügel.* Stuttgart/Berlin, Fritz Pfenningstorff, 6. Aufl. 1950.

HAMERTON, A. E.: Diseases of aviary birds. Vet. J. *89:*5, 1933.

HASHOLT, J.: *Fuglesygdomme.* Aa. Poulsen:Prydfjerkræ, Skibby bogtrykkeri, 1959.

HASHOLT, J.: Current diseases of cage birds. J. small anim. Pract. *2:*97, 1961.

HILBRICH, P.: *Krankheiten des Geflügels.* Schwenningen am Neckar, Verlag Hermann Kuhn, 1963.

HODKIN, A. L.: *The Conduction of the Nervous Impulse.* The Sherrington Lectures VII, Liverpool University Press, 1964.

JONES, O. G.: Common diseases of cage birds and other less usual pets. Vet. Rec. *68:*918, 1956.

KEMNA, A.: *Krankheiten der Stubenvögel.* Minden, Philler Verlag, 1959.

KEYMER, I. F.: The diagnosis and treatment of common psittacine diseases. Mod. Vet. Pract. *39*(21):22, December 15, 1958.

KEYMER, I. F.: The diagnosis and treatment of some diseases of seed-eating passerine birds. Mod. Vet. Pract. *40(7):* 30, April 1, 1959.

LESBOUYRIES, G.: *Pathologie des oiseaux de basse-cour.* Paris, Vigot Frères, 1965.

LESKIEN, I.: Stoffwechselstörungen beim Sittich und Kanarienvogel u. i. Behandlung. Berl. u. Münch. tierarztl. Wschr. u. Wiener tierarztl. Monatsschr. 1944—254.

MARTHEDAL, H. E.: Fjerkræsygdomme I. De studerendes råd. Vet. og. Landbohøjskolen, København. 1957

PLAZIKOWSKI, U.: *Boken om Burfåglar.* London/Stockholm/New York, S. E. Berghs Förlag, 1959.

RADTKE, A.: Lähmungserscheinungen bei Wellensittichen. Gefiederte Welt 1958—64.

RAGOTZI, B.: Lähmungserscheinungen bei Wellensittichen. Gefiederte Welt 1958—166.

REINHARDT, R.: *Lehrbuch der Geflügelkrankheiten.* Hannover, M. & H. Schaper, 1950. 384 pp.

RUBNER,: Lähmungserscheinungen bei Goulds und anderen Prachtfinken. Gefiederte Welt 1957—30.

SANGER, V. L., and HAMDY, A. H.: A strange fright-flight behavior pattern (hysteria) in hens. J.A.V.M.A. *140:* 455, 1962.

SCOTT, M. L., and STOEWSAND, G. S.: A study of the ataxias of vitamin A and vitamin E deficiencies in the chick. Poultry Sci. *40:*1517, 1961.

STURKIE, P. D.: *Avian Physiology,* 2nd ed. Ithaca, N.Y., Comstock Publishing Associates, 1965.

TINBERGEN, N.: *Social Behavior in Animals.* Methuen a.co. Ltd., 1953.

WAILLY, P. DE: *L'amateur des oiseaux de cage et de voliere.* Paris, J. B. Bailliere et fils, 1964.

WIGHT, P. A. L.: Lymphoid leucosis and fowl paralysis in the quail. Vet. Rec. *75:*685, 1963.

ZWART, P.: Über einige Vogelkrankheiten und ihre praktische Bedeutung. Kleintier-Praxis *8:*7, 1963.

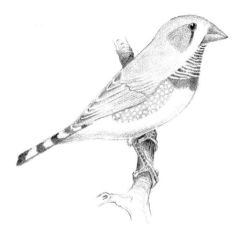

22

Diseases of the Endocrine System

David K. Blackmore

Of all the categories of disease of cage birds, probably the one about which least is known is diseases of the endocrine system, and little is known concerning the exact role of the various endocrine organs in the physiology of the normal bird. The small amount of information available on this subject is almost entirely limited to the budgerigar (*Melopsittacus undulatus*); the discussion in this Chapter is therefore biased toward this species.

The organs considered will be the pituitary, thyroid, parathyroid, and adrenal glands. However, to make the Chapter as complete as possible, mention will also be made of the pancreas, thymus, and gonads, although there is still considerable doubt as to whether the thymus has any definite endocrine function. For those who wish to know more about general avian endocrine physiology, excellent reviews have been written by Höhn[9] and Sturkie.[23]

Although it is likely that cage birds will eventually be shown to suffer from as diverse a group of endocrine diseases as other domesticated animals, at the present moment, except for thyroid and parathyroid abnormalities, neoplastic disease appears to be the most frequently diagnosed form of disease of the endocrine glands in cage birds. The budgerigar appears to be particularly susceptible to neoplastic disease, including neoplasia of the endocrine organs, and it is interesting to surmise whether this high incidence of neoplasia may itself be associated with some primary endocrine disturbance.

Cage birds exhibit many diseases of unknown etiology which future investigation may show to be of endocrine origin. Typical examples are alopecia and other feather abnormalities, certain forms of infertility, and, as already suggested, certain forms of neoplasia. Until much more basic work has been carried out, the whole subject of endocrine disease of cage birds will be rather speculative, but it is hoped that the discussions in this Chapter will help to stimulate a greater interest in and result in greater knowledge of this subject.

THE PITUITARY GLAND (HYPOPHYSIS)

The pituitary gland in birds can easily be exposed by removing the lower mandible and palate, then with a pair of blunt forceps breaking away the medial ridge of the sphenoid bone. The pituitary will be found lying in the sella turcica of the sphenoid, just posterior to the optic chiasma. In the budgerigar it is a brownish globular structure approximately 2 mm. in diameter (Fig. 22-1). The following discussion on the anatomy and physiology of the pituitary gland is taken from Höhn.[9]

The general structure of the avian pituitary gland is similar to that of mammals, except for absence of the pars intermedia. The part of the gland of pharyngeal origin consists of the anterior lobe and pars tuberalis; the smaller posterior lobe is of neural origin.

The major cells of the anterior lobe consist of chromophobe and chromophile cells, and the latter cells are subdivided into two types of acidophils and one type of basophil. The pars tuberalis consists mainly of chromophobe cells. The basophils probably produce gonadotropins; the acidophils produce prolactin, probably thyroid-stimulating hormone, adrenocorticotropic hormone (ACTH, or corticotropin), and possibly an intersititial cell–stimulating hormone. There is no definite evidence of a growth-promoting hormone in avian species.

The hormones of the posterior lobe are apparently similar to those found in mammals, that is, vasopressin (arginine vasotocin) and oxytocin. These various avian hormones will not be discussed in detail, but mention should be made of the effects of prolactin on the secretion of "crop milk" in pigeons, its effects in combination with estrogens in causing the incubation patch or laying patch in passerine birds, and its relation to broodiness. It may also be clinically important to realize that oxytocin is believed to have the same effect on the oviduct as it has on the uterus in mammals.

Neoplasia or hyperplasia of the pituitary appears to be the only disease of this organ recorded in cage birds, and all references to this condition concern budgerigars. Schlumberger,[21] in his review of tumors characteristic of certain animals, records 156 primary chromophobe adenomas or carcinomas of the pituitary among 497 tumors affecting budgerigars.

Pituitary neoplasia does not appear to be observed so frequently in other countries, and is comparatively rare in the United Kingdom. Beach[4] records only eight cases of pituitary enlargement from a series of 866 budgerigar necropsies, and was able to diagnose chromophobe adenoma, similar to those described by Schlumberger,[18] in only two cases. I have recorded only one similar case from over 900 budgerigar necropsies,[6] and Keymer,[11,12] in his articles on both psittacine and passerine birds, failed to mention the condition. Frost[7] and Arnall,[2,3] in their essentially clinical papers, do not record lesions or symptoms that are likely to be associated with pituitary neoplasia.

The signs and symptoms described by Schlumberger[18] as associated with these chromophobe adenomas or carcinomas are mainly related to the mechanical effects of enlargement of the organ and local infiltration of surrounding structures. Affected birds often exhibit a unilateral or bilateral proptosis due to retro-ocular invasion, and impaired vision or total blindness. Cerebral involvement can result in general malaise and periodic convulsions which may last for two or three days before death. Some birds show signs of diabetes insipidus in that they develop a severe diarrhea and polydipsia, presumably due to an impaired production of antidiuretic hormone. Experiments carried out by Schlumberger[20] indicate that these tumors can cause a generalized obesity, but as this latter condition is so frequently seen in birds

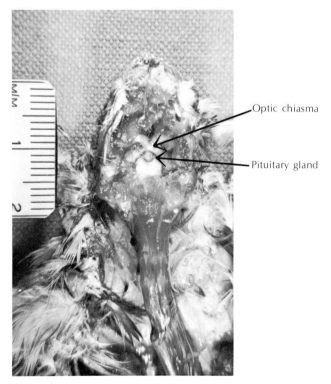

Fig. 22-1. *Normal pituitary gland of budgerigar.*

Optic chiasma

Pituitary gland

which do not have such tumors, too much emphasis should not be placed on this feature.

Postmortem examination of affected birds shows gross enlargement of the pituitary, and in a series of 50 cases examined by Schlumberger[18] 40 per cent showed as much as a 10-fold increase in weight, 56 per cent showed invasion of local structures, and 4 per cent had metastases in other organs. The only secondary changes noted in other endocrine organs, associated with neoplasia of the pituitary, were suppression of spermatogenesis and lack of developing follicles in the ovary.

THE THYROID GLANDS

The thyroid glands of birds are divided into two distinct lobes, which are situated in the lower cervical region, closely applied to either common carotid artery, ventral to the brachial plexus (Fig. 22-2). The thyroids cannot be palpated in the living bird, except in a few cases of gross pathological enlargement, as they are in

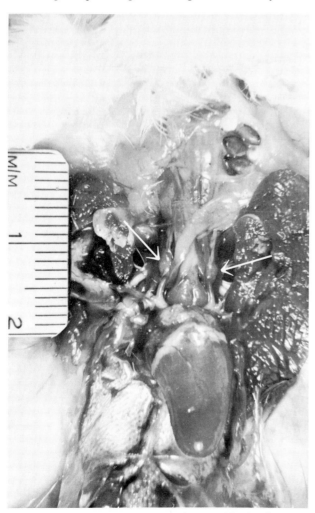

Fig. 22-2. *Normal thyroid glands of budgerigar.*

the anterior thoracic cavity enclosed by the lower cervical region dorsally and the sternum and pectoral muscles ventrally. At necropsy the two glands are easily exposed by removing the sternum and pectoral muscles with a pair of blunt-ended dissecting scissors.

Embryonically the thyroids develop from the pharyngeal pouches. The parathyroids are usually closely applied to the posterior pole of each thyroid.

The relative weight of normal thyroid glands of different species tends to vary, but in the smaller cage birds the combined thyroid weight is in the region of 0.02 per cent of the total body weight. A budgerigar of 35 gm. body weight will have normal thyroids weighing approximately 3 mg. each and measuring approximately 2 mm. in length and 1 mm. in width. The left thyroid is usually slightly larger than the right. Not infrequently one thyroid is vestigial, and when this presumably congenital abnormality occurs the remaining thyroid is enlarged, so that the relative weight of the combined glands remains constant. The thyroids of canaries and the other small passerines are more globular in shape and pinhead in size.

The avian thyroid resembles that of other vertebrates in structure, consisting of numerous acini lined with a single layer of epithelial cells and containing a homogeneous acidophilic colloid material. In the normal gland, there is little obvious interstitial tissue and few large blood vessels.

The epithelial cells preferentially absorb iodine from the circulating blood, and combine it with the amino acid tyrosine to form both mono- and di-iodotyrosine. These compounds combine to form the hormone thyroxine, which is stored in the colloid in loose combination with protein, as thyroglobulin. The thyroxine is released from the colloid into the circulating blood by enzyme activity.

The activity of the thyroid is controlled by thyroid-stimulating hormone (T.S.H.) from the anterior lobe of the pituitary. Increased activity is indicated morphologically by an increase in the size of the epithelial cells of the thyroid. The level of T.S.H. produced by the pituitary is regulated by the level of circulating thyroxine. In birds, as in other vertebrate species, thyroxine has an effect on the metabolic rate; it is also considered to have an effect on the development of the gonads and on the normal molting process.

Thyroid Dysplasia (Hyperplasia)

INCIDENCE AND OCCURRENCE

The most common thyroid disease of budgerigars is the one termed thyroid dysplasia.[5] This condition is especially common in those kept as household pets, but does not appear to be a problem in other species of cage birds.

The high incidence of the disease has been noted by Arnall,[3] Beach,[4] Blackmore,[5] and Frost[7] in the United Kingdom, and by Geyer[8] in Germany; the publication *Avian Medicine,*[1] by the American Animal Hospital Association, stresses the importance of the disease in budgerigars in America.

Analysis of the cause of death of 129 pet budgerigars examined by me[5] showed that 85 per cent of these birds were affected with varying degrees of thyroid abnormality, and 23.8 per cent had died as a direct result of thyroid dysplasia.

ETIOLOGY

This work[5] also indicated that the disease was associated with an iodine deficiency in seed mixtures normally fed to budgerigars, and that it could be prevented by iodine supplementation of the diet. Earlier work in America[19] and in Germany[8] had also indicated an iodine deficiency as the basic cause of the condition, but had related sites of occurrence of the disease to known goitrogenic areas.

The symptoms of affected birds appear to be directly related to the mechanical effects of the gross thyroid enlargement. In *Avian Medicine*[1] the condition is described as a thyrotoxicosis, but, although there is a hyperplasia of the thyroid epithelium in the early stages of the disease, there is no experimental evidence of excessive thyroxine production, and it would be more logical to expect the production of thyroxine to be reduced.

PATHOLOGY

Examination of carcasses of birds that have died as a result of thyroid dysplasia shows gross enlargement of both thyroids, with length exceeding 1 cm., and each gland sometimes weighing over 300 mg. (Figs. 22-3, 22-4). Glands that are also grossly cystic are sometimes palpable and may attain a weight of over 1 gm.

The diseased glands are brownish in color and contain yellow granular material. Similar granular material is often adherent to the internal surface of the sternum and the pericardium at the base of the heart. Many diseased glands contain cysts of varying size, filled with a brown or blood-stained fluid.

The condition starts as a typical iodine-deficiency syndrome, with hyperplasia of the epithelium of the acini. The glands then become congested, and interstitial and intra-alveolar hemorrhages occur, followed by desqua-

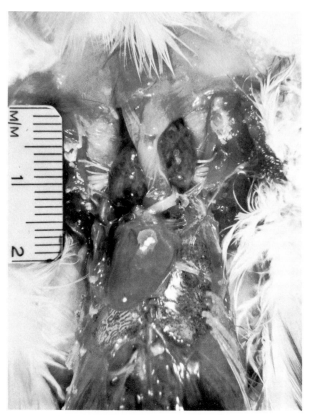

Fig. 22-3. *Thyroid glands of budgerigar showing dysplasia.*

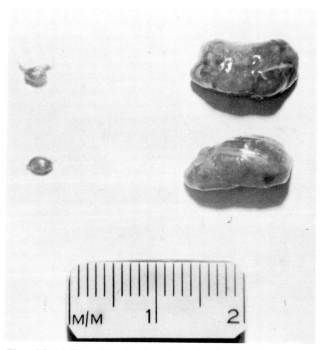

Fig. 22-4. *Thyroid glands of budgerigar: left, normal; right, showing dysplasia.*

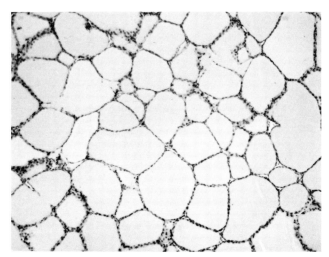

Fig. 22-5. *Section of normal thyroid gland of budgerigar.* ×98.

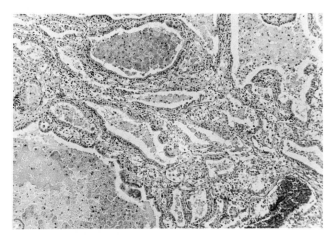

Fig. 22-6. *Section of thyroid gland of budgerigar, showing advanced dysplasia.* ×88.

mation of the epithelium, loss of colloid, and complete disruption of normal architecture. Details of these histological changes have been published elsewhere.[5]

Figures 22-5 and 22-6 reveal the difference apparent on microscopy of normal thyroid tissue and tissue from a gland showing advanced dysplasia.

SYMPTOMS

The major symptoms of this disease are respiratory and are associated with pressure on the syrinx and lower trachea, resulting in labored respiration, often accompanied by a squeaking respiratory noise. The bird that previously was able to talk will discontinue. Because of concurrent pressure on the lower esophagus, seed is unable to pass into the proventriculus, so that marked swallowing movements, regurgitation of seed, and dila-

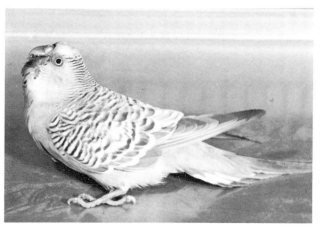

Fig. 22-7. *A typical posture seen in budgerigar suffering from severe thyroid dysplasia. (Courtesy of R. T. French Company.)*

tation of the crop may result. Associated with this esophageal constriction may be signs of gradual starvation and severe loss of weight. Some cases also show signs indicative of cardiac embarrassment due to pressure by the diseased glands on the heart and blood vessels (Fig. 22-7). These birds may develop convulsions and/or partial paralysis. Birds have been examined in which the final cause of death was rupture of the gland and internal hemorrhage.

In only a small proportion of cases is it possible to palpate an enlarged and cystic thyroid in the lower cervical region.

PREVENTION AND TREATMENT

It has been shown that thyroid dysplasia can be prevented by supplementing the diet with small quantities of iodine in the form of potassium iodide (less than 20 μg. of iodine is required per week). The condition is rare in birds whose diet is supplemented with cod liver oil, which has a high content of natural iodine, containing an average of 10,000 μg. of iodine per Kg.; canary seed seldom contains more than 30 μg. of iodine per Kg.

Lafeber[14] recommended daily injection of 0.01–0.03 ml. of a 20% solution of sodium iodide into the pectoral muscles until symptoms have regressed. The higher levels of dosage are administered in critical cases. Marked improvement should occur within three days. If no change occurs, the diagnosis should be re-evaluated.

The patient is continued on dilute Lugol's solution (2 parts of Lugol's solution and 28 parts of distilled water) in the drinking water at home. As a *therapeutic dose* one drop of *dilute Lugol's solution* is given in 1 oz. of fresh drinking water daily; as a *prophylactic measure,* one drop of *dilute Lugol's solution* is given in 1 oz. of fresh drinking water once a week. Other medications should not be mixed in the iodinated water.

I have seen only one case of a disease resembling thyroid dysplasia in another species, this being in an aviary-kept twite (*Carduelis flavirostris*). Petrak[17] reported having seen three clinical cases in Java sparrows (*Padda oryzivora*).

Other Non-neoplastic Thyroid Diseases

Iodine-deficiency diseases are recognized in poultry and can probably, in exceptional circumstances, occur in all species of cage birds.

Hollander and Riddle[10] described goiter in pigeons in America which responded to supplementation of the diet with potassium iodide. The disease was characterized by thyroid enlargement, and affected birds showed evidence of myxedema of the head, ruffled plumage, and occasionally respiratory distress, but the greatest effects were decreased hatchability of eggs, and an increased mortality of the newly hatched squabs.

I have noted hyperplastic thyroid changes of captive wild birds suffering from acute septicemic diseases (pasteurellosis and erysipelas).

One adult budgerigar with a thyroglossal cyst has been examined. The affected bird had a marked swelling in the mid-cervical region (Fig. 22-8).

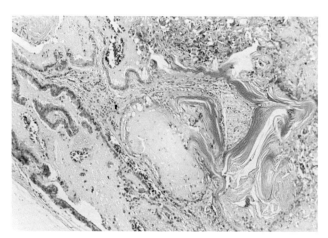

Fig. 22-8. *Section of thyroglossal cyst of budgerigar. ×88.*

Neoplastic Thyroid Disease

Schlumberger[19] stated that neoplasia of the thyroid is rare in birds, and cited references to thyroid neoplasia in a scarlet macaw (*Ara macao*) and a few cases in various species of birds kept in zoological collections. Beach[4]

recorded one carcinoma and one adenoma affecting the thyroids of budgerigars. I have seen two cases of thyroid neoplasia in budgerigars; one of these was a unilateral adenoma, and the other was bilateral with a large metastatic lesion weighing over 9 gm. in the pectoral region. Unfortunately, the tissue was too autolyzed for detailed microscopic study.

It would appear that neoplasia of the thyroid is an uncommon disease, but affected birds are likely to exhibit symptoms similar to those associated with thyroid dysplasia.

THE ADRENAL GLANDS

The adrenal glands of birds are paired yellowish structures closely applied to the anterior pole of either kidney and covered ventrally by the gonads (Fig. 22-9). In the majority of avian species, the size of the adrenals is directly related to the body weight, and they weigh

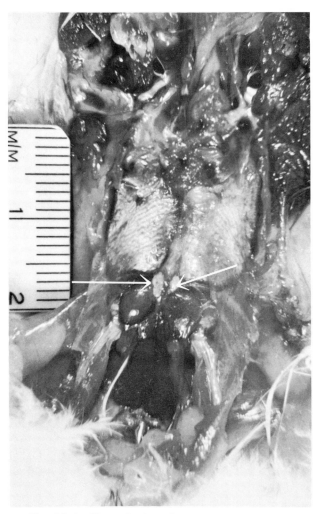

Fig. 22-9. *Normal adrenal glands of budgerigar.*

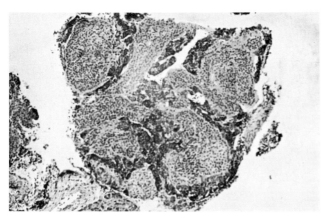

Fig. 22-10. *Section of normal adrenal gland of budgerigar. ×80. Note darker-staining medullary tissue.*

about the same as the thyroids. The glands consist of two main parts: the cortical tissue, of endodermal origin, and the medullary, or chromaffin, tissue, of ectodermal origin. In birds, the junction between these two parts of the adrenal is less definite than in mammals, and the cortex is not divided into definite zones (Fig. 22-10).

The hormones produced by the avian adrenal cortex are steroids, apparently similar to those produced in mammals, that is, mineralocorticoids (aldosterone), glucocorticoids (corticosterone), and sex hormones. The activity of the adrenal cortex is under the control of the anterior lobe of the pituitary gland through the secretion of the adrenocorticotropic hormone.

The medullary tissue is basically similar in function and structure to that of mammals, and studies in fowls and pigeons have demonstrated the production of epinephrine and norepinephrine, with physiological effects similar to those of the mammalian hormones.

No detailed study has been carried out on the diseases of the adrenals in cage birds, and the few references available mainly concern neoplasia. Sturkie[23] refers to work by Riddle which demonstrated an increase in adrenal size in pigeons affected by ascaridiasis and tuberculosis. Sturkie[23] also refers to Beznak's observation of an increase in the size of adrenals from pigeons suffering from a vitamin B$_1$ deficiency.

Beach[4] recorded a case of a budgerigar with bilateral adrenal adenomas and a budgerigar with marked adrenal cortical hyperplasia, but the clinical symptoms of the affected birds were not described. I examined one budgerigar with a unilateral adrenal adenoma, but the affected bird showed no obvious symptoms prior to death.[6] A little owl (*Athene noctua*), which had been in captivity for several months, was found to be suffering from an adrenal carcinoma with a metastatic lesion in the liver. This bird had signs of general malaise for several weeks.

Apparently the smaller cage birds and recently imported birds are extremely susceptible to various stress

factors, and it would be interesting to know how many of these birds that die have suffered from adrenal exhaustion, although no obvious lesions are revealed at necropsy. This whole problem of "stress" is of considerable importance in cage-bird practice, and every attempt should be made to minimize stressful conditions.

THE PARATHYROID GLANDS

In early embryonic development each parathyroid gland consists of two lobes, but these become fused together to form one main body closely attached to the posterior pole of each thyroid gland. Small areas of apparent parathyroid tissue can sometimes be found elsewhere within the thyroid. The tissue is made up of cords of epithelial cells with round, deeply staining nuclei.

The hormone produced by the parathyroid glands is protein in nature. It controls the serum calcium level by promoting the excretion of phosphorus by the kidney, stimulating the release of calcium from bone, and promoting the absorption of calcium from the intestine. The parathyroid is apparently not under the control of any other endocrine organ, but is stimulated by a fall in the level of serum calcium. The problem of parathyroid function in relation to the serum calcium and phosphorus levels has been excellently reviewed by Krook.[13] In poultry, there is evidence that parathyroid hormone and estrogens have a synergistic effect.

Parathyroid hyperplasia occurs frequently in cage birds, especially those that are essentially seed-eaters, but primary hyperparathyroidism due to neoplasia of the gland has apparently not been described.

Nutritional Secondary Hyperparathyroidism

Very little attention has been paid previously to nutritional secondary hyperparathyroidism of cage birds, but this condition, which is characterized by gross parathyroid enlargement (Fig. 22-11) and hyperplastic change of the cells of the gland (Fig. 22-12), together with evidence of osteodystrophy, frequently affects a wide variety of cage birds. The condition is caused by a hypocalcemia due to a nutritional deficiency of calcium, an excess of phosphorus, or a combination of both of these factors. The feeding of a seed mixture alone results in a diet in which the amount of phosphorus is far in excess of the calcium. Such circumstances are well known to produce a nutritional hyperparathyroidism in the horse, characterized by gross deformity of the bones of the jaw and commonly known as "Miller's disease."

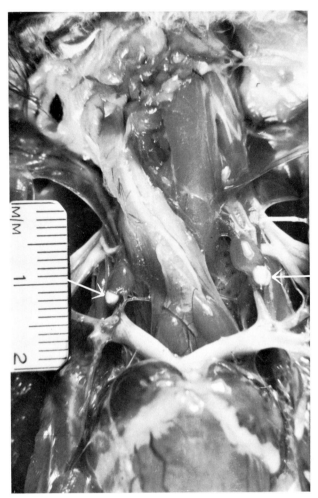

Fig. 22-11. *Parathyroid hyperplasia in an African grey parrot.*

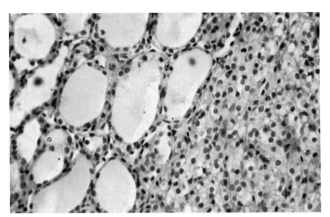

Fig. 22-12. *Section of junction of thyroid/parathyroid glands in a budgerigar, showing marked parathyroid hyperplasia. ×320.*

Cage birds such as budgerigars and other psittacines that are fed on a strict cereal diet frequently show marked enlargement and hyperplasia of the parathyroid glands, and young budgerigars that have failed to thrive have often been shown to be suffering from a parathyroid hyperplasia and generalized osteodystrophy. A similar condition is sometimes seen in older birds, in which gross parathyroid hyperplasia is often associated with a complete absence of grit in the gizzard.

Preliminary experiments in my laboratory have shown that withdrawal of the usual calcium supplements (soluble grit and cow's milk) from breeding budgerigars resulted in a marked decrease in fertility and an increase in embryonic deaths; those chicks that hatched died after a few weeks, showing marked parathyroid hyperplasia and a generalized osteodystrophy. Similar results have been produced in non-experimental aviaries by a diet which contained insufficient soluble grit.

There is a need for veterinarians interested in cage birds to pay more attention to parathyroid hyperplasia and to the levels of calcium, phosphorus, and vitamin

D_3 in the diet. These factors may also be relevant in connection with general infertility problems, as well as the osteodystrophic diseases of young birds.

Renal Secondary Hyperparathyroidism

Domesticated animals suffering from nephritis and other kidney diseases often have a renal secondary hyperparathyroidism as a result of impaired renal excretion of serum phosphorus, with a consequent decrease in the serum calcium.

Although cage birds often suffer from various forms of kidney disease there is little information concerning concurrent parathyroid changes. This is probably because birds affected with kidney disease die before clinical symptoms of parathyroid hyperplasia are evident, and because avian pathologists have often overlooked these secondary changes. No detailed analysis has been carried out, but hyperplasia of the parathyroids has been noted in budgerigars suffering from nephritis. In such cases it is difficult to know whether the hyperparathyroidism is renal or nutritional in origin.

THE PANCREAS

In birds, as in mammals, the pancreas is both endocrine and exocrine in function, and the endocrine portion is the islet tissue. In birds, the pancreas is a relatively large organ situated close to the duodenum; in budgerigars the organ consists of two main lobes placed either side of the duodenum, one lobe being within the loop of the duodenum. The general histological appearance of the pancreas in birds is similar to that of the mammalian pancreas, but the islets are less well defined

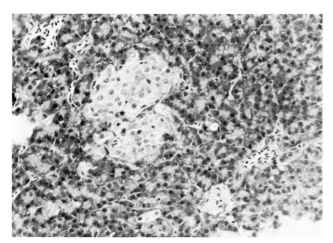

Fig. 22-13. *Section of pancreas of budgerigar, showing an islet of Langerhans.* ×320.

(Fig. 22-13). The islet cells consist of alpha and beta cells, and a third small delta cell has been described in pigeons. The hormones produced are glucagon and insulin, but the effects of insulin on the level of blood sugar are far less marked than they are in mammals, except in the carnivorous birds.[16] It would appear that adrenocorticotropic hormones and prolactin have a far greater effect on the level of blood sugar than insulin has. Thus diabetes mellitus is not to be expected in birds, with the possible exception of strictly carnivorous species. This is confirmed by experimental pancreatectomy, which in grain-eating birds results in a mild hyperglycemia for a week only, with blood sugar then reverting to normal levels.[15]

Records of endocrine disease of the pancreas in cage birds are rare, but from the previous comments it is apparent that any birds that are affected are unlikely to show symptoms of diabetes mellitus. Schlumberger[22] recorded one case of an islet cell tumor in a budgerigar; Beach[4] recorded a case of generalized pancreatic atrophy in a budgerigar, but the affected bird showed symptoms apparently associated with dysfunction of the exocrine portion of the gland. The only case of pancreatic disease I noted was a case of neoplasia of the gland in a budgerigar, but the tumor appeared to be an adenoma of exocrine origin.[6]

No articles concerning pancreatitis with involvement of either the endocrine or the exocrine portion of the gland could be found in the literature.

THE THYMUS

The function of the thymus in both mammals and birds is obscure, and whether this organ has any endocrine functions is even more obscure.

The thymus is most highly developed in young birds

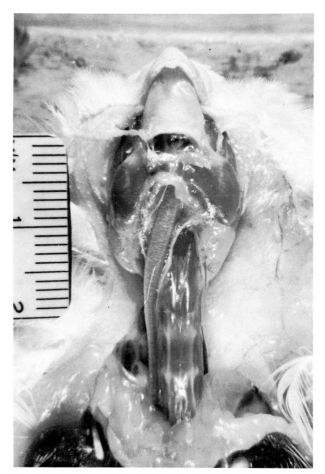

Fig. 22-14. *Mandibular lobes of thymus in a young budgerigar.*

and tends to regress with age, although in some species there is some subsequent hypertrophy during the breeding season. The gland is made up of a chain of small lobes, closely related to the jugular vein, extending from the angle of the jaw to the base of the neck. In budgerigars the gland is pale and similar in color to the surrounding subcutaneous fat; the largest lobes are in the submandibular region (Fig. 22-14), and the remaining two or three smaller lobes extend down the neck to just cranial to the thyroid glands. The structure of the gland is similar to the mammalian thymus, with the tissue divided into cortical and medullary zones. The Hassall bodies are often extremely prominent (Fig. 22-15).

Excessive atrophy of the thymus in birds has been associated with the stress of infectious disease and may be due to the influence of adrenocortical hormones.

Pathological hyperplasia or neoplasia of the thymus is sometimes recognized in cage birds, particularly in the budgerigar. This is usually characterized by a circumscribed globular mass up to 1 cm. in diameter in the upper cervical region (Fig. 22-16). I have seen two such cases of neoplasia of the thymus in budgerigars.[6]

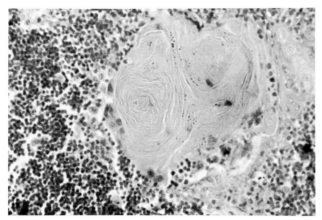

Fig. 22-15. *Section of thymus of budgerigar, showing a Hassall body. ×320.*

Beach[4] recorded a case of thymus hyperplasia in a budgerigar, and Petrak[17] saw a similar case in a canary associated with subcutaneous hemorrhage in the region of the hyperplastic thymus gland. Surgical removal of these enlarged glands would appear to be difficult, owing to the closeness of the jugular vein.

THE GONADS

The major diseases of the testes and ovaries are discussed in Chapter 20, but as these organs also have an important endocrine function they are mentioned briefly in this Chapter.

Androgens are produced by the interstitial cells of the testes and by the ovary. The ovary produces estrogens and progesterone, but in birds the exact site of production of these hormones is not known. The androgens and estrogens are responsible for the secondary sex characteristics. In the majority of avian species, sex difference in the color of plumage is due to the effects of estrogens, whereas in some species androgens are responsible for a difference in the color of the beak. In chickens, androgens are responsible for the growth of the comb in males and in females during egg production. Estrogens cause hypertrophy of the oviduct and increase in the levels of serum calcium and phosphorus and of

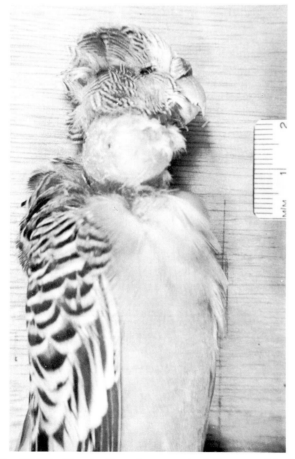

Fig. 22-16. *Neoplastic enlargement of thymus of budgerigar.*

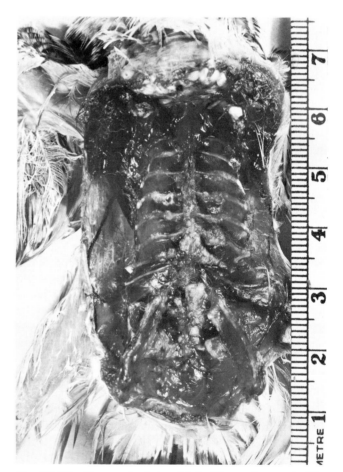

Fig. 22-17. *Hyperostosis in a bird with ovarian cysts. The viscera with the cysts have been removed, revealing the bony protuberances on the pelvic bones, vertebral column, and the ribs. (From Beach, J. E.: Vet. Rec. 74:136, 1962.)*

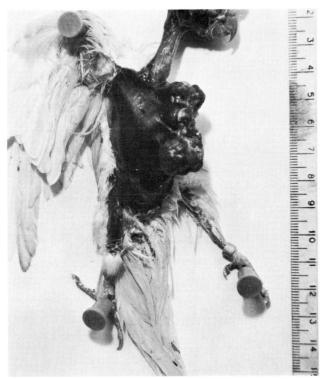

Fig. 22-18. *Hyperostosis. In this extreme case the ribs and skull bones were also affected. (From Beach, J. E.: Vet. Rec. 74:136, 1962.)*

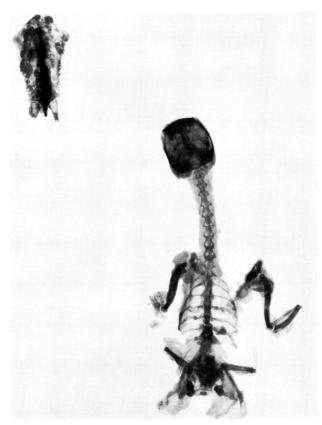

Fig. 22-19. *Radiograph of the budgerigar shown in Fig. 22-18. Note the hyperostosis of ribs, vertebrae, sternum, and humerus. (Courtesy of J. E. Beach.)*

blood lipids. Schlumberger[22] showed that stilbestrol implants in budgerigars would induce excessive medullary bone formation.

The most important group of endocrine diseases affecting the gonads are those due to neoplasia, and these conditions, which are particularly common in the budgerigar, are described in Chapters 20 and 27. They are often accompanied by an obvious change in the secondary sex characteristics. Such changes in the budgerigar include change in color of the cere, which in adult males is blue, and in females, varying shades of brown. Beach[4] records a change in the color of the cere of budgerigars affected with granulosa cell tumors, Sertoli cell tumors, and seminomas. This change of color does not always occur with these forms of neoplasm.

Another disease of budgerigars apparently associated with a disturbance in estrogen production is polyostotic hyperostosis, which is characterized by generalized gross bone deposits, especially affecting the sternum, skull,

and spine of female birds. Schlumberger[22] recorded 21 naturally occurring cases in a series of 1300 budgerigar necropsies, and was able to reproduce the disease experimentally with stilbestrol implants.

Beach[4] reported hyperostosis in a bird with ovarian cysts (Fig. 22-17); in another bird with an extreme case of hyperostosis the ribs and skull bones were involved, as well as the vertebrae, sternum, and humerus (Figs. 22-18 and 22-19).

A disease of budgerigars that frequently appears to be of endocrine origin is a generalized alopecia or loss of body feathers; this often responds to testosterone administered weekly over a six-week period.

An association between estrogens and the level of blood lipids suggests that further investigation may show that certain obese budgerigars may be suffering from a concurrent endocrine disturbance.

References

1. AMERICAN ANIMAL HOSPITAL ASSOCIATION: *Avian Medicine*. Elkhart, Indiana, 1964. 27 pp.

2. ARNALL, L.: Experiences with cage-birds. Vet. Rec. *70:* 120–128, 1958.

3. ARNALL, L.: Further experiences with cagebirds. Vet. Rec. *73:*1146–1154, 1961.

4. BEACH, J. E.: Diseases of budgerigars and other cage birds. A survey of *post-mortem* findings. Vet. Rec. *74:*10–14, 63–68, 134–140, 1962.

5. BLACKMORE, D. K.: The incidence and aetiology of thyroid dysplasia in budgerigars (*Melopsittacus undulatus*). Vet. Rec. *75:*1068–1072, 1963.

6. BLACKMORE, D. K.: The pathology and incidence of neoplasia in cage birds. J. small anim. Pract. *6:*217–223, 1965.

7. FROST, C.: Experiences with pet budgerigars. Vet. Rec. *73:*621–626, 1961.

8. GEYER, S.: Report of third international symposium of zoo animal pathology, Vet. Rec. *73:*973–974, 1961.

9. HÖHN, E. O.: Endocrine Glands, Thymus, and Pineal Body. In *Biology and Comparative Physiology of Birds,* A. J. Marshall, ed. New York, Academic Press, 1961. Vol. II, pp. 87–114.

10. HOLLANDER, W. F., and RIDDLE, O.: Goiter in domestic pigeons. Poultry Sci. *25:*20–27, 1946.

11. KEYMER, I. F.: Specific diseases of the canary and other passerine birds. Mod. Vet. Pract. *40*(17):32–35, September 1 (Part I); *40*(18):45–48, September 15 (Part II), 1959.

12. KEYMER, I. F.: Postmortem examinations of pet birds.

Mod. Vet. Pract. *42*(23):35–38, December 1, *42*(24): 47–51, December 15, 1961.

13. KROOK, L.: Metabolic Bone Disease of Endocrine Origin. Handbuch der speziellen pathologischen anatomie der haustiere (in press).

14. LAFEBER, T. J.: Thyroid dysplasia in the Budgerigar, Animal Hospital *1:*208–218, 1965.

15. MIRSKY, I. A., NELSON, N., GRAYMAN, I., and KORENBERG, M.: Studies on normal and depancreatized domestic ducks. Am. J. Physiol. *135:*223–229, 1941.

16. NELSON, N., ELGART, S., and MIRSKY, I. A.: Pancreatic diabetes in the owl. Endocrinology *31:*119–123, 1942.

17. PETRAK, M. L.: Personal communication, 1964.

18. SCHLUMBERGER, H. G.: Neoplasia in the parakeet. I. Spontaneous chromophobe pituitary tumors. Cancer Res. *14:*237–245, 1954.

19. SCHLUMBERGER, H. G.: Spontaneous goiter and cancer of the thyroid in animals. Ohio J. Sci. *55:*23–43, 1955.

20. SCHLUMBERGER, H. G.: Neoplasia in the parakeet. II. Transplantation of the Pituitary Tumor. Cancer Res. *16:*149–153, 1956.

21. SCHLUMBERGER, H. G.: Tumors characteristic for certain animal species. A review. Cancer Res. *17:*823–832, 1957.

22. SCHLUMBERGER, H. G.: Polyostotic hyperostosis in the female parakeet. Am. J. Path. *35:*1–23, 1959.

23. STURKIE, P. D.: *Avian Physiology,* 2nd ed. Ithaca, N.Y., Comstock Publishing Associates, 1965.

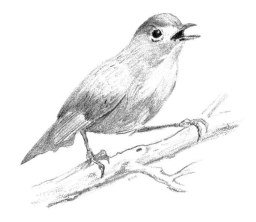

23

Diseases of the Organs of Special Sense

Erwin Small

A review of the literature reveals a paucity of information on diseases of cage birds generally, with an even greater scarcity in the area of diseases of the organs of special sense. Of the articles written, many are by breeders reporting on their individual experiences. In recent years, the increasing popularity of budgerigars, canaries, and finches as household pets has resulted in presentation of additional disease problems to the practitioners of veterinary medicine. The organs of special sense are responsible for a limited number of the difficulties, and this Chapter is devoted to discussion of the clinical signs and treatment of certain conditions affecting them.

CONDITIONS INVOLVING THE EYE

Congenital and Hereditary Anomalies

Anophthalmia is extremely rare. A case of bilateral involvement was reported in a 3-month-old budgerigar which had some difficulty in obtaining food.[2] The bird was normal in all other respects.

Cataracts have been reported in aged members of the parrot family, in the crested and crest-bred canary and cockatoo.[3,6,8] There is evidence of relation to inbreeding or local trauma. The appearance of the cataract, which is defined as any opacity of the lens or of its capsule, is identical with that in other domesticated animals. There is a serious question whether surgical correction should be attempted in birds used for breeding.

Hereditary albinism associated with a recessive gene has been reported by Sage[16] and McIlhenny,[14] and defective eyesight was detected in 12 nests of mockingbirds described by McIlhenny.[14]

Diseases of the Lids and Conjunctiva

BLEPHARITIS

Blepharitis is usually a complication of chronic ocular discharge resulting from conjunctivitis, infraorbital sinusitis, injuries, irritants, cnemidocoptic mange (Fig. 23-1), and certain bacterial or viral diseases.[1] Signs include inflammatory edema with erythema of the conjunctiva and exudates that are dry, scaly, or moist upon examination. An affected eye is often pasted shut. Treatment with bland protective preparations such as 5% boric acid ophthalmic ointment and 1% yellow oxide of mercury ophthalmic ointment, accompanied by intramuscular injection of broad-spectrum antibiotics, will usually suffice in those cases of blepharitis due to injury, conjunctivitis, or irritation. Blepharitis resulting from generalized bacterial or viral diseases is generally refractory to treatment.[5] Successful treatment of cnemidocoptic mange and infraorbital sinusitis will usually result in corresponding improvement in blepharitis.

Bird pox or variola resulting from virus infection often produces blepharitis and has been reported in pheasants, pigeons, canaries, and parakeets.[4,8,11] The reader is referred to Chapter 24 for additional discussion of this condition.

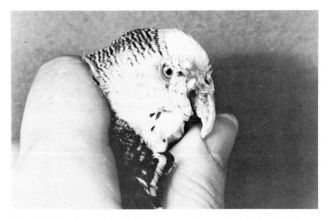

Fig. 23-1. *Cnemidocoptic mange in a budgerigar. (Courtesy of Dr. T. J. Lafeber.)*

CONJUNCTIVITIS

Keratoconjunctivitis is seen commonly in members of the parrot family.[1,3,7] It may be an aviary problem and

associated with bacterial or viral agents; more often, however, it is associated with injuries, foreign bodies, and fighting. In cases of infectious origin, the daily administration of chlortetracycline hydrochloride,* oxytetracycline hydrochloride,† or chloramphenicol succinate‡ intramuscularly at a dosage of 0.01 ml. per 30 grams body weight is recommended. Those cases resulting from irritants, foreign bodies, or trauma can be improved by removal of the offending material and the topical use of antibiotic ophthalmic preparations.

A contagious form of conjunctivitis that is often fatal has been reported in parakeets.[12] Bacteriological cultures and antibiotic sensitivity tests in two cases revealed resistant *Staphylococcus aureus*. There was mild to moderate thickening of the eyelids, ocular discharge, frequent blinking and rubbing of the affected eye, edema of surrounding tissues, and displacement of feathers with eventual pasting of the lids. Treatment should include the use of chlortetracycline hydrochloride* or chloramphenicol succinate‡ intramuscularly and the topical application of the same ophthalmic preparations which are used in the treatment of keratoconjunctivitis.

Xerophthalmia due to lack of vitamin A often causes conjunctivitis which is of gradual and insidious onset. Several species of Australian parakeets, for example, crimson-winged (*Aprosmictus erythropterus*), Bourke's (*Neophema bourkii*), and grass parakeets, and other members of the parrot family have been affected.[12] Manifestations include ocular exudation, puffiness of the upper and lower eyelids, and minute corneal ulcers. Diets rich in vitamin A, administration of cod liver oil, injectable vitamin A, 0.005 ml./30 gram, and the topical application of vitamin A ophthalmic ointments are therapeutic.

WOUNDS OF EYELIDS

Occasionally, eyelids are traumatized and torn. The lids can be sutured under proper anesthesia with 00000 gut on a swage needle.

CONJUNCTIVAL CYSTS

Cystic enlargement may involve the conjunctiva of the lower eyelid (Figs. 23-2, 23-3). Under general anesthesia, the cyst is incised, the material aspirated, and the cyst lining destroyed with either mild tincture of

*Aureomycin, intravenous (100 mg./ml.)—American Cyanamid Co., Princeton, N.J.

†Terramycin, intravenous (100 mg./ml.)—Charles Pfizer & Co., N.Y., N.Y.

‡Chloromycetin succinate (100 mg./ml.)—Parke, Davis & Co., Detroit, Mich.

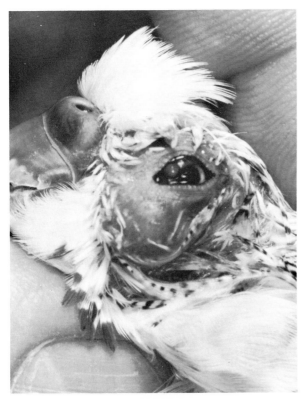

Fig. 23-2. *Conjunctival cyst in a budgerigar.*

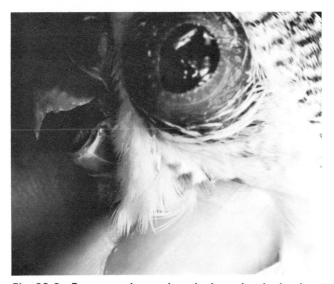

Fig. 23-3. *Postoperative conjunctival cyst in a budgerigar.*

iodine or 1% silver nitrate solution. Operative procedures should be followed by daily application of antibiotic steroid ophthalmic preparations.

LIPOGRANULOMA OF EYELID

Small pea-shaped masses, fairly solid but with fluid centers, may be seen on the eyelids of budgerigars. These are usually lipogranulomas and probably arise

as cysts of the meibomian glands.[15] Preferred treatment is surgical excision under general anesthesia.

PROLAPSE OF THE THIRD EYELID

Prolapse of the third eyelid may occasionally occur in amazon parrots. The recommended treatment is partial excision.[10] However, one must be sure to provide adequate hemostasis. A cotton-tip applicator saturated with Klot* or epinephrine and applied to the incision will prevent excessive hemorrhage.

Diseases of the Globe

Corneal disease usually involves the conjunctiva also. The signs and treatment of keratoconjunctivitis have been described under the heading Conjunctivitis.

KERATITIS

Superficial keratitis resulting from irritation or other injury can be readily treated with daily application of ophthalmic antibiotic preparations, after removal of the source of irritation and injury.[1]

IRIDOCYCLITIS

A case of iridocyclitis in a white-browed guan (*Penelope jacucapa*) was reported.[6] There was moderate conjunctivitis and marked thickening of the cornea, with complete opacity. The lens was destroyed and the retina infiltrated with gelatinous material.

OPHTHALMITIS AND PANOPHTHALMITIS

Panophthalmitis has been seen in rock peplars and amazon parrots.[1,10] The usual cause is infection or injury. Treatment of acute cases includes aspiration of the exudate under general anesthesia and topical application of ophthalmic antibiotic ointments. Enucleation of the eyeball is preferred if involvement is extensive.

Enzootic ophthalmitis of canaries has been reported in several aviaries.[8] Initially, it started as conjunctivitis and an ocular discharge which was watery and seromucous in nature. The infection later invaded the globe. The causative agent is perhaps a virus, as indicated by the rapid and acute course and high morbidity and mortality rate. Treatment may include broad-spectrum antibiotics given intramuscularly.

*Klot—a combination of 7% *n*-butyl alcohol C.P., V/V, and NaCl, 0.9% W/V, in water for injection, Warren-Teed Pharmaceuticals, Inc., Columbus, Ohio.

TUBERCULOSIS

Ocular lesions resulting from generalized tuberculosis in a parrot have been reported.[6] Semi-solid masses present in the orbit resulted in dislocation of the bulb. Also, yellowish granulating masses were present under the conjunctiva. There is no effective treatment, and euthanasia is recommended.

NEOPLASMS

Neoplasms involving the orbit of cage birds are generally malignant, with large, diffuse sarcomas predominating.[1,13] Signs and symptoms include pain, congestion and edema of the eyelids, displacement of the iris, and, on occasions, central nervous system disturbances due to pressure. Treatment may involve enucleation of the eyeball. Special care must be taken in owls because of the sclerotic ring surrounding the eyeball. Pituitary neoplasms have caused complete blindness. A case of unilateral blindness with proptosis resulted from a glioma surrounding the optic nerve.[2,7]

DISPLACEMENT OF THE EYEBALL

Rupture or prolapse of the eyeball is associated with trauma from fighting, contact with penetrating objects, or other accident. Enucleation of the involved eye is the preferred treatment.

DISEASES OF THE EARS

LABYRINTHITIS

Vertigo resulting from labyrinthitis has been reported in the budgerigar, bullfinch (*Pyrrhula pyrrhula*), canary, goldfinch (*Carduelis carduelis*), linnet (*Carduelis cannabina*), and pigeon.[9] Causes include infections of the semicircular and auditory canals, metastasizing tumors, and infestation with mites. Gray[9] stated that an exudate develops in the semicircular canals as a sequel to pox

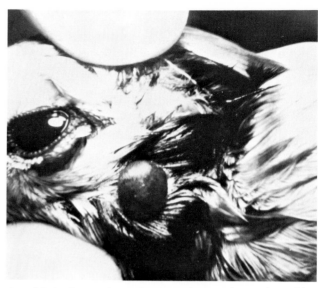

Fig. 23-4. *Protrusion of tympanic membrane in a blue jay (Cyanocitta cristata). (Courtesy of Dr. M. L. Petrak.)*

virus infection in pigeons, and recommended instillation of 1 or 2 drops of iodized glycerin in each ear twice a week; however, use of either chlortetracycline hydrochloride* or chloramphenicol succinate† intramuscularly might be more effective. In cases of vertigo associated with metastasizing tumors, euthanasia is recommended.

PROTRUSION OF TYMPANIC MEMBRANE

On rare occasions, the tympanic membrane may protrude through the auditory canal (Fig. 23-4). Aspiration of fluid through a 25-gauge needle may result in complete recession of the membrane. Probable cause is mechanical interference with drainage of the ear. Petrak[15] saw a blue jay (*Cyanocitta cristata*) that had an osteomyelitis of the jaw bone below the involved ear.

---

*Aureomycin, intravenous (100 mg./ml.)—American Cyanamid Co., Princeton, N.J.

†Chloromycetin succinate (100 mg./ml.)—Parke, Davis & Co., Detroit, Mich.

References

1. ARNALL, L.: Anaesthesia and surgery in cage and aviary birds. II. A regional outline of surgical conditions. Vet. Rec. *73:*173–178, 1961.

2. ARNALL, L.: Anaesthesia and surgery in cage and aviary birds. III. A systematic outline of surgical conditions. Vet. Rec. *73:*188–192, 1961.

3. ARNALL, L.: Further experiences with cagebirds. Vet. Rec. *73:*1146–1154, 1961.

4. BIGLAND, C. H., WHENHAM, G. R., and GRAESSER, F. E.: A pox-like infection of canaries. Can Vet. J. *3:*347–351, 1962.

5. COFFIN, D. L.: *The Care, Feeding and Diseases of Psittacine Pets.* Angell Memorial Parakeet and Parrot Book. Boston, Mass., 1953. 32 pp.

6. FOX, H.: *Disease in Captive Wild Mammals and Birds.* Philadelphia, J. B. Lippincott Co., 1923. Pp. 402–409.

7. FROST, C.: Experiences with pet budgerigars. Vet. Rec. *73:*621–626, 1961.

8. GRAY, H.: The diseases of cage and aviary birds, with some reference to those of furred and feathered game. Vet. Rec. *16:*343–352, 1936.

9. GRAY, H.: The diseases of cage and aviary birds, with some reference to those of furred and feathered game. Vet. Rec. *16:*377–386, 1936.

10. HASHOLT, J.: Current diseases of cage birds. J. small anim. Pract. *2:*97–108, 1961.

11. KEYMER, I. F.: Specific diseases of the canary and other passerine birds. Mod. Vet. Pract. *40*(17):32–35, September 1 (Part I); *40*(18):45–48, September 15 (Part II), 1959.

12. LAKE, F. B.: Parakeet eye disease. Avic. Mag. *59:*61–65, 1953.

13. LOMBARD, L. S., and WITTE, E. J.: Frequency and types of tumors in mammals and birds of the Philadelphia Zoological Garden. Cancer Res. *19:*127–141, 1959.

14. McILHENNY, E. A.: Albinism in mockingbirds. J. Hered. *31:*433–438, 1940.

15. PETRAK, M. L.: Personal communication, 1964.

16. SAGE, B. L.: Albinism and melanism in birds. British Birds *55:*201–222, 1962.

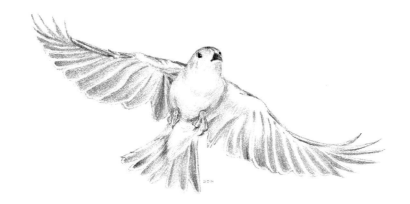

24

Infectious
Diseases

Diseases of
Bacterial Origin
R. N. T-W-Fiennes

Viral Diseases
John P. Cavill

Psittacosis and
Ornithosis
Paul Arnstein and Karl F. Meyer

DISEASES OF BACTERIAL ORIGIN

GENERAL OBSERVATIONS

The most serious clinical problems confronting persons who keep cage and aviary birds are posed by infectious diseases, the diagnosis of which is sometimes difficult, and the origin of which is often impossible to trace. In a large breeding aviary, such diseases may rapidly kill many birds before adequate steps can be taken to control them, or even to get a precise bacterial diagnosis. Or a single pet bird may suddenly die of some infectious cause, with a resultant sense of loss and bereavement to the owner. It is necessary, therefore, to understand the sources from which infectious diseases may arise, so that these may be avoided. It is similarly important to know the types of infection which are liable to occur in the different avian species, and something of the steps that can be taken rapidly to prevent the infection from spreading in an aviary or to eliminate it in a favorite pet.

The commonest source of bacterial infection in birds may well be a bird's own commensal organisms, which may cause disease when the bird is chilled or upset, or the even tenor of its life is otherwise disturbed. The avian pathologist is continually embarrassed by requests to certify that a bird has died through the negligence of a dealer from whom it was recently obtained, when in fact its death was apparently caused by an infection set up by the bird's own commensal microorganisms as a result of psychological stress associated with the change of residence and ownership.

Sometimes such a death is wrongly ascribed to infectious causes, when in fact it is the result of stress or shock. Few people realize that bowel hemorrhage is the most easily demonstrated lesion in birds dying of shock, resulting in many misdiagnoses of infectious enteritis. In addition to diseases of the alimentary system, those of the respiratory system may also result from the enhanced virulence of commensal organisms. This is the case both with the upper respiratory tract infections associated with organisms of the genus *Haemophilus,* and also with lower respiratory tract disease which may sometimes be associated with commensal organisms of the *Mycoplasma* group. Also hemorrhage into the lung often occurs agonally and sometimes leads to the mistaken diagnosis of pulmonary congestion or pneumonia.

External sources from which birds acquire infectious diseases are wild birds, rodents, and man. The food of cage or aviary birds should be protected from either direct or indirect contamination by wild birds or rodents. Direct contamination occurs when these creatures have access to the aviary or cage and can contaminate the food by their droppings or saliva; indirect contamination occurs when rodents raid and soil food stores or granaries, from which the food is subsequently fed to cage or aviary birds.

Man himself can be a danger to his captive birds in two particular ways. Any bird attendant with a respiratory infection may transmit it to the birds; the worst danger appears to be from the hemolytic staphylococci derived from throat infections. Staphylococci readily prove septicemic in cage and aviary birds and may start an epidemic. The other special danger from human beings stems from contamination of the hands with gram-negative organisms derived from the feces. The common *Bacillus coli* (*Escherichia coli*), normally present in human feces, causes fatal enteritis in many groups of birds, and it would appear that many outbreaks are associated with failures of personal hygiene and subsequent contamination of birds' food by mixing with soiled hands. The dangers of contamination by feces of rodents and birds are rather similar in that both transmit *Salmonella* (especially *S. typhimurium*), *Mycobacterium tuberculosis,* and *M. pseudotuberculosis.* All of these can cause epizootic infections that are serious and often highly fatal.

Most avian medicine is a matter for the pathologist. In aviaries where large numbers of birds are kept, birds are rarely seen to be sick and they often die when on the wing. Concealment of sickness appears to be a defense mechanism with many species of wild animals, including birds, because any animal that is seen by its companions to be sick or weak may be attacked and killed. For this reason, it is important that a full ex-

amination of the carcass of a dead bird be made; injuries and lacerations may be merely the result of a vicious terminal attack on a sick bird by its companions.

Two further precautions must not be overlooked by pathologists when they are examining dead birds. First, hemorrhages in certain sites may occur agonally at the time of death; these sites include the right atrium, the lungs, and the calvaria. Such hemorrhages have already been described in Chapter 17. Second, the pathologist must guard against throwing away the carcass of a bird because he thinks it is too putrefied for proper examination. Early putrefaction may be a clue to septicemia, and it is often worth the trouble of making cultures, even from a putrefied carcass. A bird's body must be examined particularly to see whether putrefaction affects merely the abdominal or some other organs, while the muscles and other parts of the body remain relatively fresh. Such a state is an indication that the disease is an infection of the bowel and is an important clue to the cause of the trouble. However, a bird's body is sometimes received in an advanced state of disintegration that affects the whole carcass, and nothing whatever can be done with it.

It is important also in avian pathology to discard any preconceived ideas about diseases of individual organs, for instance, that salmonellosis is a disease only of the bowel, or that other diseases affect only certain organs or systems. A bird's body is so compact, and all organs and systems are so interdependent, that no such particular division can be made. Interrelationships of organs and systems are also so reinforced by vascular anastomoses, such as that existing between the bowel and the kidneys, that infection passes readily from one organ or system to another. Thus salmonellosis in birds, although it may start in the bowel, is as much and as frequently a disease of the kidneys, and characteristic changes often occur also in the liver. Certain subdivisions will be made in this discussion for the sake of convenience in considering the diseases of cage and aviary birds, but it must be realized that these are largely for the sake of convenience and are exceedingly arbitrary.

TECHNIQUES OF POSTMORTEM EXAMINATION

Before proceeding to an account of the types of infection which may be present in the various systems of birds, it is advisable to make some remarks about techniques of postmortem examination. Birds requiring study will vary in size from that of a hummingbird to that of an ostrich, but the majority will be in the general range from that of a zebra finch to that of a pheasant or duck. In the case of birds with thick down, such as ducks, it is necessary to pluck the feathers from an area along the keel and abdomen, to expose the skin. With most birds this is unnecessary, but the feathers along the breast-bone should be wetted thoroughly to prevent feather dust from being blown about the room or inhaled by the operator. This is important, because psittacosis can be transmitted by feather dust. After such wetting, the feathers along the keel of the sternum are smoothed aside, exposing the skin along the proposed line of incision.

In most species the skin is delicate and readily cut by light strokes with the point of a sharp scalpel. When this is done, the fingers are inserted under the skin which, except in old birds, will readily separate from the underlying muscles over the sternum. An incision is now made around the caudal margin of the sternum, cutting close to the bone. This is continued around the eaveslike overhang which separates the lateral part of the sternum from the ribs. At this point the blunt end of the scalpel or some spatula-like instrument can be used to depress the ribs at the point of the costochondral junctions; in most cases the ribs will neatly and readily separate from their cartilages so that the sternum can be lifted. If they will not separate, they must, of course, be cut with strong scissors or bone forceps. The sternum can now be lifted, and the pericardial attachment to the sternal floor is separated close to the bone. There is no need to remove the sternum by section of the coracoids or clavicles. Indeed, this is best not done at this stage for fear of damaging the arteries and causing hemorrhage. The entire content of the thorax can now be viewed from the ventral surface, including the heart, lungs, the great arteries at their origin, and the brachiocephalic arteries, which are nicely exposed.

The operator now turns his attention to the abdomen, the contents of which have already been exposed by the incision in the skin. The abdominal organs are bound tightly together and to the body walls by peritoneum and by divisions of the abdominal air sacs. The carcass of the bird is placed with its head to the left; the abdominal contents are manually drawn toward the right side of the body and the attachments to the left abdominal wall are incised by quick strokes of a sharp scalpel. The bird can now be reversed in position, and the attachments to the right abdominal wall are incised by repeating the procedure in reverse. In most species of birds the abdominal contents will now be freed as a single mass in the abdominal cavity, and examination can be made of spleen, kidneys, and ovary or testes. Care should be taken to remove the cloaca intact, together with a margin of the external skin; this will release the abdominal contents for re-

moval and examination later. At this stage the operator will have a good idea of what the trouble is and can pursue his investigations along any lines indicated.

It is particularly important that smears of contents of the lower intestine be examined directly under the microscope for detection of coccidia or helminth ova. This is especially necessary in the case of trematode or *Syngamus* infections. Trematode infections are likely to be overlooked, since, particularly in water birds, the worms may be small and they may be present in obscure sites, such as the bursa of Fabricius. The finding of ova in the intestinal contents makes it mandatory for the operator to continue a thorough examination until the adult worms are discovered.

A common fault in avian pathological investigation is discontinuance of the examination at the point now reached in this description. It is essential that the pharynx and larynx, sinuses, brain, and cranial cavity be examined, unless the cause of death is already obvious. The crop must be located and its condition and contents examined; this can be done by incising the skin along the ventral surface of the neck. The crop may be the site of fungus infection due to *Candida* species, and in Columbiformes it is often the site of *Trichomonas* infection. The pharynx and larynx are next examined; this is most easily done by incising the corners of the mouth with sharp scissors; if the skin and skeleton are required intact, these structures must be dissected from the caudal end. The orifice of the trachea is discovered at the base of the tongue and this too must be incised, the contents examined, and condition of the mucous membrane noted. Sometimes, particularly in budgerigars, a small seed may be located in the tracheal entrance, accounting for choking and subsequent death. In the Anatidae (ducks, geese, and swans), the syrinx takes on many weird and wonderful shapes, becoming progressively distorted as the bird grows older. This is of no significance, but it is advisable to examine the syrinx because it is sometimes affected with *Aspergillus* or *Candida*. The nasal passages and sinuses are most easily examined by cutting away the beak with scissors at the point of the cere. Pressure can then be applied to see if they contain pus or an excess of mucous discharge. Finally, the cranium can be removed by means of a sharp scalpel and the underlying brain examined for traces of damage which might be caused either by injury or by infection. In my experience, cerebral infections usually have their origin in upper respiratory tract disease, which extends to the sinuses and thence to the base of the brain. It is, therefore, advisable to remove the entire brain to trace any such pathway of infection.

Such a necropsy on a small bird can be completed with the help of an assistant in 5 to 10 minutes, after which the operator should be reasonably satisfied as to the cause of the bird's death. If injury is suspected, the bird's skin should be removed and the internal surface examined for signs of bruising, or for the point of entry of a shot or air-gun pellet. If infection is suspected, the appropriate material from bowel, liver, kidneys, brain, or other organ can be removed for bacteriological study. If there is splenomegaly, pericarditis, or perihepatitis, or all three, ornithosis (psittacosis) may be suspected, and in this case the operator will take care to avoid infecting himself or his assistants. He may then decide to examine spleen smears for inclusion bodies, do animal inoculations, or send material to a Public Health Laboratory. Avian tuberculosis is readily diagnosed, if not evident from the nature of the lesions, because acid-fast bacilli are always present in large numbers and can be demonstrated under the microscope in smears stained with Ziehl-Neelsen stain.

REGIONAL INFECTIONS

UPPER RESPIRATORY TRACT DISEASE AND
DISEASE OF THE BRAIN

Upper respiratory tract disease may be caused by a number of different organisms, of which—as in man—streptococci and staphylococci probably predominate. It is evidenced by inflammation of the upper respiratory passages, particularly the pharynx, which may be red and raw. Alternatively, the surfaces may be covered with thick mucoid or purulent material. The sinuses are frequently blocked with mucus or pus, making a diagnosis of upper respiratory tract infection obvious. The infection may often spread to the cerebral tissues, and symptoms of encephalitis may be manifested before death. The rather typical Nelson's coryza is said to be caused by an organism of the *Haemophilus* group (*H. gallinarum*). This is easily diagnosed from the occurrence of a periorbital swelling and possibly proptosis. The condition is not ordinarily bilaterally symmetrical but usually occurs to a greater extent on one side or the other. It can often be corrected by surgical removal of the pellet of purulent cheesy material from behind the eye. It is unusual for upper and lower respiratory tract disease to be present simultaneously, and it appears that the two conditions are of entirely different causation.

Many cases of encephalitis that cannot be diagnosed by bacteriological studies will be encountered in birds. These are chiefly caused by virus infections, many of them not yet well understood. Virus infections must, of course, be borne in mind when the etiology of upper respiratory tract infections is being considered; infection of the brain may, however, be associated with the presence of *Listeria* or, particularly in Columbiformes, of *Erysipelothrix*.

LOWER RESPIRATORY TRACT DISEASE

The organs which may be affected in cases of lower respiratory tract disease are the lungs and air sacs. Probably the commonest causes of disease in these organs are *Aspergillus fumigatus* and *A. flavus*. The lesions in these infections take two distinct forms: that of felted masses of hyphae covering and thickening the air-sac surfaces, or of large, rather regular nodules throughout the lung tissue. Two other diseases, in which nodules may be present in the lung tissue, are tuberculosis and pseudotuberculosis. As stated previously, tuberculosis is readily diagnosed by examination of direct smears. The nodules of mycosis are rather characteristic, by reason of size, and to a certain extent by their even spacing throughout the lung tissue; they will not normally be confused by an experienced pathologist. There should thus be no difficulty in distinguishing these three conditions, although it may be advisable to make cultures when pseudotuberculosis is suspected.

Although the lungs of birds are unlike those of mammals, pneumonia in birds is similar in appearance and goes through the same stages as it does in mammalian lungs: congestion, red hepatization, and then grey hepatization. Affected avian lungs also sink in water, and it is advisable to apply this test to grossly distinguish true pneumonia from congestion or hemorrhage. Either of the latter conditions may be agonal and have nothing to do with the fatal disease or its development.

The organisms associated with pneumonia may be various. Mycoplasmata have been blamed in poultry, but the significance of these organisms in the etiology of pneumonia in cage and aviary birds is doubtful (see below). Ornithosis is associated with a febrile septicemia, usually accompanied by severe hemorrhagic gastroenteritis and splenomegaly. Most avian pneumonias do not show these accompanying features. To-day, at the London Zoo, ornithosis is diagnosed very rarely, and then primarily in newly imported birds sent by dealers for necropsy. It is useful, when facilities are available, to make cultures routinely in all birds dying of pneumonia. The organism usually found is *Escherichia coli;* sometimes *Salmonella* spp., *Klebsiella* (*Pneumobacillus*), *Corynebacterium pyogenes*, *Pseudomonas aeruginosa*, and *Staphylococcus* are incriminated. It is noteworthy that all of these organisms may also be associated with infections of the intestinal tract or of other abdominal organs such as the kidneys, or with conditions of septicemia. Diseases of the lungs and air sacs in birds, therefore, appear to be more those of the abdomen than of the upper respiratory passages, a situation differing greatly from that in mammals.

DISEASES OF THE ALIMENTARY SYSTEM

In avian pathology, one finds diagnoses of enteritis occurring with distressing regularity. As already stated, hemorrhage or catarrh of the bowel in birds can be a sign of stress or shock, which occurs fairly frequently in response to chilling, malnutrition, or environmental change. In many such cases, some quite innocent organism may be isolated from the bowel content and blamed for death of the bird.

The diagnosis of enteritis made frequently at the London Zoo without the isolation of possible pathogens stimulated an investigation of the normal gut flora of most groups of birds.[21] As a result, it was discovered that gram-negative organisms were not normally present in the bowels of many groups of birds. In particular, grain-eating and fruit-eating species have no gram-negative gut flora; no *Escherichia coli* occurs as in mammals, and consequently its finding in the droppings indicates the presence of a pathogen. Gram-negative organisms are present in carnivores and insectivores only. This statement must be qualified by saying that most granivorous species take insect food during the breeding season and at this time some gram-negative organisms may appear in the droppings. Formerly, the presence of *Escherichia coli* in avian species was ignored, but today we regard it as the commonest cause of infectious enteritis. Often it appears that the infection is acquired as a result of inadequate personal hygiene on the part of those who prepare the birds' food. This is a special danger when food is left in bowls in heated aviaries, allowing a diminutive level of contamination to build up to culture proportions.

In spite of this, some birds may be "carriers" of "coli" group organisms, while apparently remaining in good health. Such birds, introduced in an aviary and subjected to the stress of new surroundings, may develop overt disease and can be a danger to their companions. In such an event, prophylactic therapy must be rapidly applied to all in-contact birds.

The most important point in management is prevention of exposure of the caged birds to fecal contamination. Avoidance of contaminated water and food, contaminated floors, perches, and cages is imperative.[47]

Droppings from affected birds should be cultured and antibiotic sensitivity testing done. This is especially important because of the prevalence of *Escherichia coli* and the emergence, in recent years, of resistant strains of the microorganism. McKay *et al.*[64] reported that in 1957 approximately 60 per cent of the strains of *E. coli* isolated from pathological specimens or clinical cases were resistant to streptomycin. By 1963, over 90 per cent were resistant. A similar pattern developed with the tetracyclines. Strains resistant to neomycin increased from 10 per cent in 1957 to approximately 50 per cent in 1963. In the same period, chloramphenicol-resistant coliform bacteria increased from 8 to 22 per cent. Tests with nitrofurazone and chlorhexidine demonstrated that less than 10 per cent of the coliform strains were resistant to these chemotherapeutic agents. Brander[9] reported that ampicillin is effective against *E. coli* and is more bactericidal than chloramphenicol or tetracycline.

Other intestinal pathogens may be *Staphylococcus*, *Salmonella*, *Pseudomonas aeruginosa*, *Pasteurella multocida*, or *P. pseudotuberculosis*. In Great Britain, the incidence of staphylococcal infections in birds appears to have increased greatly[24] since the use of antibiotics in the treatment of human disease became prevalent, and staphylococci tended to gain some mastery as a result of an increase in drug-resistant strains. Salmonellae tend to become septicemic, and the organism is in any event as much a cause of nephritis in birds as it is of enteritis. The commonest species found is *Salmonella typhimurium*, and the infection is usually accompanied by hepatitis, the liver being a rich golden color and somewhat fatty. *Pseudomonas* in bird feces should always be regarded as a dangerous pathogen. In the bowel it is usually described as a commensal, but, in birds particularly, owing to the vascular links between bowel and kidneys, it can spread rapidly to start infection in the body proper. Starting with nephritis, which may prove fatal, in the later stages the infection may become septicemic. Many other odd gram-negative organisms will be found from time to time in the bowel contents of birds. In those species which normally carry gram-positive bowel flora, all gram-negative organisms should be regarded as potentially pathogenic and steps should be taken to eliminate them. The commonest of these organisms are the paracolon bacilli, but from time to time other intermediate types will be found, including organisms such as *Shigella alkalescens*.

Pasteurella pseudotuberculosis causes multiple white nodules (Fig. 24-1) throughout the bowel, liver, and other organs. Conditions that should be considered in differential diagnosis include tuberculosis, pyemic abscesses associated with staphylococcal infections,

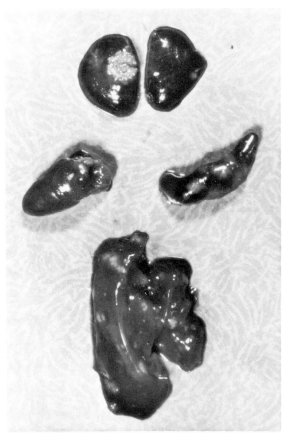

Fig. 24-1. *Lungs (top), heart (left), spleen (right), and liver (below) of a typical seed-eating passerine bird, showing necrotic lesions varying in size up to 5 mm. in diameter and caused by* **Pasturella pseudotuberculosis.** *These lesions closely resemble those seen in salmonellosis in this type of bird, but in salmonellosis they are usually smaller and confined to the liver and spleen. Note the shape of the spleen, which is approximately three times its normal size. (Keymer, I. F.: Mod. Vet. Pract. 42(24): 50, Dec. 15, 1961.)*

and, theoretically, listeriosis which produces similar lesions in chinchillas and other rodents. It must be remembered also that white deposits in the liver and other organs in birds may contain lymphoblastic tissue and be associated with leukemia.

SEPTICEMIC DISEASES

Septicemic diseases in wild birds commonly occur in association with many of the organisms already mentioned, including *Salmonella, Escherichia coli, Pseudomonas, Streptococcus,* and *Staphylococcus.* Of the recognized septicemic organisms, the most serious in cage and aviary birds are *Pasteurella multocida* and *P. tularensis.* These may be identified by means of blood smears or by bacterial culture. It is worthy of

mention that, when difficulty is experienced in isolating pasteurellae, they alone of the common infecting organisms will multiply at refrigerator temperature, and it is usually possible to culture them if a carcass is left in the refrigerator for some days.

PATHOGENIC BACTERIA

COCCI

The dearth of references in the literature to infections of birds with cocci is surprising. According to Lee,[58] an outbreak of streptococcal septicemia was described in canaries by Ruhling[76] in 1925 and by Völker[89] in 1926. Urbain[87] reported an outbreak occurring in both exotic and indigenous birds. There are two reports of pneumonia associated with *Pneumococcus,*[40,42] the earlier report[40] describing an infection in a Carolina duck (*Aix sponsa*). Reports of staphylococcal infection are very scarce, although Rowlands and Smith[75] described an outbreak in geese. Keymer,[54] in a survey of the causes of mortality in British wild birds, records *Staphylococcus* spp. in a wood pigeon (*Columba palumbus*), house sparrow (*Passer domesticus*), nuthatch (*Sitta europaea*), and blue-winged teal (*Anas discors*). The death of the blue-winged teal was thought to be due to a staphylococcal septicemia resulting from infection in a leg wound. Jennings,[49] as reported by Keymer,[54] isolated coagulase-positive staphylococci from the heart, blood, liver, and bone marrow of a green woodpecker (*Picus viridis*) and a hawfinch (*Coccothraustes coccothraustes*).

Fiennes[24] described staphylococcal infections in a number of bird species in association with enteritis. The small number of cases of disease, both local and general, recorded in the literature can hardly reflect the actual frequency with which staphylococci are associated with avian diseases. Sensitivity testing with antibiotic discs should be carried out, if possible, to determine the most effective drug to be used therapeutically.

CORYNEBACTERIUM

Very occasionally *Corynebacterium* is reported as the causal agent of disease of birds, but this appears to be rare, although possibly it is not so rare as the scarcity of reports would indicate. Urbain recorded disease in eagles and vultures caused by this organism, and also recorded *Corynebacterium ovis* in a budgerigar.[86] *Corynebacterium pyogenes* was isolated from a case of septicemia in a Chilean flamingo (*Phoenicopterus chilensis*),[24] but this bird was also mildly affected with aspergillosis and suffered from a large thrombus of the brachiocephalic artery. There is, therefore, some doubt as to the role played by *Corynebacterium* in the etiology of bird disease. Pruski[70] attributed the deaths of six ostriches in a Poland zoo to a mixed infection of *Corynebacterium pyogenes* and *Streptococcus viridans*. Fox[26] described "avian diphtheria" in three cassowaries which suffered from false membranes in the throat; from these cases he isolated an organism which he termed *Bacillus diphtheriae avium*, presumably a *Corynebacterium*.

PASTEURELLA

Pseudotuberculosis is extremely common among wild birds and rodents. There is little reason to doubt that it is spread to cage and aviary birds primarily by contamination of food by the feces of free-living species of wild birds. Chiefly incriminated are birds such as sparrows, starlings, blackbirds, pigeons, and others which frequent aviaries to steal food. Nevertheless, the literature regarding this disease among both free-living and captive wild birds is extremely sparse. Almost certainly all groups of birds are susceptible, and the following list covers most of the reports recorded thus far.

Harshfield[38] reviewed the literature with regard to infection in canaries, finches, pigeons, fowls, pheasants, and swans. Urbain and Nouvel[88] reported the disease in toucans, Beaudette[5] in a blackbird, Hulphers and Lilleengen[45] in game birds, partridge, blackcock, and hazel grouse, Appleby[3] in various tropical birds, and Clark and Locke[14] in the common grackle (*Quiscalus quiscula*). In addition, I described the following cases in the Annual Reports of the Pathologist to the Zoological Society of London: in three king penguins (*Aptenodytes patagonica*),[23] and in one gannet (*Sula bassana*), one red-vented parrot (*Pionus menstruus*), and one budgerigar (*Melopsittacus undulatus*).[25]

Keymer[55] reported that pseudotuberculosis has been observed in canaries, the amadavat, or tiger finch, (*Amadava amadava*), and the butterfly finch (*Habropya phoenicotis*), and that he diagnosed it in a Cuban finch (*Tiaris canora*) and in a wild snow bunting (*Plectrophenax nivalis*). He further reported that the disease in canaries may be acute and cause death within 3 or 4 days, but sudden death is unusual. Mortality may be high or sporadic. Symptoms are not consistent or diagnostic. Listlessness, ruffled feathers, and anorexia may occur a day or two before death; diarrhea seldom accompanies the disease.

Septicemic pasteurellosis, associated with *Pasteurella multocida,* is undoubtedly widespread in nature, although again the references to it under natural conditions are somewhat scanty. A survey of this disease in wild birds in the San Francisco Bay area was reported by Rosen and Bischoff[74]; another survey of the disease in upland game birds in the United States was made by Shillinger and Morley.[78] The disease was reported by Hudson[44] in ring-necked pheasants (*Phasianus colchicus*) and by Hulphers and Lilleengen[45] in game birds in Sweden. It was recorded by Hill[43] in a bronze-winged dove and by Fox[26] in parrots. It has also been reported by Keymer[55] in canaries, by Guerez[34] and by Quortrup et al.[72] in wild ducks, by Joest[50] in owls, by Januschke[48] in eagles, and by Hill[41] in a vulture.

There are two interesting reports of the disease in penguins. Carlson and Pennifold[12] described it in four Humboldt penguins (*Spheniscus humboldti*) which died 2 to 36 hours after termination of a long air trip. The interesting point in these cases was that the abdominal air sacs were filled either with a firm cheesy mass or with purulent exudate, suggesting aspergillosis; however, no *Aspergillus* was isolated, and the disease was diagnosed as fowl cholera because of the presence of *Pasteurella multocida*. Fiennes[23] also reported the deaths of three adult king penguins following exposure during an exceptionally cold wet night one August. The livers were pale and streakily patched with superficial and deep-splashed hemorrhages; the intestines were filled with liquid undigested blood. The carcasses showed evidence of the birds' having been fevered. Bacterial cultures revealed the presence of *Pasteurella multocida,* and the serum agglutinated the organism to a titre of 1:10,000.

Evans,[18] writing about parakeets in veterinary practice, stated that large aviaries may suffer heavy losses as a result of pasteurellosis. Such an experience would be in conformity with what occurs in other animals, perhaps particularly in rodents (chinchillas), but the literature on the subject is meager in the extreme and it may be hoped that in the future all cases will be reported. Deaths from pasteurellosis will in most cases occur rapidly, and diagnosis will be made only at necropsy.

There is little information with regard to the efficacy of fowl cholera vaccines or antibiotic treatment, but the latter should be started for all in-contact birds as soon as an outbreak is diagnosed. Experience with pasteurellosis in other animals such as rodents suggests that it could quickly sweep through an aviary, killing most of the inhabitants.

Antibiotic sensitivity testing of the strain of *Pasteurella* involved in an individual outbreak is important. Penicillin, the tetracyclines, and sulfaquinoxaline have all been effective prophylactically in certain outbreaks and in various species.[8,59,71] An exacerbation of disease frequently seems to result if the drug is not given for a long enough period of time, or even after discontinuation of long-term therapy. Culturing fecal matter for the presence of *Pasteurella* may be helpful in determining recurrence of the infection after discontinuation of the drugs. Paterson and Cook[69] have described a method for the recovery of *Pasteurella pseudotuberculosis* from feces.

The problem of tularemia appears to be limited to game birds. Grouse, partridge, quail, pheasant, sage hen, and prairie chicken are all potential sources of danger, since the disease occurs in them in the wild and associated cases in man have been recorded. It is important, therefore, in countries where tularemia is enzootic, to be careful when handling suspected cases and cultures of organisms and to arrive at a true diagnosis.

The disease was described first by Green[29] in grouse, partridge, and pheasant. In attempted experimental transmission in various birds,[31,32,33] pigeons were found to be resistant, but ruffed grouse (*Bonasa umbellus*) and ring-necked pheasants (*Phasianus colchicus*) were found to be susceptible. Green and Shillinger[30] described a natural infection in the sharp-tailed grouse (*Pedioecetes phasianellus*) and the ruffed grouse. Park *et. al.*[68] described the disease in sage hen (*Centrocercus urophasianus*) and reported human cases following contacts with quail. Brown,[10] working in Canada, reported grouse, quail, pheasants, and prairie chickens to be susceptible; and Kursban and Foshay[57] described a case of tularemia acquired from a pheasant.

SALMONELLA

In days gone by, the relationship of salmonellae to poultry diseases was simple. *Salmonella gallinarum* caused bacillary white diarrhea in chicks, and differentiation from coccidiosis was necessary; adult birds suffered from fowl typhoid caused by *Salmonella pullorum*. Occasionally it was recognized that some other serotypes might be involved, but these were a rarity and caused little concern to the veterinarian. Even with poultry this simple picture no longer prevails. In a wide survey, Bigland *et al.*[6] isolated 26 serotypes of *Salmonella* from mammals or birds, the commonest from poultry being *S. typhimurium, S. thompson, S. heidelberg, S. bareilly,* and *S. oranienburg;* these were in addition to *S. pullorum* and *S. gallinarum* isolated generally from chickens and turkeys. Today the total number of known serotypes of salmonellae approaches the 900 mark, and although we affectionately cling to the old names we know and understand, it is no longer possible to deal with so large a variety of organisms in this way.

Among free-living wild birds and birds in cages and aviaries, salmonella infections are widespread.

Jungherr[51] surveyed the known hosts, mentioning particularly chickens, turkeys, ducks, geese, pigeons, pheasants, quail, and canaries among the free-living species, and finches, siskins, titmice, gulls, and parrots among the species in captivity.

Dozsa[15] reported failure of strict control measures to eliminate *S. typhimurium* infection from birds at the Budapest Zoo. In order to discover the means of spread, 266 captured sparrows were examined for evidence of infection; *S. typhimurium* was isolated from the liver and intestinal tract in 52 and *S. anatis* was identified in 1. Forty-seven of the infected birds were captured in March when they crowded into the city from the outskirts; only 5 infected birds were found among those captured during April to September, when they dispersed to the grain fields and fed on ripening plants.

Séry and Strauss[77] examined birds in a Czechoslovakian bird sanctuary for salmonellosis and psittacosis. *S. typhimurium* and *S. london* were isolated from 13 of 188 ducks and from 10 of 25 duck eggs, from 72 of 177 gulls and from 5 of 100 gull eggs; *Salmonella* species were also isolated from 7 per cent of other bird species examined, which included gulls, pigeons, pheasants, jackdaws, collared turtle-doves, and wild birds of seven other species. Lofton *et al.,*[61] in a survey of 127 birds of seven species in Colorado, isolated salmonellae of four different serotypes from blackbirds, horned larks (*Eremophila alpestris*), and rufous-sided towhees (*Pipilo erythrophthalmus*). The authors concluded that the relatively high incidence indicated that birds might serve as an important reservoir of salmonellae in the mountain pasture and watershed areas of the State.

Faddoul *et al.*[19] reported that salmonellae were identified in 12 of the first 100 consignments of wild birds submitted during a 1-year survey in Massachusetts. Eight outbreaks of *S. typhimurium* infection were identified in brown-headed cowbirds (*Molothrus ater*), seven of the outbreaks occurring during winter months. Two outbreaks of infection by the same strain were identified in house sparrows (*Passer domesticus*) and one in a white-throated sparrow (*Zonotrichia albicollis*). One case of infection by *S. derby* occurred in a herring gull (*Larus argentatus*). In birds that died of a septicemic infection the lungs were often congested and the liver and spleen were swollen and highly congested. An abscess in the brain or abdominal cavity was not uncommon. According to Keymer,[55] the canary, bullfinch (*Pyrrhula pyrrhula*), goldfinch (*Carduelis carduelis*), and house sparrow are all reported to be susceptible to infection with *Salmonella pullorum*. Edwards *et al.*[16] (cited by Keymer[55]) described an outbreak that caused the death of 50 of 75 canaries in a single aviary. Infection was attributed to contamination by a new bird that died one week after it was placed in the collection. Birds of all ages were affected, and death occurred 12 to 24 hours after ruffled feathers, droopiness, diarrhea, and severe lethargy were noted.

Keymer[55] also stated that infection with *S. typhimurium* is often reported in canaries, and that 60 canaries from a collection of 170 reportedly died following infection by *S. suipestifer,* convulsions being one of the symptoms in this outbreak. Keymer observed infection from *S. typhimurium* in a variety of finches. He noted that the incubation period is 4 or 5 days and that birds die 2 to 4 days after symptoms of illness appear. Convulsions often precede death. Surviving birds are apparently carriers and can infect new, susceptible birds. Williams[92] reviewed the literature on salmonella infections in aviary and cage birds; Buxton[11] also reviewed this literature.

The full literature on salmonellosis cannot be surveyed here, but the preceding paragraphs will familiarize the reader with the main sources of information. The epizootiology of the disease is important, and attention may be drawn to the paper of Steiniger,[82] who described the bacteriological examination of 100,000 samples of bird feces. Salmonellae were isolated more frequently from feces found on vegetation than from feces found on stones and soil. It was suggested that the temperature and humidity of plant material are favorable to salmonellae, which survived for 28 months on plant material that was allowed to dry slowly. Since so many rodents and birds are carriers of salmonellae, plainly in any rather damp country a danger of infection must lurk for long periods in good vegetational cover. In zoos and aviaries, as is true for *Pasteurella pseudotuberculosis,* the main danger lies in contamination of food in aviary or paddock by bird droppings, and occasional outbreaks of salmonellosis resulting from such contamination are very hard to avoid. The chief infecting organism in captive birds is *S. typhimurium,* infections by other salmonellae being insignificant in comparison. Steps to be taken to avoid the trouble consist in protecting aviaries from wild birds and rodents, or in providing the birds' food in places where it cannot become contaminated by the droppings of wild birds.

All cage and aviary birds must be regarded as susceptible to salmonellosis, which is a rapidly fatal enteric and septicemic disease. Deaths have been recorded in almost all species, including penguins, pelicans, flamingos, and the smaller passeriform species. It may well be that, on occasions, a newly introduced bird in an aviary may be a carrier of some salmonella which may be transmitted to the other birds. Newly acquired birds must always be treated with respect until they are known to be healthy and not capable of transmitting

disease. When salmonellosis occurs, rapid diagnosis by postmortem examination and bacterial culture must be made; meanwhile all in-contact birds should be given antibiotic cover as in infections with *Escherichia coli.* Nitrofurazone* and furazolidone† are probably the drugs of choice in species and age groups that can tolerate them. Treated birds that are apparently recovered may be carriers and shedders of salmonellae.

SHIGELLA

The shigellae are not normally regarded as pathogens of birds. However, as with other gram-negative organisms, the possibility of trouble arising from them should not be overlooked. Gupta and Rao[35] described enteritis of ducklings caused by *Shigella alkalescens,* and the loss of a golden-fronted fruitsucker (*Chloropsis aurifrons*) from the same organism was described by Fiennes.[22] Fiennes[24] described the death of a Malachite sunbird (*Nectarinia famosa*) with a catarrhal condition of the gut, from which a strain of *Shigella flexneri* was isolated. The bird's death was associated with shigellosis, and two other bird deaths associated with *Shigella* infection were listed during the same year.

Unlike *Salmonella, Shigella* can only be passed by direct animal-to-animal contact; it cannot survive for long in vegetation or outside the vertebrate body. Therefore there is little danger from contamination of natural foodstuffs by wild birds or other animals.

OTHER GRAM-NEGATIVE BACILLI

Little need be added to what has already been said regarding the pathogenicity of other gram-negative bacilli. The matter has been reviewed by Fiennes.[21,22,24] The information in Table 24-1, showing the bird species which would normally carry gram-negative bacilli and those which do not, is reproduced from Fiennes.[21] In birds of all of the latter group listed, gram-negative bacilli found in the gut are to be regarded as pathogenic, whatever their genus, species, or strain. *Escherichia coli* infection is probably the commonest cause of death among psittacine birds, and, because *E. coli* is widely regarded as a normal gut inhabitant, such infection is often overlooked. Control measures have already been outlined. Table 24-2, reproduced from Fiennes,[24] lists the pathogenic organisms which were found to be associated with enteric and other conditions of birds dying at the London Zoo.

*Furacin Water Mix Veterinary—Eaton Laboratories, Norwich, N.Y.

†Furoxone Suspension Veterinary—Eaton Laboratories, Norwich, N.Y.

Table 24-1. Findings of the Normal Intestinal Flora in Examination of 98 Fecal Specimens of Birds of Various Groups That Were Apparently in Good Health*

Order	Number of Specimens	Gram-positive Flora	Gram-negative Flora
Passeriformes	46	Prevalent (micro- and gram-positive diplococci mainly, generally bile-inhibited, fungi, yeast, anthracoids) spec. unknown	In a number of specimens none or few coliform only; also moderate numbers of non-lethal forms, mostly *B. proteus*
Piciformes	15	No dominant factor organisms as above	Coliforms fairly numerous
Trogoniformes Cuculiformes		As in Piciformes	As in Piciformes
Coraciiformes Hornbills	8	Scarce	Coliforms dominant factor, also *B. proteus*
A roller		Staphylococci, diplococci, anthracoids	1 or 2 isolated gram-neg. bacilli
Apodiformes Hummingbirds		Exclusively gram-positive organisms	None
Psittaciformes	18	Mixture of organisms as in Passeriformes	Only in 2 specimens isolated coliforms; 16 specimens none
Strigiformes	1	Few fungi	Rich growth of coliforms
Falconiformes	1	None	*Aerobacter cloacae*
Anseriformes	1	None	Coliforms only
Sphenisciformes	1	None	Coliforms
Gruiformes	1	Anthracoids, gram-positive diplococci	Coliforms
Columbiformes A pigeon	2	Gram-positive diplococci, yeast, anthracoids	None

*From Fiennes.[21]

Table 24-2. Pathogenic Organisms of Birds (Microorganisms Found *post mortem* in Birds Dying of Enteric and Other Diseases)*

Organism	Enteric	Respiratory	Septicemic	Nervous	Others
Salmonella	35	0	0	0	0
Shigella	3	0	0	0	0
Escherichia coli	55	0	0	0	0
Pseudomonas	3	3	1	1	0
Anaerobic organisms	0	3	0	0	0
Staphylococci	5	9	1	0	2
Streptococci and Diplococci	0	3	3	0	0
Erysipelothrix	0	0	1	1	0
Aspergillus	3	9	0	1	0
Actinomyces and *Nocardia*	0	1	0	1	0

*From Fiennes.[24]

MISCELLANEOUS PATHOGENIC ORGANISMS

Brucella abortus as a cause of infection of birds may be ignored, although Emmel and Huddleson[17] described what they believed to be a case of natural *Brucella* infection in two guinea fowl.

The paucity of references to other infecting organisms, apart from tuberculosis described below, is probably due more to the scarcity of the observations made or to the inadequacy of bacteriological work possible at many zoos than to non-occurrence of infections caused by them.

It is known, for instance, that pigeons are highly susceptible to infection with *Erysipelothrix,* yet reports of infection by this organism in free-living wild birds are rare. Raines and Winkel[73] reported an outbreak of erysipelas on a commercial pheasant farm. For 10 years a large number of cock pheasants had become lame and died within a few days every autumn. However, the particular outbreak described in this report began with a flock of hens. Necropsy of three birds showed a slightly enlarged and friable liver in each one of the three, and a slightly enlarged spleen with numerous tiny necrotic foci in two. Swine were believed to be the source of infection. All birds in affected groups were given 50,000 units of procaine penicillin intramuscularly, and all birds in other groups were vaccinated. Death losses stopped almost immediately. The swine were removed from the premises, and the recommendation to vaccinate every six months was made.

Waller[91] reported on erysipelas in a quail from a game farm. Necropsy revealed small hemorrhages on and in the pectoral muscles, clear fluid in the pericardial sac, and petechiae in the myocardium; the liver was congested and swollen.

Keymer[54] recorded the infection in a crane and quoted various authors as having reported *Erysipelothrix rhusiopathiae* infection in ducks, quail, pheasant, pigeons, chickens, greenfinches (*Chloris chloris*), wild mallards (*Anas platyrhynchos*), white storks (*Ciconia ciconia*), herring gulls (*Larus argentatus*), chaffinches (*Fringilla coelebs*), and the golden eagle (*Aquila chrysaetos*). Keymer[55] reported such an infection in a bullfinch (*Pyrrhula pyrrhula*) and in zebra finches (*Poephila castanotis*).

Blackmore and Gallagher[7] described an outbreak of erysipelas in captive wild mammals and birds. Seventeen birds died over a period of one year. Birds involved were a grebe, turtle dove, moorhen (*Gallinula chloropus*), coot, loons, a guillemot, owl, pheasants, a gull, jackdaw (*Corvus monedula*), partridge, and pigeon. The source of the infection was never determined. Budgerigars infected by intraperitoneal injection or by scarification with the *Erysipelothrix* inoculum died in 48 hours.

Erysipelas may cause sporadic deaths in aviaries, but it does not appear to be widespread or of major importance. Antibiotic sensitivity testing should be done in any outbreak. Raines and Winkel[73] found their strain to be sensitive to penicillin and dihydrostreptomycin. Hall[36] and Axworthy[4] both used chlortetracycline successfully, one in the drinking water and the other in the feed. Their reports involved outbreaks in pullets and ducks, respectively.

Listeriosis is also likely to be found frequently in birds, but references are scanty. Gray,[28] describing listeriosis in fowls, reviewed the reports, which included its occurrence in parrots and canaries. Zwart and Donker-Voet[95] reviewed the incidence of *Listeria* infection in captive animals, including two diamond doves (*Geopelia cuneata*), two Swainson lorikeets (*Trichoglossus novaehollandiae*), and three canaries. Thamm[84] reported on the epizootiology of listeriosis in East Germany, finding the condition mostly in regions with loamy soil, marl, or humus. The disease occurred in cattle, pigs, goats, roe deer, cats, rabbits, guinea pigs, and fowls; the highest incidence, however, occurred in sheep. Fiennes[24] described the deaths of three crested pigeons with symptoms of coryza, sinusitis, and cerebral congestion; cultures from the brains revealed the presence of *Listeria* and *Streptothrix*. The changes were thought to be due to listeriosis, *Listeria* being a well-known pathogen of pigeons, whereas *Streptothrix* was not known to cause cerebral symptoms in them.

Waldhalm et al.[90] described magpies (*Pica pica*) as carriers of bovine *Vibrio foetus*. *Vibrio metchnikovi* was described by Allan[2] as causing the death of a hill mynah. Respiratory distress for a few hours before death was the only symptom noted.

The role of birds as carriers or distributors of *Leptospira* was investigated by Ferris et al.[20] in Australia; no birds were found infected, although infection was widespread in mammals and was found in the single snake examined. Yakunin,[93] in a study of spirochetes of wild birds, found *Borrelia anserina* in Spanish sparrows, rooks, and small doves in Kazakhstan. It would appear, therefore, that imported birds may be carriers of spirochetes, although they possibly do not play a part in the transmission of leptospirosis.

BACILLUS ANTHRACIS

It is stated in textbooks of bacteriology that the common fowl cannot be infected with *Bacillus anthracis*. From this it is frequently assumed that birds are resistant to anthrax and neither pass the disease nor are affected by it. This statement is inaccurate, since many birds, including particularly carnivorous species, succumb readily to anthrax after eating infected meat. In addition to occurring in birds of prey, anthrax has been described by Theiler[85] in ostriches, by Mollet[66] in crows, by Freese[27] in canaries, and by Menendez et al.[65] in ducks. In all cases the outbreaks apparently were caused by ingestion of infected meat; birds have not so far been incriminated as the initiators of an outbreak of anthrax.

Hamerton[37] reported an outbreak of anthrax which occurred in the London Zoo during 1941. During the outbreak, which was traced to infected cow meat, one of three golden eagles (*Aquila chrysaetos*) and one of a pair of crowned hawk eagles (*Stephanoaetus coronatus*) which ate the meat contracted anthrax and died. Heavy infection of the blood and excreta with *Bacillus anthracis* was confirmed both by microscopical examination and by cultures. The deaths occurred within 24 hours after sudden collapse.

CLOSTRIDIUM BOTULINUM

The problem of botulism in birds was well reviewed by Levine,[60] who gave a comprehensive bibliography. Botulism has been reported in chickens, ducks, geese, turkeys, swans, and pheasant chicks, and according to Levine,[60] Theiler in 1927 reported its occurrence in an ostrich. According to Kalmbach,[52] vultures are resistant to the disease. Avian botulism is usually due to the toxin of *Clostridium botulinum* type C, although type A may occasionally be involved and a further type E has been incriminated. Symptoms result from the consumption of food material contaminated with the toxin of *Clostridium botulinum*, the organism being present in the food, but not in the tissues of the affected bird. Foods incriminated, in addition to rotten meat, have included spoiled canned corn, green beans, olives, tuna fish, and apricots. In addition, infection may lurk in maggots which have been feeding on the carcasses of dead birds or mammals; infection has especially been associated with maggots of the bluebottle fly, *Lucilia caesar*.

The disease caused is known as "limberneck"; death occurs in coma following paralysis. To the student of diseases of wild birds, the most interesting manifestation of botulism is that known as "western duck sickness." In spite of its name, this disease has been known to affect a number of other species of birds, including herons, geese, hawks, sandpipers, gulls, and blackbirds. It is caused by *Clostridium botulinum* type C, which may be present in mud, decaying vegetation, fly larvae, dead fish, grasshoppers, and the livers of dead birds. The disease occurs in areas of the United States where there are shallow stagnant water and mud flats. Growth of the organism in these areas and production of toxin

is related to high temperature (37°C. is the optimum), and slightly alkaline conditions (pH 7.5–9.0). Fantastic losses from botulism sometimes occur among ducks; for instance, of 2,000,000 ducks as many as 20 per cent may die. Cheatum et al.[13] reported serious losses of privately reared pheasants also associated with botulism, which was probably derived from ingestion of blow-fly larvae. In this case 1200 of 20,000 pheasants released are believed to have died. This disease may occur at any time among collections of birds if they are able to get hold of rotting carcasses or feed on blow-fly larvae which have emerged from them. Symptoms are those of paralysis which starts in the neck; there is little to be seen at postmortem examination.

Treatment consists of administering laxatives, such as castor oil or epsom salts, although in certain cases antitoxin may be injected.

MYCOPLASMA (CHRONIC RESPIRATORY DISEASE— C.R.D.)

Literature on the occurrence of pleuropneumonia-like organisms (PPLO), or mycoplasmata, is extremely sparse. What is available has been summarized by Klieneberger-Nobel,[56] who regards the true mycoplasmata as merely commensal organisms which live in the air sacs of birds.

It was originally supposed that the cocco-bacilliform bodies found associated with the chronic respiratory disease in poultry described by Nelson[67] were mycoplasmata. Klieneberger-Nobel,[56] however, gave reasons for regarding the cocco-bacilliform bodies as being true bacteria and not belonging to the Mycoplasmataceae. To what extent these cocco-bacilliform bodies play a part in the diseases of cage and aviary birds is unknown; indeed, no attempt appears to have been made so far to isolate them from cases of chronic respiratory disease. This disease, as seen in chickens and turkeys, is a typical coryza associated with slow onset, chronic nature, and persistence of nasal discharge for two months or longer. The cocco-bacilliform bodies are present in the nasal discharge, but are not found in healthy birds. Chronic respiratory disease is an upper respiratory tract disease to be differentiated from Nelson's coryza, which is characterized by rapid onset and short incubation period, and is caused by the bacterium *Haemophilus gallinarum*.

The only reference to possible disease associated with true PPLO in cage birds appears to be that of Adler,[1] who isolated PPLO from the air sac of a budgerigar; at necropsy a mild aerosacculitis was observed. This bird was one from a large aviary in which a few birds had died each week from an unknown cause; serological work was undertaken, but no association of PPLO with the disease could be demonstrated.

RICKETTSIA

The only rickettsia to which birds appear regularly susceptible is that which causes Q fever, *Rickettsia burneti*. However, a single report[80] suggests that some birds may be incriminated in the spread of the tick typhus caused by *Dermacentroxenus sibiricus*. The evidence for this rested on the examination of blood sera from 366 birds of 35 species, 3 to 5 per cent of which showed a positive complement-fixation reaction. This rickettsiosis is transmitted by Ixodes ticks, of which larvae and nymphs were found on birds of 14 of the species. It was supposed, therefore, that birds could play a positive role in dissemination of the disease, although they did not appear to be affected themselves.

The literature with regard to the role of birds in the etiology of Q fever is reviewed by Zdrodovskii and Golinevich.[94] These authors stated that birds show some degree of susceptibility to the agent of Q fever; pigeons, geese, and turkeys can be infected experimentally by intraperitoneal injection, and positive serological reactions are later observed. Rickettsiae may also survive in the kidneys of pigeons and turkeys for six weeks or more. In experimentally infected fowls, *R. burneti* is excreted in the feces from the 7th to the 40th day after infection. It is also stated that fowls, ducks, turkeys, geese, pigeons, and many species of wild birds in Q-fever areas show natural infection with *R. burneti*. Much of the findings of this work has depended on the results of serological tests and requires more adequate confirmation; there is no suggestion that birds are clinically infected. Contrary to the views of other workers, Tarasevich and Kulagin[83] believe that fowls are resistant to *R. burneti* and cannot be infected with it more than transiently.

MYCOBACTERIUM TUBERCULOSIS

Tuberculosis due to the avian type of *Mycobacterium tuberculosis* can occur, so far as is known, in all groups of birds, and a fairly extensive literature exists which describes it. In addition to aviary birds, wild birds are commonly affected, particularly pigeons. There appears to have been no critical study made of avian mycobacteria, and the possibility exists that more than one strain may be the cause of avian tuberculosis. Karlson et al.[53] found yellow pigment in a strain of avian-type tubercle bacillus from lesions in a swan. This organism was virulent for at least one year for chickens and rabbits, but not for guinea pigs, but became avirulent 10 years after isolation. Tuberculin hypersensitivity

and cross-agglutination occurred with some but not all strains of avian tubercle bacilli. This report highlights the necessity for work on strains of avian tubercle bacilli. Tuberculosis may affect all organs in birds and a detailed description of the disease in various species is unnecessary, although it must be said that tuberculosis of skeletal tissue is very common. Tuberculosis due to avian mycobacteria is easily diagnosed, since bacilli are always present in large numbers and can be seen in smears stained by Ziehl-Neelsen stain.

Occasionally captive birds are found infected with human-type tubercle bacilli. Hutyra et al.,[46] describing tuberculosis in parrots, stated that it can be caused by all three types of organism. There is ample evidence that parrots, at least, are sometimes susceptible to human-type tuberculosis, and such infection has been described by Stableforth,[81] Lovell,[62] and Soltys.[79] It appears that birds become infected from a tuberculous human being and not vice versa, although it is conceivable that children could be infected by sick parrots. A scanty literature suggests that even when lesions are caused by human-type mycobacteria, acid-fast bacilli are easily found in them. However, in suspected cases bacteriological culture and other methods should also be adopted because of the epidemiological importance of the disease.

The situation with regard to tuberculosis in wild birds has been reviewed by McDiarmid.[63] He suggests that a number of aberrant strains of *Mycobacterium* may be present, and considers that the principal host for *Mycobacterium* in wild life in the United Kingdom is the woodpigeon (*Columba palumbus*). He draws attention to the observation of the Hon. Miriam Rothschild that affected pigeons show an interesting color variation (darkening of the plumage), possibly associated with tuberculosis of the adrenal glands. Sometimes birds are simultaneously infected with tuberculosis and aspergillosis (Fig. 24-2).

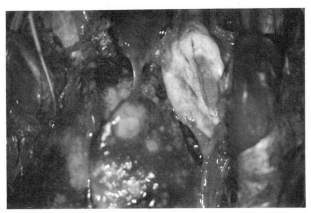

Fig. 24-2. *Tuberculosis and aspergillosis occurring simultaneously in a pigeon. Plaque of aspergillosis and liver infected with tuberculosis.*

References

1. ADLER, H. E.: Isolation of a pleuropneumonia-like organism from the air sac of a parakeet. J.A.V.M.A. *130:*408–409, 1957.

2. ALLAN, D.: *Vibrio metchnikovi* in a Hill Mynah. Vet. Rec. *75:*78, 1963.

3. APPLEBY, E. C.: A small outbreak of pseudotuberculosis in monkeys and tropical birds. Nord. Vet-Med. *14* (Suppl. 1): 213–216, 1962.

4. AXWORTHY, R. H.: An outbreak of erysipelas in ducks. Vet. Rec. *75:*674–675, 1963.

5. BEAUDETTE, F. R.: A case of pseudotuberculosis in a blackbird. J.A.V.M.A. *97:*151–157, 1940.

6. BIGLAND, C. H., WILTON, G. S., VANCE, H. N., and CARLSON, H. C.: Salmonellosis of animals in Alberta, 1949 to 1960. J.A.V.M.A. *140:*251–253, 1962.

7. BLACKMORE, D. K., and GALLAGHER, G. L.: An outbreak of erysipelas in captive wild birds and mammals. Vet. Rec. *76:*1161–1164, 1964.

8. BLAKEY, D.: Division of Preventable Disease Control, Mississippi, Weekly Morbidity Report, February 18, 1966.

9. BRANDER, G. C.: The new penicillins and their use in the control of animal disease. Animal Health *1:*43–47, 1963.

10. BROWN, J. H.: The susceptibility of fur-bearing animals and game birds to tularaemia. Canad. Fld. Nat. *58:*55–60, 1944.

11. BUXTON, A.: *Salmonellosis in Animals.* Review series no. 5 of the Commonwealth Bureau of Animal Health, 1957.

12. CARLSON, H. C., and PENNIFOLD, K. S.: Pasteurellosis in penguins. Canad. Vet. J. *2:*157–158, 1961.

13. CHEATUM, E. L., REILLY, J. R., and FORDHAM, S. C., Jr.: Botulism in game farm pheasants. Transactions of the 22nd North American Wildlife Conference, March 4, 5, 6, 1957. Washington, D.C., Wildlife Management Insitute, 1957. Pp. 169–179.

14. CLARK, G. M., and LOCKE, L. N.: Case report: Observations on pseudotuberculosis in common grackles. Avian Dis. *6:*506–510, 1962.

15. DOZSA, I.: A haziverb (*Passer d. domesticus*), mint *Salmonella typhimurium*—reservoir (The sparrow as a host of *Salmonella typhimurium*). Mag. allator. Lapja. *16:*144–145, 1961. Summaries in English and Russian.

16. EDWARDS, P. R., WEST, M. G., and BRUNER, D. W.: *Arizona Group of Paracolon Bacteria—A New Group of Bacteria Pathogenic for Animals and Probably also for Man.* Bull. Kentucky Agric. Exper. Sta., no. 499. Lexington, University of Kentucky, 1947.

17. EMMEL, M. W., and HUDDLESON, I. F.: The susceptibility of the guinea fowl to Brucella disease. J.A.V.M.A. *79:*228–232, 1931.

18. EVANS, G. A.: Parakeets in veterinary practice. J.A.V.M.A. *128:*593–595, 1956.

19. FADDOUL, G. P., FELLOWS, G. W., and BAIRD, J.: A survey on the incidence of salmonellae in wild birds. Avian Dis. *10:*89–94, 1966.

20. FERRIS, D. H., RHOADES, H. E., HANSON, L. E., GALTON, M., and MANSFIELD, M. E.: Research into the nidality of *Leptospira ballum* in campestral hosts including the hog-nosed snake (*Heterodon platyrhinus*). Cornell. Vet. *51:*405–419, 1961.

21. FIENNES, R. N. T-W-: Report of the Society's Pathologist for the year 1957. Proc. zool. Soc. Lond. *132:*129–146, 1959.

22. FIENNES, R. N. T-W-: Report of the Society's Pathologist for the year 1958. Proc. zool. Soc. Lond. *134:*297–308, 1960.

23. FIENNES, R. N. T-W-: Report of the Pathologist for the year 1960. Proc. zool. Soc. Lond. *137:*173–196, 1961.

24. FIENNES, R. N. T-W-: Report of the Society's Pathologist for the year 1961. Proc. zool. Soc. Lond. *140:*25–46, 1963.

25. FIENNES, R. N. T-W-: Report of the Society's Pathologist for the year 1962. Proc. zool. Soc. Lond. *143:*53–78, 1964.

26. FOX, H.: *Disease in Captive Wild Mammals and Birds.* Philadelphia, Lippincott, 1923. Sect. XVII, part 4.

27. FREESE, K.: Über seuchenhafte Erkrankungen mit septikämischen Charakter bei Kanerienvögeln. Dtsch. tierärztl. Wschr. *15:*501–504, 1907.

28. GRAY, M. L.: Listeriosis in fowls: A review. Avian Dis. *2:*296–314, 1958.

29. GREEN, R. G.: The problem of tularemia in game birds. Amer. Game *17:*80–81, 1928.

30. GREEN, R. G., and SHILLINGER, J. E.: Wild-life cycles and what they mean to the grouse supply. Trans. Amer. Game Conf. *20:*182–185, 1934.

31. GREEN, R. G., and WADE, E. M.: Ruffed grouse are susceptible to tularemia. Proc. Soc. exp. Biol. & Med. *25:*515–517, 1928.

32. GREEN, R. G., and WADE, E. M.: Experimental tularemia in birds. Proc. Soc. exp. Biol. & Med. *25:*637, 1928.

33. GREEN, R. G., WADE, E. M., and KELLY, W.: Experimental tularemia in ring-necked pheasant. Proc. Soc. exp. Biol. & Med. *26:*260–263, 1928.

34. GUEREZ, A.: Epidemie de cholera chez les canards marins. Encycl. vet. *4:*350, 1947.

35. GUPTA, B. R., and RAO, S. B. V.: Enteritis in ducklings caused by an organism belonging to (Shigella) Alkalascens-Dispar group. Indian Vet. J. *38*:8–10, 1961.

36. HALL, S. A.: A disease in pullets due to *Erysipelothrix rhusiopathiae*. Vet. Rec. *75*:333–334, 1963.

37. HAMERTON, A. E.: Report on the deaths occurring in the Society's Gardens during the year 1942. Proc. zool. Soc. Lond. *113:* 149–160, 1943.

38. HARSHFIELD, G. S.: Fowl Cholera. In *Diseases of Poultry*, 5th ed., H. E. Biester and L. H. Schwarte, eds. Ames, Iowa State University Press, 1965. Pp. 359–373.

39. HERMAN, C. M., and SLADEN, W. J. L.: Aspergillosis in Waterfowl. Transactions of 23rd North American Wildlife Conference, March 3, 4, 5, 1958. Washington, D.C., Wildlife Management Institute, 1958. Pp. 187–191.

40. HILL, W. C. O.: Report of the Society's Prosector for the year 1951. Proc. zool. Soc. Lond. *122*:515–533, 1952.

41. HILL, W. C. O.: Report of the Society's Prosector for the year 1952. Proc. zool. Soc. Lond. *123*:227–251, 1953.

42. HILL, W. C. O.: Report of the Society's Prosector for the year 1953. Proc. zool. Soc. Lond. *124*:303–311, 1954.

43. HILL, W. C. O.: Report of the Society's Prosector for the years 1955 and 1956. Proc. zool. Soc. Lond. *129:* 431–446, 1957.

44. HUDSON, C. B.: Fowl cholera in ring-necked pheasants. J.A.V.M.A. *104*:211–212, 1944.

45. HULPHERS, G., and LILLEENGEN, K.: Om stafylokocksjuka, pseudotuberkulos och pasteurellos hos villebråd. Medd. Veterinarhögsk. Stockh. *19*:1–54, 1946.

46. HUTYRA, F., MAREK, J., and MANNINGER, R.: *Special Pathology and Therapeutics of Domestic Animals*. London, Bailliere, Tindall and Cox, 1938. Vol. 1, p. 673.

47. JANOVSKI, N. A.: Arthropathy associated with *Escherichia coli* septicemia in caged birds. J.A.V.M.A. *148*:1517–1522, 1966.

48. JANUSCHKE, E.: Geflugelcholera beim Sperber (Accipiter nisus). Wien. tierärztl. Mschr. 272 1915.

49. JENNINGS, A. R.: Diseases in wild birds. J. Comp. Path. Therap. *64*:356–359, 1954.

50. JOEST, E.: Geflugelcholera bein Uhu (Bubo maximus Sibb). Beitr. Tierheilk. 1915, 11.

51. JUNGHERR, E.: Paratyphoid infections in birds. Vet. Med. *35*:112–116, 1940.

52. KALMBACH, E. R.: American vultures and the toxin of *Clostridium botulinum*. J.A.V.M.A. *94*:187–191, 1939.

53. KARLSON, A. G., DAVIS, C. L., and COHN, M. L.: Skotochromogenic *Mycobacterium avium* from a trumpeter swan. Am.J.Vet.Res. *23*:575–579, 1962.

54. KEYMER, I. F.: A survey and review of the causes of mortality in British birds and the significance of wild birds as disseminators of disease. I. A survey of the causes of mortality. Vet. Rec. *70*:713–720, 1958. II. A review of specific diseases not diagnosed in the survey and the significance of wild birds as disseminators of disease. *ibid.* *70*:736–739, 1958.

55. KEYMER, I. F.: Specific diseases of the canary and other passerine birds. Mod. Vet. Pract. *40*(17):32–35, Sept. 1, 1959.

56. KLIENEBERGER-NOBEL, E.: *Pleuropneumonia-like organisms (PPLO)—Mycoplasmataceae*. New York, Academic Press, 1962. 157 pp.

57. KURSBAN, N. J., and FOSHAY, L.: Tularemia acquired from the pheasant. J.A.M.A. *131*:1493–1494, 1946.

58. LEE, C. D.: Staphylococcosis, Streptococcosis, Colibacillosis, and Arthritis. In *Diseases of Poultry*, H. E. Biester and L. Devries, eds. Ames, Iowa State College Press, 1943. Pp. 343–355.

59. LEE, C. D.: Summary of practical prevention and control measures for some bacterial diseases of poultry. Proc. Book, A.V.M.A., pp. 230–232, 1951.

60. LEVINE, N. D.: Botulism. In *Diseases of Poultry*, 5th ed., H. E. Biester and L. H. Schwarte, eds. Ames, Iowa State University Press, 1965. Pp. 456–461.

61. LOFTON, C. B., MORRISON, S. M., and LEIBY, P. D.: The Enterobacteriaceae of some Colorado small mammals and birds, and their possible role in gastroenteritis in man and domestic animals. Zoonoses Res. *1*:277–293, 1962.

62. LOVELL, R.: The isolation of tubercle bacilli from captive wild animals. J. Comp. Path. Therap. *43*:205–215, 1930.

63. McDIARMID, A.: *Diseases of Free-living Wild Animals*. F.A.O. U.N. Rome 1962, No. 57, 119 pp.

64. McKAY, K. A., RUHNKE, H. L., and BARNUM, D. A.: The results of sensitivity tests on animal pathogens conducted over the period 1956–1963. Canad. Vet J. *6*:103–111, 1965.

65. MENENDEZ, N. A., REINOSO CASTRO, H., and LARDINI, H.: Infeccion espontanea por *Bacillus anthracis* en pato (Outbreak of anthrax in ducks). Rev. Med. Vet. B. Aires *43*:291–293, 1962.

66. MOLLET, F.: Die Bedeutung von Krähe und Fuchs für die Verbreitung des Milzbrandes. Cbl. Bakt. *70*:19–23, 1913.

67. NELSON, J. B.: Cocco-bacilliform bodies associated with an infectious fowl coryza. Science *82*:43–44, 1935.

68. PARKER, R. R., PHILIP, C. B., and DAVIS, G. E.: Tularaemia: Occurrence in the sage hen, *Centrocercus urophasianus*. Also report of additional cases fol-

lowing contacts with quail, *Colinus virginianus.*
Publ. Hlth Rep. Wash. *47:*479–487, 1932.

69. PATERSON, J. S., and COOK, R.: A method for the
recovery of *Pasteurella pseudotuberculosis* from
faeces. J. Path. Bact. *85:*241–242, 1963.

70. PRUSKI, S.: Krankheits- und Todesursachen bei Straussen
(Struthio camelus) in den polnischen Zoologischen
Gärten (Causes of disease and sudden death in
zoo ostriches in Poland). Kleintier-Praxis *7:*241–244,
1962. In German.

71. QUEEN, F. B., and QUORTRUP, E. R.: Treatment of
Pasteurella multocida (fowl cholera) infection in
wild ducks with autogenous bacterin and penicillin.
J.A.V.M.A. *108:*101–103, 1946.

72. QUORTRUP, E. R., QUEEN, F. B., and MEROVKA, L. J.:
An outbreak of pasteurellosis in wild ducks.
J.A.V.M.A. *108:*94–100, 1946.

73. RAINES, T. V., and WINKEL, F. H.: Erysipelas in pheasants. J.A.V.M.A. *129:*399–400, 1956.

74. ROSEN, M. N., and BISCHOFF, A. I.: The 1948–49 out-
break of fowl cholera in birds in the San Francisco
Bay area and surrounding counties. Calif. Fish
Game *35:*185–192, 1949.

75. ROWLANDS, W. T., and SMITH, H. W.: Staphylococcosis
in geese. J. Comp. Path. Therap. *55:*125–131, 1945.

76. RUHLING, R.: Eine durch Streptokokken hervorgerufene
Kanarienvogelseuche (Streptococcosis in canaries).
Inaug. Diss., Leipzig, 1925. Quoted by Lee.[58]

77. SERY, V., and STRAUS, J.: Ornitóza a salmonelóza u
volně žijících ptáků v přírodní rezervaci a u drůbeže
i lidi nejbližším okoli (Psittacosis and salmonellosis
in a bird sanctuary and in domestic poultry and
man in the neighborhood). Sborn. ces Akad.
zemedelsk. Ved vet. med. *5:*799–808, 1960. In Czech;
summaries in German and Russian.

78. SHILLINGER, J. E., and MORLEY, L. C.: *Diseases of
Upland Game Birds.* Department of the Interior
Conservation Bull. No. 21. Washington, D.C., U.S.
Government Printing Office, 1942.

79. SOLTYS, M. A.: Public health aspect of tuberculosis in
domestic animals. Brit M. J. *2:*1133–1136, 1958.

80. SOMOV, G. P., and SOLDATOV, G. M.: The role of birds
in the circulation of the tick typhus causative agent
in nature. Zhurnal Mikrobiol. Epidemiol. i. Immunobiol. Moscow *41:*126–130, 1964. In Russian.

81. STABLEFORTH, A. W.: A bacteriological investigation of
cases of tuberculosis in five cats, sixteen dogs, a
parrot, and a wallaby. J. Comp. Path. Therap. *42:*
163–188, 1929.

82. STEINIGER, F.: Wie lange halten sich Salmonellen aus
verregnetem Abwasser auf Pflanzen? (Survival of
sewage salmonella on vegetation). Berl. Munch.
tierärztl. Wschr. *74:*389–392, 1961. Summary in
English.

83. TARASEVICH, I. V., and KULAGIN, S. M.: The role of
birds in the epidemiology of Q fever. J. Microbiol.
Epidemiol. Immunobiol. *32:*809–815, 1961. Trans.
from Russian.

84. THAMM, H.: Zur Epizootologie der Listeriose. Mh. Vet.
Med. *17:*224–236, 1962.

85. THEILER, A.: Anthrax in the ostrich. Agr. J. Union So.
Africa *4:*370, 1912.

86. URBAIN, A.: Le bacille de Preisz-Nocard chez les oiseaux.
C. R. Soc. Biol. Paris *115:*1166–1167, 1934.

87. URBAIN, A.: Sur une infection streptococcique constatée
sur des oiseaux exotiques de volière et des oiseaux
indigènes. C. R. Soc. Biol. Paris *120:*285–286, 1935.

88. URBAIN, A., and NOUVEL, J.: Epidémie de pseudo-
tuberculose chez de toucans de Cuvier (*Rhamphastos
cuvieri* Gould) et des toucans ariel (*Rhamphastos
ariel* Vig.). Bull. Acad. Vet. Fr. *90:*188–190, 1937.

89. VOLKER, R.: Beitrag zur Diagnostik der Kanarienvogel-
seuchen. Dtsch. tierärztl. Wschr. *34:*803, 1926.
Quoted by Lee.[58]

90. WALDHALM, D. G., MASON, D. R., MEINERSHAGEN, W. A.,
and SCRIVNER, L. H.: Magpies as carriers of ovine
Vibrio fetus. J.A.V.M.A. *144:*497–500, 1964.

91. WALLER, E. F.: Erysipelothrix infection in a quail.
J.A.V.M.A. *95:*512–513, 1939.

92. WILLIAMS, J. E.: Paratyphoid and Paracolon Infections.
In *Diseases of Poultry,* 5th ed., H. E. Biester and
L. H. Schwarte, eds. Ames, Iowa State University
Press, 1965. Pp. 202–248.

93. YAKUNIN, M. P. L.: Spirochaetes in wild birds. Trudy. Inst.
Akad. Nauk. Kaz kh. SSR. *16:*15–22, 1962. In Russian.

94. ZDRODOVSKII, P. F., and GOLINEVICH, H. M.: *The
Rickettsial Diseases.* New York, Pergamon Press,
1960. Pp. 392 and 408.

95. ZWART, P., and DONKER-VOET, J.: Listeriosis bij in
gevangenschap gehouden dieren (Listeriosis in
animals kept in captivity). Tijdschr. Diergeneesk.
*84:*712–716, 1959. In Dutch; summaries in English,
French, and German.

VIRAL DISEASES

Birds may, during their lifetime, become infected with many different viruses. Infection is not necessarily synonymous with disease, and the viruses vary in their importance. Some cause serious disease, such as avian pox. Others, like the viruses causing encephalitis, although capable of causing serious disease in man and other animals, frequently infect birds without producing any symptoms. Improved techniques for the isolation and study of viruses have led to the discovery of still others which are known only for the effects they produce in cell culture outside the host—viruses "in search of a disease," which have come to be known as *orphan* viruses.

The diseases for which viruses are known to be responsible in cage birds are described in this Section of Chapter 24.

CANARY POX
(Kikuth's Disease, "Diphtheria")

The causal agent of canary pox is a filterable virus. It is one of a series of viruses causing pox in birds. The viruses causing avian pox appear to fall into distinct groups, and they are normally classified according to the species of the avian host. van Rooyen[53] classified canary pox virus as *Borreliota fringillae.*

Some canary pox viruses are infective only for the homologous host,[1] but the infectivity of certain strains for heterologous hosts has also been clearly demonstrated experimentally. It is usually accepted, however, that, under natural conditions, species other than the homologous host and its near relatives are not significantly affected by canary pox virus.

Canary pox is world wide in distribution, and outbreaks have been reported from the United States, Canada, South America, Japan, and European countries, including the United Kingdom. The canary (*Serinus canarius*) is the species commonly affected, but the virus has the ability to infect a number of other passerine birds, particularly those of the finch tribe. Gray[21] referred to the disease in the budgerigar (*Melopsittacus undulatus*), but this report lacks substantiation.

Most canary pox outbreaks are apparently sporadic and unconnected. Nevertheless, the disease can, in certain circumstances, assume panzootic proportions in a susceptible population. This was well illustrated in Japan in 1958. The first Japanese cases of canary pox occurred in a group of newly imported English canaries.[46] From this nidus of infection the disease spread throughout the whole country, with consequent heavy losses.

The high mortality, which often approaches 100 per cent in an outbreak, makes appearance of the disease in a flock a potential disaster for the aviculturist.

EPIZOOTIOLOGY

Several investigators have reported the transmission of avian pox by intermediary carriers, and McGaughey and Burnet,[34] in a report of avian pox in the wild sparrow, noted that the sparrows were infested with the poultry flea (*Ceratophyllus gallinae*) and the red mite (*Dermanyssus gallinae*), which was regarded as an uncommon occurrence in wild birds. Unfortunately, the part played by arthropod vectors in transmission of canary pox has not been specifically studied.

The causative agent has been successfully transmitted experimentally by the intranasal and subcutaneous routes, and also by introduction onto deplumed skin. Sato *et al.*[46] presented conclusive evidence that direct transmission is possible, but the sporadic occurrence and slow spread of canary pox suggests transmission by an intermediary carrier, as does the fact that normal isolation methods often fail to influence spread of the disease within an aviary.[11]

The house sparrow (*Passer domesticus*) has been shown to be susceptible to both the experimental and the natural disease.[9,34] Sparrows and probably wild birds of other passeriform species may therefore provide an important reservoir of infection.

CLINICAL MANIFESTATIONS

Canary pox is a slowly spreading disease, characterized by a high mortality and a course of 3 to 10 days. The incubation period as established by experimental methods varies from 3 to 16 days, depending on the route of infection. In typical cases the onset is characterized by irritation of the eyelids, which is evidenced by frequent scratching of the eyes and beak and rubbing of the head on perches and other cage fittings. An early symptom is lacrimation, and this is closely followed by the appearance of yellowish proliferative lesions on the eyelids. Over a period of 3 to 4 days the lesions may extend to the commissures of the beak, the intermandibular space, and the skin of the head and neck (Fig. 24-3); spread of the lesions into the mouth and pharyngeal area often follows. The lesions are both proliferative and inflammatory, and in addition to the tendency to scab formation, the affected areas are also frequently underrun with purulent exudate.

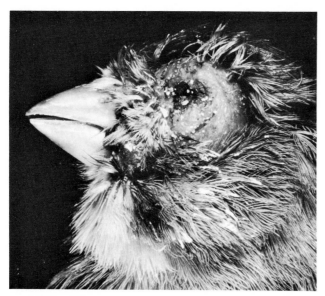

Fig. 24-3. *Canary pox: proliferative skin lesions on head. (Veterinary Record 76:464, 1964.)*

In the early stages affected birds are still active and they continue to eat until respiratory symptoms appear. At this stage illness is evident, with ruffling of the plumage, progressive lassitude, and diarrhea, with dyspnea increasing in severity until finally death occurs. When the infection is caused by virus of maximal virulence the first clinical symptom is acute respiratory distress, and death occurs without the appearance of the characteristic skin lesions. When less virulent strains of virus are involved, the external pox lesions will often spread to affect the entire body and death may not occur for several weeks.

Some even milder variants of the virus cause nonfatal disease characterized by cutaneous lesions restricted in distribution, as in "foot disease,"[55] in which they are located typically on one or more toes. These lesions consist of indurated swellings up to 5 mm. in diameter, which may regress spontaneously after a week or two unless secondary infection intervenes, in which case the toe, the foot, or even the entire tarsus may be lost.

PATHOLOGY

Birds that die of the acute viremic disease may exhibit few internal lesions except for congestion of the lungs and upper respiratory tract. More frequently signs of septicemia, with pneumonia, pericarditis, perihepatitis, and air sac lesions, are evident. The pericardium may be thickened and the pericardial cavity contain gelatinous exudate, and a thin film of exudate may also cover the liver. Lesions in the respiratory system often take the form of a discrete focal pneumonia and turbid thickening of the air sacs.

Intracytoplasmic inclusions of the type associated with all avian poxes can be demonstrated in hematoxylin–eosin–stained sections of various tissues, such as the skin, trachea and bronchi, and the proventriculus. Many of the cells in affected tissues contain these eosinophilic inclusions, which are granular, with eosinophilic material particularly evident around the periphery. The largest inclusions occupy almost the whole of the cytoplasm and are vacuolar in character, with a central unstained area. Their development is accompanied by degeneration and ultimate destruction of the nucleus of the cell.

The proliferative character of the skin lesions is due partly to an increase in the number of epithelial cell layers and partly to an increase in the size of the individually affected cells.

DIAGNOSIS

In aviaries the appearance of a slowly spreading, highly fatal acute disease, in which skin lesions are evident, particularly around the eyes, and respiratory symptoms are a feature, usually justifies the diagnosis of canary pox. Unfortunately, in individual cases and even in aviary epizootics, the pathognomonic cutaneous lesions may be absent, and in these and other atypical cases the only satisfactory diagnostic criterion is the isolation of the causal agent.

Canary pox virus can regularly be recovered from infected birds by inoculation of material prepared from the skin lesions or respiratory tract onto the chorio-allantoic membrane (CAM) of embryonated hen eggs. The technique is one which requires few additions to even a small laboratory (Fig. 24-4). Material for egg inoculation is prepared by grinding infected tissues with sterile saline solution in a mortar (Fig. 24-4 A), sand being added to assist in breakdown. Antibiotics to a concentration of 1,000 to 5,000 units of penicillin and 1 to 10 mg. of streptomycin per ml. are added to control bacterial contamination. Eggs incubated for 10 to 13 days are used, and they should be candled to ensure that the embryo is alive (Fig. 24-5). After the shell is washed with spirit a small hole is drilled into the air space. A small equilateral triangle is then cut from the shell (Fig. 24-4 C) in an area where the CAM is clear of large blood vessels. The cuts are made with a glass file or a dental drill equipped with a small cutting wheel, care being taken not to damage the shell membrane. A drop of sterile saline solution is then run onto the exposed membrane and gentle suction is applied by rubber teat to the hole into the air space. This produces an artificial air cell over the CAM. The inoculum is now deposited through the shell membrane onto the CAM, using a small syringe to deliver 0.05

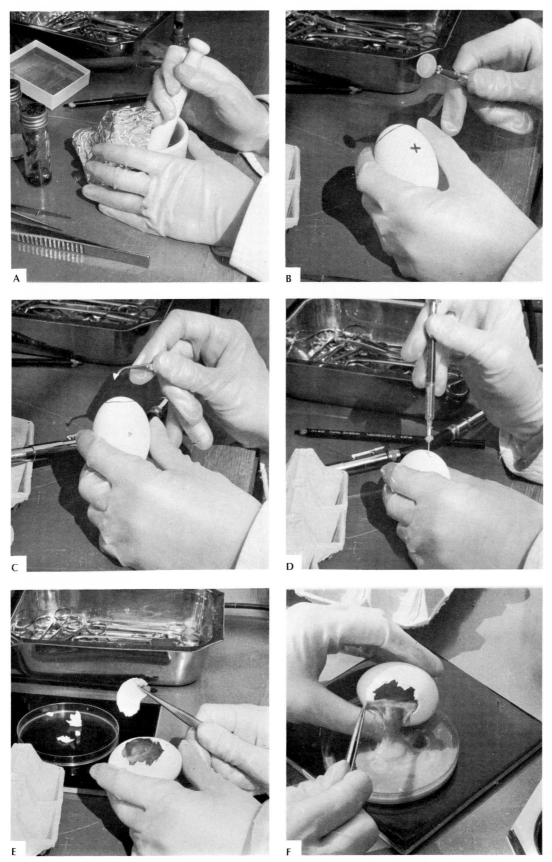

Fig. 24-4. *Canary pox virus isolation. A. Preparation of the inoculum. B. Site of cut into shell over chorio-allantoic membrane. C. Removal of cut shell. D. Injection of inoculum. E, F. "Harvesting" of the chorio-allantoic membrane.*

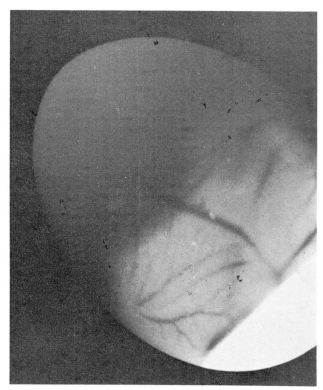

Fig. 24-5. *Ten-day embryonated hen egg candled with mercury lamp, showing blood vessels on chorio-allantoic membrane.*

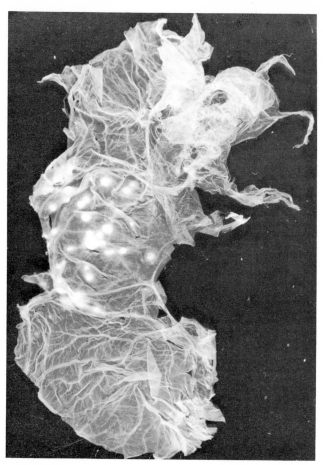

Fig. 24-6. *Pock lesions on chorio-allantoic membrane due to canary pox virus.*

to 0.1 ml. (Fig. 24-4 D), and the holes in the shell are then sealed with melted paraffin. The inoculated eggs are rocked gently to spread the inoculum and returned to the incubator for 4 or 5 days.

When the membrane is harvested the shell is cut away from the boundary of the air space (Fig. 24-4 E) and the egg contents are poured out (Fig. 24-4 F). The CAM which has remained attached to the shell membrane can now be removed, washed in saline, and examined for lesions. Large yellowish plaques, edematous swellings, or a clouding of the membrane together with scattered yellowish pocks is evidence of positive results (Fig. 24-6).

CONTROL

Precautionary measures should be designed to prevent contact with possible sources of infection and all new birds added to an aviary should be maintained in strict isolation for at least two weeks in mosquito-proof quarters. Aviaries and flights should be made mosquito-proof, with additional steps being taken to control other external parasites if necessary.

Recovered canaries appear to be solidly immune,[18] and in the hands of some workers[3,14] preventive vaccination has given favorable results. Methods of modification

of the virus and vaccination with such modified viruses have been described[4]; the isolation of natural strains of virus of low virulence has also given rise to the hope that some of these may be of value in active immunization.[6] Hartwigk and Lange[25] produced immunity in canaries by use of a field strain passed six times in chick-embryo fibroblast culture, diluted 1:1,000 and applied onto the wing web.

TREATMENT

Treatment of both the acute and the subacute disease is unlikely to succeed, and any birds showing symptoms during an outbreak should be killed and burned. Individual cases of the cutaneous form have been treated successfully by local application of antiseptics and bacteriostatics. Coulston and Manwell[14] used 1 to 3% merbromin* in 70% alcohol containing a trace of acetone applied once or twice daily to the infected pox areas. Highly successful results were reported.

*Mercurochrome in aqueous-alcohol solution—Hynson, Westcott & Dunning, Inc., Baltimore, Md.

NEWCASTLE DISEASE (Ranikhet Disease, Avian Pest, Avian Distemper)

Doyle[17] demonstrated the cause of a fatal disease of domestic poultry occurring near Newcastle-upon-Tyne, England, to be a filterable virus. A study of the infective agent showed it to be a previously undescribed virus, and the disease caused by it has since become generally known as Newcastle disease. Filtration studies and electron microscopy have indicated a particle size for the virus of 70 to 180 mμ, and on the basis of its behavior and the structure of its ribonucleoprotein it is usually classified with the myxoviruses. A significant property of the agent is its prolonged ability to survive under favorable conditions of humidity and temperature.

The hemagglutinating activity of Newcastle disease virus and the property of antiserum to specifically inhibit such hemagglutination were first demonstrated by Burnet.[10] The hemagglutination (HA) and the hemagglutination-inhibition (HI) tests have since proved to be of great value in diagnosis.

A fatal disease of poultry in Java described by Kraneveld[32] proved later to be identical with that described by Doyle, and Newcastle disease has since been recognized throughout the world. Usually thought of primarily as a disease of gallinaceous birds, it nevertheless has a much wider range of natural hosts, including a number of species of special interest to aviculturists. Outbreaks have been recorded involving both psittacine and passerine birds, often with high mortality. Among the Psittacidae, the natural disease has been recorded in parrotlets (*Psittacula krameri*),[56] African grey parrots (*Psittacus erithacus*),[48] yellow-headed parrots (*Amazona ochrocephala*), and a macaw (*Ara severa*)[12]; and an epidemic in central Africa involving Australian parrots (species unnamed) and red-headed lovebirds (*Agapornis pullaria*) is on record.[35] Passerine birds known to be susceptible include weaver finches and Java sparrows (*Padda oryzivora*),[28] and the fatal disease has also been reported in the canary (*Serinus canarius*).[37]

Although the incidence is not known among birds kept by aviculturists, the psittacines are probably the most susceptible.

The disease in hosts other than gallinaceous birds in some cases is due to exotic virus variants.[12] On the other hand, other outbreaks have been shown to be due to viruses closely related to recognized field strains.[37] In an outbreak in Kenya involving both domestic fowl and African grey parrots (*Psittacus erithacus*), it was shown that the virus recovered from the parrots remained fully virulent for poultry.[48] However, despite well-documented evidence indicating a wide species susceptibility to Newcastle disease, it is probably true that cage birds in general have a comparatively strong innate resistance to contact infection.

EPIZOOTIOLOGY

Important factors which influence the spread of Newcastle disease are the marked survival ability of the virus, its highly invasive property, its ability to infect a multiplicity of avian host species, and the facility with which it is air borne.

The danger to cage birds is no doubt greatest during epizootics in neighboring domestic poultry. At such times the infection of wild birds may not only facilitate spread but perhaps also result in adaptive mutation of the virus, leading to increased infectivity for new hosts. The complete natural host range is unknown, but about 20 species of wild birds have been shown to be susceptible to the natural disease; these include two species of wild sparrows (*Passer domesticus*[22] and *Passer italiae*[37]), and the starling (*Sturnus vulgaris*).[20]

CLINICAL MANIFESTATIONS

As commonly reported in cage birds, the illness is severe and results in death in the majority of cases. Respiratory involvement is the most characteristic finding. The appetite is depressed from the outset, and diarrhea is a feature. Gasping respiration is an early symptom, together with profuse ocular and nasal discharge. When an outbreak occurs in an aviary the birds may huddle together in a corner with ruffled feathers and eyes closed. The course is often short, terminating in death within 1 to 3 days; in some outbreaks, particularly in psittacine birds, sudden death is the first sign that disease is present. However, the disease in cage birds, as in other species, may be expected to vary greatly in intensity.

Birds which survive will often develop derangement of the central nervous system, resulting in a variety of abnormal attitudes and movements, including ataxia, torticollis, muscular twitching, and varying degrees of paralysis.[12]

PATHOLOGY

Not infrequently in birds that die suddenly no gross lesions are apparent. Enteritis is a common finding in others, and may be severe in some. A diffuse congestion of the mucous surface of the proventriculus is often a feature, and tracheitis may be present.

In those birds which develop nervous symptoms, microscopic lesions may be evident in the central nervous system. These take the form of areas of gliosis at various levels of the spinal cord and brain, and should be sought in the lumbar cord, medulla, and the molecular layer of the cerebellum.

DIAGNOSIS

When deaths in cage birds are associated with recognized outbreaks of Newcastle disease in gallinaceous birds, this may afford some evidence on which to base a diagnosis, but the absence of specific symptoms and gross lesions in the affected birds precludes diagnosis on clinical grounds. As with other infectious diseases, the only satisfactory diagnosis is that supported by the isolation and identification of the causal agent, or the demonstration of specific antibodies to it.

Trachea and spleen are commonly used for virus isolation, and the material should be taken from birds in the early stages of the disease. Embryonated hen eggs incubated for 9 to 11 days are inoculated with tissue suspensions prepared by grinding in a mortar with sterile sand. A small hole is drilled over the air space, and 0.25 ml. of inoculum is injected into the allantoic chamber. The needle should penetrate the egg to a depth of about 1.5 cm. The injected eggs, along with suitable controls, are then returned to the incubator and candled daily for 5 days, or until infection is revealed by death of the embryo. With virulent strains of Newcastle disease virus death of the embryo normally occurs within 36 to 72 hours. Allantoic fluid is then harvested and tested for hemagglutinating activity.

Newcastle disease virus will agglutinate red blood cells of a number of species, but fowl red cells are normally used in the test. The rapid test is carried out on a glass slide by mixing 1 drop of allantoic fluid with 1 drop of a 5% suspension of washed red blood cells; a positive result is indicated by a clumping of the red cells within 60 seconds (Fig. 24-7 A). Allantoic fluid from uninfected eggs is used as a control, and in this case no agglutination will occur (Fig. 24-7 B).

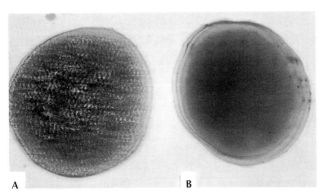

Fig. 24-7. *Rapid slide hemagglutination (HA) test for Newcastle disease virus. A. Positive agglutination. B. Negative control.*

Rapid agglutination of red cells by the allantoic fluid from eggs in which the embryos died within 36 to 72 hours of inoculation is strong evidence to support a diagnosis of Newcastle disease. If required, more precise evidence can be obtained by demonstrating that the hemagglutination is specifically inhibited by the use of Newcastle disease immune serum (HI test). Serum from affected birds can also be tested for HI activity, and this is of considerable value in diagnosis, since HI antibodies are often present as early as two days after the appearance of symptoms.

CONTROL

Newcastle disease usually occurs whenever a susceptible bird comes in contact with the virus. The measures available for control are, therefore, prevention of contact between healthy and ailing birds, and the stimulation of immunity in birds at risk by protective vaccination.

Birds are at greatest risk when the affected contacts are of the same or a closely related species. In these cases the virus will be adapted to the homologous host and there is thus greater danger of spread by contact. Even strict isolation cannot be relied on to prevent spread under most conditions, but nevertheless spread may not be particularly rapid in aviary outbreaks,[48] and vaccination of in-contacts may be of value as a means of control.

Both living and inactivated virus vaccines are used in various countries for the protection of domestic poultry, although the protection afforded by either type of vaccine is of comparatively short duration. Living vaccines have the inherent disadvantage that contamination with other infectious agents can occur. There is also some evidence that strains of reduced virulence similar to those used for vaccination of poultry may cause fatal disease in cage birds. Monda *et al.*[37] recovered a virus closely related to Asplin's "F" strain from fatal cases in the sparrow and canary.

Fortunately certain inactivated vaccines have antigenic properties equal to those of the live strains. Virus of maximal antigenicity inactivated by beta-propiolactone may be expected to stimulate a substantial degree of immunity when administered intramuscularly. Immunity develops within a week of vaccination but may wane considerably within two months.

TREATMENT

In individuals affected by mild forms of the disease, treatment with broad-spectrum antibiotics may be useful for the control of secondary bacterial infection.

THE ARTHROPOD-BORNE VIRUS ENCEPHALITIDES

Of the arthropod-borne viruses (arboviruses) two main subgroups, A and B, are recognized as important causes of disease in animals. These arbovirus infections are generally considered to be a group of diseases affecting various mammals, but closely associated with birds and a number of arthropod vectors. There are strong theoretical grounds for supposing that the earliest association is that of virus–arthropod–bird, and that mammals became involved much later in evolutionary time, following changes in habits of the hosts and vectors. With this provision of wider opportunities for dissemination of the viruses they became modified to involve new and less well adapted hosts. Since viruses were primarily known from their effects rather than for what they were, many of the viruses in this group were named after the unfortunate species in which the disease they caused was first recognized. The subgroup A arboviruses of eastern, western, and Venezuelan "equine encephalomyelitis" were thus first named for the horse.

That birds are the important vertebrate hosts for these viruses has been amply demonstrated by a number of workers.[13,26,27,31] A close association with birds has also been demonstrated for some of the group B arboviruses, for example, Japanese B and louping-ill viruses.[7,8,23,24,47,54]

Although many birds infected with these viruses remain asymptomatic carriers, clinical disease and death may occur in some species, particularly when the infecting agent is eastern encephalitis virus.[5,30]

The ring-necked pheasant (*Phasianus colchicus*), when in captivity, is highly susceptible to natural infection, and other species known to be severely affected include the red-winged blackbird (*Agelaeus phoeniceus*), the house sparrow (*Passer domesticus*), the cedar-waxwing (*Bombycilla cedrorum*), and the cardinal (*Richmondena cardinalis*).

Eastern encephalitis occurs principally in the Atlantic and Gulf Coast states of the United States, but there is evidence that closely related if not identical viruses have a much wider geographical distribution.

EPIZOOTIOLOGY

The virus is transmitted chiefly by various mosquito vectors. In these insects virus is known to multiply, and once the mosquitoes become infected they may remain so for life. Direct bird-to-bird transmission can also occur, but this is of minor importance in the over-all picture.

CLINICAL MANIFESTATIONS

In those bird species in which fatal disease occurs the predominant signs are those of central nervous system involvement and consist in muscular tremors, torticollis, and varying degrees of paralysis.

DIAGNOSIS

No diagnostic gross lesions are seen on postmortem examination. For the isolation and identification of the causal agent embryonated hen eggs can be used, and 10-day embryos are satisfactory. Tissues most likely to contain virus are brain, liver, and spleen, and the tissue emulsion is injected into the amniotic cavity. Positive results are indicated by death of the embryo within 18 to 72 hours. Identification of the virus can be confirmed by neutralization techniques, using chick embryos and mice as test hosts.

CONTROL

Anti-mosquito measures should be adopted to prevent the introduction of infection into flights and aviaries. Prophylactic vaccination has been used for the protection of pheasants and provides a useful degree of control in outbreaks of clinical disease.[51]

VIRUS HEPATITIS

Virus hepatitis was first recognized in birds in the collection of the Zoological Society of Philadelphia in 1946. The first specimens to be affected were a group of newly imported European birds, and it seems likely that either the infection was introduced by these birds or that the virus was already present and by enhancement of its virulence on passage through the new birds it became capable of causing disease in others already in the collection. The incidence is not known, and the disease has not so far been reported except from Philadelphia. The virus has a very wide host range, and the natural disease has been recorded in representatives of over 20 Orders, including not only captive birds but also free-living wild birds that have access to the Philadelphia Zoological Garden.[40,41]

A filterable agent is involved in the morbid process, and it has been transmitted experimentally by the inoculation of Seitz filtrates of liver suspension.[33] The natural disease appears to spread by direct and indirect contact and by way of infected food and water.

CLINICAL MANIFESTATIONS

Death may occur suddenly in acute cases without appearance of any previous symptoms. In the chronic form affected birds become inactive and lose both appetite and weight. The chronic course may be very protracted, and birds may either recover after a variable period of illness or may die after weeks or even months, during which time they become emaciated and distention of the abdomen may occur owing to gross enlargement of the liver.

PATHOLOGY

In the acute form the liver is usually enlarged, soft, and discolored. Microscopical examination reveals a patchy necrosis accompanied by cellular infiltrations and often by proliferation of bile duct epithelial cells.

Gross enlargement of the liver may be a feature of the chronic disease but more commonly the organ is shrunken, often to half its normal size. The surface presents a nodular appearance. Microscopically these nodules are found to consist of areas of regenerating and hyperplastic liver cells which are present throughout the diseased gland. There is also frequently extensive proliferation of bile duct epithelial cells.

In some cases malignant hepatoma develops in association with the slowly progressive form of the disease.[44]

CONTROL

The only useful control measure appears to be vaccination. Workers at the Penrose Research Laboratory of the Zoological Society of Philadelphia use a vaccine prepared from suspensions of infected tissue.[44]

LEUKOSIS COMPLEX

The leukosis complex comprises a group of diseases characterized by lesions resulting from an abnormal proliferation of blood cell precursors. The diseases have been most extensively studied in the domestic fowl, and in this species the involvement of filterable agents has long been established. Various workers have recognized diseases of this complex in species other than the domestic fowl, including both canaries (*Serinus canarius*) and psittacine birds,[2,39,42,43,52] and some are clearly of the opinion that in these birds also the diseases are caused by a virus or viruses.[52]

Transmission is thought to occur through the egg, by direct contact, and also by means of arthropod vectors.

The classification of the leukosis complex of diseases is based on the cell types involved in the pathological changes. Lymphoid leukosis, erythroblastosis, and myeloblastosis are apparently the only diseases of the leukosis complex of any consequence in cage and aviary birds.

LYMPHOID LEUKOSIS

This disease is characterized by the proliferation and infiltration of lymphoid cells into parenchymatous organs. Liver, spleen, and kidneys are most frequently involved, and all of them may be simultaneously affected. The lesions take the form of discrete white nodules of variable size, or the infiltration may be diffuse with enlargement of the whole organ. In the diffuse type the important change is alteration of the gross appearance. The affected organs are often pale pink to yellowish-tan or cream in color and granular or stippled in cross section. The enlargement may be only slight.[39] Increasing weakness, wasting, and diarrhea are characteristic symptoms, and in some cases they may be accompanied by swelling of the abdomen and pallor of the mucous membranes.

ERYTHROBLASTOSIS

A massive proliferation of erythroblasts characterizes this condition, and large numbers of these cells can be demonstrated in the circulating blood of affected birds. The disease is difficult to recognize clinically, but anemia is an important feature and often there are subcutaneous hemorrhages together with abnormal deposits of hemoglobin-derived pigments.

MYELOBLASTOSIS

This condition is also associated with an increase in circulating erythroblasts, but it can be distinguished from the erythroblastic type by the demonstration of large numbers of primitive cells of the myeloblast series in the circulating blood. Anemia and chronic wasting are features of the condition.

PATHOLOGY

In both erythroblastosis and granuloblastosis the significant changes occur in the bone marrow, which is largely replaced by the proliferating blood cell precursors. The parenchymatous organs may be moderately enlarged and altered in color and in rare cases other tissues may be involved. Petrak[39] has seen granuloblastosis in a budgerigar (*Melopsittacus undulatus*) in which there was widespread cutaneous involvement. Lesions were present involving the skin of the shank and entire head, with marked thickening producing a quilted effect, and white to yellowish discoloration of the altered skin.

Similar but smaller lesions were present over both carpal joints and small nodular lesions were present in the skin in other areas.

Diseases of the leukosis complex are progressive in character. Their diagnosis in the living subject is something of a problem unless some gross outward sign is apparent. A tentative diagnosis may be suggested by chronic wasting in the absence of any other apparent cause, but usually necropsy and tissue examination will provide the only satisfactory diagnostic proof.

No practical therapeutic measures have been found for this group of diseases in birds.

PACHECO'S PARROT DISEASE

Following the pandemic of psittacosis in man which occurred in Europe and the United States during the winter of 1929–1930, Pacheco and Bier[38] and Meyer[36] attempted to obtain evidence of the presence of psittacosis in Brazil. These workers investigated pathological conditions affecting Brazilian parrots, including the orange-winged parrot (*Amazona amazonica*), the blue-fronted parrot (*Amazona aestiva*), and the mealy parrot (*Amazona farinosa*). There was still at that time some confusion regarding the pathogenesis of psittacosis. Although the virus had been identified shortly before, the role of the *"Salmonella psittacosis"* of Nocard was still not universally clear, and some confusion no doubt attended the investigations of Pacheco and his colleagues.

It seems likely in retrospect that the conditions studied represented more than one disease entity. During the investigations, *Salmonella typhimurium* (*"Salmonella psittacosis"*) and at least one other bacterium belonging to the *Salmonella* group were isolated from dead and sick parrots. However, the isolation of a filterable agent was the main objective, and it was soon demonstrated that a filter-passing agent was involved in at least one of the morbid processes. The virus was transmitted without difficulty to Tui paroquets (*Brotogeris sanctae-thomae*), and the disease caused by it was indistinguishable from psittacosis. Attempts to transmit the infection to guinea pigs, white mice, chickens, pigeons, and monkeys failed, and on this evidence Pacheco concluded that the disease was psittacosis, but that it was due to a variant virus strictly adapted to Psittacidae.

Pacheco sent his virus to Rivers at the Rockefeller Institute, and after experimental study it was found that, although the clinical symptoms in psittacine birds were very similar to those of psittacosis, the virus was clearly not psittacosis virus. Rivers and Schwentker[45] failed to transmit the disease to mice, rabbits, guinea pigs, and canaries, although they succeeded with 10-day chick embryos, which were regularly killed within 3 to 5 days when infected by the chorio-allantoic route, and serial passage in embryonated eggs was carried out without difficulty. Budgerigars (*Melopsittacus undulatus*) were also used in transmission experiments, and in this species the clinical disease was manifested by ruffling of the feathers and progressive weakness, terminating in death in 3 to 7 days. The nasal discharge, diarrhea, and loss of weight seen in psittacosis were not particularly evident.

Foci of necrosis in the liver and spleen were the predominant gross postmortem features, and the important microscopic finding was the demonstration of intranuclear acidophilic inclusions in the liver and spleen cells.

Pacheco's disease has not been commonly reported,[19] and its incidence is unknown. It should be considered in the differential diagnosis of virus diseases in psittacines, its possible confusion with psittacosis being particularly borne in mind.

SPECIFIC OPHTHALMITIS AND CONJUNCTIVITIS

A transmissible specific ophthalmitis occurs in canaries (*Serinus canarius*) and a specific conjunctivitis of a less severe nature is also known to affect budgerigars (*Melopsittacus undulatus*) and certain other parakeets. It is not known if the two conditions are related.

Gray[21] considered that the disease in canaries was due to a filterable virus, possibly transmitted by a vector. The cause of the disease in parakeets is unknown, but an infectious agent is thought to be involved.

Clinically the two conditions are similar, with at first a serous and later a mucous ocular discharge. In the canary the disease progresses to an ophthalmitis that often leads to blindness with severe damage to the eye.

The disease in budgerigars and other parakeets has been successfully treated[28] by the use of ophthalmic preparations containing chlortetracycline.*

POLIOMYELITIS IN THE BUDGERIGAR

Inspired by a previous isolation of poliovirus type 1 from a budgerigar (*Melopsittacus undulatus*) recovering from paralysis,[50] Sommerville[49] carried out a survey of 224 families in which poliomyelitis had occurred. It was found that 56 of these families had pet budgerigars, and that in 17 instances the bird had died at about the time a child in the house had contracted poliomyelitis.

It is tempting to conclude from these observations

*Aureomycin ophthalmic ointment—American Cyanamid Company, Princeton, N.J.

not only that budgerigars can become infected with poliovirus but also that the natural disease is not particularly uncommon in this species. Experimental studies have failed to confirm this view. Dick and Dane[16] and Dane *et al.*[15] failed to infect budgerigars with a considerable number of poliovirus strains given by oral and intracerebral routes, and Sommerville[49] also failed to infect further budgerigars with his original budgerigar poliovirus type 1 isolate. Although it must be admitted that the occurrence of natural infection in the budgerigar is possible, it can only be concluded that it is comparatively rare.

References

1. ANTONIOTTO, D., and ROMAT, A.: Contribucion al estudio del epithelioma contagioso del canario. Revta Med. Vet., B. Aires *26:*326, 1940.

2. ARNALL, L.: Personal communication, 1965.

3. BEAUDETTE, F. R.: Twenty years of progress in immunization against virus diseases of birds. J.A.V.M.A. *115:*232, 1949.

4. BEAUDETTE, F. R.: The identity of canary pox and "Schnappkrankheit" with notes on vaccination and modification of the virus. Proc. U.S. Livestock Sanit. Ass. *57:*249, 1954.

5. BEAUDETTE, F. R., HOLDEN, P., BLACK, J. J., BIVENS, J. A., HUDSON, C. B., and TUDOR, D. C.: Equine encephalomyelitis in pheasants in 1952–53. Proc. U.S. Livestock Sanit. Ass. *58:*309, 1955.

6. BLANCO, A.: Estudio sobre un foco de viruela cutanea del canario. Revta Patronato Biol. Anim. Madrid. *4:*319, 1958.

7. BUESCHER, E. L., SCHERER, W. F., McCLURE, H. E., MOYER, J. T., ROSENBERG, M. Z., YOSHII, M., and OKADA, Y.: Ecologic studies of Japanese encephalitis virus in Japan. IV. Avian infection. Am. J. trop. Med. Hyg. *8:*678, 1959.

8. BUESCHER, E. L., SCHERER, W. F., ROSENBERG, M. Z., and McCLURE, H. E.: Immunologic studies of Japanese encephalitis virus in Japan. III. Infection and antibody responses of birds. J. Immun. *83:*605, 1959.

9. BURNET, F. M.: A virus disease of the canary of the fowl-pox group. J. Path. Bact. *37:*107, 1933.

10. BURNET, F. M.: The affinity of Newcastle disease virus to the influenza virus group. Aust. J. exp. Biol. Med. Sci. *20:*81, 1942.

11. CAVILL, J. P.: Canary pox:—Report of an outbreak in roller canaries (*Serinus canarius*). Vet. Rec. *76:*463, 1964.

12. CAVRINI, C., and CABASSI, N.: Pseudopeste spontanea in pappagalli della specie *Amazona ochrocephala.* Nuova Vet. *36:*123, 1960.

13. CHAMBERLAIN, R. W., KISSLING, R. E., STAMM, D. D., NELSON, D. B., and SIKES, R. K.: Venezuelan equine encephalomyelitis in wild birds. Am. J. Hyg. *63:*261, 1956.

14. COULSTON, F., and MANWELL, R. D.: Successful chemotherapy of a virus disease of the canary. Am. J. Vet. Res. *2:*101, 1941.

15. DANE, D. S., DICK, G. W. A., and DONALDSON, S. N.: Budgerigars and poliomyelitis. Lancet *1:*497, 1959.

16. DICK, G. W. A., and DANE, D. S.: Budgerigars and poliomyelitis. Lancet *1:*585, 1958.

17. DOYLE, T. M.: A hitherto unrecorded disease of fowls due to a filter-passing virus. J. Comp. Path. Therap. *40:*144, 1927.

18. DURANT, A. J., and McDOUGLE, H. C.: Investigation of pox in canaries. Proc. U.S. Livestock Sanit. Ass. *42:*181, 1938.

19. FINDLAY, G. M.: Pacheco's parrot disease. Vet. J. *89:*12, 1933.

20. GILLESPIE, J. H., KESSEL, B., and FABRICANT, J.: The isolation of Newcastle disease virus from a starling. Cornell Vet. *40:*93, 1950.

21. GRAY, H.: Diseases of cage and aviary birds. Vet. Rec. *48:*343, 1936.

22. GUSTAFSON, D. P., and MOSES, H. E.: The English sparrow as a natural carrier of Newcastle disease virus. Am. J. Vet. Res. *14:*581, 1953.

23. HAMMON, W. McD., REEVES, W. C., and SATHER, G. E.: Japanese B encephalitis virus in the blood of experimentally inoculated birds. Epidemiological implications. Am. J. Hyg. *53:*249, 1951.

24. HAMMON, W. McD., SATHER, G. E., and McCLURE, H. E.: Serologic survey of Japanese B encephalitis virus infection in birds in Japan. Am. J. Hyg. *67:*118, 1958.

25. HARTWIGK, H., and LANGE, W.: Vakzinierungsversuche bei Kanarienvogeln gegen Pocken. Dtsch. tierärztl. Wschr. *71:*180, 1964.

26. HAYES, R. O., DANIELS, J. B., ANDERSON, K. S., PARSONS, M. A., MAXFIELD, H. K., and LaMOTTE, L. C.: Detection of eastern encephalitis virus and antibody in wild and domestic birds in Massachusetts. Am. J. Hyg. *75:*183, 1962.

27. HESS, A. D., and HOLDEN, P.: The natural history of the arthropod-borne encephalitides in the United States. Ann. N.Y. Acad. Sci. *70:*294, 1958.

28. KEYMER, I. F., ARNALL, L., DALL, J. A., BRANCKER, W. M., JOSHUA, J. O., and GRAHAM-JONES, O.: *Handbook on the Treatment of Exotic Pets.* Part One: *Cage Birds.* London, British Veterinary Association, 1964.

29. KIKUTH, W., and GOLLUB, H.: Versuche mit einem filtrierbaren Virus bei einer übertragbaren Kanarien-vogelkrankheit. Zbl. Bakt. I. *125:*313, 1932.

30. KISSLING, R. E., CHAMBERLAIN, R. W., SIKES, R. K., and EIDSON, M. E.: Studies on the North American arthropod-borne encephalitides. III. Eastern equine encephalitis in wild birds. Am. J. Hyg. *60:*251, 1954.

31. KISSLING, R. E., STAMM, D. D., CHAMBERLAIN, R. W., and SUDIA, W. D.: Birds as winter hosts for eastern and western equine encephalomyelitis viruses. Am. J. Hyg. *66:*42, 1957.

32. KRANEVELD, F. C.: Over een in Ned-Indie heerschende ziekte onder het pluimves. Nederl. Ind. Blad. Diergeneesk. *38:*448, 1926.

33. LUCKE, B., and RATCLIFFE, H.: Virus hepatitis of birds and its possible relation to epidemic hepatitis of man. Trans. Ass. Am. Physicians *62:*83, 1949.

34. MCGAUGHEY, C. A., and BURNET, F. M.: Avian pox in wild sparrows. J. Comp. Path. Therap. *55:*201, 1945.

35. MALBRANT, R.: Pseudopeste aviaire au Moyen-Congo. Rev. Sci. med. Pharm. vet., Brazzaville *1:*39, 1942.

36. MEYER, J. R.: Observações anatomo e histopathologicas feitas em orgãos de Papagaios (Amazona amazonica E. A. farinosa) mortos espontaneamente e apos inoculacão de um virus que se demonstrou filtravel. Arch. Inst. Biol., São Paulo *4:*25, 1931.

37. MONDA, V., TANGA, G., and GUARINO, C.: Isolamento e studio delle caratteristiche antigeniche di due ceppi di virus di Newcastle isolati dal passero (*Passer Italiae*) e dal canarino (*Serinus canarius canarius*). Atti Soc. ital Sci. vet. *14:*736, 1960.

38. PACHECO, G., and BIER, O.: Epizootia em papagaios no Brasil e suas relações com a psittacose. Arch. Inst. Biol., São Paulo *4:*89, 1931.

39. PETRAK, M. L.: Unpublished case histories, Angell Memorial Animal Hospital, 1961-1964.

40. RATCLIFFE, H. L.: *Report of the Penrose Research Laboratory of the Zoological Society of Philadelphia,* 1952.

41. RATCLIFFE, H. L.: *Report of the Penrose Research Laboratory of the Zoological Society of Philadelphia,* 1955.

42. RATCLIFFE, H. L.: *Report of the Penrose Research Laboratory of the Zoological Society of Philadelphia,* 1956.

43. RATCLIFFE, H. L.: *Report of the Penrose Research Laboratory of the Zoological Society of Philadelphia,* 1959.

44. RATCLIFFE, H. L.: Hepatitis, cirrhosis and hepatoma in birds. Cancer Res. *21:*26, 1961.

45. RIVERS, T. M., and SCHWENTKER, F. F.: A virus disease of parrots and parakeets differing from psittacosis. J. Exp. Med. *55:*911, 1932.

46. SATO, T., SUGIMORI, T., ISHII, S., and MATUMOTO, M.: Etiologic study on an outbreak of canary pox in Japan 1958. Jap. J. Exp. Med. *32:*247, 1962.

47. SCHERER, W. F., BUESCHER, E. L., and MCCLURE, H. E.: Ecologic studies of Japanese encephalitis virus in Japan. V. Avian factors. Am. J. trop. Med. Hyg. *8:*689, 1959.

48. SCOTT, G. R., and WINMILL, A. J.: Newcastle disease in the Grey Parrot (*Psittacus erithacus* L.). J. Comp. Path. Therap. *70:*115, 1960.

49. SOMMERVILLE, R. G.: Type-1 poliovirus isolated from a budgerigar. Further studies. Lancet *1:*495, 1959.

50. SOMMERVILLE, R. G., MONRO, I. C., and CUTHBERT, C. C.: Poliovirus type 1 isolated from a budgerigar. Lancet *1:*512, 1958.

51. SUSSMAN, O., COHEN, D., GERENDE, J. E., and KISSLING, R. E.: Equine encephalitis vaccine studies in pheasants under epizootic and pre-epizootic conditions. Ann. N.Y. Acad. Sci. *70:*328, 1958.

52. VACARRI, J., BALLARINI, G., PIERESCA, G., BERTONI, L., and SEMELLINI, L.: *Argomenti di pathologica e clinica degli uccelli da gabbia e da voliera,* Faenza: Edizioni La Nuova Veterinaria, 1959.

53. VAN ROOYEN, C. E.: A revision of Holmes's classification of animal viruses, Suborder III (Zoophagineae). Canad. J. Microbiol. *1:*227, 1954.

54. WILLIAMS, H., THORBURN, H., and ZIFFO, G. S.: Isolation of louping ill virus from the red grouse. Nature, Lond. *200:*193, 1963.

55. WORTH, C. B.: A pox virus of the Slate-colored Junco. Auk *73:*230, 1956.

56. ZUYDAM, D. M.: Isolation of Newcastle disease virus from the osprey and the parakeet. J.A.V.M.A. *120:*88, 1952.

Suggested Reading

BIESTER, H. E., and SCHWARTE, L. H., eds.: *Diseases of Poultry,* 5th ed. Ames, Iowa State University Press, 1965.

O'CONNOR HALLORAN, P.: A Bibliography of References to Diseases in Wild Mammals and Birds. Am. J. Vet Res., vol. *16,* October, 1955. Part 2.

PSITTACOSIS AND ORNITHOSIS*†

Before the turn of this Century, astute medical clinicians observed an illness apparently transmitted from sick parrots to man. Since the observed human syndrome was a severe pneumonia with a relatively high mortality rate, the early designation of the illness was "pneumotyphus"; the term "psittacosis" was introduced in 1895 because this human illness seemed to follow contact with psittacine birds.[7]

There is now excellent evidence that the etiological agents of this and related infections belong to a distinct group of microorganisms which are not satisfactorily described as either viral, rickettsial, or bacterial. Collectively, these agents are often called the "psittacosis-lymphogranuloma group," or the "psittacosis-lymphogranuloma-trachoma (P-L-T) group." Because these are somewhat cumbersome expressions, the simple and euphonious term "bedsoniae," recommended by Meyer,[6] will be used here to designate the agents responsible for psittacosis, ornithosis, and related infections. The name gives credit to Sir Samuel Bedson, who was the first to adequately describe and typify the causative agent of psittacosis.[4]

The bedsoniae are obligate intracellular parasites. In purified suspensions they show the presence of the nucleic acids, RNA and DNA. They appear to multiply by fission; characteristic clusters of elementary bodies develop in infected cells. The individual spherical elementary body is the smallest viable infective unit; it is 200 to 400 mμ in diameter. A single infected cell may contain over 100 elementary bodies. Unlike the true viruses, bedsoniae are susceptible to tetracycline antibiotics, which act by arresting the maturation and multiplication of individual particles.[5,8,10]

When classified on the basis of their principal hosts, the bedsoniae fall into three groups: human, other mammalian, and avian. Psittacosis and ornithosis, avian bedsonial infections, are true zoonoses, or, more specifically, zoo-anthroponoses, that is, they are directly transmissible from the infected animal to man.

The usual term applied to bedsonial diseases in birds is "psittacosis" if the patient is of the family Psittacidae (parrots, parakeets, cockatoos, macaws, etc.)

*Supported in part by Grant No. A1-04406, National Institutes of Health, Department of Health, Education, and Welfare, Public Health Service, United States.

†*Disclaimer:* Trade names are provided as information only, and their inclusion does not imply endorsement by the Public Health Service or the U.S. Department of Health, Education, and Welfare.

and "ornithosis" if the patient belongs to any other avian family. When the avian bedsoniae cause disease in man, it is commonly termed "psittacosis," regardless of the reservoir host from which man acquired the organism.

PATHOGENESIS

Two known variables determine the course of bedsonial infections in birds after the effective initiation has occurred. The first of these is the relative susceptibility of the host. Of the common cage birds, parrots, parakeets, and pigeons may be considered relatively resistant. Generally, these same species are also accepted as natural reservoirs of bedsoniae. The other cage birds, such as canaries, finches, rice birds, and mynahs—although highly susceptible to ornithosis—usually contract it from a known reservoir host.

The second influencing variable is the pathogenicity and virulence of the infecting bedsonial strain. Numerous bedsonial strains have been tested in the laboratory to determine their relative infectivity and pathogenicity for various species of birds, and they have been proved to vary quite significantly. Strains originating in natural outbreaks have been used to infect laboratory birds and mammals experimentally. These tests have demonstrated that avian bedsoniae may range in pathogenicity from some that almost invariably produce lethal infections to others that usually produce subclinical infections. Most of the field isolates exhibit levels of pathogenicity between these two extremes.[1]

Bedsonial infections in birds cause systemic disease, with septicemia and fecal excretion of bedsoniae common during the acute phases. Outward signs of psittacosis or ornithosis are no different from those of other febrile systemic illnesses in birds: ruffled feathers, depression, "sleepiness," lack of appetite, watery feces, and rapid loss of weight have been observed in a majority of susceptible birds. Later there is commonly a reduction in the quantity of feces, which tend to become extremely dark and tenacious. If the disease persists beyond the 20th day, stools usually become copious again—very watery and whitish in color. At this time, a sticky exudate may appear at the nares.

In collections of small birds that are not ordinarily observed closely the first evidence of psittacosis or ornithosis can be sudden and high mortality. This is especially true in newly infected finches, rice birds, and canaries, and also among parakeets of disease-free ancestry. Other less common birds in which mortality is usually very high are lorikeets, rosellas, and some of the South American parrots. Of the more common cage birds, cockatoos and the various breeds of pigeons

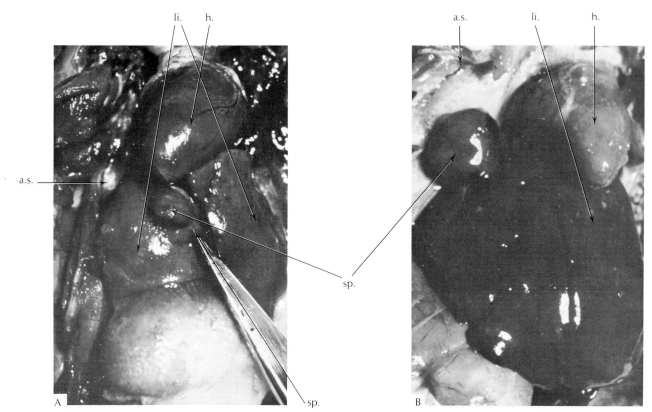

Fig. 24-8. *Viscera of yellow-headed amazon* (Amazona ochrocephala). a.s., *Thoracic air sac;* h, *heart;* li., *liver;* sp., *spleen. The spleen has been moved from its usual position in each specimen so that it may be visualized adjacent to the heart. A. Organs of normal bird. B. Organs of bird with advanced psittacosis. Note opacity and exudate in thoracic air sac; turbid exudate in pericardial sac; swelling, engorgement, and pinpoint foci of necrosis of the liver, and enlargement of the spleen.*

are relatively resistant hosts in which mortality is low—10 to 30 per cent.

The lesions which can be grossly observed in the advanced cases of psittacosis or ornithosis often form a characteristic pattern in the host; although the infectious agent is systemic in its distribution, the obvious abnormalities tend to show the following localization: (1) significant enlargement of the spleen, sometimes accompanied by softening, grey discoloration, and pearly foci on this organ; (2) liver abnormality, particularly swelling, fragility, yellowish discoloration, rounded edges, and focal necroses; (3) exudate, cloudiness, and yellowish "clots" in the air sacs; (4) purulent, serous, or fibrinous pericarditis; (5) congestion of the intestinal tract. Some of these abnormalities may be seen in the specimen shown in Figure 24-8.

The lungs in most terminal cases of psittacosis or ornithosis in cage birds are remarkably free from gross pathologic lesions.

DIAGNOSIS

Confirmation of psittacosis or ornithosis is difficult in the live patient, since symptoms resemble those of other avian diseases. Usually only a tentative diagnosis is possible, based on association of the bird with an infected or suspected reservoir host, and absence of confirmed diagnosis of other disease. Since psittacosis and ornithosis may be transmitted to man, it is probably wise to treat suspected cases as positive, even though the diagnosis is tentative. Many suspected cases could be confirmed by appropriate serologic or microbiologic tests; results are obtained usually after treatment has already begun. Nevertheless, such confirmation is of great scientific value. *Specialized laboratory training and facilities are essential for reliable serological examination, propagation of the etiological agent, and confirmation of the diagnosis of bedsonial infections.*

Since psittacosis and ornithosis are zoo-anthroponoses, departments of public health as well as of animal industry will assist the practitioner in diagnostic and control procedures. In some instances, City, County, and State Health Department or Department of Agriculture laboratories will perform the entire diagnostic procedure; otherwise, state laboratories may request confirmation by a specialized institution. All results become available to the practitioner. Some private laboratories also perform the procedures necessary to establish diagnosis.

Specimens to be submitted to the microbiological laboratory include samples of blood and feces and smears or samples of various material from the carcass.

BLOOD

Puncture of the jugular vein or wing vein may be used for collection of blood. The method preferred by us is pictured in Figure 24-9, and is a useful technique to master also for obtaining samples for blood counts, chemical determinations, and other laboratory analyses. The shallowness of the angle of approach to the vessel is shown in Figure 24-10.

Serum may be tested for complement-fixing antibody by the direct or indirect complement fixation (CF) method.[9] Most species of birds tested produce a vigorous CF antibody response following non-fatal bedsonial infection; a titer of 1:8++++ or higher indicates such infection existing at some time but not necessarily causing the current illness. Titers may rise to 1:4096 or higher. The demonstration of significant antibody-titer rise (4-fold or greater) in paired sera, collected at intervals of 10 to 30 days, suggests very recent bedsonial infection. Two species of birds are known to produce CF antibody irregularly: the common domestically propagated budgerigar (*Melopsittacus undulatus*) and the African grey parrot (*Psittacus erithacus*). The CF test is therefore not diagnostically reliable in these species.[1]

The etiological agent may be isolated by inoculation of mice or of embryonated eggs with whole blood (red blood cells or the clot from a sample drawn for serological examination may also be used) from acutely ill birds before chemotherapy is begun. This is an excellent and fully confirmatory test. The specimen should be sent refrigerated or frozen to the microbiological laboratory

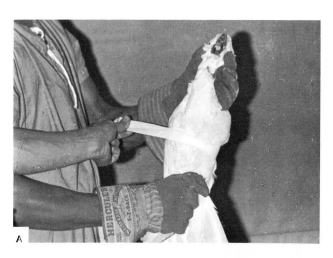

A

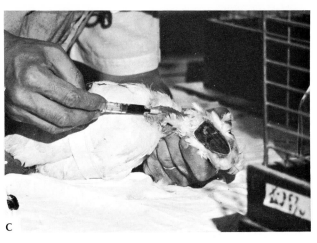

C

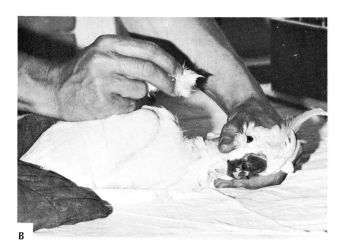

B

Fig. 24-9. *Technique of puncture of jugular vein for collection of blood for various laboratory tests. A. Adhesive tape is wrapped around the wings and completely around the body at the level of the highest point of the sternum. The bandage should be snug and should overlap. B. The operator holds the head and the catcher restrains the feet and body. The right side of the neck is plucked (the right jugular vein is considerably larger and easier to enter than the left). C. The neck is arched and the skin manipulated with the left hand until the vein is in view. The area of puncture is thoroughly swabbed with iodine–alcohol. The plastic syringe with a large flange permits one-handed operation.*

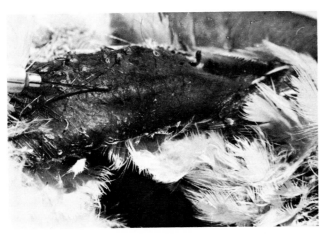

Fig. 24-10. *Dissection specimen showing close-up of right jugular vein punctured by a 25-gauge disposable needle. Note shallowness of angle.*

by the most rapid mode of transport, accompanied by a complete history of the case.

FECES

Fresh fecal samples can be obtained by irrigation and aspiration of the cloaca with nutrient broth. Samples should be immediately refrigerated or frozen if they are to be submitted for examination for bedsoniae. Bedsoniae can be isolated from feces of birds with acute and chronic psittacosis and ornithosis even after the organisms have disappeared from the blood. Isolation and identification of bedsoniae from the feces constitute an excellent confirmatory procedure.

THE CARCASS

In birds that have died of the disease or been euthanatized when it was far advanced, the typical lesions (see section on Pathogenesis, above) and a bedsonia-positive microscopic smear will prove the diagnosis of psittacosis (or ornithosis). The best diagnostic smears are made from the air-sac membranes or the pericardium, if exudate is present. The smears are stained by Macchiavello's method.[9] Briefly, the procedure is to air-dry and fix the smear by very gentle heat; the smear is then stained 5 to 10 minutes in 0.25% basic fuchsin, decolorized momentarily in 0.25% citric acid, and counterstained 20 to 30 seconds with 1% methylene blue. Bedsoniae are seen under the high-power (1,000X) oil-immersion objective as clusters of red spherules, approximately 250 to 400 mμ in size (Fig. 24-11). Intracytoplasmic red colonies are the most characteristic. Host cells and background should stain blue. Additional laboratory work is necessary for final confirmation;

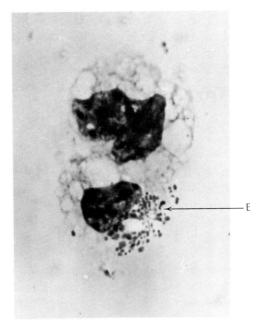

Fig. 24-11. *Macrophages from exudate of experimental psittacosis infection. Approx. 1200×; Macchiavello's stain. E, intracytoplasmic cluster of bedsonial elementary bodies.*

frozen or refrigerated samples of tissue from liver, spleen, and intestine can be submitted for bedsonial isolation and antigenic studies in specialized microbiological laboratories.

Arrangements can sometimes be made for submitting the entire carcass for laboratory diagnosis. In such instances, the animal is dipped in a soapy or detergent germicide which will disinfect feathers and skin, wrapped in disinfectant-impregnated cloth and then an impervious outer wrapper, and delivered to the laboratory immediately or shipped in a manner which will assure arrival of a frozen or well-refrigerated specimen.

EPIZOOTIOLOGY AND CONTROL

Natural transmission of the infection in birds usually occurs as a result of intimate contact of infected and susceptible individuals. Feces of infected individuals, especially during the acute disease, are rich in infective bedsoniae: up to 10,000 infectious units per gram may be present in such droppings. The susceptible birds may acquire the infection by way of either the respiratory or the gastrointestinal tract; in a crowded environment, both routes are probably involved.

In the infected bird flocks, a great diversity of epizootiological patterns may be observed. For example, parakeet aviaries in which the disease is enzootic usually have a history of somewhat elevated mortality and morbidity, particularly among the very young, but the losses do not exceed 10 to 20 per cent. In contrast, when the infection is introduced into a disease-free flock, the mortality may be extremely high for birds of all ages, and up to 90 per cent of the parakeets may succumb within a few weeks. A typical contact-spread disease mortality curve will be seen in such newly infected flocks; if the flock is untreated, the peak mortality occurs about two or three weeks after introduction of the infection (depending on the degree of crowding). Because of widespread but haphazard use of antimicrobials in many parakeet aviaries, the epizootiological pattern is often not clear cut due to modification by psittacosis-inhibitory drugs.

Parrot collections may experience exceedingly explosive contact-spread epizootics with mortality around 90 per cent. The various species of the genus *Amazona* from Latin America are especially susceptible; in general, untreated outbreaks among parrots native to the Western hemisphere have terminated only when most of the infected individuals have died. The few long-term (over 4-month) survivors usually demonstrate permanent impairment and shed infectious droppings for many months.

In contrast, among the Australian cockatoos (*Kakatoe galerita* and *Kakatoe roseicapilla*), psittacosis tends to be more benign. The experimental epizootic observed at the Hooper Foundation among 85 cockatoos was initiated by a native Australian bedsonial strain; it was readily transmitted from the shedders to the uninfected within a few weeks of close contact, but the mortality was less than 20 per cent, and spontaneous and complete elimination of the infection was the usual outcome.[1]

The prevalence of natural ornithosis among the various domestic pigeon varieties is not precisely known, but pigeon ornithosis is certainly quite common world wide. Most bedsonial strains isolated from pigeons are not particularly virulent for either pigeons or man, but some notable exceptions are on record. The highest mortality is among the very young squabs, the infection probably having been acquired from the infected mother via the regurgitated "pigeon milk." Among the adults, transmission probably also occurs by the gastrointestinal or respiratory route. The serological evidence of previous or current ornithosis infection in enzootically infected flocks is usually in the range of 20 per cent. Exceptionally, 80 per cent of the mature birds among some flocks may be serologically positive. Meyer's review[7] fully summarized the records on pigeon ornithosis.

The various finches, canaries, and mynahs do not seem to be natural reservoirs of bedsoniae. When infected by contact or aerosol from other species, flocks invariably experience an explosive, rapid die-off, and if the birds are not treated the mortality will be near the 100 per cent level.

Psittacosis is readily transmissible from the infected bird to man, by aerosols of fecal material, exudates, down, and other particles contaminated by bedsoniae. Since the human illness may range in severity from a subclinical state to an extremely serious pneumonia with septicemia, it is imperative that control measures be instituted when a diagnosis of psittacosis or ornithosis is made.

Suspected or proved cases of psittacosis and ornithosis should be reported to local or state public health authorities. In some states, such notification is required by specific regulation, but it is universally desirable, even in the absence of such laws.

Once the decision has been made to treat a single individual or a flock infected with psittacosis, avoidance of aerosols from the infected birds is of prime importance. Disinfection with a cleansing-type germicidal agent, such as saponated cresol solution, or a strong detergent is recommended rather than dry sweeping or brushing. If a group of birds is involved in a suspected outbreak of bedsonial disease, they must be immediately separated, preferably into single cages, in order to reduce transmission to a minimum. Agitation of the patients must also be avoided. Provided the owner is adequately warned and instructed, therapy may be prescribed and administered at the home or aviary. When only a few birds are involved and children are present, or when there is evidence of failure of provision of adequate safeguards, hospitalization of the affected birds for a minimum of one or two weeks may be advised. Extreme care should be exercised to avoid production and inhalation of infective aerosols. All persons near the infected birds should wear effectively applied surgical masks. Early administration of antimicrobial therapy is important, and usually results in a favorable outcome.

Experimental vaccination of birds has given promising results, but the vaccines tested to date would not be of practical value in clinical practice; immunized birds usually survive psittacosis challenge but remain carriers and shedders for a long time. Additional investigations of the use of vaccines are in progress.

TREATMENT

All strains of avian bedsoniae tested are readily inhibited by the tetracyclines. Because of the ready availability of chlortetracycline (CTC) in convenient formulations and also its most extensive history of efficacy against the bedsoniae, it is the current drug of choice. Administration of the antibiotic in the feed requires a minimum of manipulation of infected birds, thus reducing the risk of infection for the therapist; it is also a very effective method and is the one chosen under usual conditions. Parakeets, parrots, and pigeons are probably the most frequently encountered psittacosis (or ornithosis) suspects in veterinary practice. Procedures for their treatment will be described in detail.

PARAKEETS

Antibiotic medication, in the form of chlortetracycline-impregnated millet (0.5 mg. CTC per gram of seed*) is being administered to parakeets by several cooperating wholesale centers for 15 days, just prior to consignment of the birds to retail channels. It is estimated that about 75 per cent of the parakeets offered for retail sale in the United States have at one time undergone this treatment. As a result, parakeet psittacosis occurs much less frequently than it did as recently as 5 to 10 years ago.[11]

There is no easy method of ascertaining whether any one specific parakeet may or may not be a psittacosis hazard for its owner. Treated birds cannot be differentiated from untreated; in addition, psittacosis can be contracted by a bird after previous chemotherapy. Therefore, the recommendation to the pet owner should be that all his parakeets receive an effective antibedsonial regimen at least once after purchase. The easiest method is the feeding of the CTC-impregnated millet seed. This formulation is readily available and effectively controls psittacosis if it is fed exclusive of all other feed for 15 to 30 consecutive days. It should be borne in mind that after the treatment is terminated the bird can be re-infected, so the treated birds should be kept isolated from potential sources of infection.

If a parakeet suspected of having psittacosis is very ill and refuses to eat, tetracyclines (chlortetracycline, oxytetracycline, or tetracycline) may be given intramuscularly for the first few days. (This should be done only if the owners are particularly fond of the pet; otherwise the safest course under these circumstances is probably euthanasia.) Injections can be made into the pectoral muscles; 5 to 10 mg. a day contained in a 0.5-ml. inoculum can be given for up to 5 days. By then the bird should be able to eat the medicated millet; at least 15 full days of treatment with the medicated millet should be given after the bird's daily consumption returns to normal (30 days is preferable if the original illness was severe). Of course, if there is

*Keet Life—Hartz Mountain Products Corporation, New York City.

more than one bird in the same household, all should be treated prophylactically at the same time. If new parakeets are to be added to the household, they should undergo the prophylactic oral regimen before being placed in contact with the previously treated birds. Contact with possible sources of psittacosis or ornithosis should be avoided, because parakeets will be susceptible shortly after the medicated feed is replaced by the usual ration. Other small seed-eating birds such as canaries, finches, and rice birds may be fed the CTC-impregnated millet prophylactically or therapeutically if they are exposed to psittacosis or if the infection is diagnosed in an early phase.[3]

PARROTS

At the present time, importation of parrots into the United States is not very great, and psittacines larger than parakeets do not reproduce successfully outside their natural habitats. Nevertheless, some parrots are imported under special permits as personal pets and for purposes of public exhibit. Knowledge of practical chemotherapy for these species is therefore important.

As a rule, parrots do not relish a diet consisting exclusively of millet. A satisfactory feed base for incorporation of CTC is cooked rice and hen scratch; a convenient source of drug is a 22% mixture in soybean meal (chlortetracycline hydrochloride,* 100 grams per pound of soybean meal).

The actual ration is prepared as follows: The cooked mash is prepared by first mixing rice, hen scratch feed, and water in a weight ratio of $2:2:3$, respectively (e.g., 1 pound of rice, 1 pound of hen scratch, and $1\frac{1}{2}$ pints of water). This mixture may be cooked in a pressure cooker, autoclave, or similar cooking utensil until soft but not mushy. Cooking for 10 to 15 minutes in a pressure cooker produces about the right consistency. The mash base must be allowed to cool. The chlortetracycline–soybean meal mixture is then added. If the 22% CTC formula is used, a simple procedure is to weigh the needed quantity of feed first, and then add an amount of soybean meal mixture equivalent to 2 per cent of this weight. Mixing must be very thorough, and a small amount of brown sugar may be added last, to improve palatability. If these directions are followed, the final concentration of chlortetracycline will be 4.4 mg. per gram of cooked feed. This is the minimum effective concentration for the large birds.

As much of the medicated feed should be portioned out as the bird will consume in 24 hours. A rough guide is that a bird, once it has become used to the diet, will

*Aureomycin SF66—American Cyanamid Company, Princeton, New Jersey.

need an amount equivalent to about a fifth of its weight a day. Consumption will differ, and the amount offered should be varied accordingly. On this formulation, birds tested have built up, within a few days, blood levels of 2 to 10 micrograms of CTC per ml. of blood. Other feed should not be offered during the treatment period. A small supply of coarse sand or fine gravel is given in a separate dish, preferably mixed half and half with a vitamin-rich poultry powder such as broiler chow; fresh water should be available to the birds at all times. It is recommended that the medicated mash be offered to the birds for *45* consecutive days. The ration must be prepared fresh daily.[3] The long-term administration of the medication is essential. In a few instances, parrots treated only 30 days have relapsed and died of psittacosis shortly after returning to unmedicated feed.[1]

Intramuscular administration of tetracyclines (chlortetracycline, oxytetracycline, or tetracycline) may save birds with advanced psittacosis that are too ill to eat the medicated feed. Doses of 40 to 50 mg. a day in a 1-ml. inoculum are given until the bird is well enough to eat the CTC ration. Birds should be handled with care; production and inhalation of infective aerosols should be avoided, and the operator must wear a mask to avoid contracting psittacosis.

It is strongly urged that all newly acquired parrots or parrots whose psittacosis status is unknown be given the 45-day CTC chemotherapy regimen on a prophylactic basis in order to eliminate the possibility of latent subclinical infection. This applies both to individual pets and to collections in zoos, aviaries, and the like. Of course even after the prophylactic regimen is completed, the treated birds must be protected from potential sources of infection.

Dry stable pellets containing essential daily nutrients and 0.5% chlortetracycline have been developed and tested. They are accepted by all seed-eating parrots and effectively control psittacosis in known infected groups. Administration is the same as described for the cooked mash, but daily preparation is unnecessary since the pellets maintain potency at least 6 months and probably longer. This medicament is not available for commercial distribution at this time, but may become available in the near future. Requests for information regarding current availability may be addressed to: Hartz Mountain Products Corp., Research Dept., 1961 No. Nashville Ave., Chicago, Ill. 60635.

Fruit- and nectar-feeding parrots (lories, lorikeets) may be treated with chlortetracycline by incorporating 0.05% of the drug into liquid ration containing water, honey, and dietary supplement ("Metrecal" or "Nutrament").

PIGEONS

Uncooked hen scratch is the best feed base for preparing a chemotherapeutic ration for pigeons. The drug source may be the same soybean meal mixture used for parrots (chlortetracycline hydrochloride, 100 grams per pound). The steps of preparation are as follows: (1) weigh out the needed amount of scratch feed; (2) add an amount of the CTC–soybean meal mixture equivalent to 4 per cent of this weight; (3) moisten with just enough water to cause the soybean meal mixture to stick to the seeds of the hen scratch feed; (4) mix very thoroughly.

The final concentration of chlortetracycline will be 0.89%. Usually, the pigeons will eat only 10 to 15 grams of this mix for the first few days; when they become accustomed to it, the consumption will average 50 grams daily. The levels of CTC in the pigeons' blood will be between 2 and 4 micrograms per ml., which is adequate for ornithosis control if maintained about 45 days.[2] The expense of this treatment may be too high for large flocks, but individual birds that are specially prized, or small groups of pigeons, may be worth the expense.

The dry stable nutrient pellets with 0.5% CTC, mentioned above, have been fed to small numbers of pigeons; consumption and resulting levels of CTC in the blood were adequate for ornithosis control. When this product becomes readily available, its use should be practical, particularly on a prophylactic basis.

If intramuscular therapy is required, daily administration of 40 to 50 mg. of one of the tetracyclines, as for parrots, is adequate.

IMPORT REGULATIONS

Current regulations of the Department of Health, Education, and Welfare permit the importation of only those parrots which have been treated adequately with effective antibiotics for at least 45 days. Details are available upon request from the U.S. Department of Health, Education, and Welfare, Foreign Quarantine Program, National Communicable Disease Center, Atlanta, Georgia 30333.

The U.S. Department of Agriculture regulates the importation of birds belonging to the Orders Anseriformes, Columbiformes, and Galliformes. Ducks, geese, pigeons, doves, the domestic chicken, and related birds belong to these Orders. A 21-day period of quarantine is required at the U.S. Department of Agriculture facilities in Miami, Honolulu, and New York. Details concerning the importation procedures on these birds may be obtained from the U.S. Department of Agriculture, Agricultural Research Service, Animal Inspection and Quarantine Division, Federal Center Building, Hyattsville, Maryland 20781. At present, the importation of finches and canaries is not officially regulated, except for customs and general sanitation rules; in addition, Department of Agriculture inspectors visually examine *all* imported birds at the port of entry for clinical signs of disease. Birds that are obviously ill are not released to the importer.

References

1. ARNSTEIN, P.: Unpublished data.

2. ARNSTEIN, P., COHEN, D. H., and MEYER, K. F.: Medication of pigeons with chlortetracycline in feed. J.A.V.M.A. *145:*921–924, 1964.

3. ARNSTEIN, P., and MEYER, K. F.: Psittacosis-ornithosis. In *Current Veterinary Therapy 1966–1967,* R. W. Kirk, ed. Philadelphia, W. B. Saunders Company, 1966. Pp. 543–546.

4. BEDSON, S. P., and BLAND, J. O. W.: A morphological study of psittacosis virus, with the description of a developmental cycle. Brit. J. Exp. Path. *13:*461–466, 1932.

5. DOHERTY, R. L., CARLEY, J. G., LEE, P. E., MEYER, K. F., and EDDIE, B.: The effect of chlortetracycline on Australian parrots naturally infected with psittacosis. Med. J. Aust. *2:*134–139, 1961.

6. MEYER, K. F.: Psittacosis group. Ann. N.Y. Acad. Sci. *56:*545–556, 1953.

7. MEYER, K. F.: Ornithosis. In *Diseases of Poultry,* 5th ed., H. E. Biester and L. H. Schwarte, eds. Ames, Iowa State University Press, 1965. Pp. 675–770.

8. MEYER, K. F., and EDDIE, B.: Chemotherapy of natural psittacosis and ornithosis. Field trial of tetracycline, chlortetracycline, and oxytetracycline. Antib. & Chemo. *5:*289–299, 1955.

9. MEYER, K. F., and EDDIE, B.: Psittacosis-lymphogranuloma Venereum Group (Bedsonia Infections). In *Diagnostic Procedures for Viral and Rickettsial Diseases,* 3rd ed., E. H. Lennette and N. J. Schmidt, eds. New York, American Public Health Association, Inc., 1964. Pp. 603–639.

10. QUAN, S. F., MEYER, K. F., and EDDIE, B.: Attempts to cure parakeet psittacosis carriers with aureomycin and penicillin. J. Infect. Dis. *86:*132–135, 1950.

11. United States Public Health Service: Zoonoses Surveillance Report, 1964: Psittacosis. Atlanta, Ga., Communicable Disease Center.

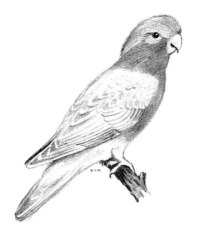

25

Parasitic Diseases

I. F. Keymer

Birds such as budgerigars and canaries, which have been bred in captivity away from all other species and normally kept in indoor cages or aviaries, are seldom troubled with parasitic diseases. In recent years, however, especially in North America and Europe, the popularity of keeping tropical birds has increased considerably. Hundreds of different species, particularly passerines and psittacines, are now imported annually from various parts of South America, Africa, and Asia, and native birds of the temperate regions are also often kept.

Owing to the considerable variety of birds which are involved, it is clearly impossible in this Chapter to deal with all the parasites to which they are subject. Likewise, no attempt will be made to deal with all the species of birds. Parasites of budgerigars and canaries, however, are dealt with in some detail, especially those that are known to be pathogenic, not only to the captive birds but also to free-living species, particularly if birds of the species are often kept in captivity or commonly occur near human habitations, where they may be a source of infection to captive birds. House sparrows (*Passer domesticus*) and starlings (*Sturnus vulgaris*) are good examples of such species and are a potential source of many diseases in birds kept in aviaries, especially in zoos where they are attracted by the readily accessible supply of food.

Parasite morphology and life history are not described in detail, being dealt with only sufficiently for a practicing veterinarian to diagnose the type of parasite present, and enable him to adopt appropriate measures of prevention, control, and treatment.

In all cases an indication of the host range of the parasite is given when this is known, because sometimes a disease may be common in domestic birds, such as poultry and pigeons, or in some species of wild birds, and therefore these species may be potential sources of infection. Often the disease, although almost unknown in cage and aviary birds, may have been well investigated in domestic birds, in which case textbooks on poultry diseases should be consulted for further information.

Although the pathogenicity of some parasites in free-living birds is well known, there is little doubt that the majority are quite harmless under natural conditions. Even in well-managed collections of birds in outdoor aviaries, a relatively high parasite burden may be supported by the inmates and the normal host-parasite relationship be maintained. Should an outbreak of disease occur in such a collection, however, or should there be any marked alteration in environmental conditions, such as excessive fluctuations in temperature, or a change of food, as is frequently brought about by the sudden subjection of wild birds to the artificial conditions of captivity, then this delicate host-parasite balance may be upset and sickness or death due to parasitic disease may occur. This is undoubtedly one of the reasons for the high morbidity and mortality in recently imported tropical birds, which have usually been captured shortly before export and kept in overcrowded, unhygienic conditions.

Attempts are also often made, especially by townspeople, to rear fledglings which they have found in the garden and which they imagine to be deserted by the parent birds. The fact that these youngsters have usually been fed a diet containing a high proportion of arthropods, earthworms, or molluscs, many of which are the intermediate hosts for helminths, means that they often carry a high parasite burden. In the wild state a young bird is usually able to tolerate a certain number of helminths without much trouble, but when a sudden change is made to an artificial diet—especially, as is so often the case, if it is as unsatisfactory as bread soaked in milk and water—the result is usually disastrous. In fact, for controlling the pathogenic effect of helminths inhabiting the alimentary tract, the importance of correct feeding cannot be emphasized too strongly.

In addition to the high incidence of parasitic diseases in wild-caught and hand-reared birds, those kept in outdoor aviaries are more commonly infected than birds kept in cages and aviaries indoors. Outside, not only are they exposed to infection by free-living wild birds by way of their excreta or molted feathers, or by direct contact, but they are also more liable to be bitten by the insect vectors of blood parasites. Birds kept in elaborate aviaries well provided with growing vegetation and pools of water may also contract helminth infections by eating the intermediate hosts mentioned earlier. These environmental conditions, by providing shelter for vectors, may help to maintain the life cycle and infection rate of some internal parasites which under more artificial conditions, such as those provided in aviaries with concrete floors, would sooner or later be eradicated.

Finally, in view of the fact that healthy birds can carry a heavy burden of parasites, sometimes of several different kinds, caution is needed when making a diagnosis. The temptation to attribute to a large population of parasites clinical signs or lesions which are unlikely to have been produced by their presence should be resisted and care should be exercised. Even when the clinical signs and lesions appear to be produced by the parasites, caution is needed because often in such cases there is evidence that the parasite may be of only secondary importance, and the condition may well be primarily of bacterial, viral, or nutritional origin. On the other hand, of course, the converse may sometimes be true.

PROTOZOA

The Phylum Protozoa contains an enormous variety of parasitic organisms, many species of which occur in birds, although only a few are known to be pathogenic to the passerine and psittacine species, with which this book is mainly concerned. In poultry and other gallinaceous birds, however, two of the most important diseases, namely, coccidiosis and histomoniasis, are caused by protozoa.

Detailed morphology and taxonomy will not be discussed here, but a simplified classification, which is based on those of Honigberg et al.[81] and Levine,[111] and which includes all the protozoa likely to be encountered in cage and aviary birds, is given below. The parasites are dealt with not in systematic order, but according to the part of the body they mainly infect.

CLASSIFICATION

Phylum	Protozoa
Subphylum	Sarcomastigophora
Superclass	Mastigophora
Class	Zoomastigophorea
Order	Rhizomastigida

Characteristics: Pseudopodia and usually one to four flagella present simultaneously, or at different times in trophozoites; most species free-living.

Family	Mastigamoebidae

With one to three, rarely four flagella.

Example: *Histomonas*

*   *   *   *

Order   Kinetoplastida
Suborder   Trypanosomatina

Characteristics: One flagellum, either free or attached to the body by means of an undulating membrane; all species parasitic.

Family   Trypanosomatidae

Example: *Trypanosoma*

*   *   *   *

Order   Diplomonadida

Characteristics: Body bilaterally symmetrical with two karyomastigonts, each with six flagella and a set of accessory organelles; most species are parasitic.

Family   Hexamitidae

With six or eight flagella and two nuclei.

Examples: *Giardia* and *Hexamita*

*   *   *   *

Order   Trichomonadida

Characteristics include four to six flagella, of which one is recurrent. True cysts are unknown. Nearly all species are parasitic.

Family   Trichomonadidae

With an undulating membrane associated with a recurrent flagellum.

Example: *Trichomonas*

*   *   *   *   *   *

Superclass   Sarcodina
Class   Piroplasmea
Order   Piroplasmida
Family   Babesiidae

Characteristics: Relatively large, piriform, round or oval non-pigmented parasites occurring in erythrocytes. It should be noted, however, that the systematic position of the piroplasms is doubtful and they are placed here for convenience.

Example: *Aegyptianella*

*   *   *   *   *   *   *

Subphylum   Sporozoa
Class   Telosporea
Subclass   Coccidia
Order   Eucoccida
Suborder   Eimeriina
Family   Eimeriidae

Characteristics include intracellular development, and oocysts without sporocysts, or with one, two, four, or many sporocysts, each with one or more sporozoites.

Examples: *Dorisiella, Eimeria, Isospora,*
                 and *Wenyonella*

Family   Lankesterellidae

Characteristics include intracellular development, and oocysts without sporocysts, but with eight or more sporozoites. Sporozoites in red or white blood cells, or both, are transferred by, but do not develop in, an invertebrate.

Example: *Lankesterella*

*   *   *

Suborder   Haemosporina
Family   Plasmodiidae

Characteristics include independent development of macrogametocytes and microgametocytes as in the Eimeriidae. Schizogony and gametocytes in peripheral blood and also schizogony in tissue cells of vertebrate host; sporogony in invertebrate. Pigment is formed from the host cell hemoglobin.

Example: *Plasmodium*, avian parasites being grouped in the subgenera *Haemamoeba, Giovannolaia, Novyella,* and *Huffia*

Family   Haemoproteidae

Characteristics similar to those of Plasmodiidae, but only gametocytes are found in the peripheral blood, schizogony occurring elsewhere in the vertebrate host.

Bennett *et al.*[25] have split the Haemoproteidae into the two genera of *Haemoproteus* and *Parahaemoproteus*. The characteristics of *Haemoproteus* include sporogony in hippoboscids, whereas in *Parahaemoproteus* this part of the life cycle occurs in *Culicoides* midges. Many parasite species formerly included in *Haemoproteus* occur in birds of the types dealt with here and which do not normally harbor hippoboscids. It is likely, therefore, that these will be shown to be transmitted by *Culicoides* spp. and therefore will prove to belong to the genus *Parahaemoproteus*.

Family   Leucocytozoidae

Characteristics similar to Haemoproteidae, but the parasites are not pigmented.

Bennett *et al.*[25] have also divided the Leucocytozoidae into two genera: *Leucocytozoon* and *Akiba*. The genus *Leucocytozoon* includes all the parasites transmitted by simuliid flies, and *Akiba* all those transmitted by *Culicoides* midges. So far as is known all the parasites of this Family affecting birds that are dealt with in this Chapter belong to the genus *Leucocytozoon*.

* * * * *

Class	Toxoplasmea
Order	Toxoplasmida
Family	Sarcocystidae

Characteristics include absence of true spores and the formation of cysts containing many naked trophozoites. Multiplication by binary fission.

Example: *Sarcocystis*

Family   Toxoplasmatidae

Characteristics similar to Sarcocystidae, but pseudocysts formed in addition to true cysts.

Example: *Toxoplasma*

PARASITES OF THE ALIMENTARY SYSTEM
Trichomonas and Trichomoniasis

SPECIES AND HOSTS

The two most important trichomonads of birds are *Trichomonas gallinae,* which inhabits the upper digestive tract, and *T. gallinarum,* which appears to be confined to the lower digestive tract. *T. gallinarum,* however, is not considered here, as it seems to occur only in the turkey and domestic fowl. *T. gallinae,* which is variously referred to as *T. columbae, T. hepaticum, T. diversa,* or *T. halli,* also occurs in turkeys. It is probably best known, however, as the cause of "canker," an important disease of pigeons, and in falcons it causes a similar condition called "frounce"—a disease which has been known to falconers for hundreds of years. Natural infections of *T. gallinae* have been encountered in canaries in England, and have been recorded in the Java sparrow (*Padda oryzivora*) by Callender and Simmons,[32] and in zebra finches (*Poephila castanotis*) and orange-cheeked waxbills (*Estrilda melpoda*) by Zwart.[181] Callender and Simmons[32] also experimentally transmitted *T. gallinae* to the Tovi parakeet (*Brotogeris jugularis*), and Levine *et al.*[112] transmitted the organism to the canary and house sparrow, but failed to infect a starling by feeding it cultures of the organisms.

DISTRIBUTION AND INCIDENCE

T. gallinae is a widespread organism, occurring in America, Europe, Japan, and South Africa. The incidence of trichomoniasis in cage birds is unknown,

however, and the disease may well be overlooked occasionally.

LIFE HISTORY

Unknown.

CLINICAL SIGNS OF TRICHOMONIASIS

Strains of *T. gallinae* are known to vary considerably in virulence, and it is not uncommon for pigeons and doves to be healthy carriers of the organism. This probably is true also of passerine birds. Sometimes, however, the disease can cause serious losses.

The clinical signs, which are not diagnostic, include lassitude, inappetence, ruffled feathers, diarrhea, and dyspnea. In an acute case there may be little indication that the bird is sick, and death may occur quite suddenly.

DIAGNOSIS

The live flagellates can be found associated with the lesions at necropsy for as long as 48 hours after death; they are best demonstrated by examining microscopically, beneath a cover slip, a small amount of material from a lesion which has been crushed on a slide and warmed to body temperature. The organisms will then be seen swimming rather slowly in a jerky fashion, with the aid of their flagella.

In the laboratory *T. gallinae* can be cultured easily from fresh postmortem material.

T. gallinae and *T. gallinarum* are morphologically very similar, and staining techniques are necessary to distinguish them. Both organisms have four anterior flagella and a backwardly directed flagellum. In *T. gallinae* this flagellum extends with its undulating membrane for only about three-fourths of the length of the body; in *T. gallinarum* it projects posteriorly as a free-trailing flagellum.

DIFFERENTIAL DIAGNOSIS. The necrosis of the esophageal and crop epithelium, first reported in budgerigars by Keymer[95] and subsequently described further by Keymer[97] and by Beach,[19] closely resembles the lesions of trichomoniasis in passerines. So far, however, trichomoniasis has not been recorded in budgerigars or other psittacines, apart from the experimental infection in a Tovi parakeet referred to above.

TREATMENT

One gram of 2-amino-5-nitrothiazole* should be dissolved in one liter of water, and provided as the only

*Enheptin—American Cyanamid Co., Princeton, N.J.

source of drinking water for a period of six successive days.[47]

POSTMORTEM FINDINGS AND PATHOLOGY

These have been described in passerines by Callender and Simmons,[32] and by Levine *et al.*[112]

Lesions occur in the pharynx, esophagus, and crop, usually appearing as whitish and later as yellowish, rather hard caseous, necrotic foci, which tend to become contiguous and extend in furrows along the epithelium (Fig. 25-1). A small amount of fluid is often present in the crop, and in a chronic case produced experimentally by Levine *et al.*[112] the entire crop wall was greatly thickened and the epithelium covered by a single dry, caseous lesion.

Giardia and Giardiasis

Inclusion of giardiasis here is based entirely on a report of the condition in a parakeet (presumably a budgerigar) by Leibovitz[109] in North America.

SPECIES AND HOSTS

Giardia intestinalis (syn. *G. lamblia*) is sometimes associated with intestinal disorders in man and is a common cause of disease of chinchillas. The parasite also occurs in other mammals and, in addition to the occurrence in a parakeet reported by Leibovitz,[109] it has also been reported in herons, avocet, shrike, and the black-winged kite (*Elanus caeruleus*).[73]

LIFE HISTORY

Multiplication is by longitudinal binary fission and, unlike the case with *Trichomonas*, cysts are formed which pass out of the host in the feces, where they can remain viable for 3 weeks if kept moist. When the cysts are swallowed, trophozoites (Fig. 25-2) are liberated in the small intestine of the host; these then migrate to the large intestine, and the cycle is repeated.

CLINICAL SIGNS OF INFECTION

Leibovitz[109] stated that the 2-year-old parakeet that was infected had never been in good health, and was in poor condition when it died, after exhibiting chronic diarrhea and leg weakness.

DIAGNOSIS

Diagnosis is based on identification of the organisms from the intestine, associated with lesions observed at

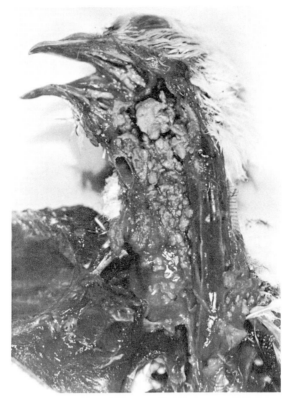

Fig. 25-1. *Extensive and advanced lesions of trichomoniasis in a domestic pigeon* (Columba livia) *involving the epithelial lining of the buccal cavity, and esophagus. Massive necrosis is present, with the formation of a considerable amount of yellowish white caseous material. (Keymer, I. F.:* Mod. Vet. Pract. *vol. 42, 1961.)*

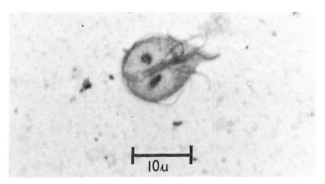

Fig. 25-2. *Trophozoite of Giardia sp. The large sucking disc which is applied to the intestinal epithelium appears as a pale area in the rounded anterior half of the body. There are two dark oval nuclei, two slender "axostyles" in the midline, and eight flagella in four pairs, although these are not all clearly visible. The first pair of flagella arise from basal granules in the midline between the nuclei, pass forward, cross each other, and then are deflected posteriorly, lying on either side of the parasite. The other flagella are all directed posteriorly. (Courtesy of T. Dennett.)*

necropsy or on detection of the thick-walled oval-shaped cysts in the excreta.

In fresh preparations the organisms swim vigorously in a characteristic undulating fashion, by means of their flagella.

The cysts are 9–14 microns long, and are not entirely filled by the encysted parasite, an empty space being present at each end. Richardson and Kendall[148] stated that two nuclei are originally situated at one pole of the cyst, but that they soon divide to produce four nuclei. A comma-shaped parabasal body and the remains of flagella are also prominent structures.

Leibovitz[109] described the protozoa he found as shaped like a tennis racket without a handle. These trophozoites were 9–15 microns long and bilaterally symmetrical. Two nuclei with their respective karyosomes were also present, and a possible parabasal body.

PREVENTION AND TREATMENT OF INFECTION

As the disease is spread *via* the feces, strict attention must be paid to hygiene to avoid the spread of infection. Cerva[33] has found that 2–5% phenol or saponated cresol solution will kill the cysts, and these disinfectants are therefore recommended. In man, the infection is satisfactorily treated with quinacrine or chloroquine.[111]

POSTMORTEM FINDINGS AND PATHOLOGY

Leibovitz[109] reported that at necropsy the lower two-thirds of the small intestine was distended with a creamy semi-solid material.

Histological examination of the intestinal wall showed distortion due to internal pressure. The crypts of Lieberkühn between the villi contained great numbers of trophozoites and cystic forms.

Hexamita and Hexamitiasis

Hexamitiasis causes catarrhal enteritis in turkeys and pigeons, and appears to be restricted to pigeons and gallinaceous birds. Hinshaw and McNeil[80] failed to find the organisms in various passerines, a hawk, and an owl in North America, on or near premises where turkeys were infected. The organisms involved are *Hexamita meleagridis* in turkeys, and *H. columbae* in pigeons. The disease is mentioned here because, as the organisms are found in the intestinal tract, the condition might be confused with giardiasis or trichomoniasis. *Hexamita* spp. occur mainly in the upper intestinal tract and, unlike *Giardia,* do not form cysts. In addition to the different habitat, they also differ from trichomonads, when examined microscopically in a fresh prep-aration, by their very rapid movement and the presence of six anterior flagella.

Histomonas and Histomoniasis

Although histomoniasis, or blackhead, is an important disease of turkeys and occurs also in other gallinaceous birds, there is no reliable evidence that *Histomonas meleagridis* naturally infects other species of birds. The report of the disease in one psittacine bird by Hasholt[72] cannot be accepted as authentic in the absence of any detailed information concerning the infection.

Coccidia and Coccidiosis

Coccidiosis is also a disease of great importance to the poultry industry but of little significance to aviculturists and owners of pet birds, although in the past it has, on the flimsiest of evidence, been blamed for sickness in psittacines and passerines.

SPECIES AND HOSTS

In gallinaceous birds and pigeons, coccidiosis is mainly caused by organisms belonging to the genus *Eimeria.* Pellerdy,[140] in his check list and host index of the Eimeriidea, listed only one passerine host of *Eimeria,* namely, the starling, which may be infected with *E. balozeti,* and the budgerigar is the only psittacine in his list. Keymer[94] reported coccidiosis in budgerigars, the condition being found by Davies to be caused by an *Eimeria* sp.; two years later, Farr[57] described *E. dunsingi* n.sp. in the budgerigar. Weidman[176] appears to have given the first and only other record of coccidiosis in these birds, but he provided no details of the infection or of the species of parasite involved.

Eimeria spp. have also been reported from birds belonging to the Orders Pelecaniformes, Anseriformes, Gruiformes, and Charadriiformes.

Isospora is the genus occurring mainly in passerines, but it is also found in birds in the Orders Struthioniformes, Falconiformes, Galliformes, Coraciiformes, Charadriiformes, Psittaciformes, Strigiformes, and Piciformes. As far as is known, *Isospora* spp., unlike *Eimeria,* are not host specific.

Pillers[142] referred to the presence of *I. lacazei* of the house sparrow in canaries and other finches, and Gray[66] regarded the parasite as being pathogenic to canaries and other aviary birds, such as linnets (*Carduelis cannabina*) and goldfinches (*C. carduelis*).

Coccidia of the genus *Dorisiella* have also been recorded in passerine birds, such as *Munia* spp. and the avadavat (*Amandava amandava*).

Bedford[21] described clinical signs attributed to coccidiosis in budgerigars, but produced no evidence to prove that the disease was in fact caused by coccidia. Similarly, the report by Harwood[71] must be regarded with skepticism, in view of the rarity of the disease in budgerigars.

DISTRIBUTION AND INCIDENCE

Both *Eimeria* and *Isospora* are very widespread in wild birds occurring in many parts of the world, and are therefore likely to be encountered in many species which have been trapped and introduced into captivity.

In domesticated cage birds such as the canary, coccidiosis now appears to be rather uncommon, and in all species of psittacines it appears to be extremely rare, the reports by Weidman[176] and Farr[57] in the U.S.A., and by Keymer[94] in England probably being the only authentic records.

LIFE HISTORY

This is similar for both *Eimeria* and *Isospora*. The bird becomes infected by ingesting oocysts, which on reaching the intestine release sporozoites that invade the epithelial lining. Once inside a tissue cell, the sporozoite becomes a trophozoite, and this gradually develops into a mature schizont containing numerous merozoites.

When the schizont ruptures, motile merozoites are released, and these then penetrate other epithelial cells to become trophozoites and form a second generation

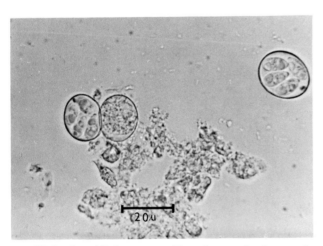

Fig. 25-3. *Coccidial oocysts,* Eimeria *sp., in feces of a Swinhoe's pheasant (Phasianus swinhoi). Two oocysts have sporulated and contain four sporocysts, each of which, when mature, contains two sporozoites. The middle, unsporulated oocyst is the form which is always seen in the feces and which is expelled by the host, sporulation taking place only under suitable conditions outside the body of the host. (Courtesy of T. Dennett.)*

of schizonts. This process of asexual reproduction may be repeated several times before some of the merozoites that are released penetrate other epithelial cells and develop into either microgametocytes or macrogametocytes. The microgametocyte undergoes multiple division to produce a large number of motile microgametes (males), whereas the macrogametocyte enlarges and eventually develops into a single macrogamete (female). Fertilization takes place when a microgamete penetrates a macrogamete, producing a zygote. The zygote then secretes a cyst wall around itself and becomes an oocyst (Fig. 25-3). This encysted and relatively resistant stage is passed out in the feces, and matures on the ground to form sporocysts, still within the confines of the cyst wall. Within the sporocysts, sporozoites are produced which invade the epithelial cells of the intestine when the oocyst is ingested.

CLINICAL SIGNS OF INFECTION

Keymer[94] recorded loss of condition, extreme lethargy, insatiable appetite for grit, and attempted regurgitation of the crop contents in a budgerigar that was heavily infected; in an experimental infection Farr[57] reported diarrhea, loss of appetite, and ruffled feathers on the sixth day after the injection of sporulated oocysts, followed by death on the seventh day.

In passerines, Gray[66] recorded convulsions and sudden death. In less acute infections he stated that the birds are listless and have ruffled plumage and inappetence and diarrhea, which result in emaciation and death. Keymer,[96] however, pointed out that some passerines, such as house sparrows and greenfinches (*Chloris chloris*), may harbor large numbers of *Isospora* parasites and yet remain in. perfect health, so care is needed in diagnosis.

DIAGNOSIS

During life the infection may be diagnosed by microscopical examination of a drop of the excreta on a slide beneath a cover slip, when the oocysts are clearly visible as more or less spherical, distinct walled objects. The oocyst wall can be seen to have a double contour if the objective of the microscope is focused up and down. In *Eimeria* spp. four sporocysts can be seen within the oocyst, but in the oocyst of *Isospora* spp. (Fig. 25-4) only two sporocysts are present. *Eimeria* sporocysts each contain two sporozoites, and *Isospora* four sporozoites. At necropsy, Keymer[94] found *Eimeria* oocysts mainly confined to the duodenum in budgerigars. Farr[57] pointed out that the oocysts of *E. dunsingi* are larger than most of those described from other birds.

It should be noted that Schwalbach[156] found that in passerines there is a rhythm of excretion of *Isospora*

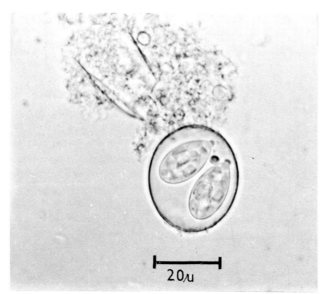

Fig. 25-4. *Coccidial oocyst,* Isospora *sp., in feces from an azure jay (Cyanocorax cyaneus). After sporulation in potassium dichromate, two sporocysts which have well developed "knobs" or Stieda bodies are visible. In all* Isospora *spp. each mature sporocyst contains four sporozoites. (Courtesy of T. Dennett.)*

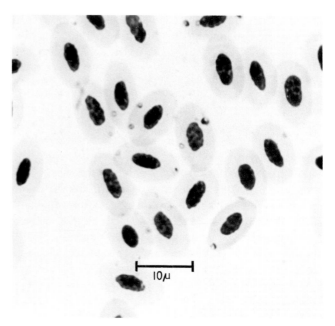

Fig. 25-5. Aegyptianella *sp. in blood smear. The piroplasms show as almost round signet ring–like structures in the erythrocytes of the peripheral blood. (Courtesy of T. Dennett.)*

oocysts, which are passed mainly in the evening when the birds go to roost for the night.

TREATMENT

For the disease in budgerigars Keymer[94] suggested about 10 drops of 16% solution of sulphadimidine* in each ounce of drinking water for three days, then two days without, followed by medicated water for another three days. No opportunity arose, however, to determine the effectiveness of this therapy, and it has the obvious disadvantages of all treatment administered in this way.

POSTMORTEM FINDINGS

In the cases recorded by Keymer,[94] congestion of the duodenal mucosa of varying degrees was observed; in the case reported by Farr[57] the duodenal loop was somewhat enlarged.

PARASITES OF THE CIRCULATORY SYSTEM

Aegyptianella and Avian Piroplasmosis

Very little is known about this tick-borne infection caused by *Aegyptianella* spp. in passerines. It is primarily

*Sulphamezathine, or sulfamethazine, U.S.P.

a disease of domestic poultry, but, according to Levine,[111] *A. moshkovskii* occurs in the Indian house crow (*Corvus splendens*) and *A. pullorum* has been transmitted experimentally to the canary.

Huchzermeyer[84] in Rhodesia has also encountered an *Aegyptianella* sp. in Nyasa lovebirds (*Agapornis lilianae*) kept in an aviary and in contact with poultry. Deaths occurred, associated with a low parasitemia (Fig. 25-5) and anemia characterized by polychromasia. He stated that in poultry he has observed that a high parasitemia precedes this type of anemia.

Huchzermeyer was able to transmit the infection to poultry by blood inoculation.

Lankesterella (Atoxoplasma) and Lankesterellosis

This organism has been found so far only in birds and amphibians. The parasites, which usually occur in the lymphocytes and monocytes of birds, were formerly regarded as hemogregarines or *Toxoplasma,* until Garnham[61] showed that they were not *Toxoplasma* and called the parasite *Atoxoplasma.* Lainson,[102,103] however, subsequently showed the life cycle to be essentially that of *Lankesterella,* a genus which was originally created in the last century for a parasite of the frog.

SPECIES AND HOSTS

Lainson[102] stated that there is no reason why *Lankesterella* should not have a wide range of hosts, and he described two new species, namely *L. serini* in the canary and *L. garnhami* in the house sparrow. However, he subsequently proved that these organisms are identical, and *L. serini* is therefore a synonym of *L. garnhami*.[103] He also re-named three other parasites: *L. paddae* in the Java sparrow (*Padda oryzivora*), *L. argyae* in the rufous babbler (*Argya rubiginosa*), and *L. adiei* in the Indian sparrow (presumably *Passer domesticus indicus*), which had previously been known as *Atoxoplasma avium*, *A. argyae*, and *Haemogregarina adiei*, respectively. *L. corvi* has been described in the English rook (*Corvus frugilegus*) by Baker *et al.*[16] Zasukhin *et al.*[180] have also reported *Atoxoplasma* in fringillines, emberizines, and other passerines.

DISTRIBUTION AND INCIDENCE

This parasite may well be widespread and common in view of the fact that all of 99 adult house sparrows examined by Lainson[102] were infected, and he subsequently failed to find non-infected canaries in England; Levine[111] also quoted Meyers and Manwell as reporting in 1957 that *Lankesterella* was common in house sparrows in parts of the U.S.A.

The parasite has also been recorded in France,[105] India,[1] East Africa,[61] U.S.S.R.,[180] and Australia.[117]

LIFE HISTORY

The only species whose life cycle is known is *L. garnhami*, having been described by Lainson,[101,103] who found all stages of schizogony in the lymphoid-macrophage cells of the spleen, bone marrow, and liver of house sparrows. As the schizogonic cycle abated, male and female gametocytes, formed by some of the merozoites liberated from mature schizonts, appeared. They were found in the liver, lungs, and kidney, apparently in the lymphoid-macrophage cells. Fertilization of a macrogametocyte leads to the formation of a zygote within a prominent oocyst wall. In the sporogonic cycle no sporoblasts are formed, but the zygote divides repeatedly to give rise to a large number of sporozoites. When this asporocystic oocyst ruptures, the large number of naked sporozoites invade lymphocytes and monocytes (Fig. 25-6) and enter the circulating blood. The sporozoites are the infective stage, and are ingested by red mites (*Dermanyssus gallinae*) when these feed on the infected bird. As is characteristic of the genus *Lankesterella*, no development occurs in the mites, and Lainson[103] showed that the infection is

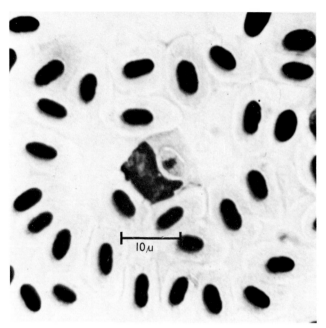

Fig. 25-6. *Sporozoite of* Lankesterella garnhami *in a monocyte in the peripheral blood of a house sparrow (Passer domesticus). The parasite is situated in the cytoplasm of the host cell, and is surrounded by a clear area. A prolonged search is often necessary before these intra-leukocytic forms can be found in blood smears. (Courtesy of R. Lainson.)*

transmitted when birds ingest the infected mites. Baker *et al.*[16] considered that the mite *Ornithonyssus sylviarum* may transmit *L. corvi*. The length of time taken for the sporozoites to give rise to schizonts is unknown, but Lainson[102] found schizonts in the spleen and bone marrow of 6-day-old nestlings.

CLINICAL SIGNS OF LANKESTERELLA INFECTION

No clinical signs have been described, although Lainson[102] reported that several trapped house sparrows "died from massive infections," and Zasukhin *et al.*[180] also reported that heavy infections may cause death. The difficulty of rearing young house sparrows has been well known for a long time, and it is tempting to suggest that some of the high mortality in young canaries is due to *Lankesterella* infection.

DIAGNOSIS

Diagnosis is based on discovery of the intra-lymphocytic or intra-monocytic parasites in smears of the spleen (Fig. 25-7) or liver, or of the blood. The infection in adult birds is usually light, and a prolonged search may be necessary before parasites are found. *L. corvi*, however, also occurs in the erythrocytes, thrombocytes,

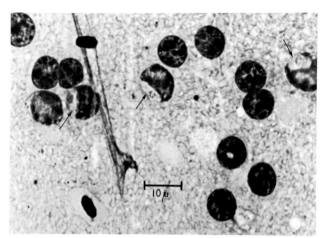

Fig. 25-7. Lankesterella garnhami *in impression smear of the spleen of a house sparrow* (Passer domesticus). *The parasites appear as pale ovoid structures containing faint pink-staining chromatin when stained with Giemsa's stain, and they are situated in the cytoplasm of lymphoid-macrophage cells, often causing an indentation in the side of the nucleus of the host cell. These stages in splenic smears are usually found more easily than those in blood smears. (Courtesy of T. Dennett.)*

and polymorphonuclear leukocytes. Microscopical examination of tissue from various internal organs may also reveal organisms in other stages of the life cycle.

DIFFERENTIAL DIAGNOSIS. Although the parasite has frequently been confused with *Toxoplasma* in the past, *Toxoplasma* is crescent-shaped and is not known to occur in erythrocytes. *Lankesterella* can also be distinguished from *Plasmodium* and *Haemoproteus* by the absence of pigment; it can also be further distinguished from *Plasmodium* by its failure to undergo division, that is, schizogony, in the intra-erythrocytic stage.

TREATMENT

It should be possible to control the disease by complete eradication of red mites. There is no available information on the use of specific drugs.

POSTMORTEM FINDINGS AND PATHOLOGY

Lainson[100] reported congestion and hemorrhage of the blood vessels and inflammatory foci in the liver and lungs of infected sparrows, and Lainson[102] and Baker et al.[16] described the microscopic appearance of the parasite in various internal organs. Lainson[101] found the liver in infected birds to be enlarged, pale, and often marbled in appearance, and the spleen was twice its normal size. Manwell[120] also recorded enlargement of these organs in house sparrows. Although he referred to

the infection as toxoplasmosis, according to Levine[111] it was in fact *Lankesterella* infection.

Plasmodium and Malaria

About 40 different species of avian malarial parasites have been described. For many years these parasites were placed in the genus *Plasmodium,* then more recently they were transferred to the genus *Haemamoeba* by some protozoologists. However, it has been suggested by Corradetti et al.[41] that the genus *Plasmodium* should be retained and four subgenera created. A tremendous amount of work has been done on bird malaria by medical research workers, but the disease—except in the domestic fowl, pigeons, and the avian species considered in this book—is of little importance in veterinary medicine. Garnham[62] has given detailed descriptions of the malarial parasites of birds and other animals.

SPECIES AND HOSTS

Less than half of the species of *Plasmodium* described from birds are considered valid by most authorities, and as they occur in a very wide variety of avian hosts and are not strongly host specific, there is little point in listing here all the species that have been described, together with their hosts. Coatney and Roudabush[39] and Berson,[27] however, have published lists of species and hosts.

The two malarial parasites of the domestic fowl, namely *P. (Haemamoeba) gallinaceum* and *P. (Novyella) juxtanucleare,* are apparently not transmissible to passerine birds. The best-known species which occur in numerous passerines, including the canary and house sparrow, are *P. (Giovannolaia) circumflexum, P. (H.) cathemerium, P. (Huffia) elongatum, P. (N.) hexamerium, P. (N.) rouxi,* and *P. (Haemamoeba) relictum* (syn. *P. [H.] praecox*). The last-named species occurs in many passerines, and the closely related *P. (H.) matutinum* is chiefly responsible for malaria in pigeons and doves.

Malaria in psittacines seems to be rare. Coatney and Roudabush[39] reported the infection in the red and blue macaw (*Ara chloroptera*); Berson[27] listed *Plasmodium* spp. in four other species of psittacines; and Garnham[62] recorded *P. (N.) nucleophilum, P. (G.) circumflexum,* and *P. (H.) relictum* in the blue-headed parrot (*Pionus menstruus*). There appears to be no report, however, of *Plasmodium* in the budgerigar.

There are a number of reports in the literature of *P. (H.) relictum* being pathogenic to several species of penguins in zoological gardens. Parasites of these birds, however, are not dealt with in this Chapter, and the reader should consult Lindt and Hörning,[113] who described the disease in penguins and provided references to reports of other outbreaks.

DISTRIBUTION AND INCIDENCE

The parasites are by no means confined to the tropics, *P. (H.) relictum* and *P. (N.) rouxi,* for example, being world wide in distribution. Several species infect wild birds in parts of Europe and North America.

Surveys on the blood parasites of wild birds in North America show that the percentage infected with *Plasmodium* spp. varies in different areas and also according to the season, as well as the species of bird. The figures given for percentages of birds infected vary considerably, for example, from 1.6 per cent[70] to 44 per cent.[86] Although Hart[70] found the incidence lowest (1.6 per cent) in the summer months and highest (4.9 per cent) in the winter, Micks[132] reported the opposite to be the case. Micks,[132] reviewing the literature, recorded an over-all incidence of infection of approximately 7 per cent in 9,577 birds representing many different species.

LIFE HISTORY

The life cycle has been shown to vary somewhat in those species of avian *Plasmodium* which have been studied, but it is basically the same in all.

Sporozoites are released into the subcutaneous tissues and to a lesser extent into the blood stream of the bird when it is bitten by an infected mosquito, this usually being a *Culex* or *Aedes* or sometimes, as in mammalian malarias, an *Anopheles* mosquito. Within an hour or so the sporozoites commence the exo-erythrocytic stage of schizogony in either the endothelial cells (for example, *P. [H.] relictum, P. [H.] cathemerium, P. [G.] circumflexum,* and *P. [N.] hexamerium*) or, mainly, in the hematopoietic cells (for example, *P. [H.] elongatum* and *P. [N.] rouxi*).

On maturity these schizonts, derived from sporozoites, release merozoites known as cryptozoites, which repeat the exo-erythrocytic schizogony in fixed cells, giving rise to merozoites called metacryptozoites, which enter the blood stream and infect the erythrocytes. The early stage of the parasite in a red blood corpuscle is known as a trophozoite, this developing into a schizont within the erythrocyte (Fig. 25-8). The merozoites released into the blood stream by these schizonts either re-infect other red cells, to give rise to an indefinite number of erythrocytic schizogonic cycles, or enter the tissue cells to produce a further exo-erythrocytic cycle. In this event the merozoites so formed are referred to as phanerozoites. When an infection has been present for some time,

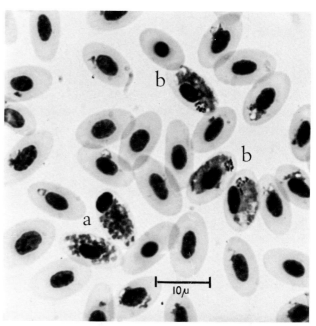

Fig. 25-8. Plasmodium *sp. in peripheral blood. The parasites labeled a are virtually mature schizonts. In one example, the nucleus of the host cell is displaced, while both parasites clearly show the dark, well-defined masses of chromatin which stain a reddish color with Giemsa stain. The pigment granules do not show in this photograph of these two parasites, although they are clearly visible as clumps of small very dark-staining dots in the less mature schizonts labeled b. The pigment which also occurs in* Haemoproteus *sp. is refractile, usually yellowish in color, and cannot be stained. The smaller, irregularly shaped parasites represent trophozoites and, like the later schizogonic stages, do not occur in the peripheral blood in* Haemoproteus *infections. (Courtesy of T. Dennett.)*

however, the merozoites produced by erythrocytic schizogony enter other erythrocytes and develop into either macrogametocytes or microgametocytes. When the gametocytes are taken up by a mosquito, they develop into gametes in its stomach, and the microgametes swim actively about to find and fertilize the macrogametes. The resultant zygote or ookinete penetrates the stomach wall and forms an oocyst, the nucleus of which divides to produce sporozoites, which break out of the oocysts into the body cavity to migrate to the salivary glands, from which they are injected into the blood stream of another host when the mosquito feeds.

CLINICAL SIGNS OF MALARIA

Fatal infections in canaries are usually caused by *P. (H.) cathemerium,*[20,76,85,126] but *P. (H.) relictum* sometimes causes disease and occasionally death.[157,169] Canaries are also highly susceptible to experimental infections with some species of plasmodia, for example,

P. (Haemamoeba) giovannolaia of the European blackbird (*Turdus merula*).[42]

Sergent *et al.*[160] appear to have been the first to describe what was probably a natural infection in canaries, the parasite involved being *P. (N.) rouxi*. In the natural infection described by Herman and Vail,[76] the affected bird had ruffled feathers and showed difficulty in maintaining its balance. Death occurred 36 hours after the appearance of clinical signs. In the outbreak described by Mathey,[126] however, the canaries were visibly sick for only a few hours.

Sometimes swelling[126] and other lesions of the eyelids are associated with various types of malarial infections in different avian hosts. Al-Dabagh[3] believed that these symptoms may be caused by pantothenic acid deficiency, it being "likely that they result from competition between the malarial parasites and the host for pantothenic acid." In view of the fact that swollen eyelids may occur in acute passerine pox and ornithosis, these diseases should always be excluded before the lesions are attributed to malaria, especially as the outbreak of malaria in canaries reported by Hudson[85] was known to be associated with pox.

DIAGNOSIS

Intra-erythrocytic pigmented schizonts and gametocytes are present in blood smears. In *P. (H.) relictum* and *P. (H.) cathemerium* infections the gametocytes are round, whereas in *P. (G.) circumflexum, P. (N.) hexamerium, P. (N.) rouxi*, and *P. (H.) elongatum* infections they are elongate. Microscopical examination of the bone marrow in infections caused by the two last-named organisms may also reveal the exo-erythrocytic schizonts.

DIFFERENTIAL DIAGNOSIS. If no intra-erythrocytic schizonts can be found in blood smears, then the infection cannot with certainty be differentiated from that caused by a *Haemoproteus* species, even with histological examination of exo-erythrocytic stages combined with a critical examination of the erythrocytic gametocytes, although, typically, those of *Haemoproteus* are halter-shaped.

The clinical signs and the lesions observed at necropsy are not diagnostic and can be confused with those of acute passerine pox, ornithosis, or pantothenic acid deficiency as discussed above.

TREATMENT

Mosquitoes should be controlled (see page 423), and the birds protected with mosquito-proof netting.

Mathey[126] successfully treated *P. (H.) cathemerium* infection in canaries with quinacrine (mepacrine) hydro-chloride,* at the dosage rate of 0.24 mg. per gram of body weight per day. For a canary weighing 1 ounce, this works out to 7.5 mg. per day. Losses stopped one week after treatment was begun. Vaccari *et al.*[169] also discussed treatment of *P. (H.) relictum* infection in canaries with quinacrine hydrochloride and other drugs. In fact, as all the synthetic anti-malarial drugs used in human medicine have been selected as a result of screening them against avian malaria, it is likely that any of them will be of value in the treatment of infections caused by avian parasites of the Suborder Haemosporina.

POSTMORTEM FINDINGS AND PATHOLOGY

Herman and Vail[76] and Mathey[126] reported marked enlargement of the spleen and liver, and Hewitt[77] found splenic infarcts in 47 per cent of his experimentally infected canaries after the third day. Subcutaneous hemorrhages may also be seen.[126]

Heavy infections result in anemia, the drop in the number of erythrocytes and decrease in hemoglobin content being proportional to the intensity of the infection.[2] Hemolytic anemia, normocytic and normochromic in type, was observed by Al-Dabagh[2] in *P. (H.) cathemerium, P. (H.) elongatum*, and other infections.

Haemoproteus and Haemoproteus Infections

Like *Plasmodium* spp., these organisms are also widespread and infect numerous species of birds. None are of medical or veterinary importance; only the two parasites of pigeons, that is *H. columbae* and *H. sacharovi*, so far as is known, are slightly pathogenic to domestic birds, although *H. lophortyx* is apparently very pathogenic to the California quail.[72] These parasites are all known to be transmitted by hippoboscids and therefore they definitely belong to the genus *Haemoproteus*.

SPECIES AND HOSTS

The parasites occur in many passerine birds as well as in pigeons and gallinaceous species. Coatney[37] published a check list of *Haemoproteus* spp. with a host index, and a similar host–parasite list has been compiled by Berson[27]; these lists give a good idea of the wide variety of birds that may be infected.

Passerine species that may harbor the parasites (probably, in many cases, *Parahaemoproteus*), and therefore are of interest here, include the mynah (*Acrido-*

*Atabrine dihydrochloride—Winthrop Laboratories, 90 Park Ave., New York, N.Y.

theres tristis), goldfinch (*Carduelis carduelis*), chaffinch (*Fringilla coelebs*), cut-throat finch (*Amadina fasciata*), weaver finches (*Hyphantornis* and *Munia* spp.), house sparrow, and Java sparrow. Sergent and Sergent[159] recorded an interesting outbreak of *H. wenyoni* infection in canaries in Algeria, which was probably due to exposure to infected wild sparrows (*Passer hispaniolensis*).

The parasites are less common in psittacines, however, and apparently have not been reported in the budgerigar. Coatney[37] listed Salle's amazon parrot (*Amazona ventralis*), the eclectus parrot (*Lorius roratus*), the red and yellow macaw (*Ara macao*), *Palaeronis* spp., and other genera as hosts. Maqsood[123] described the new species *H. handai* from the Indian blossom-headed parakeet (*Psittacula cyanocephala*), and Mackerras and Mackerras[117] reported *Haemoproteus* sp. in an Adelaide rosella parakeet (*Platycercus adelaidae*) and white cockatoo (*Kakatoe galerita*). Although Berson[27] listed a further 18 species of psittacines, the list is short compared with the number of passerines that may be infected. In most cases the parasite involved will probably be shown to be *Parahaemoproteus*.

DISTRIBUTION AND INCIDENCE

These are similar to those of *Plasmodium* and *Plasmodium* infection, the parasite being world-wide in distribution and frequently encountered during surveys of blood parasites of wild birds; examples of infection rates reported are 81 per cent[86] and 15 per cent[177] in America, and 26 per cent[24] in Canada.

LIFE HISTORY

The life history is basically the same as that of *Plasmodium*, except that only exo-erythrocytic schizogony occurs, taking place in the endothelial cells of blood vessels, particularly in the lungs; also, the known vectors are not mosquitoes, but *Culicoides* midges in the case of *Parahaemoproteus* and louse flies (Hippoboscidae) for *Haemoproteus* spp.

CLINICAL SIGNS OF INFECTION

There is virtually no evidence that the parasites are pathogenic to wild birds or to passerine and psittacine species kept in captivity, although Maqsood[123] believed that a heavy infection of *H. handai* caused the death of a blossom-headed parakeet. The clinical signs and postmortem lesions that he described, however, could well have been due to some other cause.

DIAGNOSIS

Diagnosis is based on the presence of pigmented intra-erythrocytic halter-shaped gametocytes in blood

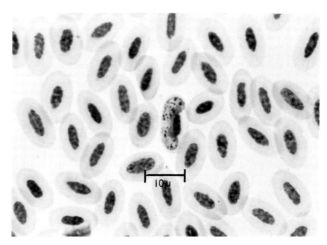

Fig. 25-9. *Gametocyte of* Haemoproteus *sp. in a blood smear from an owl, showing the typical halter-shaped appearance. Approximately two-thirds of the erythrocyte is occupied by the organism. The dark spots in the cytoplasm represent the pigment granules derived from the hemoglobin of the erythrocyte. With Giemsa stain the nucleus of the parasite stains red and the cytoplasm stains blue. (Courtesy of T. Dennett.)*

smears (Fig. 25-9), together with the absence of schizonts.

DIFFERENTIAL DIAGNOSIS. Malaria due to *Plasmodium* species.

TREATMENT

See section on Treatment under "*Plasmodium* and Malaria."

POSTMORTEM FINDINGS

Maqsood[123] reported emaciation, congestion of the lungs, and soiling of the vent feathers, with whitish droppings, in a blossom-headed parakeet.

Leucocytozoon and Leucocytozoonosis

In some parts of North America and Europe leucocytozoonosis is an important disease of ducks and geese. Some species of *Leucocytozoon* are also pathogenic to domestic fowls and turkeys, and, so far as is known, the genus is confined to birds.

SPECIES AND HOSTS

Leucocytozoon spp. have been found in many passerines and other birds, and the hosts include the house sparrow, starling, and wild canary. Coatney[38] and Berson[27] did not list any psittacines, and the only case in this group of birds appears to be that reported by Frank,[60] who found the infection in a young Pennant's parakeet (*Platycercus elegans*) in Germany.

DISTRIBUTION AND INCIDENCE

Like *Plasmodium*, *Parahaemoproteus*, and *Haemoproteus*, some species of *Leucocytozoon* are world wide in distribution and the incidence of the infection they cause, as shown by surveys on blood parasites of wild birds, may be seasonal and may also vary according to the species of bird. The surveys seem to indicate that in North America *Leucocytozoon* is about as common as *Haemoproteus* and *Parahaemoproteus*, and is more frequently encountered than *Plasmodium*. In Egypt, however, Mohammed[133] found the incidence of infection to be only 0.55 per cent in the birds he examined.

LIFE HISTORY

The life cycle of most species of *Leucocytozoon* is unknown, but that of *L. simondi* in ducks has been studied in some detail and is basically similar to that of *Haemoproteus*, *Parahaemoproteus*, and *Plasmodium*, except that, unlike in *Plasmodium*, there is no schizogonic cycle in the circulating blood cells. As the name suggests, the gametocytes occur in leukocytes (Figs. 25-10, 25-11), although in some species only the erythrocytes are infected. Schizogony occurs in the parenchyma of the liver, heart, kidney, brain, spleen, and

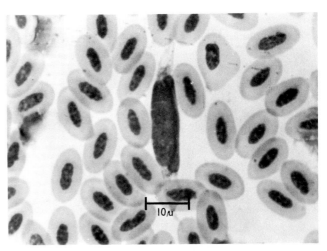

Fig. 25-11. *Elongate gametocyte of* Leucocytozoon *sp. in a blood smear from an owl. Note the extreme distortion of the host leukocyte and its nucleus, which shows as a narrow band with rounded ends lying to one side of the parasite. The gametocyte stains darkly, is elongated and also has rounded ends, but is much wider than the host cell nucleus. (Courtesy of T. Dennett.)*

other organs, and in *L. simondi* two different types of schizonts occur, namely small hepatic schizonts, and megaloschizonts, which are much larger and not confined to the liver. Frank[60] found schizonts mainly in the heart of a parakeet, but also in the liver and lung.

Sporogony is probably confined to dipterous insects, occurring in simuliids, or black flies.

CLINICAL SIGNS OF INFECTION

Garnham[61] recorded deaths in wild 3-week-old weaver bird nestlings (*Sitagra jacksoni*) in Kenya, which he believed were due to *Leucocytozoon* infection, as the blood of dead and dying birds was heavily infected. The intensity of the infection decreased with age, and adult birds in the colony were found to be only slightly infected.

Frank[60] considered that the infection was responsible for the death of two young parakeets, although he supplied little convincing evidence.

DIAGNOSIS

Round (Fig. 25-10) or elongate (Fig. 25-11) gametocytes are observed in the leukocytes and sometimes in erythrocytes. No true pigment is present, and no schizonts occur in any of the circulating blood cells.

TREATMENT

No satisfactory treatment has yet been described, although Frank[60] treated a suspected infection in a

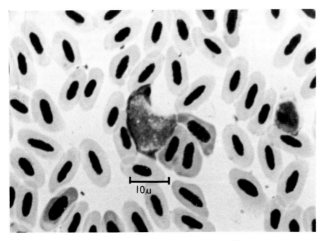

Fig. 25-10. *Round type of gametocyte of* Leucocytozoon dubreulli *in a blood smear from the European blackbird (Turdus merula). The leukocyte is almost obliterated by the parasite and shows as a darker staining band around one side of the parasite. The pale semilunar area to one side of the gametocyte represents the reddish-staining nucleus, while the cytoplasm stains blue with Giemsa stain. (Specimen provided by Dr. J. R. Baker.)*

young parakeet with a coccidiostatic drug. Sulfonamides would probably be effective, and also anti-malarial drugs.

POSTMORTEM FINDINGS

Garnham[61] found gross enlargement of the spleen in heavily infected young weaver birds.

Trypanosoma and Trypanosomiasis

Trypanosomiasis is a well-known disease of man, and of domestic and game animals in some tropical regions, but not an important infection of domestic poultry, in spite of the fact that a wide variety of wild birds may harbor the parasites in their blood, even in temperate zones.

SPECIES AND HOSTS

Several species of avian trypanosomes have been described, for example, *Trypanosoma avium majus, T. avium minus, T. fringillinarum, T. paddae, T. confusum,* and *T. corvi.* Baker,[13] however, was not convinced that these are valid species, and considered that bird trypanosomes should be classified as one species, namely, *T. avium,* which was the name proposed by Danilewsky in 1885 when he first described this parasite.

Trypanosomes have been found in a wide variety of birds, especially passerines, including canaries and other finches, as well as in members of the Corvidae and Turdidae. The parasite has also been found in gallinaceous birds, waterfowl, pigeons, and owls, but seems to be either rare or non-existent in psittacines.

DISTRIBUTION AND INCIDENCE

Avian trypanosomes appear to have an almost worldwide distribution, being found in both tropical and temperate regions. Very little is known, however, about their incidence, and the comparatively low infection rates recorded in some surveys of blood parasites of wild birds may be due to such factors as species or seasonal incidences, especially as Baker,[15] working in England, has shown that the parasites are found in the peripheral blood only during the summer months.

LIFE HISTORY

The life history of trypanosomes in passerine birds has been worked out by Baker,[15] and he[14] has shown that in England the louse fly (*Ornithomyia avicularia*) is a natural vector for the parasite of wild birds, the trypanosome undergoing cyclical development in the alimentary canal of the fly. The parasite multiplies in the crithidial stage and in the hindgut the crithidia change into metacyclic trypanosomes. When a bird eats an infected louse fly, the metacyclic trypanosomes probably invade the lymph system and develop into the large typical forms that are seen in the bird's blood 18 to 24 hours later. Baker found that the trypanosomes persist in their natural hosts (but not in canaries) throughout the winter, being more or less restricted to the bone marrow.

Macfie and Thomson[116] produced strong evidence that red mites transmit trypanosomes to canaries, and Manwell and Johnson[122] also believed that *Dermanyssus gallinae* might be a vector of the parasites for these birds, as the infection developed in one canary after it had been given an intraperitoneal injection of an emulsion of mites taken from a cage containing infected birds. Obviously more investigations are necessary, because red mites are much more likely to be vectors of the parasites to canaries than are louse flies, with which canaries seldom come in contact.

Bennett[23] has shown that simuliids and *Aedes aegypti* mosquitoes may act as intermediate hosts, and he considered simuliids to be the natural vector of the parasites to wild birds in Canada.

CLINICAL SIGNS OF INFECTION

There is little evidence of pathogenicity, although Macfie and Thomson[116] said that "heavy infections were associated with illness," and Manwell and Johnson[122] reported that at the height of infection in canaries one or two birds appeared to be a little sick, although they were not certain that this was due to the parasites.

Normally, infections in all birds are light.

DIAGNOSIS

Parasites are evident in Giemsa-stained smears of the blood (Fig. 25-12) or bone marrow. The organism can also be cultured from these tissues on N.N.N. medium.

TREATMENT

Manwell and Johnson[122] reported that quinine had no effect on the infection, but that plasmochin* probably had a curative value, although they gave no dosage rates.

POSTMORTEM FINDINGS

No lesions appear to have been described.

*Pamaquine Naphthoate—Winthrop Laboratories, 90 Park Ave., New York, N.Y. 10016.

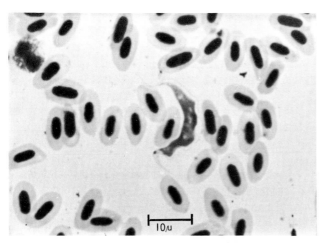

Fig. 25-12. Trypanosoma avium *in a blood smear from a canary* (Serinus canarius). *Note the relatively short, anteriorly directed free flagellum, the fairly well developed undulating membrane terminating near the small round darkly staining kinetoplast, and the slender tapering posterior end. (Specimen provided by Dr. J. R. Baker.)*

Toxoplasma and Toxoplasmosis

Toxoplasmosis has a worldwide distribution and is best known as an infection of children and less frequently of adults. Many other species of animals are also infected, although there are far fewer reliable records of infection in birds.

The literature on the subject is vast, but useful accounts of the disease are given by Manwell *et al.,*[121] Jacobs,[89] and Levine.[111]

SPECIES AND HOSTS

Owing to the fact that *Lankesterella* infection in birds has until recently often been incorrectly diagnosed as due to *Toxoplasma gondii,*[61] it is sometimes difficult to determine which reports of toxoplasmosis presented prior to 1950 are valid. The only avian hosts in which the natural infection is believed to have been confirmed are the pigeon and domestic fowl,[58] penguins,[146] canary,[151] and the American crow (*Corvus brachyrhynchos*).[58] Sergent and Poncet[158] also diagnosed the infection in the canary.

DISTRIBUTION AND INCIDENCE

Very little is known about the distribution of *Toxoplasma* in birds, although when more research has been carried out it may prove to be cosmopolitan.

Finlay and Manwell[58] stated that in some areas there appears to be a high incidence of toxoplasmosis in pigeons.

LIFE HISTORY

In spite of a great deal of research, the life cycle of *Toxoplasma* remains unknown, and no vector has been conclusively incriminated.

CLINICAL SIGNS OF INFECTION

The clinical signs of infection are indefinite. There is evidence that strains of the organism vary considerably in pathogenicity, and infected birds may remain quite healthy.

DIAGNOSIS

The disease cannot be diagnosed without the use of laboratory methods such as inoculation of experimental animals and histological techniques. Serological tests, however, are available, including a dye test developed by Sabin and Feldman.[153]

DIFFERENTIAL DIAGNOSIS. As stated previously, the infection has been confused frequently with that caused by *Lankesterella.*

TREATMENT

Owing to the lack of reliable information on the disease in birds and the difficulty of diagnosis, no treatment has yet been devised.

POSTMORTEM FINDINGS

Ratcliffe and Worth[146] stated that the central nervous system is primarily involved, and described necrotic foci in the liver, lungs, and spleen. On microscopical examination they usually found the crescent-shaped parasites associated with the lesions.

Sarcocystis and Sarcocystis Infection

Very little is known about *Sarcocystis* infection, which occurs not only in birds, but in man and numerous other species of mammals in many parts of the world.

The disease has been recorded in many species, including waterfowl and passerines, but there appears to be no record of the infection in the canary or in psittacines.

Occasionally the crescent-shaped "spores" are found in blood smears as the result of rupture of a cyst in striated or in cardiac muscle when blood is taken to prepare the smear. Sometimes the cysts can be recognized at necropsy as small yellowish white areas, about

4 mm. long and less than 0.5 mm. wide, located in muscle tissue, especially in the leg and pectoral muscles.

For fuller accounts of the disease the reader should consult Chute,[34] Clark,[35] and Levine.[111]

HELMINTHS

NEMATODES, OR ROUNDWORMS

All roundworms belong to the Class Nematoda and are unsegmented, cylindrical, and elongate worms, covered with a tough but flexible non-cellular cuticle. Bird nematodes may vary in length, according to the species, from a few millimeters to several centimeters. The worms taper at both ends. They have no respiratory system, but have well-developed reproductive organs and a relatively simple tubelike alimentary canal. The mouth is situated at the extreme anterior end and is usually surrounded by sensory organs known as lips; the anus opens near the posterior end of the body. Most nematodes are sexually distinct, the male usually possessing two chitinous spicules near the posterior end, but in some cases possessing only one. The male genital organs open into the cloaca alongside the anus, but the vulva of the female is variable in position and usually opens in the anterior half of the body.

Nematodes occur mainly in the intestinal tract of the host, but may occur also in many other parts of the body, and it is probably easier here to deal with them according to the part of the body where they may be found, rather than in taxonomic order. A simple classification of the most important bird parasites, however, is presented before the species are considered separately.

Classification of Nematodes Found in Birds

Phylum	Nemathelminthes
Class	Nematoda
Order	Strongyloidea

Characteristics: Males possess a copulatory bursa. Buccal capsule is well developed. The mouth is usually fringed by leaf-crowns.

Family	Strongylidae
Example:	*Syngamus*

* * * *

Order	Ascaroidea

Characteristic: Mouth possesses three lips—one dorsal and two subventral. In the Families listed below, no buccal capsule or bursa is present.

Family	Ascaridae
Example:	*Porrocaecum*
Family	Heterakidae
Examples:	*Ascaridia* and *Heterakis*

* * * *

Order	Trichinelloidea

Characteristics: The body is divided into a relatively thin esophageal portion and a thicker posterior portion containing the organs. This characteristic, however, is more marked in the whipworms of mammals than in many of the avian nematodes, such as *Capillaria*. The male has a single spicule.

Family	Trichinellidae
Example:	*Capillaria*

* * * *

Order	Spiruroidea

Characteristics: Usually small worms with two lateral lips and an esophagus which is divided into a short anterior muscular portion and a long glandular posterior portion. The spicules of the male are unequal in size, and the posterior end is usually spiral in form.

Family	Acuariidae
Examples:	*Spiroptera, Dispharynx,* and *Habronema*
Family	Thelaziidae
Example:	*Oxyspirura*

* * * *

Order	Filaroidea

Characteristics: Threadlike worms without a buccal capsule and the mouth devoid of lips. The esophagus is similar to that seen in the Spiruroidea. The male is much smaller than the female, and the genital opening of the female is near the anterior end of the body; the spicules of the male are unequal in size.

Family	Filariidae
Example:	*Diplotriaena*

NEMATODES OF THE RESPIRATORY SYSTEM

Syngamus and Syngamiasis, or Gapes

Adult gapeworms are found in the trachea or bronchi. They appear as bright red nematodes attached to the mucous membrane, and, if they are not properly examined, they can be mistaken for elongated clots of blood. The female reaches a length of 40 mm.; at the anterior third of the body, permanently attached to the vulva, is the smaller male, which does not exceed 6 mm. in length.

SPECIES AND HOSTS

Syngamus trachea is the only species of gapeworm likely to be encountered in passerine birds, *S. parvus, S. gracilis,* and *S. merulae* all being regarded by Madsen[118] as synonyms of *S. trachea. S. trachea* has been reported in a vast number of species, representing the Orders Passeriformes, Psittaciformes, Piciformes, Apodiformes, Strigiformes, Columbiformes, Charadriiformes, Gruiformes, Falconiformes, Galliformes, and Anseriformes. There is little doubt that almost any species of cage or aviary bird is liable to be affected if exposed to infection. Both Hamerton[69] and Gray[66] reported syngamiasis in aviary birds, and Gray[66] also reported deaths in aviary-reared "nestling ornamental thrushes," the king bird of paradise (*Cicinnurus regius*), and other species. Appleby[4] reported the death of a rosy pastor (*Pastor roseus*) in the Edinburgh Zoological Gardens, caused by a heavy infection with the parasite.

DISTRIBUTION AND INCIDENCE

Before poultry were kept under intensive methods of husbandry, *S. trachea* was an important parasite of the domestic fowl in many parts of the world, but it is seldom reported in that species nowadays. It does, however, cause trouble occasionally where turkeys are extensively kept, is quite common in game birds, and is encountered very frequently in wild birds in Great Britain[99] and other parts of the world. Mettrick[131] also found it to be widespread in Britain, reporting 55 per cent of nestling and fledgling starlings (*Sturnus vulgaris*) to be infected, 86–93 per cent of jackdaws (*Corvus monedula*), and 100 per cent of young rooks (*Corvus frugilegus*). Adult birds are affected less frequently, however, Mettrick giving figures of 32 per cent for starlings and 33 per cent for rooks.

LIFE HISTORY

Fertilized eggs deposited in the trachea of the host by the female worm are coughed up and either swallowed and passed in the feces (Fig. 25-13), or directly expelled onto the ground from the trachea. In either event, after an incubation period of 1 or 2 weeks under optimal conditions, the third-stage infective larva is reached, still within the egg. These infective larvae hatch from the eggs and are either eaten directly by the avian host or

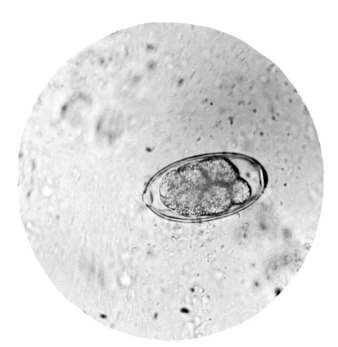

Fig. 25-13. Syngamus trachea *ovum in the excreta. Note the presence of an operculum at each pole. Magnification X410. (Benbrook and Sloss:* **Veterinary Clinical Parasitology,** *3rd ed. Ames, Iowa State University Press, 1961.)*

are ingested by transport hosts such as earthworms, slugs, or snails, in which they become encysted. The encysted larvae in such transport hosts will remain infective for a bird which eats them, for at least a year. The larvae are believed to penetrate the intestinal wall of the definitive host to enter the blood stream and be carried to the lungs which, as has been shown, they can reach 6 hours after ingestion by the bird. A further molt occurs in the lungs, and then the young worms migrate up the bronchi to the trachea. Eggs are produced by the worms in the trachea, about two weeks after ingestion of the infective larvae.

CLINICAL SIGNS OF INFECTION

Young birds of all species are mainly affected, resistance appearing to develop as the birds mature. The severity of the disease depends mainly on the degree of infection, although small birds with a narrow tracheal lumen are more severely affected than large hosts. The worms cause partial or complete obstruction of the trachea, resulting in dyspnea and eventually asphyxia. Affected birds open the mouth widely, at the same time stretching out the neck to give the characteristic "gape." They may also cough and shake the head in an effort to dislodge the worms from the trachea. In severe cases, birds refuse to eat, lose condition, and die as the result of starvation and anemia caused by the blood-sucking habits of the parasites.

DIAGNOSIS

Diagnosis is based on the clinical signs and demonstration of *Syngamus* worms in the trachea, by removal during life or at necropsy, or by discovery of the eggs on microscopical examination of the droppings.

DIFFERENTIAL DIAGNOSIS.   Respiratory acariasis, aspergillosis, or the acute form of passerine pox must be considered in differential diagnosis.

TREATMENT

Generally speaking, treatment is unsatisfactory, especially in small birds, and the inhalation of barium antimonyl tartrate powder in an enclosed box[175] has, until recently, been the treatment usually recommended for gapes in gallinaceous birds.

Kelley[93] experimented with the use of a solution of disophenol (2,6-diiodo-4-nitrophenol), containing 35 mg. disophenol per ml., by subcutaneous injection, for the disease in pheasants. He found this drug to be highly efficacious, but unfortunately toxic, causing an 11 per cent loss when administered at the dosage rate of 10.5 mg. per kg. According to Kelley,[93] Boisvenue had found the same drug to be effective when given by mouth; Kelley believed that he might have had more success if he had added the drug to the diet at a lower level and administered it for a longer period of time. With many species of aviary birds, however, administration of drugs in the diet is impractical.

There is reason to believe that thiabendazole* is effective when it is administered orally in tablet form,

*Thibenzole—Merck & Co., Rahway, N.J. 07065

based on the usual dosage of 44 mg. per kg. body weight.

Fardell[56] recorded the successful treatment of a raven (*Corvus corax*) by administering thiabendazole at the dosage rate of 1 gm. per day for 10 days, combined with removal of the worms from the trachea every 3 days by spay forceps. Although this drug was not toxic, its therapeutic effect in this case remains unknown, because recovery may have been due entirely to mechanical removal of the worms. On the other hand, Leibovitz[108] found the drug to be effective in the treatment of syngamiasis in pheasants.

Mechanical removal of worms by passing a cotton-wire pipe cleaner down the trachea and twisting it around two or three times before withdrawing it was recommended by Gray.[66] Although this often seems to be a satisfactory method for birds no smaller than a mynah, it is likely to cause asphyxiation or produce irreparable damage to the larynx and trachea of smaller species.

The disease can be controlled to a certain extent in outdoor aviaries by excluding the entry of wild birds and by covering the top of the aviary with some material that will prevent contamination by their droppings. Such precautions are particularly advisable if the aviary is in the vicinity of a rookery or starling roost. Exclusion of transport hosts, however, is likely to be more difficult, especially in an aviary with an earth floor.

POSTMORTEM FINDINGS

Findings at necropsy may vary from only a small amount of mucus formed in the trachea to fairly severe tracheitis, bronchitis, and areas of congestion in the lungs. The lungs are also often edematous. The trachea

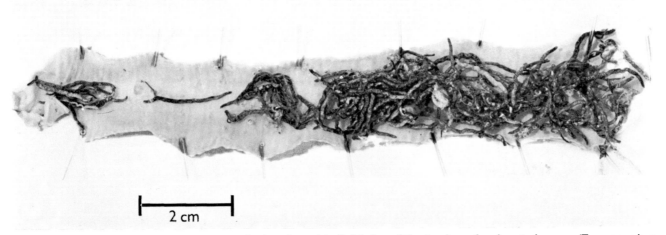

Fig. 25-14. **Syngamus trachea** *worms attached to the epithelial lining of the trachea of a pinnated grouse* (Tympanuchus cupido), *causing almost complete obstruction of the trachea. The worms are red in color, the female being much larger than the male, which is permanently attached to the vulva of the female. Both sexes attach themselves to the epithelium, causing an inflammatory reaction around the point of attachment. (Courtesy of T. Dennett.)*

is sometimes found to be almost completely obstructed by the mass of worms attached to its epithelical lining (Fig. 25-14).

NEMATODES OF THE RESPIRATORY AND CIRCULATORY SYSTEMS

Filarial Roundworms and Filariasis

Filarial roundworms are long, thin, threadlike nematodes, the larvae of which (microfilariae) are found in the host's blood or tissues.

SPECIES AND HOSTS

A large number of species of filariae, many of which have not been named, occur in a wide variety of birds, including representatives of the Orders Passeriformes, Psittaciformes, and Falconiformes. Members of the Families Corvidae and Coraciidae, in particular, may harbor several species.[119] *Diplotriaena* spp. are commonly found in North American crows, thrushes, and grackles (Wetmore,[177] quoting Wehr).

DISTRIBUTION AND INCIDENCE

These worms are practically world wide in distribution. In North America, where several surveys have been carried out on wild birds, infection rates as high as 8 per cent have been found in samples covering a wide range of species.[150] In England, James[90] found 1 to 2 per cent of imported Java sparrows showed microfilariae in their blood, and Markbreiter[124] reported the parasites in 12 per cent of 183 birds of 21 different species which had died in the London Zoological Gardens.

LIFE HISTORY

Manson-Bahr[119] pointed out that the life cycle of filarial worms as it occurs in birds is mainly unknown, although it has been studied in man and other mammals.

The adult worms of both sexes live in the lymph, blood, and connective tissues of the bird. The female produces many ova, which give rise to larvae, or microfilariae. Large numbers of these enter the blood stream (Fig. 25-15), where they may remain for several months. When blood-sucking insects such as simuliids, *Culicoides* midges, or even some species of lice feed on the bird, microfilariae are taken up in the blood and pass into the stomach of the insect, where they bore through the wall, eventually to reach and encyst in the thoracic muscles. Three ecdyses occur in the insect, and under favorable conditions of temperature and humidity the larvae

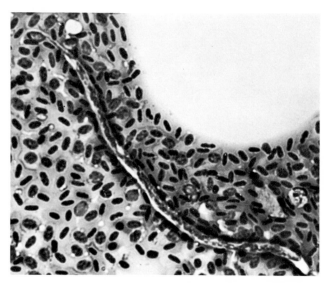

Fig. 25-15. *Microfilaria in the blood of a cordon bleu finch* (Uraeginthus bengalis). *(Courtesy of T. Dennett.)*

may become fully developed in 14 days, at this stage possessing alimentary, excretory, and reproductive systems. They then become very active and work their way through the tissues of the insect host to reach the head and penetrate the proboscis sheath. When the insect bites its victim, the larvae emerge onto the skin. In the definitive host the worms reach maturity after a few months, produce ova, and the cycle is then repeated.

CLINICAL SIGNS OF FILARIASIS

Wetmore[177] drew attention to the fact that little is known about the effect of avian types of filarial worms on the host. Hamerton,[69] however, regarded *D. tricuspis* as pathogenic to jays, causing pneumonia and consolidation of the lungs, and Plimmer[143] reported "fits" and sudden death in birds due to microfilariae plugging the cerebral capillaries.

DIAGNOSIS

The infection can be diagnosed in the live bird by finding the microfilariae in the blood, by examination either of a wet preparation under the low power of the microscope, when the larvae will be seen wriggling actively, or of a thick blood smear stained with Giemsa's stain. It must be remembered, however, that the microfilariae may exhibit a periodicity, so that a series of examinations at approximately 8-hour intervals is necessary.

At necropsy, diagnosis is made by identifying the worms in the air sacs or thoracic and abdominal cavities. On rare occasions, when great numbers of intestinal or proventricular nematodes are present, some of these may perforate the wall of the intestines or proventriculus, especially after death, and enter the abdominal cavity or air sacs, so care is needed to check that this has not occurred.

DIFFERENTIAL DIAGNOSIS. In examination of wet blood preparations, trypanosomes because of their movement may be confused with microfilariae. The latter are in fact much larger and more active, and can actually be seen with the low-power objective of the microscope, whereas trypanosomes cannot be seen at such low magnification, only the movement of the erythrocytes in their vicinity being detectable.

TREATMENT

None. Control of possible vectors such as simuliids and *Culicoides* spp. is very difficult, and no method of treatment appears to have been recorded.

PATHOLOGY AND POSTMORTEM FINDINGS

The adult worms are found coiled under the serosa of the air sacs, especially around the proventriculus, which in some cases they may actually penetrate to reach the lumen.[176] Weidman also stated that they may rupture the inferior vena cava, producing severe anemia, and be associated with subserosal cysts in the intestine.

Hamerton[69] stated that the microfilariae sometimes concentrate in great numbers in the capillaries and bronchi of the lungs, probably being responsible for the congestion and edema with which they are associated. Vast numbers of worm eggs may also be found in the lung tissue of jays infected with *D. tricuspis*, being easily seen on microscopical examination.

NEMATODES OF THE ALIMENTARY SYSTEM

Proventricular and Gizzard Worms

The avian nematodes that are dealt with here all belong to the Order Spiruroidea, and are found in the "stomach" and occasionally in the esophagus.

SPECIES AND HOSTS

Spiroptera incerta (syn. *Habronema incertum*), the most important species attacking cage and aviary birds, has been recorded by Weidman[176] in numerous psittacine birds, including various Old World parrots and lovebirds, amazon parrots, cockatoos, crested ground parakeets, lories, macaws, conures, rosehill (rosella)

parakeets, Pennant's parakeets, and a budgerigar. In addition to psittacines, Weidman[176] recorded the worm in toucans, pigeons, starling, quail, thicknee, and barbet.

Dispharynx nasuta (syn. *Dispharynx spiralis, Disphaáragus spiralis, Acuaria spiralis*), besides being found in poultry and other gallinaceous birds, also occurs in a number of passerines, including the house sparrow and starling.[65]

DISTRIBUTION AND INCIDENCE

S. incerta has been reported in North America and Great Britain, and Goble and Kutz[65] stated that *D. nasuta* occurs in Europe, Asia, Africa, North and South America, and Australia.

There is very little information regarding the incidence of *S. incerta,* but the findings at postmortem examination of 774 birds of over a dozen different species of psittacines recorded by Weidman[176] may give some idea of the susceptibility of various species, assuming that all were equally exposed to infection. The highest infection rate, 41.6 per cent, was recorded in rosella parakeets, with 34.6 per cent in macaws, 28.5 per cent in Pennant's parakeets, and only 8.9 per cent in crested ground parakeets and 5.8 per cent in cockatoos. The lowest incidence of all was 0.8 per cent in budgerigars, among 121 examined.

LIFE HISTORY

The life cycles of all species are indirect, and the intermediate hosts are arthropods.

Wehr,[174] quoting Cram,[44] stated that in North America the pillbug (*Armadillidium vulgare*) and the sowbug (*Porcellio scaber*) can act as intermediate hosts of *D. nasuta*. These crustaceans ingest embryonated eggs (Fig. 25-16) passed in the droppings of the bird, and the larvae are subsequently found in their tissues. The infective third larval stage is reached in the arthropod, and birds become infected by eating the intermediate hosts.

Beetles and ants are the intermediate hosts of some worms, but the life cycle of *S. incerta* is unknown.

CLINICAL SIGNS OF PROVENTRICULAR AND GIZZARD WORMS

Weidman[176] stated that mucus may appear in the droppings, and parrots either die after an acute attack or become emaciated. Goble and Kutz,[65] in a survey of birds for *Dispharynx* infection in New York City, found that although the worm was pathogenic to gallinaceous birds, the catbird (*Dumetella carolinensis*) was the only passerine species that was obviously adversely affected by infection with *Dispharynx*.

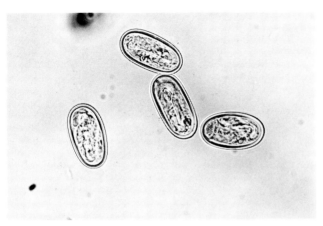

Fig. 25-16. *Ova of* Dispharynx nasuta. *The ova are embryonated when passed in the droppings of the bird. Magnification X410. (Benbrook and Sloss:* Veterinary Clinical Parasitology, *3rd ed. Ames, Iowa State University Press, 1961.)*

DIAGNOSIS

Diagnosis is based on the presence of eggs on microscopical examination of the droppings, or worms found in the proventriculus or gizzard at necropsy.

DIFFERENTIAL DIAGNOSIS. The identification of worms which are found in the air sacs is necessary, in case there is a concomitant infection with Filariidae.

PREVENTION AND TREATMENT

There is no known treatment. Access to the aviary floor of ants, beetles, and other arthropods should be prevented, if possible.

POSTMORTEM FINDINGS

Weidman[176] stated that as many as 100 *S. incerta* worms may be found in the proventriculus, causing swelling of the mucous membrane and interfering with the passage of food. The worms burrow into the mucosa and occasionally penetrate through the proventricular wall into the air sacs. He stated that on one occasion this produced an adenomatous hyperplasia of the mucous membrane, associated with peritonitis. Immature worms are also occasionally found beneath the horny lining of the gizzard.

Intestinal Worms

Porrocaecum and Porrocaecum Infections

SPECIES AND HOSTS

Porrocaecum worms of several species are commonly found in the small intestine of wild birds in Great Brit-

ain.[91] *P. ensicaudatum* has a wide distribution among crows and thrushes, and is also found in many other passerine species.

DISTRIBUTION AND INCIDENCE

Porrocaecum spp. are world-wide in distribution, *P. ensicaudatum* being particularly widespread in the northern hemisphere.

LIFE HISTORY

Unlike that of other members of the Ascaroidea dealt with here, the life history of *Porrocaecum* is indirect, and the intermediate hosts vary according to the species. The intermediate host for *P. ensicaudatum*, according to Baer,[10] is the earthworm *Allolobophora chlorotica*. When infected worms were fed to blackbirds, the nematode larvae were found 48 hours later beneath the horny lining of the gizzard, this being where the third larval molt occurs. It is believed that the fourth-stage larvae pass into the gut lumen to become adults, and Baer did not think that the presence of the fourth larval stage in the intestinal mucosa which he observed was a normal phase of the life cycle, but that it occurred because of host reaction to successive infections. After two further molts, the fourth stage gives rise to the fifth larval stage and finally the adult.

CLINICAL SIGNS OF PORROCAECUM INFECTION

Baer[10] described ruffled feathers, obvious sickness, and inability to maintain balance in a heavily infected young blackbird.

DIAGNOSIS

Presence of larvae beneath the horny lining of the gizzard or attached to the intestinal epithelium, associated with fibrous tumors on the peritoneal surface of the intestine.

TREATMENT

No treatment has been described. Prevention is by control of intermediate hosts.

POSTMORTEM FINDINGS AND PATHOLOGY

Baer[10] found the fourth-stage larvae—which are 10 to 11 mm. long—attached by their anterior extremity to the intestinal epithelium at different levels of the intestine. In one heavily infected blackbird, fibrous tumors were present on the peritoneal surface of the intestine. Baer found that the tumors consisted of a cavity lined by a syncytium of giant cells and enclosed by fibrous connective tissue. Within the cavity he found the fifth larval stage, partly surrounded by the fourth molt, whereas in later stages the larvae had been destroyed.

Ascaridia and Ascaridiasis

Although ascaridiasis is a common condition in the domestic fowl, caused by *Ascaridia galli,* this species of roundworm rarely occurs in passerines. *A. hermaphrodita,* however, which has been described by Cram,[43] is found in many psittacine birds.

SPECIES AND HOSTS

Cram[43] listed 19 different species of psittacines as hosts of *A. hermaphrodita,* whereas Swierstra *et al.*[166] recorded the worm in the budgerigar. Blackmore,[29] in England, also found this worm in budgerigars, 16 other species of parakeets, a blue-fronted amazon parrot (*Amazona braziliensis*), and a lorikeet. Weidman[176] recorded intestinal roundworms in amazon parrots, but did not state the species of the parasites, although they were probably ascarids.

In England Fowler[59] found *A. numidae* in an elegant grass parakeet (*Neonanodes elegans*) and *A. columbae* in a Barraband's parakeet (*Polytelis swainsonii*).

DISTRIBUTION AND INCIDENCE

A. hermaphrodita occurs in Australia and Europe, as well as in South America and probably also in North America.

Out of 774 psittacines examined after death by Weidman,[176] only three harbored roundworms.

The canary does not appear to be affected.

Very little information on incidence is available, but nowadays *Ascaridia* spp. seem to be less rare in psittacines than had been thought.

LIFE HISTORY

The life cycle is direct. Eggs are passed in the feces (Fig. 25-17), and larvae then form within them. When these are ingested by the host, the larvae are released in the small intestine, and some of the larval stages are actually spent in the intestinal mucosa, in addition to being present in the lumen of the small intestines with the adults (Fig. 25-18).

CLINICAL SIGNS OF INFECTION

There appear to be no published accounts, but Blackmore[29] encountered loss of condition and paralysis of the legs in parakeets.

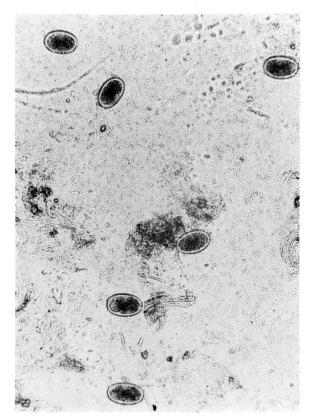

Fig. 25-17. *Ova of* Ascaridia *sp. in the excreta of a parakeet. Magnification approximately X120. (Courtesy of D. K. Blackmore.)*

DIAGNOSIS

Presence of adult worms or eggs in the feces.

DIFFERENTIAL DIAGNOSIS. Other intestinal helminth infections.

TREATMENT AND PREVENTION

No completely satisfactory treatment has been found, although Fowler[59] had some success dosing birds with piperazine *per os* by means of a stomach tube. He uses a solution containing 50 mg. per ml. and recommends a dose in the range of 1 ml. per 100 grams of body weight. Treatment can be repeated if necessary. Birds should not be regarded as free from infection until a minimum of two fecal samples, taken at an interval of 10 days, have been found negative on microscopical examination. The worms most frequently cause trouble when present in large numbers, and are often difficult for the bird to pass because the lumen of the lower part of the small intestine in parakeets is smaller than that of the duodenum, and piperazine only paralyzes the worms. For this reason administration of a lubricant, such as liquid paraffin, or a vermifuge about 12 to 24 hours after dosing with piperazine is indicated.

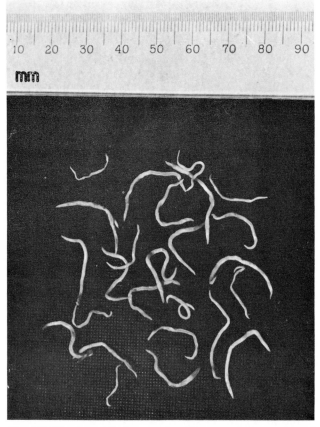

Fig. 25-18. Ascaridia hermaphrodita *nematodes removed from the duodenum of a splendid parakeet* (Neophema splendida). *(Courtesy of T. Dennett.)*

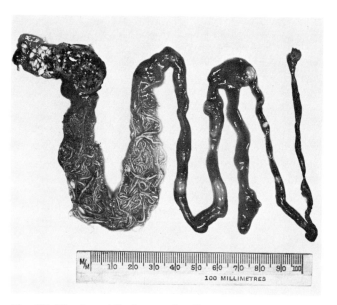

Fig. 25-19. Ascaridia hermaphrodita *worms causing impaction of the duodenum of a splendid parakeet* (Neophema splendida). *(Courtesy of T. Dennett.)*

Heterakis and Heterakis Infections

Heterakis gallinae, the well-known cecal worm of poultry and other gallinaceous birds, is of no importance in passerines, psittacines, and other common types of cage and aviary birds.

Capillaria and Capillariasis

Capillaria spp., commonly known as threadworms, are frequently found infecting poultry and game birds.

SPECIES AND HOSTS

Numerous species have been described from a large variety of wild passerine birds, but practically nothing has been published regarding *Capillaria* worms in cage and aviary birds, although Pillers[142] stated that canaries may harbor great numbers of these nematodes.

Mortelmans[134] has seen heavy infections in budgerigars in Belgium, and Blackmore[29] encountered the nematodes in rosella parakeets (*Platycercus eximus*) in England.

DISTRIBUTION AND INCIDENCE

Many species of *Capillaria* have been reported from poultry and wild birds in various parts of the world, but nothing is known of the incidence of capillariasis in cage birds.

Swaenepoel and Swaenepoel[165a] recommend giving 100 mg. of piperazine per 100 grams of body weight in small progressive doses instead of one massive dose so that too many worms will not be evacuated at once and cause bowel obstruction. They state that since piperazine has no effect upon the larvae in the intestinal mucosa the treatment should be repeated in 2 to 3 weeks after the initial therapy.

In heated aviaries there is likely to be a greater risk of heavy infections with ascarids, because warmth increases the rate of embryonation of the eggs. Embryonation of eggs is also stimulated by moisture, and care is therefore necessary to prevent leakage from drinking vessels. Any litter, such as sawdust, on the floor should be renewed every week, especially from around the water receptacles.

POSTMORTEM FINDINGS

Birds may die when heavily infected, due to obstruction of the duodenum (Fig. 25-19) and small intestine with the worms.

LIFE HISTORY

The life cycle may be direct or indirect, depending on the species.

The eggs are expelled from the host in the feces. Infective larvae develop in the eggs after a period which varies from species to species; they are then ingested by birds, to develop into adult worms in the crop or small intestine, or the eggs are swallowed by earthworms. In the latter event, birds become infected by eating the earthworms.

CLINICAL SIGNS OF INFECTION

According to Gray,[66] capillariasis not infrequently causes death among canaries and other aviary birds, although he described no specific clinical signs.

DIAGNOSIS

Diagnosis is based on microscopical examination of the excreta, revealing the typical eggs with bi-polar plugs (Fig. 25-20), or the threadlike worms are found at necropsy, adhering to the crop or intestinal mucosa.

DIFFERENTIAL DIAGNOSIS. See discussions on *Porrocaecum* and *Ascaridia* (*supra*).

TREATMENT

Mortelmans[134] reported the successful treatment of capillariasis in budgerigars, passerines, and other species with methyridine.* The drug is given subcutaneously at the dosage rate of 200 mg. per kg. body weight. Piperazine should also be effective at the dosage rate recommended above for ascaridiasis.

Preventive measures similar to those recommended for ascaridiasis should be instituted.

POSTMORTEM FINDINGS

Gray[66] stated that when the worms are present in large numbers they cause swelling of the bowel wall and distention of its lumen.

NEMATODES OF THE EYE

These are small slender worms which occur beneath the nictitating membrane or in the conjunctival sacs and lacrimal duct of birds and mammals.

---

*Promintic—Imperial Chemical Industries Limited, Alderley Park, Macclesfield. Cheshire, England.

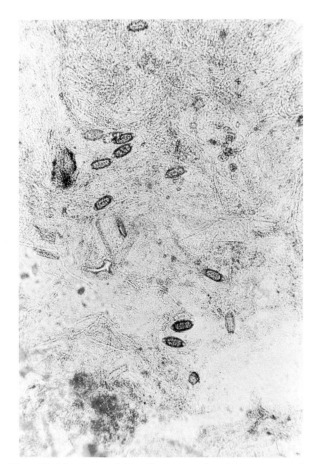

Fig. 25-20. *Ova of* Capillaria *sp. in the excreta of a rosella parakeet* (Platycercus eximus). *Note the presence of bi-polar plugs. Magnification, approximately X120. (Courtesy of D. K. Blackmore.)*

SPECIES AND HOSTS

Oxyspirura mansoni is the only parasite of importance in this category. It occurs in the domestic fowl, turkey, duck, and peafowl,[174] and also naturally in the mynah, house sparrow, Chinese dove, Japanese quail, and pheasant.[155] Several passerines and the pigeon (*Columba livia*) have also been experimentally infected.

DISTRIBUTION AND INCIDENCE

Confined to the southern states of America, Hawaii, and other tropical areas.

LIFE HISTORY

Sanders[154] stated that the adult female worm lays its eggs in the eye of the host, and these are washed down the lacrimal duct, swallowed, and passed out in the excreta. For the next stage to develop, the eggs must be ingested by the cockroach (*Pycnoscelus* [*Leucophaea*] *surinamensis*), in the body cavity of which the mature larvae are found; larvae may also form cysts in the alimentary tract and adipose tissue. When an infected cockroach is eaten by a bird, the larvae escape into the crop, migrate up the esophagus, and enter the nasolacrimal duct by way of the mouth, to reach the eye.

CLINICAL SIGNS OF NEMATODES IN THE EYE

Wehr[174] described conjunctivitis and swelling of the nictitating membrane. Sometimes the eyelids become adherent to each other and caseous material forms under them. Affected birds are restless and continuously scratch the affected eye, while the nictitating membrane flicks constantly in an effort to remove the parasite. If no treatment is carried out, Wehr stated that severe ophthalmia and eventual loss of the eyeball may occur.

DIAGNOSIS

Clinical signs and discovery of the nematode in the eye lead to the diagnosis. In advanced cases of the disease, however, Wehr[174] stated that worms are seldom found.

TREATMENT

If worms are present in the eye, they should be removed—if necessary under a general anesthetic. This is followed by the usual therapy for eye diseases, using antibiotics, cortisone preparations, or analgesics as indicated.

ACANTHOCEPHALIDS, OR THORNY-HEADED WORMS

These worms are usually classified with the nematodes and placed in the separate Class Acanthocephala, in the Phylum Nemathelminthes.

The worms are found in the intestinal tract of birds as well as that of other vertebrates, and appear as rather elongate, mainly cylindrical forms with a retractile, oval or cylindrical proboscis. This proboscis is armed with transverse and longitudinal rows of hooks, which vary in number and arrangement, according to the species. The hooks become attached to the intestinal mucosa and the worm feeds by absorption through the body wall, no alimentary tract being present.

CLASSIFICATION

The following taxa include some of the acanthocephalids found in birds.

Phylum	Nemathelminthes	
Class	Acanthocephala	Thorny-headed worms.
Order	Echinorhynchidea	
Family	Polymorphidae (Parasites of vertebrates, especially birds and mammals.)	
Example:	*Polymorphus*	
Family	Plagiorhynchidae (Parasites of reptiles and birds. All the bird parasites are confined to the subfamily Plagiorhynchinae.)	
Example:	*Plagiorhynchus*	
Family	Fillicollidae (Parasites of aquatic birds.)	
Example:	*Filicollis*	
Order	Gigantorhynchidea	
Family	Prosthorhynchidae (Parasites of birds and mammals.)	
Example:	*Prosthorhynchus*	
Family	Centrorhynchidae (Parasites of birds and mammals.)	
Example:	*Centrorhynchus*	

SPECIES AND HOSTS

Polymorphus boschadis occurs mainly in waterfowl, but has also been reported from some passerines, including the starling and members of the thrush family in England.[99]

Plagiorhynchus formosus has been reported from passerines in North America by Wehr,[174] but *Filicollis anatis* appears to be confined to water birds. Rothschild and Clay[152] stated that the birds most commonly infected with acanthocephalids are the ducks (Anatidae), birds of prey, and thrushes. *Prosthorhynchus* spp. and *Centrorhynchus* spp. are common in passerines.

DISTRIBUTION AND INCIDENCE

The species mentioned above occur in North America and Europe.

There is little information regarding the incidence of acanthocephalids in either free-living or captive birds, but Mettrick[131] carried out a survey in England of 571 wild birds from Hertfordshire and found that 26.5 per cent of the helminth-infected birds also carried acanthocephalids; the worms were found in birds of 7 (31.7 per cent) of the 22 species examined.

LIFE HISTORY

It is believed that all species require development in an intermediate host before they can become infective for the final host, and birds become infected by ingesting intermediate hosts infected with the larval stages.

The intermediate host of *Polymorphus boschadis* is the fresh-water shrimp *Gammarus pulex,* and that of *Filicollis anatis* is the fresh-water isopod *Asellus aquaticus;* birds therefore become infected by drinking water containing these crustaceans. The worm then develops in the intestine, and the eggs are eventually passed out in the feces. Species affecting passerines utilize annelids and terrestrial insects as intermediate hosts.

PATHOLOGY OF ACANTHOCEPHALID INFECTION

Inflammatory areas and nodules develop on the intestinal mucosa at the site of attachment of the worms, and anemia and cachexia may follow.

DIAGNOSIS

Diagnosis is not possible in the living bird, but only by finding the worms at autopsy.

TREATMENT

None. Appropriate preventive measures should be taken, such as elimination of fresh-water crustaceans from the water supply, and the control of annelids and other likely intermediate hosts.

CESTODES, OR TAPEWORMS

Tapeworms are flattened, segmented helminths belonging to the Class Cestoda in the Phylum Platyhelminthes. The tapeworms which are likely to be found in birds dealt with in this book belong to the Order Cyclophyllidea, although a comparatively small number of avian cestodes belong to the Order Pseudophyllidea. Those occurring in birds, when mature, may vary in length, according to species, from 2 to 35 cm. or more.

All tapeworms consist of a scolex, followed by a neck which produces a variable number of segments, known singly as proglottids and collectively as the strobila. The retractile organ known as the rostellum, which is present in most taenioid tapeworms, is armed with crook-shaped hooks in worms of the Family Davaineidae, and usually also in those of the Hymenolepididae and Dilepididae

families. The size, shape, and number of these hooks vary considerably in the different species, and are important taxonomically. The youngest proglottids, nearest to the neck, are broad and short, but their length increases as they mature. Those in the middle of the strobila usually show two distinct sets of genital organs, so that each proglottid is a hermaphroditic unit. The excretory and nervous systems are continuous throughout the strobila. An alimentary system is absent, and the tapeworm feeds by absorption through the body wall. In older segments, at the posterior end of the strobila, the egg sacs become increasingly conspicuous.

Practically all adult tapeworms are found in the small intestine of the host, attached to the intestinal mucosa by the scolex, and different species are often located in particular portions of the intestine. In very heavy infections, however, the worms may be present throughout almost the entire length of the small intestine.

SPECIES AND HOSTS

Below is a simple classification of the tapeworms most likely to be found in passerine and psittacine birds. In view of the vast number of tapeworms occurring in birds, it is only possible to give here a few examples of the common ones, and to point out that most of the genera have representatives infecting a wide variety of hosts. Some species are confined to certain Orders or Families of birds, but show no host specificity.

Phylum	Platyhelminthes
Class	Cestoda
Order	Cyclophyllidea Tapeworms

Characteristics: The scolex bears four cup-shaped suckers; the rostellum may be present or absent.

Family	Dilepididae (Especially common in passerines.)
Examples:	*Dilepis, Amoebotaenia, Choanotaenia, Anomotaenia,* and *Anonchotaenia*
Family	Davaineidae (Found in a wide variety of birds, including passerines and psittacines.)
Examples:	*Davainea, Raillietina, Ophryocotyle, Cotugnia,* and *Ophryocotyloides*
Family	Hymenolepididae (Found chiefly in the Anatidae, but also in passerines and other birds.)
Example:	*Hymenolepis*

Family   Biuterinidae

Examples: *Biuterina* and *Deltokeras*

Family   Anoplocephalidae (Mainly parasitic in mammals, but a few occur in psittacines.)

Examples: *Triuterina, Hemiparonia, Aporina, Moniezoioides, Paronia,* and *Cittotaenia*

Baylis[18] described a new cestode, *Raillietina taylori,* in the African grey parrot (*Psittacus erithacus*), and even then—nearly 40 years ago—eight species of *Raillietina* had been recorded in parrots, including *R. leptosoma, R. psittacea,* and *R. aruensis.* Weerekoon[172] described a new tapeworm (*Cotugnia platycerci*) from Stanley's rosella parakeet (*Platycercus icterotis*), and Meggitt,[129] a tapeworm of the same genus (*C. brotogerys*) in the all-green parakeet (*Brotogerys tirica*). Other species have also been recorded from psittacines.

Numerous species, too many to list here, are found in passerines, especially in insectivorous species and so-called "softbills." *Dilepis undula* is one very widespread example which, in addition to *Anomotaenia heterocoronata* and *Paricterotaenia magnicinosa,* occurs in mynahs,[141] members of the thrush family (Turdidae), and numerous other passerines.

It must be appreciated that new species of cestodes are being described constantly, and even the provisional identification of a cestode requires careful fixation and staining techniques and microscopical examination.

DISTRIBUTION AND INCIDENCE

Avian tapeworms have a worldwide distribution and, because they require an intermediate host, are less frequently encountered in predominantly seed- or fruit-eating birds, such as psittacines and finches, than in insectivorous or flesh- and fish-eating species. It is not uncommon to find tapeworms in the nestlings of "seed-eaters," since these are frequently fed with insects and do not eat the adult diet until the post-fledgling period.

LIFE HISTORY

The cyclophyllidean bladderworms occur in a wide variety of intermediate invertebrate hosts, such as aquatic and terrestrial arthropods, molluscs, and annelids. If a bird eats an intermediate host harboring a fully developed bladderworm, when the worm reaches the intestine, the scolex evaginates and attaches itself to the epithelium and commences growth and development. When sexual maturity is reached and fertilization has occurred, the eggs are passed in the feces. Their resistance to factors such as desiccation is usually not good, and therefore they must be swallowed fairly soon by a suitable intermediate host if the life cycle is to be completed. The hexacanth embryo penetrates the intestinal wall of the invertebrate and eventually settles down in a suitable part of the body, which varies for different species of cestode and in different invertebrates, in order to develop into the cysticercus, or bladderworm stage. The mature cysticercus is a spherical cyst containing fluid, and it has an outer cuticle and an inner germinal layer which gives rise to one or more scoleces. When the hooks and suckers are fully developed, the cysticercus is capable of infecting the avian host.

CLINICAL SIGNS OF TAPEWORM INFECTION

Clinical signs of cestode infection are indefinite and may range from general debility to diarrhea, resulting in weakness and death.

Sometimes a bird may harbor vast numbers of cestodes without apparent ill effect, whereas at other times the presence of only a few tapeworms seems to be pathogenic. It is not possible, in the present state of knowledge, to state which species of cestodes are most pathogenic to particular species of birds.

DIAGNOSIS

Diagnosis is based on discovery of proglottids or eggs in the feces on microscopical examination, or on the postmortem findings.

TREATMENT

Therapeutic procedures are seldom effective, and often do more harm than good. Special attention should be paid to correct feeding, and suitable precautions should be taken to eliminate intermediate hosts when this is practicable.

Bithionol* has recently been used successfully as an anthelmintic against cestodes in poultry, and might on occasion be worth trying in other birds.

POSTMORTEM FINDINGS

Heavy infections may be associated with varying degrees of enteritis, sometimes catarrhal or hemorrhagic, and at times thickening of the intestinal mucosa may be present. Large numbers of cestodes may also cause intestinal obstruction.

*Actamer—Monsanto Chemicals Ltd., Monsanto House, Victoria St., London, S.W.I.

TREMATODES, OR FLUKES

Flukes are parasitic flatworms belonging to the Class Trematoda in the Phylum Platyhelminthes. The Class is divided into three Orders, but the flukes which parasitize domestic animals and birds all belong to the Order Digenea, and all bird flukes belong to the Suborder Prosostomata, which is a further division of this Order.

Bird flukes are usually leaflike or roughly cylindrical in shape, with the mouth at or near the anterior end of the body. A sucker usually surrounds the mouth, and a second sucker is often present on the ventral surface, usually near the middle of the body, which is frequently covered with scalelike spines. Different species vary considerably in size, but many are 1 cm. or more long.

The bird flukes are usually hermaphroditic, except for the blood flukes (Schistosomatidae), and, in addition to reproductive systems, are provided with relatively simple digestive, nervous, and excretory systems.

Flukes may be found parasitizing almost any part of the body, for example, the circulatory, respiratory, alimentary, reproductive, and excretory systems, the skin, and the eye.

CLASSIFICATION

The following taxa include some of the trematodes found in birds.

Phylum	Platyhelminthes
Class	Trematoda Flukes
Order	Digenea
Suborder	Prosostomata
Family	Troglotrematidae (Parasitic in carnivorous birds and mammals. Mainly infect organs such as lungs, kidney, skin, or nasal sinuses of the definitive host, rather than the intestine.)

Example: *Collyriculum*

Family	Schistosomatidae (Parasitic in birds and mammals, living in the blood vessels.)

Examples: *Trichobilharzia* and *Gigantobilharzia*

Family	Plagiorchidae (Parasitic in the intestines of vertebrates.)

Example: *Prosthogonimus*

Family	Psilostomatidae (Parasitic in the alimentary tract of birds and mammals.)

Example: *Psilostomum*

SPECIES AND HOSTS

The species of flukes number in the hundreds, but they are unlikely to be encountered in cage and aviary birds unless these have been recently captured or are kept in elaborate outdoor aviaries, especially those which may contain stagnant water, such as goldfish ponds. *Prosthogonimus ovatus* occurs in passerines such as the house sparrow, rook, jackdaw, and starling, and also in the domestic fowl and geese; *Collyriculum faba* is also found in house sparrows, starlings, and poultry, in addition to other species of birds. The canary has been experimentally infected with *Trichobilharzia stagnicolae* and *Psilostomum ondatrae;* Riggin[149] reported infecting the parakeet (presumably the budgerigar) with the latter species, thus demonstrating that this proventricular fluke of fish-eating birds is, like many other flukes, capable of infecting a wide range of species. Najim[136] described a new species of blood fluke, *Gigantobilharzia huronensis,* in the North American goldfinch (*Spinus tristis tristis*) and succeeded in experimentally infecting canaries. The cardinal (*Richmondena cardinalis*) is also a natural definitive host of this parasite.[137]

Members of the Family Plagiorchidae occur chiefly in passerines, and the genus *Prosthogonimus* occurs in the oviduct of these birds.

DISTRIBUTION AND INCIDENCE

Flukes are world-wide in distribution, although some species appear to be confined to certain areas; *G. huronensis* has so far been identified only in the U.S.A.; *C. faba* and *P. ovatus* occur both in North America and in Europe.

The incidence of flukes is highest in waterfowl and other aquatic birds.

LIFE HISTORY

The developmental cycle of many bird flukes is unknown, but in those species in which it has been described, for example, the blood fluke *Gigantobilharzia huronensis,*[137] it is so complicated that there is little danger that all of the conditions will be attained, in even the most elaborate outdoor aviary.

Typically, the eggs from mature flukes are passed in the bird's excreta; if these reach water, either they hatch, producing a free-living miracidium, or the miracidium is liberated when the egg is ingested by the snail intermediate host. In the snail, the miracidium develops into a sporocyst, which, according to the species of fluke, may give rise to daughter sporocysts and cercariae (in the Schistosomatidae) or to redia and then cercariae. The free-living cercariae swim about in the water. In the case of the Schistosomatidae, on meeting the avian definitive host, the cercariae penetrate the skin and develop into the adult fluke in the circulatory system, but in flukes of the other families the cercariae become encysted, giving rise to metacercariae. Either these encysted forms are eaten directly by the definitive host, or the cercariae penetrate secondary intermediate hosts such as snails, tadpoles, dragonfly nymphs, and fish, before becoming encysted; the final development into the fluke takes place when these are eaten by the bird.

In the case of flukes affecting passerines, the intermediate host is often a terrestrial snail or, more frequently, an insect which has become infected either by eating the metacercariae or by being penetrated by the cercariae in the larval state, the infection persisting through to the imago.

CLINICAL SIGNS OF INFECTION WITH FLUKES

The clinical signs are not diagnostic, except that two flukes are contained in each of the skin cysts caused by *Collyricum faba.* These cysts are 4 to 6 mm. in diameter.

Petrak[141] reported obstruction of the cloaca due to a large cluster of *C. faba* cysts, apparently resulting in the death of two wood thrushes (*Hylocichla mustelina*).

DIAGNOSIS

In the case of *C. faba,* demonstration of the cysts in the skin, or identification of flukes at postmortem examination.

PREVENTION AND TREATMENT

The usual precautions should be taken to prevent access of possible intermediate host. There is no treatment.

ARTHROPODS

The Phylum Arthropoda includes jointed-limbed, invertebrate animals, and most of those which are parasitic have respiratory systems based on tracheal tubes opening on the exterior surface of the body, which is provided with a chitinous exoskeleton. Most of the vast variety of arthropods which attack birds are ectoparasites, but a few burrow into the skin and others are actually found in some of the viscera.

Many avian ectoparasites transmit diseases of various types, and as some of these arthropods are not markedly host-specific, it will be appreciated that such infestation makes foreign birds potentially dangerous carriers of disease, both when they are imported by man and when they are natural migrants.

The commonest and most important arthropods in each main Order which are likely to be encountered in the types of birds under discussion are listed in a simplified classification before they are dealt with in more detail.

CLASS INSECTA: INSECTS

The insects are arthropods in which the body is divided into three main parts, namely, head, thorax, and abdomen. The head bears one pair of antennae, and the thorax bears three pairs of legs and usually one or two pairs of wings. There are no appendages arising from the abdomen.

Order Diptera

The Order Diptera includes insects with only one pair of wings and suctorial mouthparts. The prothorax and metathorax are smaller than the mesothorax and are fused to it.

Insects of this Order are important to cage and aviary birds mainly as vectors of protozoan and other diseases. For detailed descriptions and life histories, the reader should consult textbooks on entomology.

CLASSIFICATION

Phylum	Arthropoda
Class	Insecta
Order	Diptera
Suborder	Nematocera
Family	Culicidae
Examples:	Mosquitoes and gnats—*Anopheles, Culex,* and *Aedes*
Family	Simuliidae
Example:	Blackflies, or buffalo gnats
Family	Ceratopogonidae
Example:	Biting midges—*Culicoides*
Suborder	Cyclorrhapha
Family	Calliphoridae
Example:	Blowflies
Family	Hippoboscidae
Example:	Louse flies—*Stenepteryx, Ornithomyia,* and *Pseudolynchia*

Mosquitoes and Gnats

Representatives of the family Culicidae are found practically all over the world, but are commonest in the tropics.

Except where they are present in very large numbers, mosquitoes are unlikely to cause anemia by their blood-sucking habit, but some species are capable of transmitting diseases. They may, as is well known, be vectors of *Plasmodium* spp., the cause of malaria, trypanosomes,[23,48,145] fowl pox virus (several publications, *e.g.,* Matheson *et al.*[125]), and certain viruses of the "arbor" group, such as that causing eastern equine encephalomyelitis, which is a virus that may result in actual clinical disease in such species as house sparrows.[162]

CONTROL

Cage and indoor aviary birds may be protected by being kept in mosquito-proof netted buildings, but it is hardly practical to provide complete protection for outdoor aviaries. The insects can, however, be prevented from breeding in outdoor aviaries by frequent replacement of the water provided for bathing and drinking, which sometimes is allowed to become stagnant.

A safe and satisfactory spray for controlling the insects is pyrethrum synergized with piperonyl butoxide.

Blackflies, or Buffalo Gnats

Simuliids are widely distributed throughout the world, but occur most frequently in the northern temperate zone and in tropical Africa. They are potentially dangerous to birds kept in outdoor aviaries, especially in Canada, because in late spring and early autumn they may swarm, particularly near well-aerated running streams in which the aquatic larvae live. Quite apart from causing considerable irritation, they are vicious blood suckers. They have also been reported by various workers to transmit different species of *Leucocytozoon* to poultry, waterfowl, and other birds, and Bennett and Fallis[24] suggest that they may also be vectors of avian trypanosomes in Canada. They are known to be vectors of certain filariid nematodes to man and domestic mammals and ducks; they may therefore transmit these helminths to some species of aviary birds.

CONTROL

As control of these insects is extremely difficult, keeping birds in outdoor aviaries should be avoided in areas where simuliids occur, especially near running water.

Biting Midges

The females of species in the Family Ceratopogonidae, like mosquitoes and simuliids, are blood suckers. They occur on the North American continent, and transmit *Parahaemoproteus* to certain species of wild birds. In the tropics they are known to be intermediate hosts for filariae which infect man, and they may therefore also transmit microfilariae to certain species of birds.

CONTROL

As the insects breed in stagnant pools of water, control should be on lines similar to those recommended for control of mosquitoes.

Blowflies

The Family Calliphoridae contains a very large number of species, which are almost world-wide in distribution.

Myiasis, or the invasion of the flesh by the larvae or maggots of blowflies, is not as common in birds as it is in mammals. Aviary birds are less prone to attack than domestic poultry, which not infrequently develop cannibalistic habits when kept in overcrowded conditions and produce open lesions which may attract the adult flies. Nevertheless, on rare occasions, birds in outdoor aviaries are affected with myiasis, and the nests of wild birds sometimes become infested with the larvae of various species of blowflies, so that nestlings of birds in outdoor aviaries are in potential danger of being attacked by the insects.

Some species lay eggs, whereas others are viviparous and deposit the larvae directly on either living or dead tissue. Nestlings, being unable to escape from the flies, are especially prone to attack when affected with diarrhea. In addition to the irritation and destruction of tissue which these larvae cause, such wounds are particularly prone to secondary bacterial infections.

The larvae of certain blowflies breed on decomposing carcasses and may ingest toxins produced by the bacterium *Clostridium botulinum*. If these larvae are eaten by some species of birds, such as domestic poultry or waterfowl, then death from botulism may result. A number of different species are known to be susceptible to this disease, although vultures have been shown to be resistant.

TREATMENT AND CONTROL

Larvae should be removed manually from affected birds and nests, and wounds should be cleaned and dressed. The birds and nests should also be sprayed lightly with a safe insecticide, such as pyrethrum synergized with piperonyl butoxide.

Hippoboscid, or Louse, Flies

Hippoboscid flies are practically cosmopolitan, and besides attacking domestic mammals are quite frequently found on numerous species of wild birds.

These flies are often, but not always, wingless. The head and body are flattened, and the short legs are each provided with a pair of strong claws, enabling the fly to cling to feathers of the birds.

Louse flies usually move rapidly through the feathers and, in spite of their relatively large size, are easily overlooked. Any bird in an outdoor aviary that shows signs of periodic irritation should be caught and carefully searched for these parasites. When a recently captured wild bird is first acquired, it is particularly important to look for the flies as they suck blood, and just one or two on a small bird may be sufficient to kill it, especially when it is being subjected to the sudden additional stress of living in captivity.

Baker[13] showed that the hippoboscid *Ornithomyia avicularia* can transmit *Trypanosoma avium* of corvid birds in Great Britain, and Benbrook[22] stated that another species, *Pseudolynchia canariensis,* is a vector of *Haemoproteus columbae* to pigeons in North America. *O. avicularia,* in addition to attacking wood pigeons, has also been reported from many species of birds, including the European blackbird (*Turdus merula*) and the chaffinch (*Fringilla coelebs*), and is carried by migrating birds to many parts of the world.

It is quite likely that, as investigations proceed, hippoboscids may well be found to transmit *Haemoproteus* to several species of birds, especially as neither the insects nor the protozoa are markedly host specific.

TREATMENT AND CONTROL

Manual removal of the flies, and periodic inspection in case the bird becomes re-infested. As some species of louse flies breed in birds' nests, old nests should be destroyed and the surroundings cleaned and treated with an insecticide.

Order Mallophaga: The Biting or Chewing Lice

These lice are probably the most common and widespread avian ectoparasites. They are mainly parasites of birds, whereas the sucking lice, Order Siphunculata, are confined to mammals. All lice are small, swiftly moving, wingless insects, with bodies which are flattened dorso-ventrally. Eyes are absent or much reduced, and the legs are short. The Order is usually divided into two main Suborders, namely, Amblycera and Ischnocera. Although the insects are known as biting lice, in actual fact they do not bite the skin of their hosts, the majority having mouthparts especially adapted for chewing and eating epithelial structures such as sloughed-off bits of skin and feathers. Some species, such as *Menacanthus stramineus,* the body louse of domestic fowl, puncture the soft base of young feather quills and ingest the blood which escapes.[45] Infective filariid larvae have been found in one species of bird louse, thus providing additional evidence that some species of Mallophaga feed on the blood of their host.

Non-parasitic book-lice (Order Psocoptera) may occasionally be found on cage birds (*e.g.,* the budgerigar) and in birds' nests, and may lead to confusion if they are not properly examined and identified.

SPECIES AND HOSTS

There are a vast number of different species of avian lice, many of which have not even been described.

Most species are strictly host specific, although a single bird may harbor several different species, sometimes representing more than one genus. Fortunately for the veterinarian, however, most of these species affect their hosts in a similar way and all may be controlled by the same methods. The exact identification of the biting lice is therefore mainly of academic interest, and only those which are usually found on cage and aviary birds are listed and classified below in a simplified form, based on the check list of Hopkins and Clay[82] and the classification of Imms.[88]

CLASSIFICATION AND CHARACTERISTICS

Order   Mallophaga. The Biting or Chewing Lice.

Suborder   Amblycera. Usually not closely adapted to particular habitats on the bird's body. Nearly all are fast runners and not specialized for life on particular feathers.

Family   Menoponidae

Colpocephalum spp. have been reported from 11 Orders of birds, including passerines.[152] *Menacanthus* spp. occur on several Orders of birds, including passerines, for example, the canary (*Serinus canarius*), house sparrow (*Passer domesticus*), and starling (*Sturnus vul-*

garis). *Myrsidea* spp. are also found on passerines, including the canary, house sparrow, and starling.

Eomenopon spp. and *Psittacomenopon* spp. occur on psittacines.

Family   Ricinidae

Ricinus spp. occur on numerous passerines.

Suborder   Ischnocera. Many of these lice are especially adapted to a particular environment, for example, the head and neck, or wings and back. Those on the head and neck are usually out of reach of the bird's beak and therefore are often sluggish parasites, having no need for rapid movement.

Family   Philopteridae

Brüelia spp. are found on passerines, including the canary and house sparrow. *Sturnidoecus* spp. also occur on passerines, including the starling. *Penenirmus* spp. occur on some passerines, and *Philopterus* spp. have been reported from several Orders, including many passerines, for example, the house sparrow. Clay[36] considered that *Docophorus communis*, referred to by Gray[66] on the canary, should be regarded as being a *Philopterus* sp.

Echinophilopterus, Neopsittaconirmus, Psittaconirmus, Psittoecus, and *Paragoniocotes* spp. all occur on psittacines.

DISTRIBUTION AND INCIDENCE

Lice are frequently found on recently captured wild birds in all parts of the world. The heaviest infestations usually occur on birds which are sick or injured,[8,99] especially if they have deformed mandibles, and Ash[8] reported a peak infestation prior to the breeding season in wild birds. Lice are commoner on canaries and other passerines (which are known to harbor at least 14 genera) than on psittacines; lice from budgerigars (which are rarely infested) do not appear to have been described. Hasholt[72] in Denmark, in a survey of diseases of cage birds comprising 1,221 psittacines (1,032 of which were budgerigars), 298 canaries, and 371 other passerines, listed pediculosis in 18 of the passerines but in only 8 of the psittacines. Arnall[6] recorded lice on parrots, but they do not commonly occur on pet birds.

Rothschild and Clay[152] pointed out that the distribution of lice is mainly a host distribution rather than a geographical one, and Meinertzhagen and Clay[130] stated that the proportion of Amblycera to Ischnocera lice tends to be higher on captive than on wild birds, it appearing that Ischnocera are not able to survive so successfully on captive birds.

LIFE HISTORY

The entire life cycle of lice is spent on the host. The eggs, which are often known as nits, are usually attached in clusters to the feathers (Fig. 25-21 A). Within each egg a single nymph develops, which is structurally similar to the adult louse. This first nymph hatches from the egg, feeds and grows, undergoes ecdysis to become the second nymph, which in turn develops similarly to become the third nymph. After a third and final ecdysis, the fourth nymph grows into a sexually mature adult (Fig. 25-21 B and C). The adults can live for several months on the bird, but can survive only a few days away from the host.

CLINICAL SIGNS OF INFESTATION BY BITING LICE

Signs of the presence of biting lice include evidence of irritation, such as restlessness, and continuous preening and ruffling of feathers.

Debility and loss of condition in heavy infestations are often associated with malnutrition or some other disease. Arnall[6] recorded malaise and debility in a parrot due to lice, and Gray[66] reported the parasites to be particularly troublesome in heavily plumaged canaries, such as the Norwich and Lancaster breeds. Even in heavy infestations, however, the plumage does not appear to become damaged.[130]

DIAGNOSIS

Diagnosis is established by discovery of eggs, nymphs, or adults in the feathers. More than one species of louse may be present on a single bird, and the head and vent regions are often attacked, although, as previously stated, some species of lice have a predilection for certain sites to which they are mainly confined; hence the common names of head, fluff, wing, body, or shaft lice applied to different species found on poultry. *Philopterus* spp. found on passerines mainly inhabit the head region.[152]

TREATMENT

As lice do not normally leave the bird and are transmitted from one bird to another by direct contact, such as during mating or when roosting and huddled together in cold weather, it is essential to dust the birds thoroughly and regularly every week with an insecticide powder. When heavy infestations are present, it is also advisable to clean and disinfest the accommodations, paying particular attention to perches and nest boxes. For dusting small birds, Buxton and Busvine[31] recom-

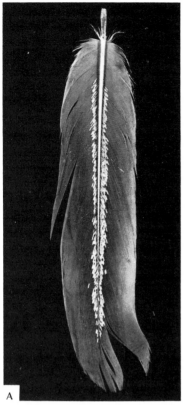
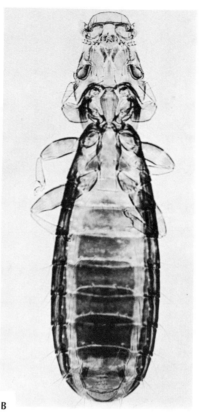
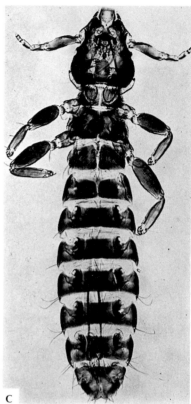

Fig. 25-21. *Louse eggs and adult lice. A. Secondary feather, showing eggs of lice. B. Biting louse,* Ricinus *sp.; example of Suborder Amblycera. C. Biting louse,* Pectinopygus *sp.; example of Suborder Ischnocera. (A, Bradbury, 1952; B and C, Pollen, 1952; all in "Fleas, Flukes and Cuckoos." By courtesy of the Hon. Miriam Rothschild.)*

mended the use of a finely powdered insecticide, such as pyrethrum containing 0.5% pyrethrins. Small species are often very susceptible to the toxic effects of the more persistent types of modern insecticides, and, although D.D.T., for example, may be safe to use for dusting perches, etc., it is inadvisable to use the other insecticides which are now in common use.

Order Hemiptera: Bugs

The insects in this Order that parasitize birds and other animals have mouthparts adapted for piercing the skin and sucking body fluids.

The bugs parasitic on birds belong mainly to the family Cimicidae, the best-known representative of which is the bedbug *Cimex lectularius* (Fig. 25-22). These bugs are flattened dorso-ventrally, and measure 2–5 mm. in length. The color varies according to the species, and may be brownish, yellow, or red. The wings are rudimentary, the pigmented eyes prominent, and the abdomen segmented. The bedbug is provided with stink glands, which give the insect and its surroundings an unpleasant odor.

CLASSIFICATION

The following taxa include some of the bugs that parasitize birds.

Phylum	Arthropoda
Class	Insecta
Order	Hemiptera Bugs
Suborder	Heteroptera
Family	Cimicidae ("Bedbugs" parasitic on mammals and birds.)

Examples: *Cimex* and *Oeciacus*

SPECIES AND HOSTS

Examples: *Cimex lectularius* attacks man and many other mammals, and poultry, and a closely related species, *C. columbarius,* is found on pigeons. *Oeciacus vicarius,* according to Myers,[135] is commonly found in the nests of barn swallows (*Hirundo erythrogaster*), from which it may spread to poultry and undoubtedly also to other species of birds kept in aviaries.

adults are capable of withstanding starvation for at least two months, the adults even for as long as a year. The minimal time from hatching of the nymph from the egg to mature adulthood is said to be about 40 days.

CLINICAL SIGNS OF INFESTATION

Heavy infestations, especially on small or young birds, can cause anemia, and perhaps even death. The bites often produce swelling and irritation, and birds may become restless, especially at night.

DIAGNOSIS

Diagnosis depends on the finding of nymphs or adult parasites on birds or hiding in cracks and crevices of cage or aviary. As these bugs usually feed at night, they are most easily detected at this time, after the birds have been left in the dark for an hour or so.

DIFFERENTIAL DIAGNOSIS. The *Dermanyssus* mites are also nocturnal blood-suckers, but they are considerably smaller than bugs.

TREATMENT

Eradication is extremely difficult, owing to the ability of the bugs to withstand starvation for long periods, and the effective manner in which they conceal themselves when not feeding. Ideally, infested cages and aviaries should be burned, but if this is not practical, then they must be left unoccupied for as long as possible; they should be kept free from vermin which could provide an alternative supply of food, and be fumigated or sprayed very thoroughly with a persistent insecticide such as D.D.T., particular attention being paid to all crevices and cracks. In addition, the birds themselves should be dusted or sprayed with pyrethrum, as recommended for the control of lice and blowflies, respectively.

Order Siphonaptera: Fleas

Fleas are small brownish or black insects with laterally compressed bodies enabling them to run rapidly through the feathers. The adults, although devoid of wings, have well-developed legs and are able to leap considerable distances as well as run. The mouthparts are especially adapted for piercing the skin of their host and for sucking blood.

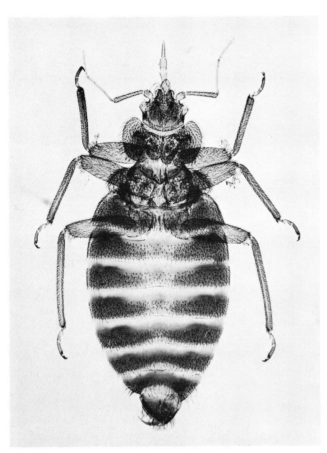

Fig. 25-22. *The bedbug* Cimex lectularius, *approximately X14. (Bradbury, 1952; in "Fleas, Flukes and Cuckoos." By courtesy of the Hon. Miriam Rothschild.)*

DISTRIBUTION AND INCIDENCE

Bugs are most prevalent in temperate and subtropical countries and can be particularly troublesome in artificially heated laboratory animal houses where a variety of animal species are kept. They seldom, however, attack cage and aviary birds, and Rothschild and Clay[152] stated that few wild birds are attacked by bugs because the bugs can survive only if the host is the type which returns to its old nest. The nest must be in a situation where it will remain fairly dry.

LIFE HISTORY

Large numbers of eggs are laid and cemented down in crevices and cracks of the building or cage in which the birds are kept. In the case of *C. lectularius,* the eggs hatch within about 10 days in a warm temperature. The young nymphs which hatch from the eggs resemble the adults, and undergo five molts before reaching maturity. At each stage they feed on the blood of their host, then drop off the bird and hide in crevices to undergo ecdysis. The nymphs and, especially, the

CLASSIFICATION

The following taxa include some of the fleas that parasitize birds.

Phylum	Arthropoda
Class	Insecta
Order	Siphonaptera Fleas
Family	Ceratophyllidae

Examples: *Ceratophyllus* and *Dasypsyllus*

Family   Pulicidae

Example: *Echidnophaga*

SPECIES AND HOSTS

There are several hundred species of fleas, many of which attack birds. Unlike lice and some other types of ectoparasites, fleas are very adaptable and show comparatively little host specificity. Most species prefer a specific host but are quite capable of feeding on animals which are only remotely related. The commonest avian flea, *Ceratophyllus gallinae* (European chicken flea), for instance, will feed not only on domestic poultry but on many species of wild birds and even on man. Probably no species of cage or aviary bird, therefore, is likely to be immune to its attacks. Another important flea is *Echidnophaga gallinacea,* the stick-tight or tropical chicken flea. This flea has perhaps an even wider range of avian and mammalian hosts than has *C. gallinae.*

Owing to the versatility of fleas, there is little point in giving a long list of species and hosts; the following species are some of the common ones which might be encountered, especially in birds in outdoor aviaries.

Dasypsyllus gallinulae mainly attacks passerine birds, especially those which build their nests on or near the ground; *C. gallinae,* on the other hand, prefers nests that are built higher and in dry situations. The situation of the nest, rather than the species of bird to which it belongs, is the important factor and seems to govern the species of flea likely to be found in it. *C. fringillae* may occur on various species of finches and sparrows kept in captivity.[142]

DISTRIBUTION AND INCIDENCE

Fleas are cosmopolitan, although they mainly occur in temperate and tropical climates. *C. gallinae* is found throughout Europe and also in North America, but *E. gallinacea* is chiefly confined to subtropical and tropical areas, being absent from Great Britain and most of Europe.

Fleas only rarely attack cage birds, but domestic poultry or the nests of wild birds near aviaries are potential sources of infection.

LIFE HISTORY

The white, glistening, almost spherical eggs (Fig. 25-23 A) may be laid while the adult is on the host, and fall to the ground; or, as is probably more often the case, they are laid directly in cracks or crevices. Eggs are laid more or less continuously throughout life, but the rate at which they hatch varies with the species of flea, the temperature, and the degree of humidity—dampness being essential for their development. When the egg hatches, a small maggot-like larva (Fig 25-23 B) is released; this feeds on various types of organic matter, including the feces of adult fleas, which are rich in products originating from the blood of the hosts. The larva is yellowish white in color and, although it somewhat resembles a dipterous maggot, it can be identified by the rather chitinous head followed by 13 bristle-bearing segments. The larva feeds and grows, usually molting twice before becoming a white, opaque third-stage larva. This spins a silken cocoon around itself, through which the developing pupa can easily be seen (Fig. 25-23 C). This stage of development may take approximately 2 weeks to 6 months or more, depending on environmental conditions. Similarly, the duration of the pupal stage may vary, sometimes lasting as long as a year. On emerging from the cocoon, the young flea seeks a host, feeds, and reaches maturity within a few days.

CLINICAL SIGNS OF INFESTATION

Evidence of irritation, characterized by periodic ruffling of the feathers and intermittent preening, and blood loss are observed when infestations are heavy, leading eventually to dejection and weakness, especially in young birds.

DIAGNOSIS

Diagnosis depends on identification of the eggs and larvae, which are most likely to be found in nests or nest boxes. The adult fleas are easily recognizable although they are difficult to find on a living bird, and are seldom found on a dead one, since they usually leave the body soon after the bird's death. The adult flea may feed during the day or night, and as it remains on the host for only short periods, examination of a bird's plumage after dark is not such a useful means of detection as when searching for bugs or red mites (*Dermanyssus* spp.).

Unlike other fleas, the adult stick-tight flea (*Echidno-*

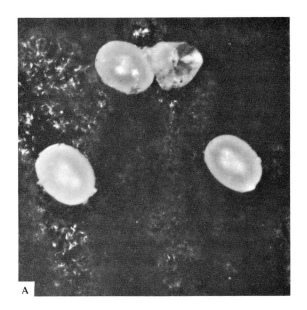

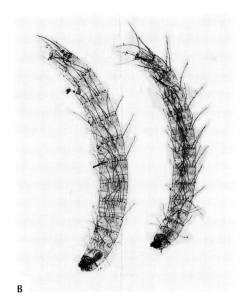

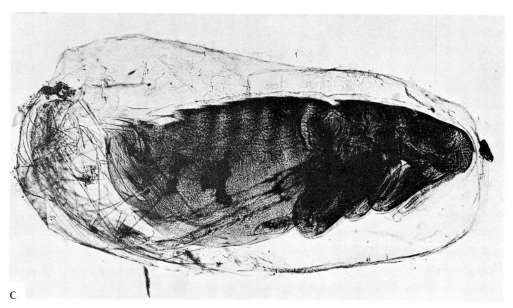

Fig. 25-23. Life cycle of flea. *A. Eggs of flea, X42.5. B. Larvae of flea, approximately X30. C. Pupa within cocoon, X44. (Bradbury, 1952; in ''Fleas, Flukes and Cuckoos.'' By courtesy of the Hon. Miriam Rothschild.)*

phaga) is easily detected on the host because fleas of this species usually attach themselves to the bird's head and form clusters, with the mouthparts deeply embedded in the skin, so that they are difficult to dislodge.

TREATMENT

Similar to that recommended for bugs. In addition, particular attention should be paid to the destruction of all old nests in the vicinity, whether they are those of poultry or of wild birds, or actually in the aviary. Nests in use should also be disinfested if at all possible.

Domestic animals, such as poultry, dogs, and cats, should be kept away from the birds, as they are potential sources of re-infestation.

Order Coleoptera: Beetles

Beetles are mentioned here not because they are important parasites of birds, but simply to remind the reader that numerous species—both adults and larvae—may serve as intermediate hosts for many species of tapeworms and some acanthocephalids. Beetles are commonly eaten by birds, and it is hardly worth while, or even desirable, to attempt eradication of this source of live food, unless there is definite evidence of an outbreak of helminthiasis in which beetles may be playing a rôle as intermediate hosts.

CLASS ARACHNIDA: TICKS AND MITES

Members of the Class Arachnida show considerable variation. A true head and antennae are absent from all arachnids, and the bodies of ticks and mites show no obvious external signs of segmentation. The first and second pairs of appendages, the chelicerae and pedipalps, respectively, are modified for feeding, whereas those of parasitic ticks and mites are especially adapted for sucking blood or tissue fluids and for attaching to their hosts. Also, in ticks and some mites, these mouthparts are borne on a chitinous plate called the capitulum, and collectively these constitute the false head. The nymphs and adults of all arachnids have four pairs of walking legs behind the pedipalps. This Class also contains scorpions, spiders, and marine king-crabs, which are not considered here.

The Subclass Acari includes all the ticks that are relatively large and easily seen with the naked eye, and the much smaller mites which, in cage and aviary birds, are the most important of all types of ectoparasites. The structures at the ends of the legs are of special taxonomic importance in this Subclass. Typically two claws are present on each leg, although the number varies in different species and sometimes on different legs of the same species. In addition to claws, a transparent sucker-like caruncle or pulvillus may be present, and many members of the Family Trombidiformes have a bristle or empodium between the two claws. For details on how to distinguish the many families and genera, the reader should consult a textbook which deals with acarology.

Before ticks and mites are discussed in detail, a simplified and summarized classification will be presented, based on those of Baker and Wharton,[12] Evans et al.,[51] Radford,[144] and Strandtmann and Wharton.[164]

CLASSIFICATION

Class	Arachnida
Subclass	Acari
Order	Metastigmata Ticks
Family	Argasidae. Soft ticks

Examples: *Argas* and *Ornithodoros*

Family   Ixodidae. Hard ticks

Examples: *Haemaphysalis, Ixodes, Boophilus,* and *Hyalomma*

*   *   *   *

Order   Mesostigmata   Mites

(A useful list of hosts for this group is provided by Strandtmann and Wharton.[164])

Family   Laelaptidae (syn. Dermanyssidae). Pathogenic feather mites

Examples: *Dermanyssus* and *Ornithonyssus* (syn. *Liponyssus*) (Radford[144] includes *Protonyssus* in this family.)

Family   Rhinonyssidae. Visceral mites (respiratory system)

Examples: *Sternostoma, Ptilonyssus, Rhinonyssus,* and *Speleognathus* (This genus is placed in the Order Prostigmata, Family Speleognathidae by Baker and Wharton.[12])

*   *   *   *

Order   Prostigmata   Mites

Family   Trombidiidae

Example: *Picobia,* Quill mite.

Family   Trombiculidae. Chiggers, or harvest mites

Example: *Trombicula*

Family   Cheyletidae

Example: *Neocheyletiella,* Mange mite.

Family   Myobiidae. Quill and feather follicle mites

Examples: *Syringophilus* and *Harpyrhynchus* (syn. *Sarcopterinus*)

*   *   *   *

Order   Astigmata   Mites

Family   Analgesidae.*   Non-pathogenic feather mites

Examples: *Analges, Mesalges, Megninia, Diplaegidia, Protonyssus, Protalges,* and *Pteronyssoides*

Family   Dermoglyphidae.* Feather and quill mites

*There is disagreement among some taxonomists regarding the members of these two families—Analgesidae and Dermoglyphidae. Radford[144] recognized the family Falculiferidae and placed in it the genera *Dermoglyphus, Sphaerogastra,* and *Trouessartia.*

Examples: *Dermoglyphus, Falculifer, Protolichus, Pteronyssus, Pseudalloptes, Pterolichus,* and *Kramerella*

Family Proctophyllodidae. Feather mites

Examples: *Pterophagus* and *Proctophyllodes*

Family Heteropsoridae. Skin mites

Example: *Heteropsorus*

Family Epidermoptidae[53a] Mange, skin, and feather mites

Examples: *Epidermoptes, Microlichus, Dermatophagoides, Rivoltasia,* and *Myiales*

Family Laminosioptidae. Subcutaneous mites

Example: *Laminosioptes*

Family Cytoditidae (syn. Cytoleichidae). Visceral mites

Example: *Cytodites* (syn. *Cytoleichus*)

Family Sarcoptidae. Mange mites

Example: *Cnemidocoptes* (syn. *Knemidocoptes*)

Family Acaridae. Forage mites

Examples: *Tyroglyphus* and *Tyrophagus*

Family Glycyphagidae. Forage mites

Example: *Glycyphagus*

Ticks

All members of the order Metastigmata are parasitic and are easily recognized as relatively large, bean-shaped parasites which appear flat when unfed but become distended when engorged with the blood of their host. They are most conspicuous when engorged and attached to the host.

Birds are attacked mainly by soft ticks. These can be recognized by their fairly soft and leathery cuticle, which in some species bears raised, small tubercles, called mammillae. The bodies of hard ticks lack these tubercles, the cuticle being harder and more rigid. Members of the Family Ixodidae are easily distinguished from the Argasidae by their possession of a shieldlike chitinous plate on the dorsal surface.

Argas persicus is the vector of the poultry piroplasm,

Aegyptianella pullorum, but the tick vectors of other species of *Aegyptianella* are unknown.

SPECIES AND HOSTS

Few species of ticks are host specific, so that all species of birds kept in captivity are susceptible to attack. *Argas persicus,* the fowl tick, occurs on all types of domestic poultry, pigeons, canaries, and various species of wild birds and man. Although Rothschild and Clay[152] stated that *A. reflexus* of the pigeon is the best-known example of the Argasidae in Great Britain, various species of *Ornithodoros* and the hard ticks *Haemaphysalis, Ixodes,* and *Hyalomma* occur on wild birds. *Ixodes ricinus* (Fig. 25-24), the well-known sheep tick, attacks many species of birds, particularly passerines, as well as domestic animals and man.

DISTRIBUTION AND INCIDENCE

Ticks have a worldwide distribution, the most important bird tick, *Argas persicus,* being found in many tropical and temperate regions, including North America. *Ixodes ricinus* covers a wider area, also being found in North America, in many European countries, including Great Britain, and in parts of Asia.

In spite of the wide distribution of these species and many other bird ticks, they are not important parasites of birds. They are most likely to be encountered in recently captured wild birds and outdoor aviary birds, especially those kept near sheep pastures or free-ranging poultry.

LIFE HISTORY

The life cycle is basically the same in all species. The soft ticks lay hundreds or even thousands of eggs at a time, and remain in the habitation (*e.g.,* the nest) of the host, usually engorging rapidly on the bird at night. Hard ticks, however, lay only a few eggs, at intervals, wander, and depend on chance meetings with the host, on which they feed for extended periods.

Following copulation, the male tick dies, and the female engorges with blood and then drops from the host. After a pre-oviposition period, the eggs are laid, usually near the ground, on soil, in humus or litter. When egg laying is completed, the female dies. Minute, six-legged larvae hatch from the eggs after a variable incubation period, and then, following a feed of blood on a suitable host, they molt and emerge as eight-legged nymphs superficially resembling the adults. After a further blood meal and molt, they become mature

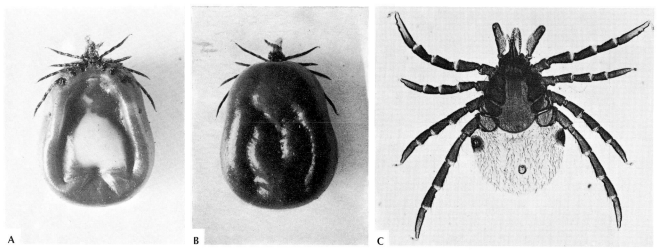

A   B   C

Fig. 25-24. *The sheep tick* Ixodes ricinus. *Engorged adult and nymph. A. Adult; ventral surface. X5. B. Adult; dorsal surface. X5. C. Nymph; ventral surface. X12. (A and B, Tams. C, Barron, 1952; in ''Fleas, Flukes and Cuckoos.'' By courtesy of the Hon. Miriam Rothschild.)*

adults or there may be another nymphal instar before maturity is reached.

With some ticks, for example *Ixodes* spp., each phase of the life history requires a separate host; such ticks are known as three-host ticks. The larvae and nymph of a two-host tick, for example, *Hyalomma* spp., feed and molt on the same host, but the adult feeds on another. With one-host ticks, for example, *Boophilus* spp., all three stages feed and molt on the same host.

The length of the cycle, which may in some cases be as much as two years, varies considerably and depends on the species of tick, and on the availability of hosts and the climatic conditions.

CLINICAL SIGNS OF INFESTATION

Loss of blood can result in the death of small species and young birds, especially if more than one tick is present, and the parasites also frequently cause irritation. According to Rothschild and Clay,[152] the saliva which is poured into the host's flesh can be highly toxic, and the eggs contain poisonous substances which may prove fatal, whereas blindness sometimes follows attachment of the ticks near the eye.

DIAGNOSIS

Diagnosis is established by the discovery of larval, nymphal (Fig. 25-24 C), or adult (Fig. 25-24 A and B) stages on any part of the bird, although they are usually found near the beak or the eye.

TREATMENT

Individual ticks may be removed by applying alcohol to the parasite, then pulling suddenly, while at the same time levering the tick away from the skin, preferably with fine-pointed curved forceps. Care must be taken, however, to ensure that the mouthparts are not left embedded in the skin.

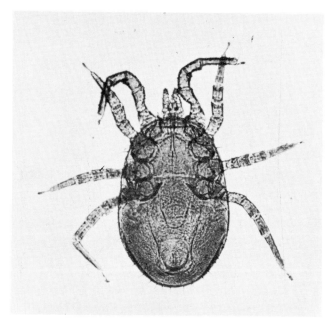

Fig. 25-25. Dermanyssus gallinae. *Ventral view of mite, showing the anus situated on the posterior half of the anal plate. In* Ornithonyssus sylviarum *the anus is situated on the anterior half of this plate. This picture is greatly enlarged;* Dermanyssus, *like* Ornithonyssus, *is approximately 1 mm. long. (Courtesy of W. P. Beresford-Jones.)*

If heavy infestations should occur in an aviary, more drastic measures are necessary, such as those recommended for the control of bugs.

Mites

Owing to the fact that different mites which inhabit the same areas of the host's body may belong to different Orders and exhibit no close taxonomic relationship, it is easier to deal with them according to their normal habitat and effect upon the host, rather than on the basis of their taxonomic classification. They will therefore be considered as listed below.

(1) pathogenic feather mites;
(2) non-pathogenic feather mites;
(3) quill and feather follicle mites;
(4) mange and skin mites;
(5) subcutaneous mites;
(6) visceral mites;
(7) chiggers, or harvest mites;
(8) forage mites.

Pathogenic Feather Mites

Pathogenic feather mites include some of the most important and most pathogenic ectoparasites found on cage and aviary birds, the best known being *Dermanyssus gallinae,* the red mite, and *Ornithonyssus sylviarum* (syn. *Liponyssus sylviarum*), the Northern fowl mite.

The bodies of these mites are flattened dorso-ventrally, and are roughly ovoid or circular in outline (Fig. 25-25). To the naked eye, mites of both genera appear as tiny, rapidly moving, greyish white specks, about 1 mm.

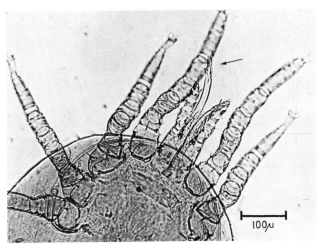

Fig. 25-26. Ornithonyssus sylviarum *mite, showing the relatively short pincer-like chelicerae which are present in both sexes. (Courtesy of T. Dennett.)*

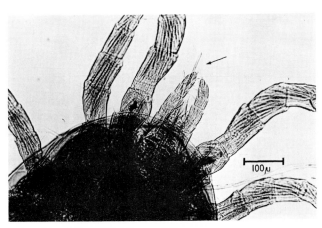

Fig. 25-27. *Female* Dermanyssus gallinae *mite, showing the long, pointed chelicerae. (Courtesy of W. P. Beresford-Jones.)*

long. After a blood meal, they appear reddish in color. Microscopically, *Dermanyssus* can be distinguished from *Ornithonyssus* by the possession of a large dorsal shield with a rounded posterior end, that of *Ornithonyssus* being smaller and the posterior end being tapered and not rounded. The chelicerae are pincer-like in *Ornithonyssus* mites of both sexes (Fig. 25-26), whereas in *Dermanyssus* those of the females are pointed, like needles (Fig. 25-27).

Dermanyssus spp.

D. gallinae transmits *Lankesterella garnhami* infection to house sparrows and canaries,[103] and according to Macfie and Thomson[116] and Manwell and Johnson[122] there is strong evidence that the mites may also transmit trypanosomes to canaries.

The virus of eastern equine encephalomyelitis (E.E.E.) has also been isolated from the mites by Howitt *et al.*[83]

SPECIES AND HOSTS

D. gallinae, the red mite of domestic poultry, is the best known mite in this genus. In addition to poultry, it also attacks canaries, budgerigars, pigeons, and many species of wild birds, including house sparrows and starlings; therefore, virtually all species of cage and aviary birds are potential victims. The closely related species, *D. passerinus,* occurs on the house sparrow, greenfinch (*Chloris chloris*), and other passerines.

DISTRIBUTION AND INCIDENCE

D. gallinae is practically world wide in distribution, and a common parasite of the domestic fowl and canary, but it appears to be less frequently found on pigeons and budgerigars.

LIFE HISTORY

D. gallinae does not breed on its host, but lays its eggs in cracks and crevices of the cage or nest boxes.

The female lays eggs 12 to 24 hours after her first blood meal, and when the temperature is warm these may hatch within 48 to 72 hours, producing the six-legged larvae. The larvae do not feed, but molt after 24 to 48 hours, becoming first-stage nymphs with eight legs. These nymphs, however, do require a blood meal before molting to become second-stage nymphs, which also feed and soon after become adult mites. Under optimal conditions the whole cycle can be completed in only one week, and adults can survive for several months without feeding.

CLINICAL SIGNS OF INFESTATION

Clinical signs include restlessness at night caused by irritation. Infestations are often heavy, so that anemia usually occurs, frequently resulting in the death of young birds, and of small species, such as canaries.

DIAGNOSIS

Diagnosis is established by discovery of nymphs or adults in the plumage, or larvae, nymphs, or adults in the cage or aviary. Both the nymphs and adults are nocturnal feeders, and leave the host after a meal, so that they are most easily detected on the bird after dark. A useful method of detecting the mites in a cage bird is to cover the cage at night with a white cloth; if mites are present, they will normally be found quite easily in the morning on the under surface of the cloth. Favorite haunts of the parasite are in the cracks of nest boxes and beneath the bottom of the cage, especially between the base and the sliding sand tray, if one is present.

TREATMENT

As the parasites seldom attack their hosts during the day, the birds should be removed from their quarters, which should be very thoroughly cleaned and scalded with boiling water or washed with a 5% solution of washing soda, special attention being paid to all cracks and crevices where the parasites might hide. This should be followed by spraying with gamma benzene hexachloride, with the entire procedure repeated at 10-day intervals until the mites have been eradicated.

It should be unnecessary normally to treat the birds themselves if the above measures are taken during the day time. If mites are found on the birds, then the birds should be dusted with an insecticide as recommended for lice.

POSTMORTEM FINDINGS

The carcass is obviously anemic, and ingested mites can often be found in the crop and sometimes in the trachea.

Ornithonyssus (syn. Liponyssus) spp.

SPECIES AND HOSTS

Ornithonyssus sylviarum is the best-known species and according to Benbrook[22] has been reported from 22 species of birds, including domestic poultry and house sparrows. Reeves *et al.*[147] reported isolation of western equine encephalomyelitis (W.E.E.) virus from these mites found in the nest of a wild yellow-headed blackbird (*Xanthocephalus xanthocephalus*). Baker *et al.*[16] thought that *O. sylviarum* may also transmit *Lankesterella corvi* infection of rooks (*Corvus frugilegus*).

O. bursa, the tropical feather mite, is a very closely related species, occurring on poultry, pigeons, sparrows, mynah birds,[11] and canaries.[164] Benbrook[22] stated that this mite carries W.E.E. virus, as shown by Sulkin and Izumi,[165] who found the parasites in a house sparrow's nest.

DISTRIBUTION AND INCIDENCE

O. sylviarum is a widespread species occurring in North America, Europe (including Great Britain), and some subtropical countries. It does not appear to be as common on cage birds as *D. gallinae,* although Swierstra *et al.*[166] recorded it from the Netherlands in a cardinal (*Richmondena cardinalis*) kept in a zoo.

O. bursa is also found in North America and occurs in Africa, China, India, and South America.

LIFE HISTORY

The life cycle of *O. sylviarum* differs from the life cycles of *O. bursa* and *Dermanyssus* in that all stages, including egg laying, may actually take place on the host; in other respects it is similar to that described for *D. gallinae.* According to Baker *et al.,*[11] *O. bursa* can only survive for about 10 days away from the host.

CLINICAL SIGNS OF INFESTATION

Similar to those of *Dermanyssus,* although often more severe, as nymphs and adults cause constant irritation and feed both day and night.

DIAGNOSIS

The eggs, larvae, nymphs, and adults of *O. sylviarum* may be found on the host at any time, and, like *D. gallinae,* when the bird is handled they usually transfer themselves rapidly to the examiner's hands and arms.

TREATMENT

Accommodations should be disinfested as described for *Dermanyssus,* and the birds treated as recommended for lice. It may, however, be necessary to use a more potent parasiticide, such as gamma benzene hexachloride, on the birds. Owing to the risk of toxicity to some small birds, it should be used sparingly and with care, in the form of a powder not exceeding 0.2% of the active principle.[47]

Non-pathogenic Feather Mites

SPECIES AND HOSTS

Non-pathogenic feather mites belong to the families Analgesidae, Dermoglyphidae, Proctophyllodidae, and Epidermoptidae, which contain a large number of species found on a very wide range of avian hosts.

Accurate identification of many feather mites is difficult and beyond the scope of this book; for lists of hosts of the numerous species, the reader should consult Radford,[144] who stated that *Diplaegidia columbae* occurs on the canary, *Protolichus lunula* and *Kramerella lunula* on the budgerigar, and species of *Protonyssus, Protalges* (Figs. 25-28, 25-29), *Protolichus, Pterolichus, Pseudalloptes,* and *Mesalges* on a variety of psittacines, such as macaws, parrots, lorikeets, and various parakeets. The canary, according to Lesbouyries,[110] is also a host for *Analges passerinus, Proctophyllodes glandarinus,* and *Megninia columbae.* Radford[144] also listed *Megninia* and *Proctophyllodes* species on passerine birds, and *Rivoltasia dermicola* on house sparrows.

Some species, such as *Kramerella lunula* of the budgerigar, are stated to be host specific, but many are not.

DISTRIBUTION AND INCIDENCE

These types of mites are widespread and relatively common, especially on wild birds or on captive birds kept in overcrowded conditions.

LIFE HISTORY

For many species the life cycle is unknown, although Baker *et al.*[11] described briefly that of *Megninia,*

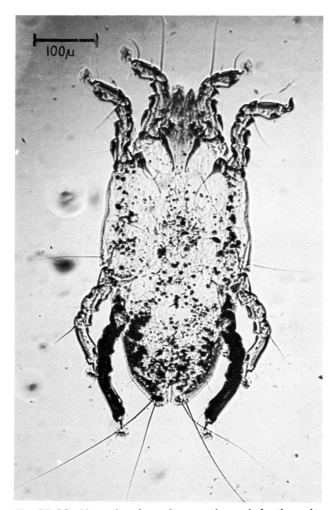

Fig. 25-28. *Ventral surface of non-pathogenic feather mite of the genus* Protalges. *(Courtesy of T. Dennett.)*

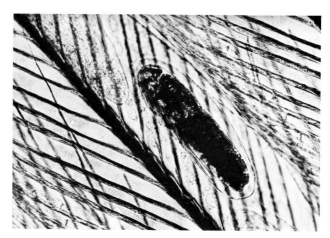

Fig. 25-29. *Egg of non-pathogenic feather mite (Protalges sp.) in feather of splendid parakeet (Neophema splendida). These eggs are much smaller than those of lice (see Fig. 25-21). X216. (Courtesy of T. Dennett.)*

Falculifer, Pterolichus, and *Pterophagus,* stating that either eggs or live larvae may be produced and that in some species the eggs are attached to the feather barbs. At least two nymphal stages occur before the adult is produced.

CLINICAL SIGNS OF INFESTATION

According to Evans *et al.*[50] the analgesid mites show a certain degree of micro-habitat specificity. The majority of species occur on quill feathers, the contour feathers supporting smaller populations. Species of *Analges* and also the epidermoptid mite *Rivoltasia* inhabit the downy proximal part of the quill feathers; according to Baker *et al.*[11] *Megninia* spp. are usually found on down and contour feathers, although they may occasionally infest feathers of the tail and wings. The mites may be active when disturbed, but normally move about very little.

Study of the mouthparts indicates that the mites do not feed on blood or sebaceous fluids; Evans *et al.*[51] stated that analgesids are predominantly scavengers feeding on feather fragments, desquamated cells from the skin, and oily substances derived from the preen, or uropygial, gland. Their feeding habits, and the fact that the mites are mainly confined to the actual feathers, indicate therefore that they are harmless, except in extremely heavy infestations, when they may cause some irritation.

DIAGNOSIS

Presence of mites in the plumage.

TREATMENT

If treatment should prove necessary, that recommended for lice would probably be effective.

Quill and Feather Follicle Mites

Quill and feather follicle mites are all very small mites, having elongated bodies especially adapted for living inside feathers.

SPECIES AND HOSTS

The two best-known quill mites are *Syringophilus bipectinatus,* which attacks the domestic fowl, other gallinaceous birds, canaries, and various other passerines and pigeons, and *Dermoglyphus elongatus,* which also enters the feathers of the domestic fowl and has been recorded in the canary and other small passerines.

Coffin[40] stated that *Syringophilus* species may be found on parrots; according to Lapage[104] *S. columbae* occurs on pigeons. *Dermoglyphus* species may attack budgerigars,[142] and *D. paradoxus* is also listed by Radford[144] as occurring in the mealy amazon parrot (*Amazona farinosa farinosa*).

Lesbouyries[110] stated that *Picobia bipectinata* attacks the skin and especially the feather quills of the canary.

Harpyrhynchus nidulans has been reported from the hawfinch (*Coccothraustes coccothraustes*) by Macdonald[115] and also occurs on other passerines.

DISTRIBUTION AND INCIDENCE

Quill mites are of widespread occurrence and appear to be encountered more frequently in canaries than in other species of cage birds.

LIFE HISTORY

Very little appears to be known about the life cycle of quill mites, although Baker *et al.*[11] stated that all stages occur in the feather quills.

CLINICAL SIGNS OF INFESTATION

Benbrook[22] stated that *Syringophilus* mites appear to cause complete or partial loss of feathers, and that the quill stumps that remain contain the mites in a powdery material.

Dermoglyphus spp., however, may be more pathogenic than *Syringophilus,* as Pillers[142] found that they caused considerable irritation to budgerigars during molting; Wehr[173] described clinical signs in canaries attributed to *D. elongatus,* characterized by irritation with considerable loss of feathers, especially on the back near the base of the tail and on parts of the wings.

Macdonald[115] described a large spherical cyst, 7 mm. in diameter, containing feather debris and numerous *Harpyrhynchus nidulans* mites on the skin of a hawfinch, and Ward *et al.*[171] described skin tumors in a lanceolated warbler (*Locustella lanceolata*), which they attributed to *Harpyrhynchus* mites.

DIAGNOSIS

Diagnosis depends on clinical signs, associated with the presence of mites in the powdery material of broken quills, or in dermal cysts or tumors. The mites can be detected with the aid of a magnifying glass.

Wehr[173] stated that *D. elongatus* is not found on the skin and feathers or in the quills of fully formed feathers. However, if the contents of the interior of the quills of underdeveloped feathers (so-called "pinfeathers") are expressed or teased out with needles, the elongate, slowly wriggling mites are easily observed embedded in the gelatinous, reddish brown material. Wehr stated that as many as 16 mites may be found in one quill. Radford[144] pointed out that the mites are invariably found in the quill some distance above the skin and not in the tip below the skin.

Diagnosis should not be made without the aid of a magnifying glass or a low-power microscope, because the blood at the base of a feather quill may otherwise easily be mistaken for mites.

TREATMENT

No satisfactory treatment is known, and in severe cases of infestation it may be necessary to destroy the bird.

Most of the species of quill mites do not appear to be particularly host specific; therefore, as with many other parasitic diseases, poultry and wild birds are a potential source of infection, and aviary birds should be protected from contact with them.

Mange and Skin Mites

Most mange and skin mites can be divided into two main groups: the epidermoptic mange and skin mites, and the better known cnemidocoptic mites which are related to the sarcoptic and notoedric mange mites of man and domestic animals. Mites in the Family Heteropsoridae were also recorded once from the skin of passerine birds in Europe.[12]

Epidermoptic Mites

Lapage[104] stated that epidermoptic mites are always very small, not more than 0.4 mm. long. The bodies are soft, somewhat flattened, and roughly circular in outline.

SPECIES AND HOSTS

Epidermoptes bilobatus has been reported from the domestic fowl[12] and the canary.[63] *Microlichus avus* also occurs on the canary,[74] the house sparrow,[144] and the starling.[99] A heavy infestation of *Myialges* species has been found on a wild blue tit (*Parus caeruleus*) by Macdonald.[115] The same mite was also found on the Pekin robin (*Leiothrix lutea*) by Evans *et al.,*[51] who named it *M. macdonaldi.*

DISTRIBUTION AND INCIDENCE

E. bilobatus has been recorded from Europe and North and South America, *M. avus* from France, Great Britain, and North America, and *Myialges* from Great Britain and Belgium.

LIFE HISTORY

Very little is known about the life cycle of most of these mites, but probably all stages occur on the host.

Hippoboscid flies have been shown by Henry and Guilhon to carry *Microlichus* and *Myialges* spp. mechanically on their wings, and Evans *et al.*[50] found stages of *Myialges macdonaldi* on two different species of hippoboscids.

CLINICAL SIGNS OF INFESTATION

E. bilobatus and *Rivoltasia bifurcata,* when present in the skin, may or may not cause lesions; when lesions do occur, they are characterized at first by a fine scaly dermatitis, which is followed by the formation of thick brownish scabs of sloughed-off epithelial tissue.[22] Gelor-

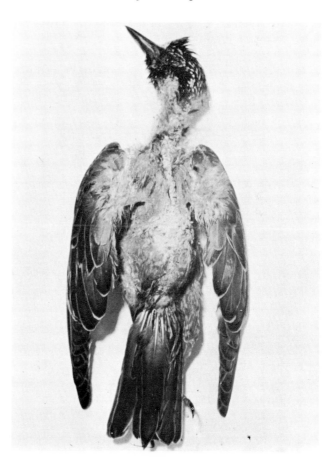

Fig. 25-30. *Starling* (Sturnus vulgaris), *showing skin lesions on the back associated with the epidermoptic mites* Microlichus avus. *The feathers have been removed to show the lesions. (I. F. Keymer et al., 1962, Vet. Rec. Crown Copyright. By permission of the Controller of Her Majesty's Stationery Office.)*

mini and Roveda[63] recorded similar lesions in canaries infested with *E. bilobatus.* Neveu-Lemaire[138] has suggested that severe lesions may be partly due to a concomitant fungal infection.

M. avus also produces similar lesions of depluming mange, with loss of feathers from the neck, throat, chest, and shoulders. Crater-like lesions around the feather roots occur, with formation of scales on the epidermis, as described in the canary by Henry and Guilhon[74] and in the starling by Keymer *et al.*[99] (Fig. 25-30).

The lesions of mange caused by *Myialges macdonaldi* are described as ruffled plumage, loss of feathers, and scaly white thickened areas of skin at the base of the beak and over the eyelids and abdomen.

DIAGNOSIS

Diagnosis rests on appearance of skin lesions associated with the presence of mites. All stages of *Microlichus avus* and *Myialges macdonaldi* may be found associated with the lesions. Keymer *et al.*[99] had little trouble in finding *M. avus* on microscopical examination of cleared skin scrapings.

DIFFERENTIAL DIAGNOSIS. Cnemidocoptic mange and depluming mange due to *Neocheyletiella* spp. or dermatomycosis.

TREATMENT

Treatment described for cnemidocoptic mange should prove satisfactory.

Cnemidocoptic Mites

Mites of the species *Cnemidocoptes pilae* (Fig. 25-31) are responsible for the so-called scaly face and scaly leg disease of budgerigars, which is probably one of the best known of all cage-bird diseases, and until a

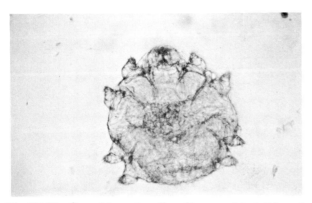

Fig. 25-31. Cnemidocoptes pilae. *Non-gravid adult female. X125. (D. K. Blackmore: Vet. Rec. 75:592, 1963.)*

few years ago was considered by bird fanciers to be caused by a fungus.

SPECIES AND HOSTS

C. pilae, although predominantly a parasite of the budgerigar, has also been reported from the Alexandrian parakeet (*Psittacula nipalensis*)[139] and the canary.[6] *C. mutans,* the cause of scaly leg in domestic fowls, has obviously been confused in the past with *C. pilae,* and early reports of its causing scaly leg disease in canaries should be treated with some skepticism, especially, as pointed out by Lavoipierre and Griffiths,[106] in the case described by Kaschula.[92]

Other species have also been described, for example, *C. jamaicensis* of the golden thrush (*Turdus aurantiacus*) by Turk,[168] and *C. fossor* from the white-headed munia (*Munia maja*), one of the Malaccan weaver birds.[49]

DISTRIBUTION AND INCIDENCE

Cnemidocoptic mites are undoubtedly world-wide in distribution, it being definitely known that *C. pilae* occurs in various parts of Europe (including Great Britain), North America, South Africa, and Australia.

Little is known of the incidence of the various species, with the exception of *C. pilae,* which is very common in budgerigars.

LIFE HISTORY

The life history of *Cnemidocoptes* is not accurately known, but the parasite apparently develops entirely within the skin of the host, while feeding on keratin,[179] and the method of transmission from one host to another is obscure. Wichmann and Vincent[178] suggested that nestling budgerigars contracted the infection from their parents, but Blackmore[28] found no evidence to support this theory.

In skin scrapings ova, larvae (Fig. 25-32), nymphs, and adults can all be found readily, but males are found much more rarely than females.[28]

CLINICAL SIGNS OF INFESTATION

SCALY FACE AND SCALY LEG DISEASE OF BUDGERIGARS (C. PILAE). Lesions have been described by several workers, but in most detail by Arnall.[5,7] Birds of both sexes and all ages may be affected, and some are infected without showing obvious lesions. In the early stages, lesions are usually confined to the region of the cere and base of the beak, at first appearing simply as a beige bloom, whereas later whitish, scaly

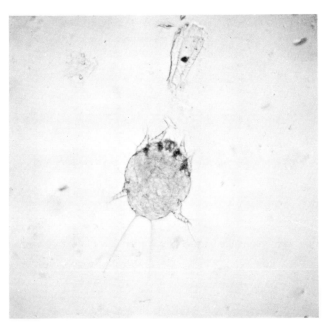

Fig. 25-32. Cnemidocoptes pilae. *Larva.* ×125. *(Courtesy of D. K. Blackmore.)*

epithelial proliferations develop. These form raised, thickened, yellowish, crater-like encrustations, in which can be seen minute holes caused by the mites burrowing into the keratinized epithelium and forming contiguous tunnels beneath the surface of the lesions (Fig. 25-33). In advanced cases there is interference with growth of the beak, especially the upper mandible, which eventually results in deformity (Fig. 25-34), and the commissures of the mouth may also show lesions. Lesions similar to those described above may also occur on the legs, feet, and the skin on almost any part of the body, but particularly around the eyes and vent. In chronic cases affecting the face, horny protuberances (Fig. 25-35), as much as 1 cm. long, sometimes develop.

Pruritus is seldom a marked feature, and when the feet are affected lameness is usually noticed only in advanced chronic cases, when the nail "beds" may become swollen and the claws displaced and twisted. Yunker and Ishak[179] pointed out, however, that in early cases of foot involvement there are no obvious gross lesions.

C. pilae infestation in the parakeet *Psittacula nipalensis* described by Oldham and Beresford-Jones,[139] unlike that typically occurring in the budgerigar, was associated with feather picking and loss of feathers around the neck, and on the ventral and dorsal aspects

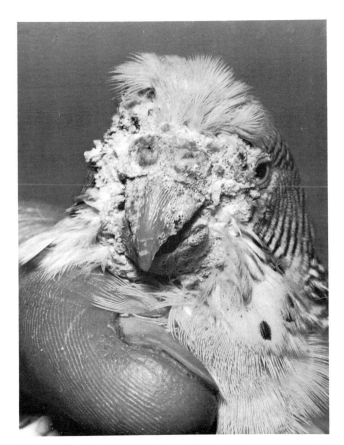

Fig. 25-33. *Head of budgerigar* (Melopsittacus undulatus), *showing typical extensive and advanced lesions of scaly face caused by* Cnemidocoptes pilae. *(Courtesy of L. Arnall.)*

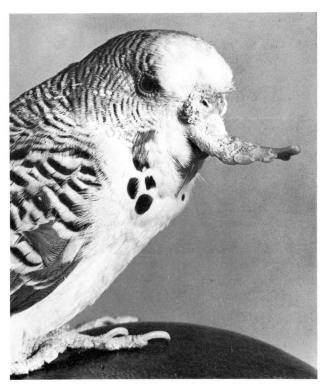

Fig. 25-34. *Budgerigar* (Melopsittacus undulatus), *with malformation of the beak associated with infestation with* Cnemidocoptes pilae. *(Arnall: Vet. Rec. 73:1146, 1956.)*

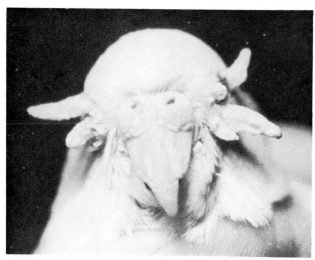

Fig. 25-35. *Head of budgerigar* (Melopsittacus undulatus), *showing bizarre horny growths arising from the skin, between the commissures of the mouth and the external auditory meatus. The upper mandible is broad and poorly arched. The lesions are believed to be caused by* Cnemidocoptes pilae. *(Arnall: J. small anim. Pract. 6:135, 1965.)*

of the body. Dermatitis and feather picking are common in caged psittacines, and it is possible that more cases may be due to the mite than is generally realized.

SCALY LEG DISEASE OF CANARIES. This disease has been known for many years by canary breeders and,

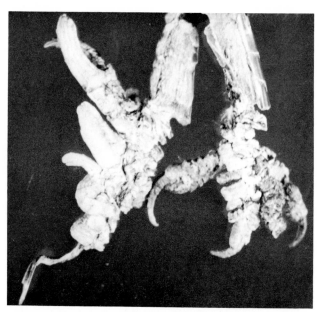

Fig. 25-36. *Lesions of pelvic limbs of red-winged blackbird* (Agelaius phoeniceus) *due to cnemidocoptic mite infestation. (Kirmse: Bulletin of Widlife Disease Association 2:89, 1966.)*

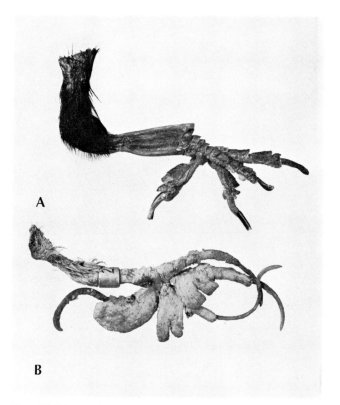

Fig. 25-37. *Lesions of pelvic limb of birds. A. The foot of a scarlet tanager* (Ramphocelus brasilius), *showing proliferation of the scales of the digits and tarsometatarsus. The lesions are common in old passerine birds and are not parasitic in origin. B. The foot of a goldfinch* (Carduelis carduelis), *showing typical advanced lesions of* Cnemidocoptes *infestation, the so-called "tassle-foot." Note the grossly distorted and overgrown nails. (Courtesy of T. Dennett.)*

as stated above, it is probably caused more often by *C. pilae* than by *C. mutans.* Lesions in canaries are usually confined to the legs and, more particularly, to the digits, a condition which Kaschula[92] referred to as "tassle-foot" (Fig. 25-36 and Fig. 25-37 B). The lesions differ from those seen in the budgerigar by commencing as crusts which form on the plantar surfaces of the feet and gradually get thicker. According to Kaschula,[92] the considerable flexion and mobility of the joints results in division of the encrustations into segments corresponding to the different segments of each digit, and this eventually leads to the formation of long tassle-like scabs extending the length of the toes. Marked lameness results, and the bird is also unable to perch comfortably.

Although the pathogenic effects of *C. pilae, C. mutans,* and *C. gallinae* of poultry are well known, all species of *Cnemidocoptes* produce scab-like formations on the bills and legs of birds, according to Turk.[168]

HISTOPATHOLOGY

Yunker and Ishak[179] described in detail the histopathology of cnemidocoptic mange in budgerigars, showing that the mites invade feather follicles, skin folds, and the epidermis by direct penetration, causing pouch-like cavities and also producing secondary pouches, resulting in a lesion "honeycombed" by many cavities.

Blackmore[28] found that *C. pilae* mites occur in the deeper layers of the *stratum corneum*, causing hyperkeratosis, sloughing of superficial keratin, and a certain degree of acanthosis.

DIAGNOSIS

In advanced cases in budgerigars, the lesions caused by *C. pilae* are so characteristic that a diagnosis can safely be made on the macroscopical appearance alone. In other species of birds, and in suspected early infections in budgerigars, however, liberal skin scrapings should be taken and crushed in 10% potassium hydroxide solution, in order to clear the material and make it suitable for microscopical examination. If the mites are present, they are easily recognized, although a fairly prolonged search is necessary in some cases. Differentiation of the different species, however, can be difficult, but according to Lavoipierre and Griffiths[106] *C. pilae* can be distinguished from *C. mutans* mainly by its smaller size and a relatively more heavily chitinized dorsal shield with distinct edges. The edges of the shield in *C. mutans* are indistinct, and the anterior part of the shield is devoid of the minute punctiform dots which completely cover the shield of *C. pilae*.

DIFFERENTIAL DIAGNOSIS. In budgerigars, the condition may occasionally be confused with carcinoma of the cere and beak.[7]

Skin lesions in birds other than the budgerigar may be confused with those caused by epidermoptic mites, species of *Neocheyletiella* mites, or dermatophytes. Lesions on the eyelids or feet can also be confused with passerine pox or papillomas, as pointed out by Keymer and Blackmore.[98]

Proliferation of the scales of the feet, which accompanies aging in passerine birds (Fig. 25-37 A), should not be confused with lesions produced by mites (Fig. 25-37 B).

TREATMENT

Wichmann and Vincent[178] discussed treatment of budgerigars with *N*-ethyl-*o*-crotonotoluidide or 25% emulsion of benzyl benzoate. These preparations were effective and apparently were non-toxic. Benoit,[26] however, successfully treated the disease in budgerigars with 0.2% gamma benzene hexachloride in soft paraffin and arachis oil. As there is a danger of this parasiticide being toxic to some species of small birds if used in a concentration greater than 0.02%, and there is a similar risk with high concentrations of benzyl benzoate, it is probably safer to use benzyl benzoate in the form of a 10% emulsion as recommended by Dall *et al.*[47] Before application of the parasiticide, the encrustations should be softened with arachis oil or soft paraffin and carefully removed. The benzyl benzoate should be applied daily for three days and then again once, seven days later. A further course of treatment can be given if necessary.

A very effective and non-toxic preparation for treatment of cnemidocoptic mange is Dettol,* a product which depends on *p*-chloro-sym-M-xylenol and terpineol for its acaricidal action.[9] It may be used on budgerigars and canaries. The recommended dilution is 10% (50 drops of Dettol to 1 oz. of water). This solution is applied with a cotton swab and allowed to penetrate and soften the crusts for a few minutes. Some of the crusts can be removed by gentle rotation of the swab at the first treatment. Daily treatment for a week or two should be sufficient for a cure.[9] As Arnall[7] pointed out, however, treatment is not likely to reverse the pathological changes in chronic cases.

Mites of the Genus Neocheyletiella

These appear to be the only trombidiform mites which have been reported to cause depluming mange in birds.

SPECIES AND HOSTS

Guilhon *et al.*[68] recorded *Neocheyletiella* spp. infecting eight canaries, five of which were of the crested variety, and a Pekin robin (*Leiothrix lutea*). They believed that the canaries contracted the infection from the nightingale.

DISTRIBUTION AND INCIDENCE

An outbreak of the disease in France, reported by Guilhon *et al.*,[68] appears to be the only outbreak on record.

LIFE HISTORY

Apparently unknown.

*Dettol—R. T. French Co., Rochester, N.Y.

CLINICAL SIGNS OF INFESTATION

Guilhon *et al.*[68] described loss of feathers from the neck, back, and especially from the head; also ruffled plumage and irritation of the skin. There was hyperkeratinization of the skin, particularly on the lateral and posterior aspects of the body, where the feathers are less numerous, the skin being covered with greyish white scales.

DIAGNOSIS

Diagnosis is based on the skin lesions, associated with the presence of mites, which, according to Guilhon *et al.*,[68] are most numerous in the head region.

DIFFERENTIAL DIAGNOSIS. Epidermoptic depluming mange due to *Epidermoptes* and *Microlichus* spp.

TREATMENT

Guilhon *et al.*[68] stated that the disease is contagious, because canaries kept in the same cage as an infected Pekin robin, separated only by a wire grill partition, became infected. Infected birds should, therefore, be separated from healthy ones.

Guilhon *et al.* mentioned no treatment, but probably that recommended for cnemidocoptic mange would be satisfactory.

Subcutaneous Mites

Lapage[104] stated that all laminosioptid mites are very small, measuring no more than about 0.3 mm. in length. The bodies are soft, elongated, and slightly flattened.

SPECIES AND HOSTS

The Laminosioptidae family is represented by *Laminosioptes cysticola*, which has been reported from the domestic fowl, turkey, pheasants, geese, and pigeons, but apparently not from passerine and psittacine birds, which are the main types kept in cage and aviary. Nevertheless, because so little is known about this mite, it is worth looking for at necropsy in all species of birds.

DISTRIBUTION AND INCIDENCE

The mite has been recorded from many parts of the world.

LIFE HISTORY

Nothing is known of the life history of *Laminosioptes*, except that the female lays embryonated eggs,[22] and all stages of development take place in the deeper tissues of the host.[138]

CLINICAL SIGNS OF INFESTATION

No clinical signs of infestation have been recorded.

DIAGNOSIS

Diagnosis is possible only at necropsy.

TREATMENT

None.

POSTMORTEM FINDINGS

Round or oval yellowish brown nodules, reaching several millimeters in diameter, are observed in the subcutaneous tissues, especially over the thorax and abdomen. The caseous or calcareous nodules are believed to be formed by the host around the mites after they die in the tissues. Benbrook[22] stated that in addition to being found in the loose connective tissue, the mites have also been seen in the muscles, lungs, and abdominal viscera of the pigeon.

Visceral Mites

The visceral mites can be divided into two main types, namely, the rhinonyssid mites, which attack the respiratory system, and the cytoditid mites, the best known of which (*Cytodites nudus*) may be found in the abdomen as well as in the respiratory system.

Rhinonyssid Mites

SPECIES AND HOSTS

Sternostoma tracheacolum, originally described in the canary by Lawrence in 1948,[107] has been reported in this species on many occasions since then. It also attacks various wild birds, such as the yellow-throated longclaw (*Macronyx croceus*) and house sparrow,[55] and has been recorded in the following birds in captivity: budgerigar, by Fain[52]; Gouldian finches (*Poephila gouldiae*) by Cumming[46]; Madagascar lovebird (*Agapornis cana*) by Keymer (unpublished); goldfinches (*Carduelis carduelis*) by Medda[128]; and sugar birds (*Cyanerpes cyanea*) by Fain and Hyland.[55] Fain and

Hyland consider *S. castroae, S. meddai, Agapornyssus faini, Ptilonyssus madagascariensis,* and *Neonyssus marcandrei* to be synonyms of *S. tracheacolum.*

Other species of mites recorded in passerine birds include *S. sialiphilus* in the Eastern bluebird (*Sialia sialis*) and *S. spatulatum* in the olive-backed thrush (*Hylocichla ustulata*) by Hyland and Ford[87]; *S. cryptorhyncheum* and *Ptilonyssus nudus* in sparrows by Lapage[104]; *S paddae* in the Java sparrow (*Padda oryzivora*) by Fain[52] and in starlings (*Speleognathus sturni*) by Boyd.[30]

DISTRIBUTION AND INCIDENCE

Since *S. tracheacolum* was first reported in South Africa by Lawrence,[107] it has been found in Brazil,[167] Sardinia,[128] Belgium,[54] Germany,[64] Madagascar,[67] the Netherlands,[182] and in England by Keymer. *Sternostoma* sp.—probably *S. tracheacolum*—was reported in Italy by Ballarini and Pieresca,[17] and it occurs in the U.S.S.R. and Ruanda-Urundi, according to Fain and Hyland.[55] The mite described by Higby[78] as *Cytodites nudus,* infecting canaries in the U.S.A., was, in the opinion of Fain and Hyland, probably *S. tracheacolum.* In spite of the fact that the mite was not described until 1948, it is obviously very widespread and probably has frequently been overlooked.

LIFE HISTORY

The life cycle appears to be unknown, and according to Stephan *et al.*[163] male mites are much less frequently found in the respiratory system than are females. Vaccari and Ballarini[170] have discussed the ecological aspects of *S. tracheacolum* in some detail.

CLINICAL SIGNS OF INFESTATION

Infestations due to *S. tracheacolum* have been described by Lawrence,[107] Stephan *et al.,*[163] Torres *et al.,*[167] Medda,[128] Zwart,[182] and others.

In mild or chronic infestations, canaries lose condition and show evidence of respiratory distress, death occurring about three weeks after the dyspnea first develops.[46] Zwart,[182] however, recorded sudden death in birds in good condition without any previous clinical signs. The disease is more rapidly fatal in Gouldian finches than in canaries, according to Cumming.[46] Frequently, loss of voice occurs in the early stages, and male canaries cease singing completely. Stephan *et al.*[163] described ruffled feathers and sleepiness, followed by characteristic "sucking" or "smacking" sounds, which they said were usually made twice in succession. Other reports also refer to this type of respiratory distress and describe frequent coughing, sneezing, gasping for breath, and attempts to clear the throat. This dyspnea results in lack of sleep, loss of condition, weakness, and eventually in death if no treatment is given. Boyd[30] stated that starlings infected with the nasal mite *S. sturni* have more nasal secretion or mucus than nonparasitized birds, although in wild birds the presence of nasal mites is not always associated with clinical signs.

DIAGNOSIS

Diagnosis is based on the clinical signs and discovery at necropsy of the mites in any part of the respiratory system, together with the lesions described below. A tentative diagnosis may also be made in the live bird, if there is a response to the treatment recommended below.

Although mites may be found in any part of the respiratory tract, Fain and Hyland[55] stated that they appeared to be present in the higher passages, namely, the nasal cavities, more frequently in wild birds than in canaries. When the lumen of the trachea is opened, the mites appear as minute black specks, the dark color being due to the ingested blood.[163] As many as 60 mites may be found in the trachea, usually congregated near the syrinx. The mites are not fixed to the mucous membrane, but may be seen to move about not only in the trachea but also in the air sacs. The parasites may also be found encysted in the external surface of the lungs, each mite being surrounded by a zone of congestion.

DIFFERENTIAL DIAGNOSIS. The clinical signs may be confused with those occurring in other types of pneumonia caused by such diseases as syngamiasis, aspergillosis, or the acute form of passerine pox.

TREATMENT

Respiratory acariasis was reported by Stephan *et al.*[163] to be communicable; the disease can probably be controlled to a certain extent, therefore, by separating healthy birds from those showing evidence of the disease. It was also suggested that parent birds may infect their young while feeding them with regurgitated food.

A satisfactory treatment appears to be the inhalation of malathion powder, Cumming[46] recommending 5% and Zwart[182] 4% concentration. Malathion is relatively non-toxic and is much safer and efficacious than sulfur dust, barium antimonyl tartrate, or a mixture of D.D.T. and benzene hexachloride, all of which were tried by Stephan *et al.*[163]

Inhalation treatment is accomplished either by placing each bird in a small paper box measuring about 10 × 11 × 15 cm.,[182] or by putting all the birds in a small cage with a wire front and covered with a towel.[46] The malathion powder is then pumped into the box or cage with an ordinary "puffer" type dispenser, in order to produce a dense "fog."

Zwart[182] simply introduced 0.5 gm. of powder (4%) into the box and then relied upon the fluttering of the bird to cause further dispersion. The bird was exposed to the treatment for 5 minutes, and the treatment was repeated at weekly intervals for 6 weeks. Cumming[46] introduced the powder (5% concentration) into the cage every 60 seconds for a period of 5 minutes, and repeated the treatment at weekly intervals for 4 weeks. Zwart's method of treating birds individually is probably the safer, since if there is more than one bird in a cage they might injure each other while fluttering about.

Cumming stated that his treatment proved very successful both with canaries and with Gouldian finches, and Zwart also reported the gradual disappearance of the respiratory distress during the course of treatment. Even young birds only 6 weeks of age showed no signs of discomfort either during or after exposure to the malathion dust.

Huchzermeyer[84] claimed that the treatment with malathion powder does not always have a lasting effect, and he prefers intramuscular injection of metriphonate* suspension. For canaries, he recommended 0.2 ml. of a 2 in 1,000 suspension in distilled water, which represents approximately 10 mg. per kg. of the active principle dimethyl 2,2,2-trichloro-1-hydroxyethyl-phosphonate. A second injection at the same dosage level is given 10 days later. He has seen no evidence of toxicity, although some local irritation appears to be produced at the site of injection in the pectoral muscles and the bird may droop its wings.

POSTMORTEM FINDINGS

Most reports describe pneumonia in canaries with *S. tracheacolum* infestations. Both lungs, only one, or just part of a lung may show marked congestion. Aerocystitis, varying from slight thickening and cloudiness or redness of the air sacs, to marked thickening associated with the formation of yellowish gelatinous fluid[182] or of pus[163] may occur. Varying degrees of tracheitis are also seen, often associated with an excessive amount of mucus, which in some cases may be blood-stained, while yellowish pus may occur in the nasal cavity. Although the lesions are normally confined to

*"Dylox"—Chemagra Corporation, Kansas City, U.S.A.

the respiratory system, Zwart[182] recorded slight enlargement of the spleen.

Cytoditid Mites

SPECIES AND HOSTS

Cytodites nudus has been recorded from the domestic fowl, turkey, pheasant, and pigeon,[22] and Fain and Hyland[55] stated that it also occurs in wild birds, having found it in the European bee-eater (*Merops apiaster*) and the black-faced babbler (*Turdoides melanops*). Higby[78] reported serious disease caused by the mite in canaries, but as Fain and Hyland[55] pointed out, the lesions described by Higby were probably caused by *Sternostoma tracheacolum,* which in 1946 had not been described. Fain[53] has also described the mite *C. psittaci* in the lung of a Meyer's parrot (*Poicephalus meyeri*).

DISTRIBUTION AND INCIDENCE

C. nudus has been reported from many parts of the world, but nothing is known of its incidence in cage and aviary birds. If it were specifically looked for at necropsy, however, it might well be found in many more species.

LIFE HISTORY

The life cycle is unknown. Benbrook[22] stated that possibly *C. nudus* produces larvae in the lower respiratory tract, which are coughed up and probably swallowed, passing through the body and reaching the ground in the feces.

CLINICAL SIGNS OF INFESTATION

These mites are probably harmless, as they are sometimes seen at necropsy in healthy birds, unassociated with any lesions. According to Benbrook,[22] however, *C. nudus* has been thought by some to cause emaciation, pneumonia, peritonitis, or obstruction of the respiratory passages, and heavy infestations have definitely been associated with loss of weight and weakness.

DIAGNOSIS

The condition is diagnosed only by identification of the mites at necropsy.

DIFFERENTIAL DIAGNOSIS. *Sternostoma tracheacolum* infestation.

TREATMENT

Probably that recommended for *S. tracheacolum* would be satisfactory.

POSTMORTEM FINDINGS

Benbrook[22] reported that close examination of the carcass of an affected bird shortly after death will reveal the presence of slow-moving, whitish dots on the surface of the air sacs, and that if these are examined under a dissecting microscope the mites can be seen. Mites may also be found in the abdominal cavity or on the surface of the liver and other viscera.

Chiggers, or Harvest Mites

All the members of the Family Trombiculidae are parasitic only in the larval stage.

The six-legged larvae are red, orange, or yellow in color; they are less than 0.5 mm. in diameter and may be difficult to see unless they have just become engorged with tissue fluid.

SPECIES AND HOSTS

The best-known species include *Trombicula alfreddugèsi, T. autumnalis,* and *T. batatas.* The larvae of these mites are not host specific, and they attack a wide variety of animals, including man, domestic and wild animals, poultry, and wild birds.

DISTRIBUTION AND INCIDENCE

The mites occur in many parts of the world. *T. alfreddugèsi* occurs in North America, *T. autumnalis* in Great Britain and parts of continental Europe, and *T. batatas* in the southern U.S.A. and tropical areas of South America.

The larvae are most likely to attack birds in an outside aviary, but there is no evidence that they are common parasites of aviary birds.

LIFE HISTORY

In a typical life cycle, eggs are laid on the ground; before the egg hatches the embryo within becomes enclosed in a membrane, forming the stage known as the deutovum. This takes about six days to develop, and after a further six days the six-legged larva emerges. The larva feeds on a host, drops to the ground again, and molts, producing the stage known as the nymphochrysalis. Within the remains of the molted skin the non-parasitic eight-legged nymph develops into the pre-adult imagochrysalis, which after a period of a few days becomes the free-living eight-legged adult mite.

CLINICAL SIGNS OF INFESTATION

Larvae attach themselves to the host by their mouthparts, puncture the skin, and inject a salivary secretion which lyses it. The larvae then feed, not on blood but on the liquefied tissue of the host. Usually the lesion which is made by a larva produces intense irritation and a firm papule or vesicle forms, surrounded by an area of hyperemia.

Gray[66] stated that harvest and other mites may sometimes enter the auditory canal of birds and cause *"labyrinthine vertigo."*

DIAGNOSIS

Diagnosis is based on discovery of the typical lesions associated with the presence of larvae on the skin.

TREATMENT

It is suggested that the ground in the aviary and in the vicinity should be sprayed with D.D.T. and individual birds be treated in the same manner as recommended for lice.

Forage Mites

Forage mites are free-living, occurring on a variety of foodstuffs, such as cheese, grain, dried fruit, flour, and other products. Many species also act as scavengers in birds' nests. They are minute, slow-moving, and usually pearly grey in color. The larvae and eggs also are barely visible to the naked eye. A striking feature is the absence of respiratory organs in practically all species.

SPECIES AND HOSTS

There are many species representing a large number of genera, but *Tyroglyphus farinae* is the one that has been mentioned most frequently for its possible pathogenicity. Other common species are *Tyrophagus dimidiatus, Glycyphagus cadaverum,* and *G. domesticus.*

DISTRIBUTION AND INCIDENCE

Solomon[161] stated that *T. farinae* is cosmopolitan. Many other species are also widespread.

LIFE HISTORY

The basic life cycle appears to consist of an egg, then a larval stage, followed by three nymphal stages, leading to the adult.[161]

CLINICAL SIGNS OF INFESTATION AND POSTMORTEM FINDINGS

A number of species are believed to cause an allergic type of dermatitis in man when they come into contact with the skin. Intestinal and urinary disorders have also been reported in man and animals when mite-infested food has been eaten. Hinman and Kampmeier,[79] however, stated that it is not known whether the pathogenicity of the mites is due to a toxic substance produced by them or to mechanical irritation, or if the symptoms are an allergic manifestation in the host.

There is very little information regarding the effect of the mites on birds, although Pillers[142] stated that they may cause irritation of the skin, natural orifices, and alimentary tract. It is possible that *Tyroglyphus* spp. and *Tyrophagus* spp. may at times be pathogenic to birds, numerous larvae, nymphs, and adults having been found on the plumage and in the mouth of a blue-winged parrotlet (*Forpus vividus*) which at necropsy showed no macroscopic lesions other than congestion of the kidneys, and from which no pathogenic organisms were isolated.

Much more evidence, however, is obviously necessary before definite conclusions can be drawn regarding the significance of the mites when found in association with lesions.

Tyroglyphus and other mites were at one time thought to cause French Molt in budgerigars, but subsequent investigations have shown that this is incorrect.

DIAGNOSIS

Solomon[161] rightly pointed out that most of the medical and veterinary reports of forage mites being pathogenic require confirmation by experimental studies; therefore, great care should be exercised when diagnosing disease in birds as due to these mites. Obviously clinical signs or lesions must always be associated with heavy infestation of mites before they can seriously be considered as pathogenic, and the condition of the birds should improve when the mites are removed and destroyed.

PREVENTION AND TREATMENT

The removal and destruction of all mite-infested food, nesting material, and litter is essential. It is worth remembering that the motile forms are adapted for distribution by insects, whereas non-motile resistant hypopi are believed to be carried by wind and mechanically in various ways.[161]

As humidity is essential to survival of the mites, all foodstuffs must be kept dry; in fact, desiccation is the most effective of all the methods of control. Insecticides that are safe to use on small birds, such as pyrethrum, are ineffective.

ACKNOWLEDGMENTS

I am indebted to Professor P. C. C. Garnham, C.M.G., F.R.S., M.D., D.Sc., Department of Parasitology, London School of Hygiene and Tropical Medicine, for advice and also to J. R. Baker, B.Sc., Ph.D., and R. Lainson, D.Sc., Ph.D., of the same department, for reading and checking the section on Protozoa.

G. Varma, B.Sc., Ph.D., Department of Entomology, London School of Hygiene and Tropical Medicine, kindly checked the section on Arthropods, and B. Elce, Ph.D., B.Sc., D.A.P.E., Brunel University, Uxbridge, Middlesex, the section on Helminths.

References

1. Adie, J. R.: Note on a parasite in the sparrow. Indian med. Gaz. *43:*176–180, 1908.

2. Al-Dabagh, M. A.: Mechanisms of death and tissue injury in malaria. VII. Malarial anemia. J. Fac. Med., Baghdad *2:*141–161, 1960.

3. Al-Dabagh, M. A.: Eyelid lesions in chicks infected with *Plasmodium gallinaceum.* Trans. R. Soc. trop. Med. Hyg. *55:*351–354, 1961.

4. Appleby, E. C.: Some observations on the diseases of finches and parrot-like birds kept in aviaries. Proc. 1st Ann. Congr. Br. small Anim. vet. Ass., 1958. Pp. 25–30.

5. Arnall, L.: Experiences with cage-birds. Vet. Rec. *70:*120–128, 1958.

6. Arnall, L.: Further experiences with cagebirds. Vet. Rec. *73:*1146–1154, 1961.

7. Arnall, L.: Conditions of the beak and claw in the budgerigar. J. small anim. Pract. *6:*135–144, 1965.

8. ASH, J. S.: A study of the Mallophaga of birds with particular reference to their biology and ecology. Ibis *102*:93–110, 1960.

9. BACHRACH, A.: Skin and Feather Problems of Caged Birds. In *Current Veterinary Therapy 1966–1967*, R. W. Kirk, ed. Philadelphia, W. B. Saunders Co., 1966. Pp. 549–553.

10. BAER, J. G.: Host reactions in young birds to naturally occurring superinfestations with *Porrocaecum ensicaudatum*. J. Helminth., R. T. Leiper Suppl., pp. 1–4, 1961.

11. BAKER, E. W., EVANS, T. M., GOULD, D. J., HULL, W. B., and KEEGAN, H. L.: A Manual of Parasitic Mites of Medical or Economic Importance. New York, National Pest Control Association, Inc., 1956. 170 pp.

12. BAKER, E. W., and WHARTON, G. W.: *An Introduction to Acarology.* New York, The Macmillan Company, 1952. Pp. 373–374.

13. BAKER, J. R.: Studies on *Trypanosoma avium* Danilewsky 1885. I. Incidence in some birds of Hertfordshire. Parasitology *46*:308–320, 1956.

14. BAKER, J. R.: Studies on *Trypanosoma avium* Danilewsky 1885. II. Transmission by *Ornithomyia avicularia* L. Parasitology *46*:321–334, 1956.

15. BAKER, J. R.: Studies on *Trypanosoma avium* Danilewsky 1885. III. Life cycle in vertebrate and invertebrate hosts. Parasitology *46*:335–352, 1956.

16. BAKER, J. R., LAINSON, R., and KILLICK-KENDRICK, R.: *Lankesterella corvi,* n. sp., a blood parasite of the English rook, *Corvus f. frugilegus* L. J. Protozool. *6*:233–237, 1959.

17. BALLARINI, G., and PIERESCA, G.: Attività svolta dal "Centro Ricerche Malattie Uccelli (FOI)" Durante il Triennio 1959–60–61. Nuova Vet. *38*:136–146, 1962.

18. BAYLIS, H. A.: A new cestode from the grey parrot. Ann. Mag. Nat. Hist. *4*:381–384, 1929. 10th series.

19. BEACH, J. E.: Diseases of budgerigars and other cage birds. A survey of post-mortem findings. Vet. Rec. *74*:10–17 (Part I), 63–68 (Part II), 134–140 (Part III), 1962.

20. BEAUDETTE, F. R.: A natural case of canary malaria. J.A.V.M.A. *105*:91–92, 1944.

21. BEDFORD, The Duke of: Parrots and Parrot-like Birds. Fond du Lac., Wis., All-Pets Books, Inc., 1954. P. 175.

22. BENBROOK, E. A.: External Parasites of Poultry. In *Diseases of Poultry*, 5th ed. H. E. Biester and L. H. Schwarte, eds. Ames, Iowa State University Press, 1965. Pp. 925–964.

23. BENNETT, G. F.: On the specificity and transmission of some avian trypanosomes. Canad. J. Zool. *39*:17–33, 1961.

24. BENNETT, G. F., and FALLIS, A. M.: Blood parasites of birds in Algonquin Park, Canada, and a discussion of their transmission. Canad. J. Zool. *38*:261–273, 1960.

25. BENNETT, G. F., GARNHAM, P. C. C., and FALLIS, A. M.: On the status of the genera Leucocytozoon Ziemann, 1898 and Haemoproteus Kruse, 1890 (Haemosporidiida: Leucocytozoidae and Haemoproteidae). Canad. J. Zool. *43*:927–932, 1965.

26. BENOIT, P. L. G.: Cnemidocoptes-schurft van de parkeit *"Melopsittacus undulatus"* in Belgie. Vlaams diergeneesk. Tijdschr. *27*:240–243, 1958.

27. BERSON, J. P.: Les protozoaires parasites des hématies et du système histiocytaire des oiseaux. Essai de nomenclature. Rev. élev. Méd. vét. Pays. trop. *17*:43–96, 1964.

28. BLACKMORE, D. K.: Some observations on *Cnemidocoptes pilae* together with its effect on the Budgerigar (*Melopsittacus undulatus*). Vet. Rec. *75*:592–595, 1963.

29. BLACKMORE, D. K.: Personal communication, 1965.

30. BOYD, E. M.: A new mite from the respiratory tract of the starling (*Acarina, Speleognathidae*). Proc. ent. Soc. Wash. *50*:9–14, 1948.

31. BUXTON, P. A., and BUSVINE, J. R.: Pests of the Animal House. In *UFAW Handbook on the Care and Management of Laboratory Animals*, 2nd ed., A. N. Worden and W. Lane-Petter, eds. London, Universities Federation for Animal Welfare, 1957. Chap. 5, p. 74.

32. CALLENDER, G. R., and SIMMONS, J. S.: Trichomoniasis (*T. columbae*) in the Java sparrow, Tovi parrakeet and Verraux's dove. Am. J. trop. Med. Hyg. *17*:579–585, 1937.

33. CERVA, L.: Resistence cyst *Lamblia intestinalis* vuči zevním saktorum. Čslká. Parasit. *2*:17–21, 1955.

34. CHUTE, H. L.: Sarcosporidiosis. In *Diseases of Poultry*, 5th ed., H. E. Biester and L. H. Schwarte, eds. Ames, Iowa State University Press, 1965. Pp. 507–511.

35. CLARK, G. M.: *Sarcocystis* in certain birds. J. Parasit. *44*(4, §2, Supplement):41, August, 1958.

36. CLAY, T.: Personal communication, 1964.

37. COATNEY, G. R.: A check-list and host-index of the genus *Haemoproteus*. J. Parasit. *22*:88–105, 1936.

38. COATNEY, G. R.: A catalog and host-index of the genus *Leucocytozoon*. J. Parasit. *23*:202–212, 1937.

39. COATNEY, G. R., and ROUDABUSH, R. L.: A Catalogue of the Species of the Genus *Plasmodium* and Index of Their Hosts". In *Malariology,* M. F. Boyd, ed.

Philadelphia, W. B. Saunders Co., 1949. Vol. I, pp. 29–53.

40. COFFIN, D. L.: Diseases of Parrots. In *Parrots and Parrot-like Birds,* by the Duke of Bedford. Fond du Lac, Wis., All-Pets Books, Inc., 1954. Pp. 24–44.

41. CORRADETTI, A., GARNHAM, P. C. C., and LAIRD, M.: New classification of the avian malaria parasites. Parassitologia (Rome) *5:*1–4, 1963.

42. CORRADETTI, A., VEROLINI, F., and NERI, I.: *Plasmodium* (*Haemamoeba*) *giovannolai,* n. sp. parassita di *Turdus merula.* Parassitologia (Rome) *5:*11–18, 1963.

43. CRAM, E. B.: *Bird Parasites of the Nematode Sub-orders Strongylata, Ascaridata and Spirurata.* Bull. U.S. natn. Mus. 140. Washington, U.S. Government Printing Office, 1927. P. 80.

44. CRAM, E. B.: *Developmental Stages of Some Nematodes of the Spiruroidea Parasitic in Poultry and Game Birds.* U.S.D.A. Tech. Bull. n. s. 227. Washington, D.C., U.S. Government Printing Office, 1931. 28 pp.

45. CRUTCHFIELD, C. M., and HIXSON, H.: Food habits of several species of poultry lice with special reference to blood consumption. Fla. ent. *26:*63–66, 1943.

46. CUMMING, R. B.: Respiratory acariasis of canaries and Gouldian finches. J. S. Afr. vet. med. Ass. *30:*31–32, 1959.

47. DALL, J. A., BRANCKER, W. M., GRAHAM-JONES, O., JOSHUA, J. O., and KEYMER, I. F.: Handbook on the Treatment of Exotic Pets. London, The British Veterinary Association, 1964. Part I. Cage Birds. 83 pp.

48. DAVID, A., and NAIR, C. P.: Observations on a natural (cryptic) infection of trypanosomes in sparrows (*Passer domesticus* Linnaeus). I. Susceptibility of birds and mammals to the trypanosomes. Indian J. Malar. *9:*95–98, 1955.

49. EHLERS, E.: Die Krätzmilben der Vögel. Ein Beitrag zur Kenntniss der Sarcoptiden. Z. Wiss. Zool. *23:* 228–253, 1873.

50. EVANS, G. O., FAIN, A., and BAFORT, J.: Découverte du cycle évolutif du genre *Myialges* avec description d'une espèce nouvelle (Myialgidae: Sarcoptiformes). Bull. Annls. Soc. r. ent. Belg. *99:*486–500, 1963.

51. EVANS, G. O., SHEALS, J. G., and MACFARLANE, D.: *The Terrestrial Acari of the British Isles,* London, Printed by order of the Trustees of the British Museum, 1961. Vol. I, Introduction and Biology. 219 pp.

52. FAIN, A.: Acariens parasites nasicoles chez les oiseaux du Zoo d'Anvers, Description de trois espèces nouvelles. Bull. Soc. r. Zool. d'Anvers *9:*1–13, 1958.

53. FAIN, A.: Révision du genre *Cytodites* (Mégnin) et description de deux espèces et un genre nouveaux dans la famille Cytoditidae Oudemans (Acarina: Sarcoptiformes). Acarologia *2:*238–249, 1960.

53a. FAIN, A.: *A Review of the Family Epidermoptidae Trouessart Parasitic of the Skin of Birds (Acarina: Sarcoptiformes).* Vehr. K. vlaarm. Acad. Wet. Klasse der wetenschappen, *27,* Part I, 176 pp. Part II, 144 pp. Brussel, Paleis der Acalemiën, 1965.

54. FAIN, A., and CARPENTIER, J.: Acariase pulmonaire mortelle chez des canaris du zoo. Bull Soc. r. Zool. d'Anvers *9:*21–24, 1958.

55. FAIN, A., and HYLAND, K. E.: The mites parasitic in the lungs of birds. The variability of *Sternostoma tracheacolum* Lawrence, 1948, in domestic and wild birds. Parasitology *52:*401–424, 1962.

56. FARDELL, M. D.: *Syngamus trachea* in the raven. Vet. Rec. *76:*590, 1964.

57. FARR, M. M.: *Eimeria dunsingi* n. sp. (Protozoa. Eimeriidae) from the intestines of a parakeet, *Melopsittacus undulatus* (Shaw). Libro homenage al Dr. Eduardo Cabberol y. lal. Jubileo, 1930–1960. Mexico D.F. (Instituto Politechico Nacional) 1960, pp. 31–35.

58. FINLAY, P., and MANWELL, R. D.: *Toxoplasma* from the crow, a new natural host. Exp. Parasit. *5:*149–153, 1956.

59. FOWLER, N. G.: Personal communication, 1966.

60. FRANK, W.: Eine Leucocytozoon—Infektion bei Pennantsittichen (*Platycercus elegans*). Die Gefied. Welt, 193–194, 1965.

61. GARNHAM, P. C. C.: Blood parasites of East African vertebrates, with a brief description of exo-erythrocytic schizogony in *Plasmodium pitmani.* Parasitology *40:*328–337, 1950.

62. GARNHAM, P. C. C.: *Malarial Parasites and Other Haemosporidia.* Oxford, Blackwell, 1966. 1114 pp.

63. GELORMINI, N., and ROVEDA, R. J.: Sarna epidermóptica en el canario, Rev. Fac. Agron. Vet. B. Aires *9:*143–146, 1941.

64. GEYER, S.: Klinische Erfahrungen bei Krankheiten der Stubenvögel. Tierärztl. Umsch. *14:*234–238, 1959.

65. GOBLE, F. C., and KUTZ, H. L.: The genus *Dispharynx* (Nematoda: Acuariidae) in galliform and passeriform birds. J. Parasit. *31:*323–331, 1945.

66. GRAY, H.: The diseases of cage and aviary birds, with some reference to those of furred and feathered game. Vet. Rec. *16:*343–352 (Part I), 377–386 (Part II), 417–427 (Part III), 1936.

67. GRÉTILLAT, S., CAPRON, A., and BRYGOO, E. R.: Acariens *Rhinonyssidae* de Madagascar. Acarologia *1:*375–384, 1959.

68. GUILHON, J., EUZÉBY J., and OBRY, J.: Une nouvelle affection cutanée parasitaire, chez les oiseaux de volière. Bull. Acad. vét. Fr. *25:*167–168, 1952.

69. HAMERTON, A. E.: Diseases of aviary birds. Vet. J. *89:* 5–12, 1933.

70. HART, J. W.: Observations on blood parasites of birds in South Carolina. J. Parasit. *35:*79–82, 1949.

71. HARWOOD, P. M. A.: Management and diseases of cage birds. J. Dep. Agric. W. Aust. *5:*225–237, 1956.

72. HASHOLT, J.: Current diseases of cage birds. J. small anim. Pract. *2:*97–108, 1961.

73. HEGNER, R. W.: *Giardia felis* n. sp. from the domestic cat and giardias from birds. Am. J. Hyg. *5:*258–273, 1925.

74. HENRY, A., and GUILHON, J.: Gale déplumante déterminée par *Microlichus avus* Tr. chez un serin. C. R. Soc. Biol. (Paris) *130:*431–432, 1939.

75. HERMAN, C. M., and BISCHOFF, A. I.: The duration of *Haemoproteus* infection in California quail. Calif. Fish Game *35:*293–299, 1949.

76. HERMAN, C. M., and VAIL, E. L.: A fatal case of spontaneous malaria in a canary. J.A.V.M.A. *101:* 502, 1942.

77. HEWITT, R.: Splenic enlargement and infarction in canaries infected with a virulent strain of *Plasmodium cathemerium*. Am. J. Hyg. *30*(C):49–63, 1939.

78. HIGBY, W. E.: A new canary plague. All Pets Mag. (Dec.) pp. 8–9, 1946.

79. HINMAN, E. H., and KAMPMEIER, R. H.: Intestinal acariasis due to *Tyroglyphus longior* Gervais. Am. J. trop. Med. *14:*355–362, 1934.

80. HINSHAW, W. R., and McNEIL, E.: Carriers of *Hexamita meleagridis*. Am. J. vet Res. *2:*453–458, 1941.

81. HONIGBERG, B. M., BALAMUTH, W., BOVEE, E. C., CORLISS, J. O., GOJDICS, M., HALL, R. P., KUDO, R. R., LEVINE, N. D., LOEBLICH, A. R., JR., WEISER, J., and WENRICH, D. H.: A revised classification of the Phylum Protozoa. J. Protozool. *11:*7–20, 1964.

82. HOPKINS, G. H. E., and CLAY, T.: *A Check-List of the Genera and Species of Mallophaga*. London, Printed by order of Trustees of the British Museum, 1952. 362 pp.

83. HOWITT, B. F., DODGE, H. R., BISHOP, L. K., and GORRIE, R. H.: Virus of eastern equine encephalomyelitis isolated from chicken mites (*Dermanyssus gallinae*) and chicken lice (*Eomenacanthus stramineus*). Proc. Soc. Exp. Biol. Med. *68:*622–625, 1948.

84. HUCHZERMEYER, F.: Personal communication, 1965.

85. HUDSON, C. B.: Spontaneous malaria in canaries. J.A.V.M.A. *104:*158, 1944.

86. HUFF, C. G.: A survey of the blood parasites of birds caught for banding purposes. J.A.V.M.A. *94:*615–620, 1939.

87. HYLAND, K. E., and FORD, H. G.: *Sternostoma sialiphilus* n. sp. (Acarina: Rhinonyssidae) from the nasal cavities of the Eastern Bluebird, *Sialia sialis* (Linnaeus). J. Parasit. *47:*101–104, 1961.

88. IMMS, A. D.: *A General Textbook of Entomology*, 9th ed., revised by O. W. Richards and R. G. Davies. London, Methuen & Co. Ltd., 1957. 886 pp.

89. JACOBS, L.: The biology of *Toxoplasma*. Am. J. trop. Med. Hyg. *2:*365–389, 1953.

90. JAMES, S. P.: Microfilariae in the blood of Java sparrows. Trans. R. Soc. trop. Med. Hyg. *33:*7, 1939.

91. JENNINGS, A. R., and SOULSBY, E. J. L.: Diseases of wild birds. Fourth report. Bird Study *4:*216–220, 1957.

92. KASCHULA, V. R.: "Scaly-leg" of the canary [*Serinus canaria* (Linn)]. J. S. Afr. vet. med. Ass. *21:*117–119, 1950.

93. KELLEY, G. W.: Removal of *Syngamus trachea*, gapeworm, from pheasants with subcutaneously injected Disophenol. Poult. Sci. *41:*1358–1360, 1962.

94. KEYMER, I. F.: Some ailments of cage and aviary birds. Proc. 1st Ann. Congr. Br. small Anim. vet. Ass., 1958. Pp. 18–24.

95. KEYMER, I. F.: The diagnosis and treatment of common psittacine diseases. Mod. Vet. Pract. *39*(21):22–30, December 15, 1958.

96. KEYMER, I. F.: Specific diseases of the canary and other passerine birds. Mod. Vet. Pract. *40*(18):45–48, September 15, and *40*(24):16, December 15, 1959.

97. KEYMER, I. F.: Postmortem examinations of pet birds. Mod. Vet Pract. *42*(23):35–38, December 1, and *42*(24):47–51, December 15, 1961.

98. KEYMER, I. F., and BLACKMORE, D. K.: Diseases of the skin and soft parts of wild birds. Brit. Birds *57:*175–179, 1964.

99. KEYMER, I. F., ROSE, J. H., BEESLEY, W. M., and DAVIES, S. F. M.: A survey and review of parasitic diseases of wild and game birds in Great Britain. Vet. Rec. *74:*887–894, 1962.

100. LAINSON, R.: Some observations on the life-cycle of *Atoxoplasma*, with particular reference to the parasite's schizogony and its transmission by the mite *Dermanyssus gallinae*. Nature, Lond. *182:*1250–1251, 1958.

101. LAINSON, R.: *Atoxoplasma* Garnham, 1950, in an English sparrow (*Passer domesticus domesticus* Linn.). Trans. R. Soc. trop. Med. Hyg. *52:*15–16, 1958.

102. LAINSON, R.: *Atoxoplasma* Garnham, 1950, as a synonym for *Lankesterella* Labbé, 1899. Its life cycle in

the English sparrow (*Passer domesticus domesticus* Linn.). J. Protozool. *6:*360–371, 1959.

103. LAINSON, R.: The transmission of *Lankesterella* (=*Atoxoplasma*) in birds by the mite *Dermanyssus gallinae.* J. Protozool. *7:*321–322, 1960.

104. LAPAGE, G.: *Veterinary Parasitology,* Edinburgh & London, Oliver & Boyd, 1956. P. 674.

105. LAVERAN, A.: Au sujet de l'hématozoaire endoglobulaire de *Padda oryzivora.* C. R. Soc. Biol. (Paris) *52:*19–20, 1900.

106. LAVOIPIERRE, M., and GRIFFITHS, R. B.: A preliminary note on a new species of *Cnemidocoptes* (Acarina) causing scaly leg in a budgerigar (*Melopsittacus undulatus*) in Great Britain. Ann. trop. Med. Parasit. *45:*253–254, 1951.

107. LAWRENCE, R. F.: Studies on some parasitic mites from Canada and South Africa. J. Parasit. *34:*364–379, 1948.

108. LEIBOVITZ, L.: Thiabendazole therapy of pheasants affected with gapeworms. J.A.V.M.A. *140:*1310–1313, 1962.

109. LEIBOVITZ, L.: Unusual bird-parasite cases and over-all parasite incidence found in a diagnostic laboratory during a five-year period. Avian Dis. *6:*141–144, 1962.

110. LESBOUYRIES, G.: *La pathologie des Oiseaux.* Paris, Vigot Frères, 1941. Vol. 2.

111. LEVINE, N. D.: *Protozoan Parasites of Domestic Animals and of Man.* Minneapolis, Burgess Publishing Co., 1961. 412 pp.

112. LEVINE, N. D., BOLEY, L. E., and HESTER, H. R.: Experimental transmission of *Trichomonas gallinae* from the chicken to other birds. Am. J. Hyg. *33*(C): 23–32, 1941.

113. LINDT, S., and HÖRNING, B.: Über Malaria bei Pinguinen. In VIII International Symposium on Diseases in Zoo Animals in Leipzig from 20th–23rd April, 1966. Organized by the Institute for Comparative Pathology at the German Academy of Sciences in Berlin. Pp. 223–231.

114. MACDONALD, J. W.: Blue Tit with acarine mange. Brit. Birds *56:*221–222, 1963.

115. MACDONALD, J. W.: Mortality in wild birds. Bird Study *12:*181–195, 1965.

116. MACFIE, J. W. S., and THOMSON, J. G.: A trypanosome of the canary (*Serinus canarius* Koch). Trans. R. Soc. trop. Med. Hyg. *23:*5–6 and 185–191, 1929.

117. MACKERRAS, M. J., and MACKERRAS, I. M.: The Haematozoa of Australian birds. Aust. J. Zool. *8:*226–260, 1960.

118. MADSEN, H.: On the systematics of *Syngamus trachea* (Montagu 1811) Chapin, 1925. J. Helminth. *24:*33–46, 1950.

119. MANSON-BAHR, P.: The life history of avian filaria parasites. Bull. Br. Orn. Club *74:*75–77, 1954.

120. MANWELL, R. D.: Avian toxoplasmosis with invasion of the erythrocytes. J. Parasit. *27:*245–251, 1941.

121. MANWELL, R. D., COULSTON, F., BINCKLEY, E. C., and JONES, V. P.: Mammalian and avian *Toxoplasma.* J. Infect. Dis. *76:*1–14, 1945.

122. MANWELL, R. D., and JOHNSON, C. M.: A natural trypanosome of the canary. Am. J. Hyg. *14:*231–234, 1931.

123. MAQSOOD, M.: *Haemoproteus handai* (sp. nov.) occurring in Indian Parakeet (*Psitticula cyanocephala*). Indian vet. J. *20:*109–111, 1943.

124. MARKBREITER, R.: Some microfilariae found in the blood of birds dying in the Zoological Gardens, 1920–1921. Proc. zool. Soc. Lond. 1923, pp. 59–64.

125. MATHESON, R., BRUNETT, E. L., and BRODY, A. L.: The transmission of fowl pox by mosquitoes, preliminary report. Rep. N.Y. St. vet. Coll. (1930–31), pp. 177, 1932.

126. MATHEY, W. J., Jr.: Malaria in canaries. Vet. Med. *50:*369–370, 1955.

127. MEDDA, A.: Acariasi delle vie respiratorie in *Serinus canarius canarius* Linn. ed in *Carduelis carduelis tschusii* Arrig. Atti. Soc. ital. Sci. vet.*7:*731–736, 1953.

128. MEDDA, A.: Il dimorfismo sessuale dello *Sternostoma meddai* Lombardini. Veterinaria ital. *8:*763–768, 1957.

129. MEGGITT, F. J.: A new species of tapeworm from a parakeet, *Brotogerys tirica.* Parasitology *8:*42–55, 1915.

130. MEINERTZHAGEN, R., and CLAY, T.: List of Mallophaga collected from birds brought to the Society's prosectorium. Proc. zool. Soc. Lond. *117:*675–679, 1948.

131. METTRICK, D. F.: Helminth parasites of Hertfordshire birds. IV. Survey results. J. Helminth. *34:*267–276, 1960.

132. MICKS, D. W.: Malaria in the English sparrow. J. Parasit. *35:*543–544, 1949.

133. MOHAMMED, A. H. H.: *Systematic and Experimental Studies on Protozoal Blood Parasites of Egyptian Birds.* Cairo University Press, 1958. Two volumes, 298 pages.

134. MORTELMANS, J.: Personal communication, 1965.

135. MYERS, L. E.: The American swallow bug, *Oeciacus vicarius* Horvath (Hemiptera, Cimicidae). Parasitology *20:*159–172, 1928.

136. NAJIM, A. T.: *Gigantobilharzia huronensis* sp. nov., a bird blood-fluke from the goldfinch. J. Parasit. *36:* p. 19, December supplement No. 6, 1950.

137. NAJIM, A. T.: Life history of *Gigantobilharzia huronen-*

sis Najim, 1950. A dermatitis-producing bird blood-fluke (Trematoda-Schistosomatidae). Parasitology *46:*443–469, 1956.

138. Neveu-Lemaire, M.: Traité d'Entomologie Médicale et Vétérinaire. Paris, Vigot Frères, 1938. P. 279.

139. Oldham, J. N., and Beresford-Jones, W. P.: Observations on the occurrence of *Cnemidocoptes pilae* Lavoipierre and Griffiths, 1951 in budgerigars and a parakeet. Brit. Vet. J. *110:*29–30, 1954.

140. Pellérdy, L. P.: Catalogue of Eimeriidea (Protozoa: Sporozoa) Budapest, Akadémiai Kiadó, 1963.160 pp.

141. Petrak, M. L.: Personal communication, 1964.

142. Pillers, A. W. N.: Notes on parasites of fur animals and cage birds. Vet. J. *88:*543–547, 1932.

143. Plimmer, H. G.: Report on deaths which occurred in the Zoological Gardens during 1909. Proc. zool. Soc. Lond. Part I. June: 131–136, 1910.

144. Radford, C. D.: The mites (*Acarina: Analgesidae*) living on or in the feathers of birds. Parasitology *42:*199–230, 1953.

145. Ramakrishnan, S. P., David, A., and Nair, C. P.: Observations on a natural (cryptic) infection of trypanosomes in sparrows (*Passer domesticus* Linnaeus). III. Morphology of the developmental forms in *C. fatigans.* Indian J. Malar. *10:*313–315, 1956.

146. Ratcliffe, H. L., and Worth, C. B.: Toxoplasmosis of captive wild birds and mammals. Am. J. Path. *27:* 655–667, 1951.

147. Reeves, W. C., Hammon, W. McD., Furman, D. P., McClure, H. E., and Brookman, B.: Recovery of western equine encephalomyelitis virus from wild bird mites (*Liponyssus sylviarum*) in Kern County, California. Science *105:*411–412, 1947.

148. Richardson, U. F., and Kendall, S. B.: *Veterinary Protozoology,* 3rd ed. Edinburgh and London, Oliver & Boyd, 1963. P. 81.

149. Riggin, G. T., Jr.: A note on *Ribeiroia ondatrae* (Price 1931) in Puerto Rico. Proc. helminth. Soc. Wash. *23:*28–29, 1956.

150. Robinson, E. J., Jr.: Incidence of microfilariae in some Ohio birds and data on the habits of a possible vector. J. Parasit. *47:*441–444, 1961.

151. Rosenbusch, F.: Toxoplasmosis avium en los canarios. Séptima Reunión de la Socièdad Argentina de Patologia Regional Del Norte *11:*904–906, 1932.

152. Rothschild, M., and Clay, T.: *Fleas, Flukes and Cuckoos. A Study of Bird Parasites.* New York, Philosophical Library, 1952. 304 pp.

153. Sabin, A. B., and Feldman, H. A.: Dyes as microchemical indicators of a new immunity phenomenon affecting a protozoon parasite (*Toxoplasma*). Science *108:*660–663, 1948.

154. Sanders, D. A.: Manson's eyeworm of poultry. Bull. Fla. agric. Exp. Stn. *206:*565, 1929.

155. Schwabe, C. W.: Studies on *Oxyspirura mansoni,* the tropical eyeworm of poultry. II. Life history. Pacif. Sci. *5:*18–35, 1951.

156. Schwalbach, G.: Die Coccidiose der Singvögel. I. Der Ausscheidungsrhythmus der Isospora-Oocysten beim Haussperling (*Passer domesticus*). Zbl. Bakt. I (orig.) *178:*263–276, 1960.

157. Sergent, Ed.: Infection latente et prémunition dans la paludisme des passereaux a *Plasmodium relictum.* Riv. Parassit. *20:*389–395, 1959.

158. Sergent, Ed., and Poncet, A.: Longue durée d'une infection latente a toxoplasmes chez un canari. Archs. Inst. Pasteur Algér. *32:*15–17, 1954.

159. Sergent, Ed., and Sergent, Et.: *Haemoproteus wenyoni* nov. sp., parasite du moineau Algerien retrouvé chez des canaris *élevés* en cage. Archs. Inst. Pasteur Algér. *26:*394–396, 1948.

160. Sergent, Ed., Sergent, Et., and Catanei, A.: Sur un parasite nouveau du paludisme des oiseaux. C. R. Acad. Sci. (Paris) *186:*809–811, 1928.

161. Solomon, M. E.: *Tyroglyphid Mites in Stored Products. I. A Survey of Published Information.* Department of Scientific and Industrial Research London, 1943. 36 pp.

162. Stamm, D. D., and Kissling, R. E.: Influence of season on EEE infection in English sparrows. Proc. Soc. Exp. Biol. Med. *92:*374–376, 1956.

163. Stephan, S. A. R., Kaschula, V. R., and Canham, A. S.: Respiratory acariasis of canaries. J. S. Afr. vet. med. Ass. *21:*103–107, 1950.

164. Strandtmann, R. W., and Wharton, G. W.: *A Manual of Mesostigmatid Mites Parasitic on Vertebrates,* edited by C. E. Yunker. Contribution No. 4 of the Institute of Acarology, Department of Zoology, University of Maryland, 1958. 71 pp.

165. Sulkin, S. E., and Izumi, E. N.: Isolation of western equine encephalomyelitis virus from tropical fowl mites, *Liponyssus bursa* (*Berlese*). Proc. Soc. Exp. Biol. Med. *66:*249–250, 1947.

165a. Swaenepoel, L. A., and Swaenepoel, G.: Of birds and worms. Avic. Mag. *73:*51–58, 1967.

166. Swierstra, D., Jansen, J., Jr., and Broek, E. van den: Parasites of zoo-animals in the Netherlands. Survey of parasites of zoo-animals and animals not endemic in the Netherlands, identified from 1948 to 1958 inclusive. Tijdschr. Diergeneesk. *84:*1301–1305, 1959.

167. Torres, C. M., Lent, H., and Moreira, L. F.: Acarinose das vias respiratórias do canário (*Serinus canarius* L.) por *Sternostoma tracheacolum* Lawrence, 1948. Rev. brasil. Biol. *11:*399–406, 1951.

168. Turk, F. A.: A new species of parasitic mite, *Cnemid-*

ocoptes jamaicensis, a causative agent of scaly leg in *Turdus aurantiacus.* Parasitology *40:*60–62, 1950.

169. VACCARI, I., and BALLARINI, G.: Aspetti ecologici della cenosi *Serinus canaria* L. *Sternostoma tracheacolum* Lawr. in ambiente di "Gabbia e Voliera." Nuova Vet. *39:*130–142, 1963.

170. VACCARI, I., BALLARINI, G., and FERRARI, A.: Aspetti di "Terapia Clinica Associata" della plasmodiosi spontanea da *Plasmodium praecox* in canarini (*Serinus canaria* L.) di allevamenti a carattere sportivo. Nuova Vet. *38:*113–120, 1962.

171. WARD, P., LAVOIPIERRE, M., and RAJAMANICKAM, C.: A Lanceolated Warbler (*Locustella lanceolata*) bearing large tumours caused by a harpyrhynchid mite. Ibis *107:*543–544, 1965.

172. WEEREKOON, A. C. J.: A new avian cestode, *Cotugnia platycerci* from Stanley's Rosella Parakeet, *Platycercus icterotis.* Ceylon J. Sci. *22:*155–159, 1944.

173. WEHR, E. E.: *Dermoglyphus elongatus* (Mégnin 1877), a quill mite of the house canary in the United States. J. Parasit. *38:*548–549, 1952.

174. WEHR, E. E.: Nematodes and Acanthocephalids of Poultry. In *Diseases of Poultry,* 5th ed., H. E. Biester and L. H. Schwarte, eds. Ames, Iowa State University Press, 1965. Pp. 965–1005.

175. WEHR, E. E., HARWOOD, P. D., and SCHAFFER, J. M.: Barium antimonyl tartrate as a remedy for the removal of gapeworms from chickens. Poult. Sci. *18:*63–65, 1939.

176. WEIDMAN, F. D.: The Animal Parasites, Their Incidence and Significance. In *Disease in Captive Wild Mammals and Birds,* by H. Fox. Philadelphia, J. B. Lippincott Co., 1923. Pp. 633, 640–641, and 657–658.

177. WETMORE, P. W.: Blood parasites of birds of the District of Columbia and Patuxent research refuge vicinity. J. Parasit. *27:*379–393, 1941.

178. WICHMANN, R. W., and VINCENT, D. J.: Cnemidocoptic mange in the budgerigar (*Melopsittacus undulatus*). J.A.V.M.A. *133:*522–524, 1958.

179. YUNKER, C. E., and ISHAK, K. G.: Histopathological observations on the sequence of infection in knemidokoptic mange of budgerigars (*Melopsittacus undulatus*). J. Parasit. *43:*664–669, 1957.

180. ZASUKHIN, D. N., VASINA, S. G., and LEVITANSKALA, P. B.: Atoxoplasma and Toxoplasma in birds. Zool. Zh. *35:*1799–1808, 1956. (Russian, with English Summary.)

181. ZWART, P.: Trichomonas hepatica infecties bii twee zebravinken en een oranjekaakje in enn Nederlandse volière. Tijdschr. Diergeneesk. *84:*1312–1314, 1959.

182. ZWART, P.: Acariasis in canaries (A clinical report). Nord. Vet-Med. *14*(Suppl. 1):292–296, 1962.

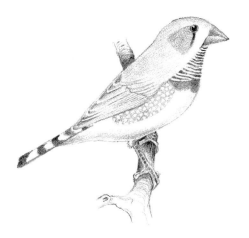

26

Mycoses

*I. F. Keymer**

With the exception of aspergillosis, which was first described in a scaup duck as long ago as 1813 by Montague, very little is known about fungal diseases of passerine and psittacine birds. Even poultry research has been confined mainly to aspergillosis and candidiasis. There is little information about candidiasis in cage birds, however, and even less about dermatomycoses, or the diagnosis of rhinosporidiosis, actinomycosis, and nocardiosis.

Kon and Linton[16] described a case of mucormycotic infection in a young rock-hopper penguin, caused by *Absidia ramosa*. In this case the left lung was found to have been destroyed and replaced by thick grey, tenacious mucoid material. Four yellow caseous nodules were present on the inner surface of the thoracic wall, and there were some pin-point hemorrhages in the cerebellum.

Ballarini and Pieresca[6] listed blastomycosis as a diagnosis in one psittacine and two canaries out of a total of 1324 birds examined, but it is not clear what they meant by this diagnosis, especially as no fungus was specified. Lesbouyries,[17] quoting from a report of Graham Smith in 1907, referred briefly to the formation of small cysts containing *Rhinosporidium kinealyi* or *R. seeberi* in the "heart and muscles" of a budgerigar. Coffin[8] vaguely implied that *Nocardia* and *Actinomyces* may cause lesions in parrots that could be confused with those of tuberculosis.

Except for the case of mucormycotic infection in

*Some of the material on aspergillosis was contributed by R. N. T-W-Fiennes, M.A., M.R.C.V.S., Head of Pathology Department, Nuffield Institute of Comparative Medicine, The Zoological Society of London.

the penguin, the reports cited must be treated with skepticism, owing to the lack of supporting evidence. Ainsworth and Austwick,[2] in their well-known review, failed to mention any records of these diseases in birds, except for a single reference to nocardiosis in the domestic fowl. At that time no authentic case of mucormycotic infection had been found in birds, although these authors stated that there was no apparent reason why such infections should not occur.

Various workers have isolated *Cryptococcus neoformans* from feces of pigeons, fowls, pheasants, housemartins, jackdaws, chaffinches, parrots, and canaries,[11,21,22,23] but cryptococcus infection in birds has so far not been confirmed. In well-managed collections of birds where the standard of hygiene is good, the fungus should have little opportunity to thrive. It is only mentioned here because *C. neoformans* can cause serious disease in man.

ASPERGILLUS AND ASPERGILLOSIS

Aspergillosis is one of the commonest of all avian diseases, and for extensive reviews of the subject Urbain and Guillot[25] and Verge[27] should be consulted.

SPECIES AND HOSTS

Aspergillus fumigatus is the usual cause of the disease, but *A. flavus, A. niger, A. nidulans,* and *A. terreus* are also listed as pathogens.[2]

It seems likely that all species of birds are susceptible to infection, the disease often being recorded in birds representing virtually all the families, especially waterfowl and penguins.[3] Parrots, parakeets, and canaries, with which this book is mainly concerned, are also frequently infected.

DISTRIBUTION AND INCIDENCE

Distribution is world-wide and the disease is common both in free-living and in captive birds. The latter, however, seem to be particularly susceptible when newly subjected to captivity, especially if this has entailed an extended sojourn in overcrowded and unhygienic conditions, as frequently happens when birds are trapped in the tropics and exported to the main bird-keeping areas of the world in North America or Europe.

CLINICAL SIGNS OF INFECTION

The clinical signs are often vague and certainly are not diagnostic. The disease may be peracute, acute, or chronic, and signs range from debility and varying degrees of dyspnea to sudden death. Occasionally symptoms of nervous involvement are also seen.

POSTMORTEM FINDINGS AND PATHOLOGY

Lesions may be found after death in almost any organ, hence the variability of the clinical signs. Primarily, the fungus attacks the respiratory tract and the lesions it produces are almost diagnostic, especially when they are confined to the lungs and air sacs (Fig. 26-1).

In the peracute pneumonic form, the only change is marked congestion of the lungs. When the disease is less acute, yellowish, miliary nodules are found throughout the lung tissue, each lesion being surrounded by an area of hyperemia. As the disease becomes more advanced, areas of consolidation occur, and often the miliary necrotic nodules coalesce to form larger nodules and masses of necrotic or granulomatous lesions. Much of the lung tissue may be replaced in this way before death occurs. Sometimes disc-shaped necrotic plaques develop, and greenish-blue or greyish patches of conidiophores may form. Plaques occur more frequently in the air sacs, where the lesions produced are similar to those seen in the lungs.

In acute cases, however, only simple inflammatory lesions may be present, the serous membrane of the air sacs gradually becoming thicker and whitish in appearance, prior to the development of necrotic plaques. Occasionally, secondary bacterial infection with *Esch-*

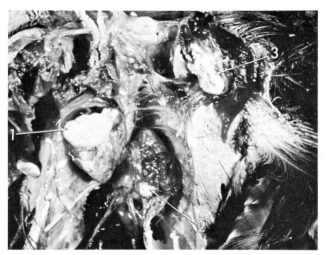

Fig. 26-1. *Lesions of aspergillosis in the rook* (Corvus frugilegus). *1, Right thoracic air sac containing a mass of necrotic material; the wall of the air sac is also thickened and opaque. 2, Granulomatous nodule on ventro-medial aspect of posterior portion of left lung; areas of congestion are also present. 3, Left axillary air sac containing a mass of necrotic material.*

erichia coli or *Mycobacterium tuberculosis* occurs, and pus formation may be seen.

Lesions are found in the upper respiratory tract less frequently than in the lungs and air sacs, and take the form of masses of necrotic material or plaques on the epithelial lining of the trachea, syrinx, or bronchi, causing asphyxia.

Plaque-like lesions occasionally occur on the mucous membrane of the mouth and even lower down in the alimentary tract, in the intestines. Sometimes peritonitis develops as an extension of lesions in the abdominal air sacs, and necrotic nodules caused by the fungus have been recorded in the liver, kidney, and other organs. Occasionally abscesses occur in the brain, and eye lesions have also been described in poultry.

DIAGNOSIS

Diagnosis is based on the presence of the typical lesions in the respiratory tract. Sometimes a tentative diagnosis can be made in birds showing dyspnea, especially if the conditions of management and hygiene are poor and presence of the disease has been established at necropsy in birds that have died previously.

If no fruiting patches of the fungus are found at postmortem examination, then necrotic nodules should be examined for hyphae. This should be done by dissecting out and crushing a portion of the lesion on a microscope slide beneath a coverslip in a drop of 20% potassium hydroxide and lactophenol–cotton blue, when the hyphae can usually be seen projecting from the edges of the fragments.

More use could probably be made of radiography in the diagnosis of chronic cases in live birds.

DIFFERENTIAL DIAGNOSIS. When the lesions in the lungs do not contain hyphae, the condition may be confused with tuberculosis or pseudotuberculosis. Pox and trichomoniasis sometimes cause lesions similar to those of aspergillosis in the buccal cavity, and granulomatous lesions in the intestine are also produced by the tubercle bacilli and by *Escherichia coli.*

PREVENTION AND TREATMENT

Hygienic methods of management are the only real safeguard against infection, because birds become infected by inhaling or ingesting the fungus spores. Fortunately the disease cannot be transmitted from bird to bird, but Wright *et al.*[28] discovered that the spores of *A. fumigatus* can penetrate embryonating chicken eggs within 8 days after contamination of the shells. Chicks hatched from such eggs developed aspergillosis when 10 days of age.

The fungus grows on damp organic material; therefore food must be clean and never allowed to become damp or stale, and it should be replaced regularly. If an outbreak of the disease occurs, all possible sources of infection should be removed and destroyed, and the cages or aviary thoroughly cleansed with a hot solution of washing soda or detergent.

Treatment is unlikely to be successful in most cases, as frequently the lesions are too far advanced by the time the disease is suspected or diagnosed. When dyspnea is present, the administration of oxygen may produce some relief. Dall *et al.*[9] suggested the use of a nystatin aerosol in a nebulizer, exposing the birds for 15 minutes twice a day; for prevention of the disease in parrots they suggested 2.5 grains (150 mg.) of potassium iodide dissolved in 2 ounces (60 ml.) of the drinking water daily or every other day. This dose can be altered at the discretion of the clinician, depending on the size and type of bird under treatment. No controlled experiments have been carried out to test the efficacy of these treatments; however, as they are unlikely to cause any harm, they are worth trying, especially when collections of valuable birds are involved.

CANDIDA AND CANDIDIASIS

Candidiasis, caused by the mycelial yeast *Candida albicans,* is also known as thrush, moniliasis, or candidosis. It is primarily a disease of turkeys and artificially reared partridges. In wild birds it occurs most commonly in pigeons, pheasants, partridges, and grouse.[18]

SPECIES AND HOSTS

The disease, although usually caused by *C. albicans,* may be associated with other species of *Candida* (syn. *Monilia* or *Oidium*), according to Ainsworth and Austwick.[2]

Most of the reports of the disease in birds refer to gallinaceous species, but there are a few records of the infection in psittacines and passerines.

Ainsworth and Austwick[1] isolated *C. albicans* from the sternum of a parrot; Keymer[13] reported the susceptibility of parrots to infection of the crop, and Austwick[4] isolated the yeast from the crop of a budgerigar.

Buckley[7] described "a black cottony growth covering the lungs" of a blue-crowned hanging parrot (*Loriculus galgulus*), from which *C. albicans* was isolated. The diagnosis of candidiasis, however, cannot be accepted without further information regarding the histopathology of the lesions, because the yeast sometimes occurs in healthy birds and it seems unlikely to have been responsible for lesions of this kind.

Ballarini and Pieresca[6] diagnosed the disease in two canaries out of a total of 1324 examined, but gave no further details of the condition. Vallée *et al.*,[26] however, described an outbreak of the disease in Gouldian finches (*Poephila gouldiae*), linnets (*Carduelis cannabina*), and Bengalese finches (*Lonchura domestica*). Although *C. albicans* was cultured from all three species, the infection killed only the Gouldian finches. It is interesting to note that the organism has been isolated from the crop and intestines of healthy wild house sparrows in Portugal.[24] Van Uden concluded that fish-eating and insectivorous birds are not suitable hosts for intestinal yeasts, but that such yeasts are most likely to be found in grain-eating and omnivorous species.

DISTRIBUTION AND INCIDENCE

Candida itself is global in distribution, but little is known regarding candidiasis in non-gallinaceous birds, and it certainly seems to be uncommon in cage and aviary species.

In Europe the disease has a seasonal incidence, being seen mainly in July.

CLINICAL SIGNS OF INFECTION

Debility has been recorded in parrots by Dall *et al.*[9] Vallée *et al.*[26] described listlessness and ruffled feathers in chronically infected passerines, whereas in the more acute condition resulting in the death of Gouldian finches the crop wall was thickened and instead of permitting visibility of the contents through the skin, as is normal in healthy birds, the wall was opaque.

POSTMORTEM FINDINGS

The infection is usually restricted to the upper part of the alimentary tract, particularly the crop. The only lesions seen in parrots by Keymer consisted of a thin layer of whitish mucus, loosely attached to the epithelial lining of the crop[9]; Vallée *et al.*[26] described classical lesions (Fig. 26-2) and the presence of a creamy substance containing numerous yeast cells and mycelial elements. McDiarmid[18] observed severe enteritis in a wild jackdaw (*Corvus monedula*), which he attributed to *C. albicans*.

The histopathology of the disease has been described by Keymer and Austwick.[14]

DIAGNOSIS

Diagnosis is possible only at necropsy, based on discovery of the lesions in the crop and the demonstration and identification of the yeast by laboratory techniques.

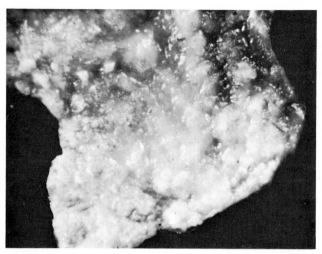

Fig. 26-2. *Candidiasis in the European partridge* (Perdix perdix). *Typical appearance of the crop, with greyish white necrotic material adhering loosely to the underlying mucous membrane.*

DIFFERENTIAL DIAGNOSIS. Lesions of trichomoniasis and necrosis of the esophageal and crop epithelium, first recorded in budgerigars by Keymer,[12] in some respects resemble the changes produced by candidiasis, but neither trichomoniasis nor necrosis of esophageal and crop epithelium has been recorded in parrots.

PREVENTION AND TREATMENT

Keymer and Austwick[14] discussed the epidemiology and predisposing causes of the infection, with particular reference to the disease in partridges, and concluded that debilitating factors and deficiencies of components of the vitamin B group may play a rôle. Strict attention should therefore be paid to correct feeding, and high standards of management should always be maintained. Aviary birds should also be protected from the excreta of house sparrows and other wild birds.

Dall *et al.*[9] suggested treatment with nystatin, but no satisfactory dose has been calculated, and there is no information regarding its effect on the disease in parrots.

Vallée *et al.*[26] experimented with the use of various medicaments, including nystatin, but had no success. They believed that the fungicides were inactivated by products in the digestive tract, because *in vitro* the isolated organisms were sensitive.

DERMATOPHYTES AND DERMATOMYCOSES

There are unreliable reports by bird fanciers of fungal diseases of the skin in cage birds under the name of favus, and recently a few cases have been confirmed in wild birds in England. However, these infections by dermatophytes or ringworm fungi of the keratinized layers of the skin and appendages are difficult to diagnose and are easily confused with other conditions.

SPECIES AND HOSTS

Pathogenic dermatophytes appear to be world-wide by Ainsworth and Austwick[2] as belonging to two genera, namely, *Trichophyton* (syn. *Achorion*) and *Microsporum;* some workers also recognize the genus *Lophophyton.* Only *Trichophyton* spp. have been recorded from birds, *T. gallinae* producing the well-known, if very rare, disease of domestic fowl known as favus. Austwick and Blackmore,[5] however, have isolated from the skin of a house sparrow a dermatophyte associated with favus-like lesions; Austwick and Keymer obtained another unidentified isolate from a European robin (*Erithacus rubecula*).[15,20] Macdonald[19] also reported a similar type of favus in a European robin.

The only apparently confirmed report of favus in a canary is that by Fischer,[10] who cultured, from skin lesions which he said were typical of favus, a fungus similar in some respects to *Trichophyton schönleinii* and in other respects to *T. rosaceum.* He called the fungus *Achorion passerinum.*

DISTRIBUTION AND INCIDENCE

Pathogenic dermatophytes appear to be world-wide in distribution, but the diseases they produce in birds are sporadic and relatively uncommon.

CLINICAL SIGNS OF DERMATOMYCOSIS

Lesions in wild passerine birds have been characterized by alopecia, especially of the head region. The skin becomes thickened and corrugated, and is dirty white in color.

It should be remembered that *T. gallinae* and other species of *Trichophyton* cause tinea (ringworm) in man and in various other mammals, both domestic and wild, and that the infection they cause is contagious.

PATHOLOGY

Lesions are limited to the epidermis, dermis, and base of the feathers, and there is little tissue reaction. The fungi grow upon and into the surface of the *stratum corneum,* which sometimes becomes thickened.

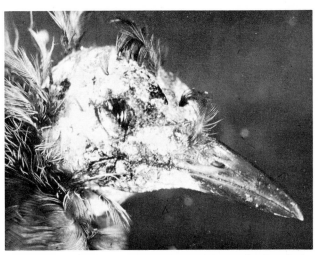

Fig. 26-3. *Chronic lesions of dermatitis on the head of a European blackbird* (Turdus merula). *Lesions of this type may be associated with either mite infestations or* Trichophyton *infection or may accompany a combination of the two conditions. Frequently it is difficult to isolate any pathogenic organisms without a detailed laboratory examination.*

DIAGNOSIS

The disease can be suspected from the macroscopic appearance of the lesions, but laboratory examination and special culture methods are necessary for confirmation of the diagnosis.

DIFFERENTIAL DIAGNOSIS. The infection is most likely to be confused with the skin lesions caused by epidermoptic, cnemidocoptic, or *Neocheyletiella* mites. There is also some evidence that faulty nutrition may be a contributory cause of alopecia in cage birds, and it should always be remembered that dermatomycosis may be encountered with a concomitant ectoparasite infestation.

TREATMENT

No information is available concerning treatment of the disease in small birds, although, if practical, oral administration of griseofulvin might be useful in some cases.

ACKNOWLEDGMENT

I am indebted to Mr. P. K. C. Austwick, B.Sc., of the Central Veterinary Laboratory, Weybridge, England, for kindly reading the text and for his helpful criticisms.

References

1. AINSWORTH, G. C., and AUSTWICK, P. K. C.: A survey of animal mycoses in Britain: General aspects. Vet. Rec. *67:*88–97, 1955.

2. AINSWORTH, G. C., and AUSTWICK, P. K. C.: *Fungal Diseases of Animals.* Review Series No. 6 of the Commonwealth Bureau of Animal Health. Farnham Royal, Bucks, Commonwealth Agricultural Bureaux, 1959. 148 pp.

3. APPLEBY, E. C.: Mycosis of the respiratory tract in penguins. Proc. zool. Soc. Lond. *139:*495–501. 1962.

4. AUSTWICK, P. K. C.: Personal communication, 1965.

5. AUSTWICK, P. K. C., and BLACKMORE, D. K.: Personal communication, 1965.

6. BALLARINI, G., and PIERESCA, G.: Attività svolta dal "Centro Ricerche Malattie Uccelli (FOI)" Durante il Triennio 1959-60-61. Nuova Vet. *38:*136, 1962.

7. BUCKLEY, F. G.: The occurrence and treatment of candidiasis in the blue-crowned hanging parrot (*Loriculus galgulus*). Avic. Mag. *71:*143–145, 1965.

8. COFFIN, D. L.: Diseases of Parrots. In *Parrots and Parrot-Like Birds,* by the Duke of Bedford. Fond du Lac, Wis., All-Pets Books, Inc., 1954. P. 26.

9. DALL, J. A., BRANCKER, W. M., GRAHAM-JONES, O., JOSHUA, J. O., and KEYMER, I. F.: *Handbook on the Treatment of Exotic Pets.* London, British Veterinary Association, 1964. Part 1. *Cage Birds.* 83 pp.

10. FISCHER, W.: Favus beim Kanarienvogel (Achorion passerinum). Derm. Wschr. *87:*1359–1361, 1928.

11. FRAGNER, P.: Naleezy kryptokoku v ptacim trusu (Isolation of cryptococcus from bird faeces). Csl. Epidem. Microbiol. Immunol. *11:*135–139, 1962. English summary.

12. KEYMER, I. F.: The diagnosis and treatment of common psittacine diseases. Mod. vet. Pract. *39*(21):22–30, December 15, 1958.

13. KEYMER, I. F.: Postmortem examinations of pet birds. Mod. vet. Pract. *42*(23):35–38, December 1, and *42*(24):47–51, December 15, 1961.

14. KEYMER, I. F., and AUSTWICK, P. K. C.: Moniliasis in partridges (*Perdix perdix*). Sabouraudia *1:*22–29, 1961.

15. KEYMER, I. F., and BLACKMORE, D. K.: Diseases of the skin and soft parts of wild birds. Brit. Birds *57:*175–179, 1964.

16. KON, V. M., and LINTON, A. H.: Mucormycotic infection of birds. Vet. Rec. *73:*1008, 1961.

17. LESBOUYRIES, G.: *La pathologie des oiseaux.* Paris, Vigot Frères, 1941. Vol. 2, p. 506.

18. McDIARMID, A.: *Diseases of Free-Living Wild Animals.* F.A.O. Working Document. Animal Health Branch Monograph No. 1. Rome, Food and Agriculture Organization of the United Nations, 1960. P. 41.

19. MACDONALD, J. W.: Another case of fungus disease affecting a robin. Brit. Birds *56:*462, 1963.

20. SOPER, E. A., and HOSKING, E.: Fungus disease affecting robins and other species. Brit. Birds *54:*289–290, 1961.

21. STAIB, F.: Vorkommen von *Cryptococcus neoformans* im Vogelmist (*C. neoformans* in bird faeces). Zbl. bakt. I. (orig.) *182:*562–563, 1961.

22. STAIB, F.: *Cryptococcus neoformans* beim Kanarienvogel (*Cryptococcus neoformans* in the canary). Zbl. bakt. I. (orig.) *185:*129–134, 1962. Summaries in English, French, Spanish, and Russian.

23. STAIB, E.: *Cryptococcus neoformans* im Muskelgewebe (*Cryptococcus neoformans* in the muscular tissue). Zbl. Bakt. I. (orig.) *185:*135–144, 1962. Summaries in English, French, Spanish, and Russian.

24. UDEN, N. van: Factors of host-yeast relationship. Recent Prog. Microbiol. *8:*641, 1962.

25. URBAIN, A., and GUILLOT, G.: Les aspergilloses aviaires. Rev. Path. comp. Hyg. gen. *38:*929–955, 1938.

26. VALLÉE, A., DROUHET, E., GUILHON, J.-C., and NAZIMOFF, O.: Un foyer de candidose (*C. albicans*) chez des oiseaux exotiques. Bull Acad. vét. Fr. *37:*153–156, 1964.

27. VERGE, M. J.: Les aspergilloses des oiseaux. Rec. Méd. vét. *103:*521–528, 1927.

28. WRIGHT, M. L., ANDERSON, G. W., and McCONACHIE, J. D.: Transmission of aspergillosis during incubation. Poult. Sci. *40:*727–731, 1961.

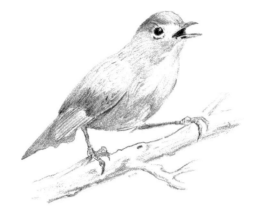

27

Neoplasms

*Margaret L. Petrak and
Charley E. Gilmore*

Neoplasia is a common cause of death in budgerigars. Beach[6] found it accounted for death in almost 25 per cent of the birds he surveyed, being the cause in 33 per cent of the pet birds and in approximately one-half of that percentage of breeders' birds. Blackmore[7] confirmed Beach's findings, citing an incidence of 30 per cent in pet budgerigars and of 9 per cent in breeders' birds.

Ratcliffe,[17] in a study of necropsies of birds and mammals at the Philadelphia Zoo, found that, in general, birds of the Order Psittaciformes had the highest incidence of neoplasms (3.5 per cent) in the Class Aves; the budgerigar (*Melopsittacus undulatus*), in particular, had a tumor incidence of 15.81 per cent, a frequency unparalleled among other birds and among mammals. On the other hand, the tumor incidence among birds belonging to the Order Passeriformes was lower than that among members of any other Order of either birds or mammals. These two Orders, Psittaciformes and Passeriformes, include the majority of species that are kept as cage and aviary birds.

Schlumberger[21] found pituitary tumors to be one of the most common neoplasms in budgerigars. We, like Beach[5] and Blackmore,[7] found a very low incidence of such tumors in our survey. The high incidence of pituitary tumors noted by Schlumberger may have been due to the fact that birds exhibiting signs of central nervous system disorder were sent to him from breeders throughout the United States. Our own studies and those of Beach and of Blackmore were based on routine postmortem examination of birds dying from many causes. The relative incidence of the various types of neoplasms noted in these different studies is graphically presented in Figure 27-1.

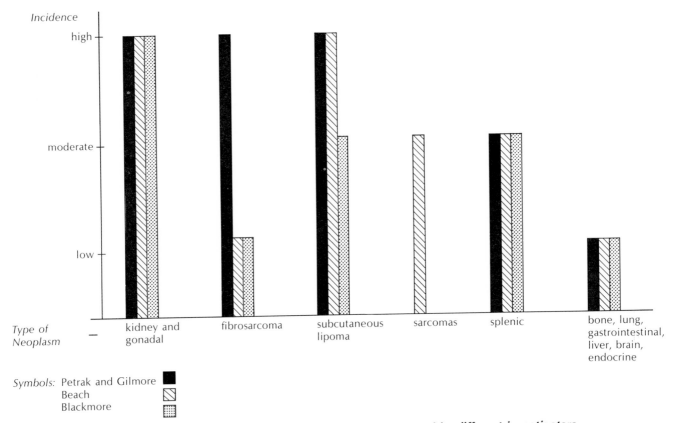

Fig. 27-1. *Incidence of various types of avian neoplasm noted by different investigators.*

This Chapter comprises a detailed report of 196 tumors (Table 27-1) in pet birds, 182 of which (93 per cent) occurred in budgerigars. Parrots, canaries, cockatoos, and cockatiels accounted for the remaining 7 per cent. The clinical examinations and gross autopsies were performed by Petrak; the histological examinations were performed by Gilmore. Discussion of the tumors is organized on a regional basis. Included in the information for each tumor is the species and, when known, the age and sex of the birds involved, pertinent clinical signs and symptoms, and a description of the gross and the microscopical appearance of the tumor. This is followed by discussion of the treatment and a review of the literature.

The ratio of malignant to benign tumors in this study was approximately 2 to 1. Of the malignant tumors, approximately 66 per cent involved the skin and subcutaneous tissue or the kidneys, being divided equally between the two groups. Seventy-five per cent of those involving the subcutis were fibrosarcomas, whereas those involving the skin were carcinomas of various types. Seventy-five per cent of the kidney tumors were adenocarcinomas, and the remainder were embryonal nephromas. The next largest group (15 per cent) comprised gonadal tumors; these were divided equally between

males and females. Seven per cent of the malignant growths involved the hemic and lymphatic system, being divided almost equally between tumors of the spleen and leukosis. The small percentage remaining involved the musculo-skeletal system, the abdominal cavity, the gastrointestinal system (including the liver), and the thyroid and pituitary glands. Approximately 90 per cent of the benign tumors involved the skin and subcutaneous tissue. Two thirds of this group were subcutaneous lipomas. Xanthomas and papillomas each contributed about 10 per cent. Tumors of the abdominal cavity and one papilloma of the larynx made up the remaining small percentage of benign tumors involving other regions.

BODY AS A WHOLE

Abdominal Cavity

Six budgerigars had neoplasms in the abdominal cavity, including five sarcomas and one lipoma. One leiomyosarcoma (Fig. 27-2) and a fibrosarcoma seemed to originate from the renal area. The source of the li-

Table 27-1. Location, Types, and Numbers of Tumors Forming Basis of This Study

Location of Tumor	Type of Tumor	Number Found	Location of Tumor	Type of Tumor	Number Found
ABDOMINAL CAVITY	sarcoma	5	DIGESTIVE SYSTEM		
	lipoma	1	Mouth	fibrosarcoma	1
SKIN AND			Crop	leiomyosarcoma	1
SUBCUTANEOUS			Cloaca	adenocarcinoma	1
TISSUE				undifferentiated	
Skin	papilloma	7		sarcoma	1
	xanthoma	9	Liver	undifferentiated	
	epidermal cysts	2		carcinoma	1
	squamous cell			fibrosarcoma	1
	carcinoma	1		hemangioendothelioma	1
	undifferentiated			adenocarcinoma of	
	carcinoma	1		intrahepatic bile	
	hemangioma	1		ducts	2
Uropygial gland	adenoma	1	UROGENITAL SYSTEM		
	adenocarcinoma	3	Kidney	adenocarcinoma	31
Subcutis	lipoma	39		embryonal nephroma	9
	liposarcoma	3	Testis	seminoma	2
	hemangioendothelioma	1		interstitial cell tumor	1
	fibroma	2		Sertoli cell tumor	5
	fibrosarcoma	23		leiomyosarcoma	1
	undifferentiated			hemangioma of	
	sarcomas	3		testicular capsule	1
MUSCULO-SKELETAL	osteosarcoma	3	Oviduct	leiomyosarcoma	2
SYSTEM	rhabdomyosarcoma	1	Ovary	granulosa cell tumor	5
RESPIRATORY				adenocarcinoma	4
SYSTEM			ENDOCRINE SYSTEM		
Larynx	papilloma	1	Thyroid glands	adenocarcinoma	4
HEMIC AND	cutaneous leukosis	2	Pituitary gland	pituitary tumor	4
LYMPHATIC	visceral leukosis	3			
SYSTEM					
Spleen	hemangioendothelioma	2			
	leiomyoma	1			
	leiomyosarcoma	2			
	lymphangioma	1			

poma and the second leiomyosarcoma and fibrosarcoma could not be determined. The remaining fibrosarcoma was proximate to the liver (Fig. 27-3). Ages of the birds ranged from 1 to 5 years, with the age of one bird being unknown. There were four females and two males.

Some signs and symptoms were evidenced in common. Five of the six birds showed obvious abdominal distention, and accordingly were dyspneic and quieter than normal. In addition, the bird with the leiomyosarcoma in the kidney region had been paralyzed in the ipsilateral leg for 3 weeks prior to examination. The tumor had metastasized to the tibio-tarsal musculature, and two areas of overlying skin were gangrenous. All birds had been noticeably ill for 2 to 6 weeks before

examination. A poor prognosis was given in all cases, and the birds were euthanatized.

The tumors varied in size from 1.5 to 4 cm. in maximal measurement. Typical gross and microscopical appearances are described under subcutaneous lipoma, subcutaneous fibrosarcoma, and splenic leiomyosarcoma (*q.v.*).

Arnall[4] recorded the occurrence of 4 intra-abdominal carcinomas and 1 liposarcoma of unknown origin among a group of 166 tumors in cage birds. Frost[10] listed 4 intra-abdominal lipomas among 199 tumors in budgerigars. Beach[5] related the finding of 9 lipomas, 2 leiomyomas, 3 spindle cell sarcomas, and 1 round cell sarcoma intra-abdominally among 210 tumors in budgerigars.

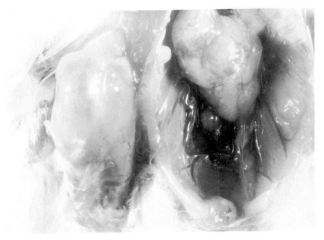

Fig. 27-2. *Leiomyosarcoma in the abdominal cavity and thigh of a budgerigar.*

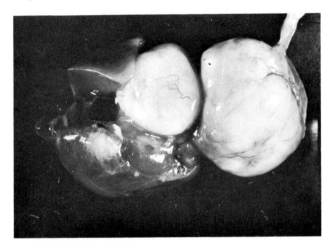

Fig. 27-3. *Fibrosarcoma in the abdominal cavity, with metastasis to the liver.*

SKIN AND SUBCUTANEOUS TISSUE

Skin

PAPILLOMA

Papillomas were encountered in seven birds representing four species: two yellow-headed amazon parrots (*Amazona ochrocephala*), one African grey parrot (*Psittacus erithacus*), one cockatiel (*Nymphicus hollandicus*), and three budgerigars (*Melopsittacus undulatus*). The parrots ranged in age from 34 to 50 years, and were of unknown sex. The cockatiel was a 1-year-old male, and the budgerigars were females, 2, 3, and 7 years old.

Symptoms and signs were related to the area involved and to the bird's proneness to pick at anything unusual on its body. Pain was evidenced by sharp screams when

the bird irritated the tumor, and at times the picking resulted in hemorrhage.

The surface of the papilloma was usually a dry, hard, irregular, brown crust unless the outer cornified layer had recently fallen off, in which event it was moist, soft, and irregular, and white, yellow, or pink. The tissue of the tumor itself was fleshy, friable, and very vascular. The tumors varied in shape from a long horn-like projection perpendicular to the skin, to an ulcerative, crusty, linear lesion. Two lesions in the parrots were perpendicular projections measuring approximately 5 × 1 × 1 cm., and the remaining ulcerous lesion was 2 cm. long, 1.4 cm. wide, and 0.9 cm. deep. Two occurred on the neck and one in the uropygial region.

The papilloma on the cockatiel was an elevated yellow-grey crust covering the second and third phalanges of the third toe. It had first appeared as a small nodule, which had been scarified and chemically cauterized intermittently for 2 months. Papillomas on two of the budgerigars were bleeding, brown, crusty ulcers, 1–2 cm. in maximal measurement, occurring in the skin

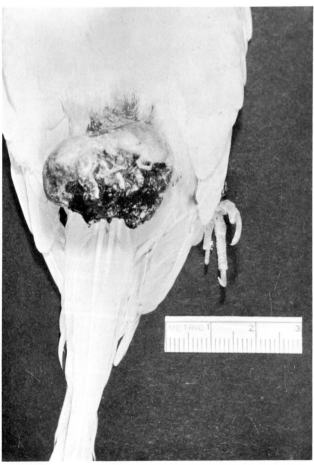

Fig. 27-4. *Papilloma arising from the uropygial gland region of a budgerigar.*

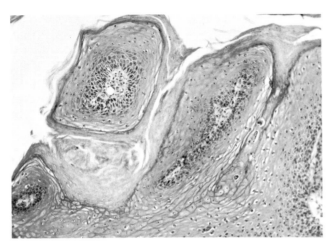

Fig. 27-5. *Papilloma of the skin. Fronds of stratified squamous epithelium are covered with a thick layer of keratin.* ×100.

over the uropygial gland (Fig. 27-4). In the third budgerigar the tumor formed a conical projection from the skin over the mandible.

Microscopically the tumors consisted of irregular fronds of squamous epithelium covered with a thick, dense layer of keratin (Fig. 27-5). Some of the fronds had a core of loose vascular connective tissue; others had a center filled with keratin and necrotic cellular debris. Cells about the periphery of the basal part of the tumor were small cuboidal; those in the projecting fronds were large polyhedral. Occasional small groups of cells within the fronds were keratinized.

The papillomas in two of the parrots and three budgerigars were removed by surgical excision. The second and third phalanges of the digit of the cockatiel were amputated, after which the bird used the foot normally. The owner of the third parrot would not permit surgery, and an unsuccessful attempt was made to treat the bird with chemical cautery. The treatment of choice is surgical excision.

In the literature reviewed, only three specific references to papillomas were found. Beach[5] recorded the occurrence of four small papillomas in budgerigars: two from the angle of the beak, one from the conjunctiva, and one from the wing. This was from a total of 210 tumors in the species. Blackmore[7] recorded the occurrence of unilateral papillomas of the feet in both free-living and aviary chaffinches (*Fringilla coelebs*). Arnall[4] listed 1 papilloma occurring on the wing of a budgerigar, among 166 tumors in cage birds.

XANTHOMA

Xanthomas were present in eight budgerigars and one roseate cockatoo (*Kakatoe roseicapilla*). The cocka-

too was 39 years old when first seen, and the budgerigars ranged in age from 1 to 11 years. There were seven males and two females.

The owner of an affected bird may seek veterinary advice when a lump is noted or when hemorrhage results from the bird's picking at the affected area or traumatizing it on perches or bars of the cage. Because of the vascularity of xanthomatous skin, hemorrhage may be clinically significant. Seemingly, pruritus may accompany this condition.

Xanthomas may occur as discrete tumor masses or as diffuse thickenings of the skin. In either event, they are yellow in color. In three of the nine cases the lesions appeared as globular yellow masses ranging from 0.2 to 1 cm. in diameter, occurring on the dorsal cervical, upper back, dorsal wing (Fig. 27-6), and uropygial regions. The condition in the other six cases occurred as xanthomatous skin reactions overlying or related to the presence of other tumors, primarily lipomas. The other underlying conditions were osteosarcoma, mucous cyst, and cutaneous leukosis. Xanthomatous skin is featherless, thickened (to as much as 0.5 cm.), yellow, friable, vascular, and often ulcerated, and presents a typically quilted appearance. It may occur anywhere on the feathered body surface. Petrak has seen this form on the hand, seemingly unrelated to any other disease condition.

Xanthomatous skin is characterized microscopically by a diffuse infiltration of large foam cells in the dermis (Fig. 27-7). The cells are reticuloendothelial cells or macrophages with abundant cytoplasm that contains tiny droplets of lipid. The cells are generally evenly distributed throughout the collagenous dermis in the affected area. The xanthoma may also contain occa-

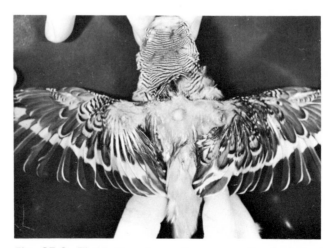

Fig. 27-6. *Three discrete xanthomas on the back and dorsal wing areas of a budgerigar. Note that one is ulcerated.*

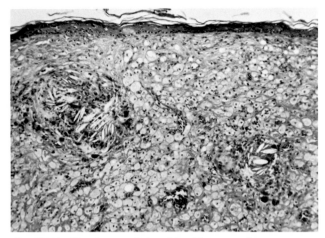

Fig. 27-7. *Xanthoma of the skin. There are foamy macrophages and cholesterol deposits in the dermis.* ×*100.*

sional elliptical spaces (cholesterol clefts), surrounded by macrophages and multinucleated giant cells (Fig. 27-8).

The treatment of choice is surgical excision. If possible, all xanthomatous skin should be removed when an underlying tumor is being excised. If this is impossible, it is helpful to crush the edges of the incision with hemostats to control hemorrhage, allowing the hemostats to remain in place until one is ready to close the incision. Sutures should be placed in normal skin, if possible, because of the friability of xanthomatous skin. At times, the extent or site of the affected area may preclude surgical intervention. Treatment in these cases consists of cautery to control hemorrhage, and use of mechanical devices such as an Elizabethan collar (see Chapters 9 and 11) to prevent self-mutilation. Euthanasia may be advisable in certain instances.

The cause of the development of xanthomatous conditions in cage birds is unknown. Sanger and Lagace[19]

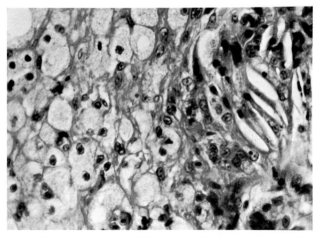

Fig. 27-8. *Higher magnification of tumor shown in Figure 27-7: vacuoles present in cytoplasm of macrophages and elliptical spaces formed by cholesterol deposits.* ×*450.*

described the occurrence of this condition in a large number of Leghorn chickens in the 3-year period from 1958 to 1960. The disease was characterized by swollen wattles, yellowish discoloration and thickening of the skin over the pectoral region and on the feathered parts of the legs, and in some instances formation of large pendulous masses. It was suggested that fat-related toxic hydrocarbons in the feed caused these cases of xanthomatosis.

EPIDERMAL CYSTS

Epidermal cysts occurred in two male budgerigars, one 5 and the other 11 years old.

An epidermal inclusion cyst had appeared several weeks earlier lateral to the uropygial gland in one bird, and a mucous cyst had been present on the lower sternal area of the other for 1 year. Both birds had picked at their lesion, causing hemorrhage.

The inclusion cyst was a firm, yellow, globular mass approximately 1 cm. in diameter, which on cross section had a creamy, yellow-brown appearance. The mucous cyst was discoid, slightly pedunculated, and measured 1 × 1 × 0.5 cm. The surface was ulcerated, granular, and tan in color. In sectioning it was found to contain a thin, clear, slightly mucoid material. An extensive area of skin surrounding the cyst was xanthomatous.

Epidermal inclusion cysts are spherical cysts within the dermis that are lined with stratified squamous epithelium and filled with thin laminations of keratin. The cyst wall is relatively thin and resembles cutaneous epidermis; the basal layer is in contact with the dermis, and the cornified layer faces the lumen of the cyst. Keratinized layers that are shed are trapped within the cyst. If the cyst is ruptured, the escaped keratin induces an intense granulomatous dermatitis.

Both cysts were removed by surgical excision. One year later, the bird that had the mucous cyst was returned for excision of a fibroma occurring at the site of the previous surgery.

Frost[10] recorded the occurrence of an apparent cyst on the leg, a caseous dorsal dermoid cyst, and a small subcutaneous cyst in the sternal region among a group of 199 budgerigars with neoplasia.

SQUAMOUS CELL CARCINOMA

One squamous cell carcinoma occurred in a 6-year-old male budgerigar. It was located in the region of the uropygial gland, and self-trauma had resulted in intermittent hemorrhage.

The tumor was irregular and firm, and measured 0.7 × 0.6 × 0.5 cm. The skin surface was ulcerated, and

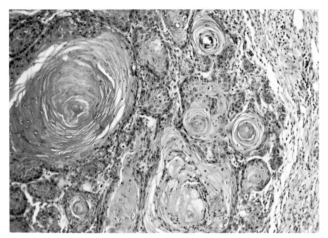

Fig. 27-9. *Squamous cell carcinoma of the skin. Nests of squamous epithelium with keratinized centers are invading the dermis.* ×*100.*

the cut surface of the tumor was grey, smooth, and glistening.

Microscopically, the tumor consisted of irregular and disorganized masses of squamous epithelium deep in the dermis. Small nests and individual cells, some of which were keratinized, were surrounded by fibrous stroma. The cells were generally large, but varied in size. Small groups of keratinized cells, sometimes in a slightly whorled pattern, formed "pearls" in the larger masses (Fig. 27-9).

Stone[23] described three squamous cell carcinomas in budgerigars, all in the region of the uropygial gland. The tumor was surgically excised in two birds; it recurred within three weeks in one bird and twice within one year in the other. Blackmore[7] listed 4 squamous cell carcinomas from a group of 168 tumors in budgerigars: 3 in the skin and 1 in the crop. Beach[5] recorded 2 such tumors among 210 tumors in budgerigars. One occurred in the skin of the neck of a 5-year-old female, and the other in the skin of the thigh of a 1-year-old male. Ratcliffe[17] listed a squamous cell carcinoma of the esophagus in a male military macaw (*Ara militaris*) that had been exhibited 56 months. This was from a group of 42 tumors discovered in 1175 postmortem examinations of psittacines. Lombard and Witte[15] reported a squamous cell carcinoma of the skin in a female bean goose (*Anser fabialis*).

UNDIFFERENTIATED CARCINOMA

A 2-year-old male budgerigar represents the only case of undifferentiated carcinoma of the dermis observed in this series. The owner of the bird had noted a small, rapidly growing mass on the lateral surface of the distal tibio-tarsus, very near the joint. The bird had picked at it slightly, but no bleeding resulted.

Grossly, the growth appeared as a soft, globular mass measuring 0.5 cm. in diameter, with a small ulcer on the surface. The cut surface was uniformly light red.

This tumor was made up of solid masses of cells of rather uniform size. Nuclei were round to oval, 8 to 10 microns in diameter, and vesicular. Each had one or two dark-staining nucleoli. Cytoplasm was scanty, and was slightly eosinophilic with hematoxylin and eosin; the cytoplasmic borders were poorly defined. There were a few fibrous trabeculae and scant blood supply in the tumor. Lack of distinguishing features accounts for its classification as "undifferentiated."

The tumor could be only incompletely excised, owing to its invasiveness.

Lombard and Witte[15] listed the occurrence of a carcinoma of the skin over the mandible in a Chapman's black thrush (*Turdus serranus fuscobrunneus*).

HEMANGIOMA

One case of hemangioma of the dermis occurred in an 8-year-old male budgerigar.

A small globular, red mass had been noted growing at the cutaneous junction of the lower mandible for 3 weeks. The bird evidenced no distress. The tumor was soft and smooth-surfaced, and measured 0.3 cm. in diameter. Its cut surface was uniformly red and glistening.

Microscopically there were endothelial-lined spaces of varying size filled with blood and plasma. The spaces were separated by a network of mature fibrous connective tissue. The entire mass was well encapsulated.

The growth was surgically excised with iris scissors, and the resultant wound was cauterized with tincture of ferric chloride.

Beach[5] recorded a subcutaneous hemangioma 2 cm. in diameter occurring in the groin area of a 5-year-old male budgerigar observed in a study of 210 neoplasms in this species.

Uropygial Gland

ADENOMA

An adenoma of the uropygial gland occurred in a 6-year-old female budgerigar. Excessive localized preening and intermittent bleeding from the area, noted by the owner for 3 weeks prior to examination, had been the only clinical symptoms and signs.

Gross examination revealed a yellow-tan, botryoid mass measuring 1.25 cm. in maximal dimension, with two short quills protruding from its surface. Cross sectioning revealed a thick-walled cyst containing yellow

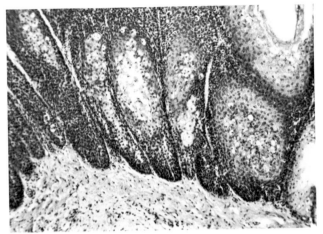

Fig. 27-10. *Adenoma of the uropygial gland. The tumor consists of lobules of poorly differentiated sebaceous type glands.* ×100.

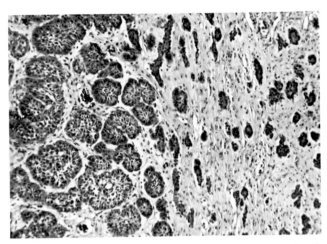

Fig. 27-11. *Adenocarcinoma of the uropygial gland. Malignant epithelium is invading the underlying stroma.* ×100.

caseated material surrounded by a soft, glossy, mottled red-and-tan periphery.

Histologically the tumor consisted of a well-circumscribed spherical mass composed of irregular lobules of epithelial cells. There was a large collection of lipid and necrotic cellular debris in the center of the mass. Some of the lobules were made up of large foamy polyhedral cells; others were composed of smaller basophilic reserve cells. There was no evidence of invasion of the surrounding stroma (Fig. 27-10).

Surgical excision is the treatment of choice. Because of the extreme vascularity of the area, a special effort must be made to control hemorrhage. A seeping-type of bleeding occurs from the large follicles of the rectrices, which is best controlled by packing absorbable gelatin sponges in the surgical area and tightly suturing the overlying skin.

Arnall[4] recorded the occurrence of an adenoma of the preen (uropygial) gland in a canary (*Serinus canarius*). This was from a group of 166 tumors in cage birds.

ADENOCARCINOMA

Adenocarcinoma of the uropygial gland occurred in three budgerigars, two males and one female, ranging from 2 to 6 years in age.

Two of the tumors had been present from 5 to 8 months before surgical excision. All birds were picking at the tumors, and hemorrhage had been noted from time to time. The gross appearance varied sufficiently to warrant separate descriptions of the three growths:

(1) An ulcerated, roughly globular, firm, yellow mass measuring 1.0 × 0.8 × 0.8 cm. The cut surface revealed a loose arrangement of papillary projections interspersed with yellow material.

(2) A firm, roughly oval, pedunculated mass measuring 1.1 × 0.8 × 0.8 cm. It had an irregular surface and was tan-white. The cut surface revealed a finely striated white mass.

(3) A hard, brown, cylindrical shell 2.0 cm. long and 1.0 cm. thick, covering a pear-shaped, white-yellow mass of viable tissue measuring 1.0 × 0.5 × 0.3 cm. The cut surface was white-yellow and smooth. This tumor recurred 4 months later as a flat ulcerous area measuring 1.0 cm. in diameter. Euthanasia was then performed.

Microscopically these tumors consisted of multiple small spherical nests of medium-sized basophilic cells in a dense fibrous stroma. Each of the nests of epithelial cells was approximately the same size; some were arranged in rosettes, and each was well separated from the others by fibrous connective tissue. Occasional larger masses contained cells with foamy cytoplasm similar to normal sebaceous cells (Fig. 27-11).

Blackmore[7] recorded the occurrence of an adenocarcinoma of the uropygial gland in a yellow-fronted parrot (*Chrysotis ochrocephala*). This was from a group of 172 neoplasms in psittacines.

Subcutis

LIPOMA

Lipomas of the subcutis occurred in 38 budgerigars and 1 roseate cockatoo (*Kakatoe roseicapilla*). The budgerigars ranged in age from 1½ to 8 years; 36 (95 per cent) of the tumors occurred in birds 2 to 7 years old. The cockatoo was a 39-year-old male. Twenty-nine of the budgerigars were males, and 9 were females. The majority of the tumors were located on the sternum (Fig. 27-12), wings, and abdomen. A small percentage

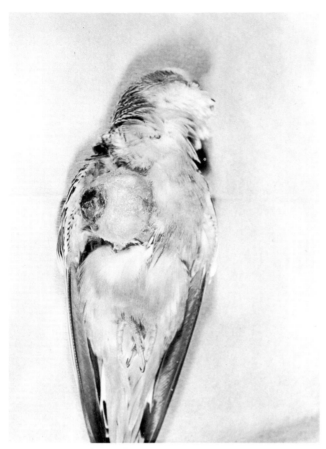

Fig. 27-12. *A large lipoma on the sternum of a budgerigar. Note the ulcerated area on the skin.*

occurred on the back, neck, and uropygium. The recurrent growths in the cockatoo were in the ischial area. Although lipomas are not malignant, a second lipoma was later noted at the same site in two birds and at different sites in three birds.

Symptoms and signs are related primarily to the size and location of tumors. Large sternal and lower cervical lipomas generally hampered flying and locomotion; they sometimes stimulated picking at the site, with resultant skin hemorrhage and drainage of fluid from the necrosing tumor. Medium-sized to large growths on the abdominal wall interfered with normal perching and climbing activities. Associated trauma resulted in abrasion of overlying skin and intermittent hemorrhage. In one case a lipoma occurred as a ring of fatty tissue around the vent, causing the bird to strain when passing its droppings. Fatty tumors on the wings and uropygium stimulated the bird to pick at the tumor in a high percentage of cases, due perhaps to the tightness of the skin in these areas and pain produced as a result of a rapidly expanding lesion. Ulceration and hemorrhage frequently resulted from the self-inflicted trauma.

Histories revealed the tumor mass had been present from 1 week to 1 year or more. Not infrequently an owner claimed that the mass had enlarged rapidly in 2 or 3 weeks. This seems to occur in lipomas undergoing central liquefactive necrosis and probably accounts for their sometimes being termed "abscesses." Lipomas occurred most commonly in obese birds, and as a consequence these birds could not be considered good surgical risks. Abnormal molting, polydipsia, loose droppings, abnormal horn with resultant overgrowth of beak and nails, and decreased vigor are all signs and symptoms that may be present in a bird with a lipoma. These factors should be kept in mind when surgery is considered.

Lipomas were typically globular, turgid, yellow, and well encapsulated. In this series, two tumors were botryoid in shape, and one was yellow-brown in color. The recurring growths in the cockatoo consisted of small, irregular, yellow, friable pieces of fatty tissue covered by ulcerated xanthomatous skin.

The tumors varied in size from 0.3 to 4 cm. in maximal measurement. Those occurring on the wing were usually nearer the minimal size, and those on the sternal, abdominal, or lower cervical area varied from 2 to 4 cm. in diameter. In one budgerigar that died following surgery, the lipoma weighed 19 grams; the bird after removal of the tumor weighed only 29 grams. The cut surface usually presented a 0.1–0.3 cm. yellow capsule surrounding a necrotic center of widely varying color and consistency. The center at times was firm and yellow-white, or soft, crumbly, and red-brown (Fig. 27-13). Sometimes the center was completely fluid and when the capsule was incised exuded varying shades of yellow to yellow-red material. Growths of this latter type grossly resembled abscesses, but when examined microscopically proved to be necrotic lipomas.

Histologically lipomas show considerable variation. Most of those in our study were well encapsulated with

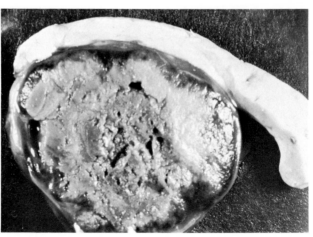

Fig. 27-13. *Cut section of a lipoma, showing a viable peripheral area and a necrotic center.*

mature connective tissue. In a few all the neoplastic fat cells were viable, and the tumor resembled normal adipose tissue. In others there was complete necrosis of the tumor, with variable amounts of hemorrhage. In these, the mass consisted of a few large foamy cells surrounded by poorly staining cellular debris and blood.

The majority of lipomas consisted of a mixture of a few viable fat cells and many large cells with foamy cytoplasm. There were usually areas of hemorrhage and necrosis within the tumors. Thin, fibrous trabeculae were found in some, but there was usually little supporting stroma. The overlying skin was likely to be xanthomatous.

If the general health of the bird and the size and location of the tumor permit, surgical excision is the treatment of choice.

Fox[9] recorded the occurrence of lipomas in six different species of birds: the palm tanager (*Tanagra* [= *Thraupis*] *palmarum*), chestnut-headed bunting (*Emberiza luteola*), roseate cockatoo (*Cacatua* [= *Kakatoe*] *roseicapilla*), parakeet (*Melopsittacus undulatus*), crested ground parakeet (*Calopsitta novaehollandiae*), and sparrow hawk (*Sparverius-Falco sparverius*). Gray[12] mentioned lipoma formation in budgerigars, cockatoos, and parrots. Ratcliffe[17] listed lipomas in two budgerigars, five roseate cockatoos (*Kakatoe roseicapilla*), and one cockatiel (*Nymphicus hollandicus*). This gave a ratio of 8 lipomas to 34 tumors of other types in psittacines. He also recorded a lipoma in a young male palm tanager (*Thraupis palmarum*) exhibited 6 months and a lipoma of the scalp in a male red-headed bunting (*Emberiza icterica*) exhibited 38 months. This was a ratio of 2 lipomas to 12 tumors of varied other types occurring in the passerines.

Gandal and Saunders[11] reported on 18 lipomas and 14 lipomas with necrosis from a collection of 45 cutaneous tumors in budgerigars. Gandal and Saunders[11] and Arnall[2] gave good descriptions of the surgical technique necessary for the removal of these tumors from various locations in the body and the indications for and contraindications to surgery. The majority of 79 extra-abdominal tumors reported by Frost[10] were sternal and abdominal wall lipomas. These were among a group of 199 tumors in budgerigars. Arnall[4] listed 62 skin and subcutaneous lipomas among 166 tumors in cage birds; the sternal area was the commonest site, with 31 tumors, and the wing was next, with 15. Central liquefactive necrosis was present in most of them. Beach[5] recorded 41 subcutaneous lipomas among 210 tumors in budgerigars. The majority occurred on the sternal and abdominal areas, with the rest distributed fairly equally among the wing, shoulder, uropygium, leg, neck, and head. The lipomas varied in size from 0.5 to 4 cm. Those between 0.5 and 1 cm. usually had dry, caseous necrotic centers.

Some of the largest were noted only 2 or 3 weeks before the birds were euthanatized. In 22 cases a fatty liver was present, but in only half of these was it extensive. One case occurred in a roseate cockatoo. Blackmore[7] listed 12 subcutaneous lipomas among 168 tumors in budgerigars.

LIPOSARCOMA

Liposarcomas occurred in two male and one female budgerigar; two birds were 5 years and one was 4 years old.

Two of the growths originated in the sternal area, and one rather spectacular mass arose in the region of the uropygial gland (Fig. 27-14). The smaller sternal tumor had been present for 3 years and had suddenly started to enlarge rapidly. This bird was 2 years old when the tumor was first noted. The skin over the sternal tumors was intact, and no specific history of excessive picking could be elicited. The three tumors are separately described:

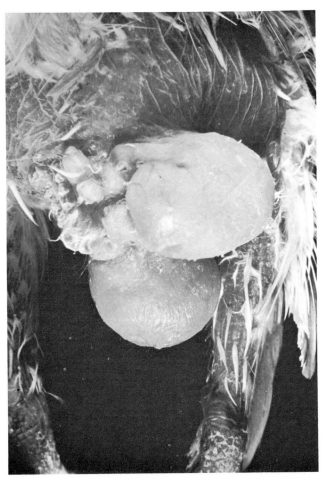

Fig. 27-14. *Liposarcoma arising from the uropygial gland region of a budgerigar.*

(1) A soft, smooth, yellow, pendulous mass originating in the region of the uropygial gland, consisting of two lobes, each measuring approximately 1 cm. in diameter, with several small ulcers in the overlying skin. The cut surface glistened and showed an intermingling of pale yellow, cream, and tan.

(2) A pale-grey, soft, globular mass measuring 1 cm. in diameter and covered on most of the surface by thin, non-adherent skin. The cut surface was dark red-brown and moist.

(3) An irregularly globular, firm, pink-grey mass occurring in the pectoral muscles and measuring approximately 4 cm. in diameter. The cut surface was homogeneously light grey with small zones of red and pale yellow.

Most of the differences in gross appearance of these tumors were caused by differences in amounts of hemorrhage and necrosis. There was, however, some variation in the histologic pattern. Two of the tumors resembled fibrosarcomas (*q.v.*), in which fat vacuoles of variable size were irregularly scattered. In addition, the cytoplasm of many of the neoplastic cells contained smaller vacuoles of lipid. There were small areas of hemorrhage and necrosis.

The other tumor consisted of an evenly distributed mixture of small fat cells and immature cells with one or two moderate-sized vacuoles in their cytoplasm. The latter cells had round to oval vesicular nuclei and were interpreted as immature fat cells. The tumor was relatively vascular, but there was little hemorrhage or necrosis (Fig. 27-15).

The small sternal tumor and the uropygial tumor were surgically excised, and there is no known history of recurrence. The large sternal tumor could not be successfully removed, and the bird died during surgery.

No reference to a liposarcoma in the subcutis could be found in the literature reviewed.

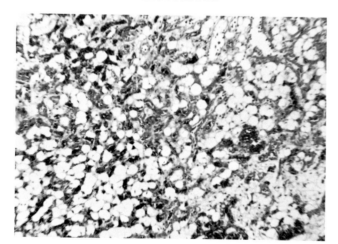

Fig. 27-15. *Liposarcoma of the subcutis. Lipid vacuoles are interspersed among malignant fat cells.* ×*100.*

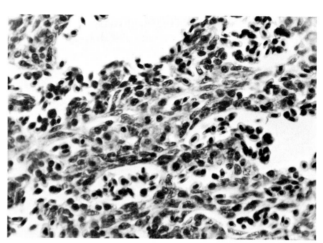

Fig. 27-16. *Hemangioendothelioma of the subcutis. Malignant endothelial cells are forming vascular spaces.* ×*450.*

HEMANGIOENDOTHELIOMA (HEMANGIOSARCOMA)

Hemangioendothelioma of the subcutaneous tissue occurred in one adult male budgerigar of unknown age. A hemorrhagic mass approximately 1 cm. in diameter had been noticed on one wing tip for 2 days.

The tumor was soft and dark red, with ill-defined borders. The cut surface was dark red, soft, and gelatinous.

The tumor was poorly circumscribed and highly cellular. It contained a few large vascular spaces, but most were small, ill-defined spaces within a mass of oval to elongate basophilic cells with indistinct cytoplasmic borders (Fig. 27-16). In most sections the cells were in short, nearly parallel rows, separated by the blood-filled spaces.

The wing tip was amputated, but the bird died while still under anesthesia.

FIBROMA

Fibromas occurred in an 8-year-old and a 12-year-old male budgerigar. Each tumor had been present for 2 or 3 months and had stimulated excessive localized preening. One growth occurred on a wing and the other on the lower sternal area at the site of earlier surgery for removal of a mucous cyst.

The wing fibroma was a small, globular, firm mass measuring 0.2 cm. in diameter. It had an irregular dark surface. The sternal mass was raised, pink, and cystlike, and measured 1.0 × 1.0 × 0.5 cm. On cut surface the tumor was firm, with an intermingling of clear, glistening areas and denser white and grey areas.

Microscopically the tumors were composed of mature, relatively avascular fibrous tissue. Cytoplasmic borders were poorly defined. Nuclei were small, dark, and elongated. They were widely separated by abundant collagen arranged in sheets and irregular fasciculi. Both tumors were surgically excised.

Beach[5] listed four fibromas, of the soft variety, occurring in female budgerigars from 4 to 10 years of age. They were located on the beak, face, wing, and thigh. This was from a study of 210 tumors in the species. Arnall[4] recorded the occurrence of 1 fibroma in a budgerigar from a group of 166 tumors in cage birds.

FIBROSARCOMA

Fibrosarcoma of the subcutis occurred in 22 budgerigars and 1 yellow-headed amazon parrot (*Amazona ochrocephala*). Eighteen (82 per cent) of the budgerigars were less than 5 years old, the youngest being 1 year and the oldest 11 years; the age of three birds was unknown. The parrot was a 45-year-old female. Sixteen of the budgerigars were males, four were females, and the sex of two birds was not recorded.

Fibrosarcomas grew many places on the body, but occurred most frequently on the extremities (Fig. 27-17). Of the 23 tumors, 6 localized on the head or beak, 7 on the wings, and 6 on the legs. One was found in each of the following regions: cervical, sternal, pelvic, and uropygial. They had a tendency to grow near or around joints, but it is of interest that none occurred distal to the tibiotarso-tarsometatarsal or carpal joints. This tumor frequently invaded underlying muscle and occasionally eroded underlying bone, such erosion occurring in four cases. The growth of this tumor in the beak led to distortion and destruction of horn.

Two of the 23 birds had metastases that were grossly apparent at necropsy. One had possible primary sites on the leg and wing, and a metastatic lesion in one lobe of the liver. The other had the primary tumor below the

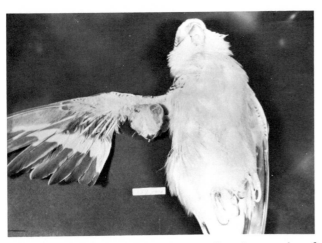

Fig. 27-17. *A large fibrosarcoma invading the muscles of the elbow region.*

ear, and metastases in the cervical and heart-base areas. This bird also had an adenocarcinoma of the kidney. Sixteen birds showed no gross metastases at necropsy. No determination could be made at the time in five birds, owing to successful surgical excision of the tumor.

Symptoms and signs were related to the location and size of the tumor. Those occurring in the beak eventually caused difficulty in eating, and at times hemorrhage resulted from beak-cleaning. The budgerigar with the growth in the auricular region was ataxic and tilted its head to the affected side. Birds with wing involvement often were unable to fly, sometimes drooped the affected wing, and not infrequently picked at the tumor. Growths on the leg resulted in lameness and occasionally paralysis, paralysis occurring especially if the thigh muscle was affected.

The maximal size of the neoplasms varied from 0.5 to 2 cm. in the budgerigars. The tumor on the parrot measured $3.5 \times 3.5 \times 2.0$ cm. The great majority were described as globular or roughly globular in shape, five as ovoid, and only one as botryoid. The surface was characteristically smooth except in the growths occurring in the beak. One was encased in a loose crust, beneath which was a moist, smooth, glistening surface.

The surface and interior colors of the tumors were varying shades and combinations of white, yellow, grey, pink, tan, and red. The majority were moderately firm, a few were soft, and one that occurred in the beak was gelatinous. The appearance of the cut surface was smooth, glistening, cellular, and slightly granular. The cut surface of the tumor on the parrot revealed a cavernous necrotic center with several round firm nodules up to 0.5 cm. in diameter scattered throughout.

The fibrosarcomas were highly cellular, compared with their benign counterparts. The cells were closely packed and usually spindle shaped. In most examples they were arranged in short interlacing fasciculi (Fig. 27-18). In some, such a pattern was not evident; in these cases the cells showed greater variation in size and shape, and were arranged with little relation to each other. The tumors were sometimes circumscribed, but were rarely encapsulated. Vascularity was variable. There was relatively little mature collagen in the tumors, and the cells had elongate to round vesicular nuclei (Fig. 27-19).

Fibrosarcomas were surgically removed from the wings of four budgerigars. In each case it was the opinion of the surgeon that some tumor tissue remained. Excision of one growth from the beak was followed by recurrence 2 months later. Surgery was unsuccessful in seven cases because of excessive hemorrhage or lack of definition of tumor borders. In the remaining 11 cases, euthanasia was performed after examination of the bird.

Ratcliffe[17] listed a fibrosarcoma of the pectoral muscles in a male all-green parakeet (*Brotogeris tirica*) that

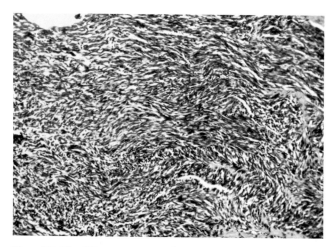

Fig. 27-18. *Fibrosarcoma of the subcutis. Malignant fibroblasts growing in interlacing fasciculi.* ×100.

had been exhibited for 69 months. This was one of 42 tumors discovered in 1175 necropsies of psittacines. Ratcliffe also recorded a fibrosarcoma of the scalp in a male masked Chinese thrush (*Dryonastis perspicillatus*), which was one of 14 tumors discovered in 2837 necropsies of passerines. This bird had been exhibited 145 months. Arnall[4] mentioned 4 fibrosarcomas of the skin and subcutis occurring in budgerigars among 166 tumors in cage birds. Beach[5] listed 1 fibrosarcoma of the beak among 210 tumors in budgerigars. Blackmore[7] recorded 2 fibrosarcomas occurring on the wings of budgerigars among 168 tumors occurring in the species. Gandal and Saunders[11] listed 5 cutaneous fibrosarcomas among 45 cutaneous tumors in budgerigars. They were located on the wing, thigh, and breast. One had metastasized to the lung and liver, causing death of the bird a few weeks after removal of the primary growth on the wing.

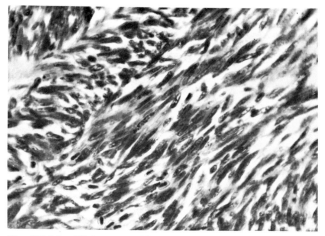

Fig. 27-19. *Higher magnification of tumor shown in Figure 27-18. The cells form little collagen and have elongate vesicular nuclei.* ×450.

UNDIFFERENTIATED SARCOMA

Undifferentiated sarcomas of the subcutis occurred in three male budgerigars, 2, 4, and 7 years old. Signs and symptoms were related primarily to the size and location of the tumor. The growths occurred on the distal tibio-tarsus, distal radius and ulna, and upper back.

The tibio-tarsal tumor caused lameness; the wing and back tumors lessened the birds' ability to fly. Each owner complained that the bird was picking at the tumor; as a result of the picking, the skin was ulcerated and bled intermittently. The general fleshing of all birds was good.

The sarcomas were generally globular or discoid and ranged from 1 to 2 cm. in maximal measurement. The consistency was soft, and the cut surface was glistening and grey or pink-yellow.

This tumor may be a variant of fibrosarcoma. Microscopically, each growth consisted of a solid cellular mass within which were a few large vascular spaces and an occasional sharply circumscribed focus of necrosis. The cells varied greatly in size and shape. Nuclei were round to lobulated and vesicular. Some cells had multiple nuclei; some had giant nuclei. Cytoplasm was scanty and eosinophilic.

Surgery was performed on the birds with tumors on the wing and back. The wing was amputated proximal to the tumor, but the bird died following surgery. The growth on the back was excised, and the bird recovered. Euthanasia was performed on the bird with the sarcoma on the leg. No metastases were seen on necropsy.

Arnall[4] listed 4 sarcomas of the subcutaneous tissue among 166 tumors in cage birds, but did not describe the growths further.

MUSCULO-SKELETAL SYSTEM

OSTEOSARCOMA

Osteosarcomas occurred in two budgerigars and one canary. The budgerigars were a 4-year-old male and a 7-year-old female. The canary was a 1-year-old male.

The tumor sites were the rib, radius, and wing-tip. The tumor on the rib wasn't noticed by the owner until the bird started picking under its wing. The radial tumor enlarged rapidly and decreased the bird's ability to fly. The wing-tip lesion had been noted as a small ulcer at the time of purchase of the bird. It had enlarged slowly over a period of 4 months, during which time the bird had picked at it and abraded it on the bars of the cage; hemorrhage resulted.

The sarcomas were firm in consistency and globular, ovoid, and botryoid in shape. They varied from 0.5 to

2 cm. in maximal measurement. The skin was ulcerated over both wing tumors, and completely so over the growth on the wing-tip. The cut surface of the rib tumor was yellow-tan and lobular and contained several cavities which had been filled with blood-tinged fluid. The cut surface of the radial tumor presented a lobulated pattern, some lobules being soft and light grey and others being mottled bright yellow and dark grey with a firm granular capsule. The wing-tip lesion was light grey and gritty when cut.

These tumors consisted of small irregular spicules of osteoid or poorly mineralized bone surrounded by immature osteoblasts (Fig. 27-20). Each cell had a round to oval vesicular nucleus with a single dense nucleolus. The cytoplasm was faintly eosinophilic and, when the borders were visible, stellate in shape. The neoplastic tissue was seldom densely cellular; it was relatively avascular, and contained a few multinucleated giant cells.

The rib tumor and the wing-tip tumor were both removed surgically, the wing being amputated distal to the carpal joint. The third bird was euthanatized; no metastases were found on postmortem examination.

Arnall[1] described 1 osteogenic sarcoma of the humerus among 54 tumors in budgerigars. A metastatic lesion occupied one-third of the thorax. In another paper[4] he recorded osteosarcoma (6 cases) in cage birds, involving the femur, stifle, tibio-tarsus, radius, elbow, orbit, and cranium. One tumor occurring in the orbit metastasized to the cervical vertebrae and sternum, although metastases generally were uncommon. These were from a collection of 166 tumors in cage birds. Arnall[3] gave the following description of the gross appearance of osteosarcomas of the limbs: "Below the stifle they appear as more or less painful fusiform or nodular swellings which are rapidly crippling. When midshaft in position, they may be mistaken for large fracture calluses or, occasionally, for granulomata, but radiography will usually demonstrate the erosion and dilation of the cortex of the diaphysis where it enters the neoplasm at either end." Beach[5] listed 1 osteosarcoma occurring at the elbow joint in a 2½-year-old female budgerigar from a group of 210 tumors in the species. Frost[10] listed 1 osteosarcoma of the elbow among 199 tumors in budgerigars.

RHABDOMYOSARCOMA

A rhabdomyosarcoma was found in a 13-year-old male budgerigar. A swelling present in the right shoulder area for 3 weeks, according to the owner, had been enlarging rapidly. As a result, the bird could no longer move the wing. Physical examination revealed a globular, moderately firm mass, about 2.5 cm. in diameter, in the region of the shoulder joint. The general fleshing was poor; the bird was weak and had loose droppings. Death occurred the following day.

Necropsy revealed a roughly oval mass measuring 2.0 × 1.5 × 1.2 cm., intimately attached at one pole to muscle and bone. The external surface was grey with opaque white to tan zones, and the cut surface was mottled grey and white. There were no metastases. The cause of death was renal gout.

The tumor was poorly circumscribed and not encapsulated, but blended with surrounding skeletal muscle. The microscopical appearance (Fig. 27-21) was similar to that of a fibrosarcoma. Most of the mass consisted of short, irregular, non-parallel fasciculi with little collagen. Cytoplasmic borders were not easily distinguished. There was great variation in size and shape of nuclei; some were very large and vesicular, and some were multiple. Occasional strap cells, with nuclei at one end

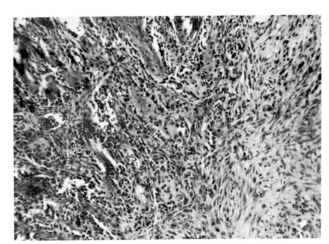

Fig. 27-20. *Osteosarcoma. Spicules of osteoid are surrounded by malignant osteoblasts.* ×*100.*

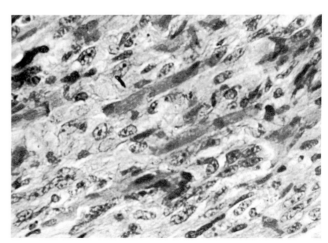

Fig. 27-21. *Rhabdomyosarcoma. The neoplastic cells are highly pleomorphic and form little collagen.* ×*450.*

had a small adenocarcinoma of the kidney. Symptoms in the female were related to the pressure effects produced by a large mass in the abdominal cavity. The bird was in good flesh but was moderately dyspneic. Marked abdominal distention was present, and the bird strained to pass droppings, which clung to the vent region. Euthanasia was performed.

Grossly the tumors were rather similar in appearance, being pink-red and soft. The tumor in the female was very large, measuring 5.0 × 5.0 × 3.5 cm. The tumor in the male was roughly triangular in outline, measuring 2.5 cm. on two sides, 1.75 cm. at the base, and 0.75 cm. in thickness. The external surface of each tumor was smooth and glistening; the cut surface of each was irregularly mottled red and white.

The microscopical features of these tumors were essentially the same as those described for hemangioendothelioma of the subcutis (*q.v.*). It is possible that a tumor of this type might be removed surgically.

LEIOMYOMA

A leiomyoma of the spleen occurred in an adult female budgerigar of unknown age. The symptoms and signs noted were related to the mechanical effects resulting from a large mass in the abdominal cavity. The abdomen bulged markedly, there was moderate dyspnea, and the wings were held slightly away from the body. Kidney disease complicated the picture, causing loose droppings, loss of appetite, and depression. The bird was euthanatized.

Necropsy revealed an irregularly globular mass, 2.0 cm. in maximal measurement, attached to a small globe measuring 0.8 cm. in diameter. The large globe was cream colored with red-brown mottlings, and the

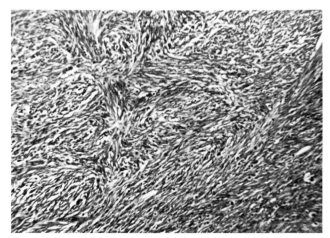

Fig. 27-25. *Leiomyoma of the spleen. Neoplastic smooth muscle cells are arranged in short interlacing fasciculi.* ×*100.*

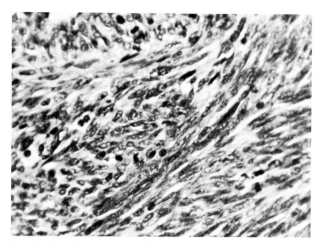

Fig. 27-26. *Higher magnification of tumor shown in Figure 27-25. The neoplastic cells have little cytoplasm and elongate, basophilic nuclei.* ×*450.*

small globe was a homogeneous red-brown. The entire mass was firm and smooth-surfaced.

The tumors were solid and highly cellular. The cells composing them were arranged parallel in groups that formed short or long fasciculi (Fig. 27-25) and occasionally small whorls. Some were in tight clusters and resembled multinucleated giant cells. The cells had uniform, elongated basophilic nuclei and scanty cytoplasm (Fig. 27-26). The tumors were relatively avascular, but apparently did not undergo necrosis. They compressed the surrounding splenic parenchyma without invading it.

If diagnosed early, this type of tumor might be removed surgically.

LEIOMYOSARCOMA

Leiomyosarcoma of the spleen occurred in two male budgerigars, 5 and 6 years old. One bird had been noticeably ill for 3 weeks, manifesting lethargy, dyspnea, and loose droppings. The second bird had difficulty in passing droppings; irritation was evident around the vent, and it picked at this area. Physical examination revealed a very distended abdomen in both birds, and euthanasia was performed.

Grossly, both tumors were roughly oval, smooth-surfaced, and pink, and measured approximately 3 × 3 × 1.3 cm. Both contained miltiloculated cysts filled with fluid which was clear in one and red-yellow in the other. The cut surface was white, moderately soft, and homogeneous in appearance, and lobulated with many cysts.

Like their benign counterparts, these tumors were highly cellular. There was little collagen, and the nuclei were more pleomorphic (Fig. 27-27). Many were round or oval, and most were vesicular. Some groups of cells

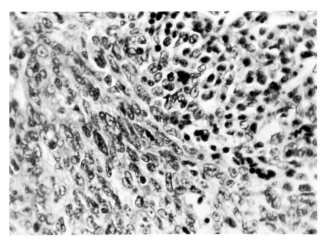

Fig. 27-27. *Leiomyosarcoma of the spleen. The nuclei of malignant smooth muscle cells are highly pleomorphic.* ×450.

were arranged parallel, but the fasciculi were short and interrupted by uniform masses of cells that did not form fasciculi. There were multiple foci of necrosis and cysts that contained proteinaceous fluid, fibrin, and cellular debris. The tumors were not sharply circumscribed from the surrounding splenic parenchyma.

Blackmore[7] recorded the occurrence of 15 leiomyosarcomas of the spleen among 168 tumors in budgerigars.

LYMPHANGIOMA

Lymphangioma of the spleen occurred in a 3-year-old female budgerigar. Symptoms manifested were slight dyspnea, difficulty in passing droppings, and picking at the vent area. Physical examination revealed good fleshing and a markedly distended abdomen. Euthanasia was performed.

Necropsy revealed a thickened peritoneum and approximately 5 ml. of clear serous fluid free in the abdominal cavity. A multiloculated cyst 3.0 × 2.0 × 1.5 cm. was attached to the spleen, which was pink and measured 0.5 cm. in diameter. The cut surface of the spleen showed intermingling of red and grey, and the cyst contained light yellow fluid with a small amount of blood.

Histologically this tumor consisted of a multiloculated cystic mass projecting from the capsule of the spleen. The cysts varied considerably in size and were separated by uniform narrow connective tissue trabeculae. Each cyst was lined with a single layer of flattened endothelium. One cyst contained blood; the others were empty after being processed for histologic study. Grossly the fluid contained in the cysts was characteristic of lymph.

Surgical removal of this type of tumor might be possible.

DIGESTIVE SYSTEM

Mouth

FIBROSARCOMA

Fibrosarcoma of the mouth occurred in a 2-year-old male budgerigar. An obviously enlarging swelling had been noticed in the region of the left commissure for 1 week. The bird was eating well. Physical examination revealed a firm, smooth-surfaced, red-yellow mass occupying two-thirds of the roof of the mouth and protruding from the left commissure. A firm swelling was also present below the left eye. Euthanasia was performed.

Necropsy revealed a firm, irregularly globular, smooth-surfaced mass measuring 1.5 cm. in maximal dimension. The cut surface was smooth, glistening pink-white, and cellular in appearance.

Microscopical features of this tumor were similar to those of fibrosarcoma of the skin and subcutis.

Crop

LEIOMYOSARCOMA

A leiomyosarcoma of the crop occurred in a 6-year-old male budgerigar. The owner had noticed a large swelling in the region of the crop for 4 or 5 days. The bird was still eating. Six to 8 weeks earlier the bird had had difficulty in swallowing food, but this had seemed to subside. Physical examination revealed a soft fluctuant mass approximately 5 cm. in diameter in the crop area. Exploratory surgery revealed a large cyst, measuring 5.0 × 5.0 × 2.5 cm., attached to the crop. The cyst ruptured, draining clear fluid, and several firm masses, white-pink in color and averaging 1 cm. in diameter, were seen to be intimately attached to the crop wall (Fig. 27-28). Euthanasia was performed.

Necropsy revealed an irregular, moderately firm, mottled yellow and grey mass measuring 2.0 × 2.0 × 0.5–0.1 cm. One surface presented smooth grey tissue, and there was a firm white mass 1.5 × 1.0 × 0.8 cm. with a swirled cut-surface between the grey tissue and the overlying skin.

Histologically this tumor resembled leiomyosarcoma of other organs (spleen). There were somewhat more collagen and greater nuclear pleomorphism in this tu-

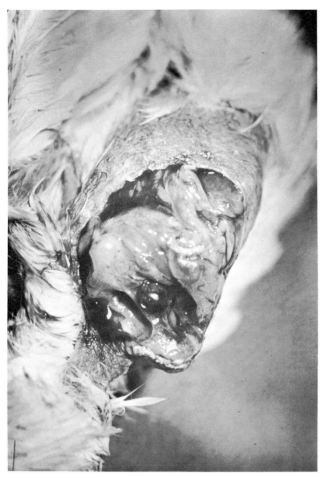

Fig. 27-28. *Leiomyosarcoma of the crop of a budgerigar.*

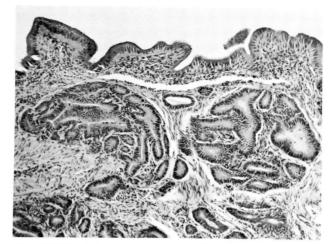

Fig. 27-29. *Adenocarcinoma of the cloaca. Malignant epithelium is invading the muscular wall of the cloaca.* ×*100.*

mor. Cells were arranged in fasciculi and small whorls. An organizing hematocyst was present in the tumor.

Cloaca

ADENOCARCINOMA

An adenocarcinoma of the cloaca in a 7-year-old female budgerigar was the only carcinoma of the digestive tract observed in this study. The bird had a history of straining to pass droppings for 2 weeks, but otherwise seemed normal. Physical examination revealed a 0.5-cm. firm, mottled-red, ulcerous mass protruding through the vent and involving about one-half of the circumference. A steroid–neomycin sulfate ointment was dispensed, to be applied to the lesion daily. The bird was returned in 2 weeks with a history of continued straining to pass droppings, decrease in activity, and some loss of appetite. The cloaca was no longer everted, but a slightly larger mass could be palpated in the area. Euthanasia was performed.

At necropsy the cloaca and vent were excised and fixed in 10% formalin. Transverse sectioning revealed firm, white, glistening tissue, 1–2 mm. thick, involving approximately one-half the circumference of the terminal cloaca.

The neoplastic tissue originated in the epithelium of the mucosa and extended through the tunica muscularis to the serosa of the cloaca (Fig. 27-29). Microscopically, the tissue was composed of acini and irregular tubules separated by bands of smooth muscle fibers and a small amount of connective tissue. The neoplastic cells were plump, columnar, basophilic-staining cells with round to oval vesicular nuclei. Most were arranged on a thin basement membrane and positioned in uniform rows to form tubules or spherical acini. Some were in small isolated nests surrounded by reactive connective tissue. Part of the tumor had replaced the mucosa of the cloaca, and on the serosal surface it had invaded the surrounding adipose tissue.

Frost[10] listed 2 sclerosing adenocarcinomas of the cloaca among 199 tumors in budgerigars. Beach[5] recorded 1 sclerosing adenocarcinoma of uncertain origin near the cloaca of a 4-year-old female budgerigar among 210 tumors in this species.

UNDIFFERENTIATED SARCOMA

An undifferentiated sarcoma of the cloaca occurred in a 40-year-old female yellow-headed amazon parrot (*Amazona ochrocephala*). Straining to pass droppings had been noted for 1 week. The droppings were loose and slightly bloody, and some adhered to the vent. Depression and decreased appetite were noted. Examination revealed a red, moist, shapeless mass, about

1.5 cm. in maximal measurement, prolapsed through the vent. Surgery was performed under general anesthesia, and the bulk of the mass was removed for biopsy. On cross section, the tumor was light grey, lobulated, and firm. The parrot continued to decline in general health and died on the fourth day after surgery.

Necropsy revealed an uneven light-grey mucosa in the affected area of the cloaca. On sectioning, a soft, white nodular area was seen in the submucosa. No metastases were evident. Intertubular nephritis and glomerulosclerosis were thought to be the cause of death.

Microscopically this tumor resembled the undifferentiated sarcoma from the skin and subcutis. Most of the mass was covered by mucosa of the cloaca. It was solidly cellular and moderately vascular. Groups of cells were divided by thin connective tissue septa that merged with the smooth muscle of the cloaca. The neoplastic cells were highly pleomorphic; most had round vesicular nuclei each with a single large nucleolus. Cytoplasm was scant and foamy, and cell boundaries were indistinct. The tumor may represent a highly undifferentiated fibrosarcoma or leiomyosarcoma.

Liver

UNDIFFERENTIATED CARCINOMA

An undifferentiated carcinoma of the liver occurred in a 2-year-old male budgerigar. One year prior to euthanasia the bird went through an episode of violently tearing at its tail feathers and mashing its primary wing feathers and tail feathers through and against the cage bars, resulting in badly broken feathers. Subsequently, the bird was lethargic for a few weeks and then seemed to return to normal. The broken wing and tail feathers seemed to be replaced much more slowly than normal.

Two weeks before euthanasia the bird went through a similar, but less violent, episode, involving the tail feathers. The bird again became lethargic and remained that way, often perching with its eyes closed and an apprehensive look on its face. The appetite was somewhat reduced. Physical examination revealed a slightly obese bird.

At necropsy the liver was seen to be slightly enlarged and uniformly yellow, with rounded edges. The brain, on cut surface, showed a spherical, red-brown focus, 0.5 cm. in diameter, in the hypothalamus. The pituitary gland was not identified, and no other lesions were noted grossly. Undifferentiated carcinoma was diagnosed in both the liver and the brain, but the primary site was not determined with certainty.

The tumor was widely disseminated throughout the liver in small, sharply circumscribed foci less than 1 mm.

in diameter. Although it may have originated elsewhere, it was thought to be an undifferentiated carcinoma of bile ducts with metastasis to the brain.

The cells were arranged in compact masses with little connective tissue stroma and few blood vessels. Nuclei were uniformly oval and moderately vesicular. Cytoplasm was scanty and slightly eosinophilic, with indistinct borders. Mitotic figures were unusually numerous. Surrounding hepatic tissue was fatty, but otherwise appeared unaffected.

Lombard and Witte[15] recorded the occurrence of a carcinoma of the liver in a female orange-headed ground thrush (*Geokichla c. citrina*) and a female hooded pitta (*Pitta cucullata*). Ratcliffe[17] listed carcinoma simplex of the liver in a male budgerigar exhibited 6 months and a female budgerigar exhibited 16 months. Arnall[1] recorded an adenocarcinoma of the liver in a 3½-year-old canary. Blackmore[7] listed 1 adenocarcinoma of the liver among 168 tumors in budgerigars.

FIBROSARCOMA

A fibrosarcoma of the liver occurred in a 4-year-old male budgerigar. Loose droppings had been noted 1 month prior to examination, but their consistency had later returned to normal. The bird had stopped talking when the loose droppings first occurred. A tremendous increase in appetite was reported. Physical examination revealed an emaciated bird with a distended abdomen. Laparotomy was performed, after which the bird was euthanatized.

Necropsy revealed a greatly enlarged left lobe of the liver, consisting of soft, pale, cellular tissue. No metastases were seen.

Histological features of fibrosarcoma vary somewhat within individual tumors and between different tumors. A general description of the microscopical features is given under fibrosarcoma of the skin.

Arnall[4] listed one sarcoma of the liver among 166 tumors in cage birds. Schlumberger[22] listed the occurrence of 159 cases of fibrosarcoma arising chiefly in the skin, spleen, and liver. This was from a collection of 497 tumors in budgerigars.

HEMANGIOENDOTHELIOMA

Hemangioendothelioma of the liver occurred in a 3-year-old female budgerigar. The bird had been considered normal until the owner found it on the bottom of the cage. It was able to perch, but seemed very weak. Death occurred within 24 hours.

Necropsy revealed a pink-tan liver of normal size, with blood vessels prominent on the surface. A pink, ovoid mass measuring 2.5 cm. in maximal dimension was attached to the liver. On cut surface, the tumor was smooth, pink, and moist.

Microscopical features of this tumor were essentially the same as those described for hemangioendothelioma of the subcutis.

ADENOCARCINOMA OF INTRAHEPATIC BILE DUCTS

Adenocarcinoma of the bile ducts occurred in a 4-year-old male and a 3-year-old female budgerigar. No history was available for the male bird. The female bird had been falling off the perch for several days, but had not lost consciousness. The appetite was poor. The bird perched with the feathers fluffed out, and some loose droppings were evident. When presented for examination, the bird was found clinging to the side of the cage. When the toes were disengaged, the bird fell to the floor and lay with outstretched wings for several minutes. The bird could perch, but could not clench the toes. Death occurred within 8 hours.

On gross examination, the liver in the female bird was normal in size, firm, and mottled cream and pink.

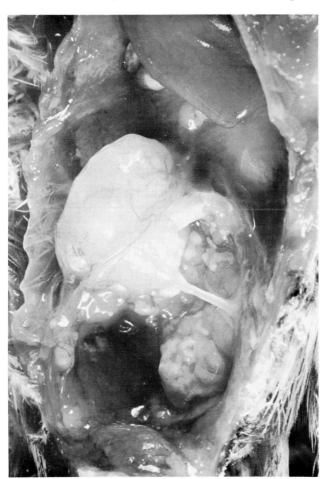

Fig. 27-30. *Adenocarcinoma of the kidney of a budgerigar.*

The liver in the male was swollen and soft, had rounded edges, and was pale red-brown with fine tan mottlings. Attached to it was a moderately firm, roughly ovoid, pink-white mass measuring 2.5 × 1.5 × 1.5 cm. The cut surface presented many well-defined, irregular, light yellow areas.

A cross section of the brain of the female bird revealed a globular, well-circumscribed grey mass measuring 0.3 cm. in diameter, located at approximately the level of the pituitary, just left of the midline in the midbrain. This mass proved to be a metastasis from the liver tumor.

In each case the tumor was distributed in multiple small, well-defined foci throughout the liver. The cells were small and basophilic, with a small amount of lightly eosinophilic cytoplasm. They were arranged in small nests or rosettes, and occasionally formed small tubules. Nuclei were uniformly round to oval and were moderately vesicular. Mitotic figures were numerous. There was little connective tissue within the tumor masses; the surrounding hepatic parenchyma contained excess fat.

Lombard and Witte[15] listed the occurrence of an adenocarcinoma of the bile ducts in a male Senegal fire finch (*Lagonosticta s. senegala*). This was from a group of 27 tumors among passerines.

UROGENITAL SYSTEM

Kidney

ADENOCARCINOMA

Adenocarcinoma of the kidney (Fig. 27-30) occurred in 31 budgerigars; 20 of the group were males, 9 were females, and in two cases the sex was not recorded. Ages varied from 1 to 8 years, with 28 (90 per cent) occurring in birds from 1 to 6 years of age. The age of one bird was not known.

There are no completely typical symptoms associated with adenocarcinoma of the kidney, but various symptoms develop, depending on the location and size of the growth. If the tumor grows in one kidney in such a location that it causes pressure on the sciatic nerve, the first symptoms noted will be paresis, usually followed by paralysis, of the ipsilateral leg. In the early stages the owner may notice that the bird is unsure when jumping from perch to perch. Differential diagnosis at this stage is very difficult, and the bird may live for weeks or even a few months with no worsening of symptoms.

When paralysis develops, differential diagnosis is not as difficult. Conditions such as a severe strain to the leg, fracture of the femur, malignant tumor in the femoral area, and avitaminosis-B should be considered. With a severe strain, there may be a history of the bird's having caught its leg in its cage or in some accouterment of the cage. This type of injury should heal in 7 to 10 days. If there is difficulty in differentiating a femoral fracture from a malignant tumor in this area, radiography will be helpful. If the history is suggestive of vitamin B–complex deficiency (basically a seed diet), the administration of vitamin B complex for 10 days should result in return of normal function of the leg.

Polyostotic hyperostosis may also be considered if the symptoms occur in a hen that has laid many eggs. The tumor may grow in such a way that bilateral paresis followed by paralysis results, or unilateral paresis may be followed by paralysis on the same side and later by bilateral paralysis. By the time the bird is paralyzed in both legs, other clinical signs and symptoms will generally have appeared, such as loose droppings, abdominal distention, dyspnea, lethargy, and weight loss, thereby making a diagnosis of malignant kidney tumor rather definite.

The tumor may also grow in such a way that symptoms related to decreased kidney function and a space-occupying abdominal mass result, with no symptoms of paresis or paralysis, or with some paresis developing as a very terminal sign. In these cases such signs and symptoms as diarrhea, weakness, loss of flesh, abdominal bulge, pasting of the vent, and dyspnea may be noted. In the cases in this study, when the presence of diarrhea was recorded, the droppings were listed primarily as green, green and white, or watery. Only once were they noted to be either grey or blood-tinged. A bulging abdomen does not result as frequently as it does from other abdominal tumors, owing to the location of the kidneys in the concavity of the synsacrum. *Thus it is possible for a bird to be in a terminal state of illness from a kidney tumor and have no perceptible bulging of the abdomen.*

The interval between onset of symptoms, as noted by the owner, and death ranged from 1 week to 8 months. Only one bird in this group of nine lived longer than $3\frac{1}{2}$ months after the onset of symptoms. In the group of 20 birds that were euthanatized, the interval between onset of symptoms and euthanasia ranged from 3 days to 6 months, with only one bird showing symptoms of illness for longer than 6 weeks. In two cases the tumors were incidental findings at necropsy.

Tumors varied from 0.25 to 3 cm. in maximal measurement, with the majority of them falling within a range of 1 to 2.5 cm. Shapes varied from irregular, to ovoid, to globular, or roughly so. The surface was almost always irregular and glistening. The consistency was typically firm unless necrosis had produced softening. Most often the color was white, or some combination of white

with yellow, grey, or pink. In a few cases, the color was noted as being yellow, tan-pink, yellow-grey, grey-tan, or light red. Not infrequently, specklings or mottlings of yellow were scattered over the surface.

The cut surface of the tumor was usually glistening and was the same color as the external surface, with the probable addition of yellow speckling. Occasionally the cut surface was opaque, granular, and necrotic or partially so, and presented some cystic areas. Two neoplasms had an attached cyst containing yellow fluid, and one was a cystic mass with firm nodules of tumor tissue scattered throughout. Metastasis to the liver occurred in five cases (16 per cent).

Although symptoms caused by these tumors, and the gross appearance of the lesions, may vary, the histological features are somewhat more consistent. There is some variation in the degree of differentiation of the tumors and the amount of connective tissue associated with them. They are composed of small nests or masses of vesicular epithelial cells separated by varying amounts of mature, or immature, fibrous connective tissue.

In the more poorly differentiated tumors, the epithelial cells form solid masses and small tubules. Larger tubules, some containing mucinous or proteinaceous fluid, and irregular fronds of epithelial cells are found in those that are more differentiated. In some, individual tubules or small groups of cells are surrounded by abundant connective tissue. In others, larger masses and groups of irregular tubules are separated by thin bands of fibrous tissue.

Individual cells are rather uniform in size and staining. Those forming tubules are cuboidal to low columnar and are always arranged in a single layer, sometimes with infolding; those in solid nests are not recognizable as glandular (Fig. 27-31).

Some of the tumors invade adjacent organs or bones; the metastatic lesions are histologically similar to the parent tumor.

Fox[9] recorded five cases of kidney neoplasia in male budgerigars. Ratcliffe[17] listed seven adenocarcinomas of the kidney, occurring in four male and three female budgerigars which had been exhibited from 14 to 62 months. These were among 28 tumors in budgerigars out of a total collection of 42 tumors in psittacines. He further listed an adenocarcinoma of the kidney in a male saffron finch (*Sicalis flaveola*) that had been exhibited 115 months, and one in a male zebra finch (*Taeniopygia* [= *Poephila*] *castanotis*) exhibited 11 months. The latter had a metastatic lesion in the lung. These were from a group of 14 tumors in passerines.

Schlumberger[22] listed 106 primary carcinomas of the kidney from a group of 497 tumors in budgerigars. Frost[10] listed the occurrence of 1 papilliform adenocarcinoma of the kidney in a female budgerigar from a

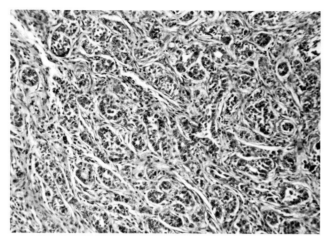

Fig. 27-31. *Adenocarcinoma of the kidney. Small nests and tubules of epithelial cells are surrounded by fibrous connective tissue.* ×*100.*

group of 199 tumors in this species. Beach[5] recorded 42 budgerigars dying or being euthanatized because of neoplasms arising in the epithelium of the kidney tubules or collecting ducts; age ranged from 1½ to 5 years, and 30 (71 per cent) of the birds were males. Beach's collection included benign and malignant tumors, but there was no numerical breakdown between them. Seven of the tumors were firmly attached to the adjoining pelvic bones, and in 10 cases there was paralysis of one leg because of pressure on the sciatic nerve roots. No metastases occurred, with the possible exception of one case. This was from a group of 210 tumors occurring in budgerigars. Blackmore[7] wrote of 44 kidney tumors among 168 tumors in the species. He described the histological appearance of the majority of the kidney neoplasms as that of nephroblastoma (embryonal nephroma). He recorded that the tumors may exceed 4 cm. in diameter, and that approximately 20 per cent are cystic and contain a brown fluid. Metastases (liver and spleen) occurred in only two cases (4.5 per cent), but local infiltration of the spinal column occurred frequently. Affected birds varied from 1 to over 10 years of age, but 77 per cent of the tumors occurred in birds under 10 years old. There were 33 males and 10 females; the sex of one bird was unknown. Incidence of the tumors was similar in both breeders' and pet birds.

EMBRYONAL NEPHROMA

Embryonal nephromas occurred in eight budgerigars and one canary, varying in age from 3 to 5 years. There were six males and three females.

Clinical symptoms associated with this tumor are similar to those associated with adenocarcinoma of the kidney (*q.v.*).

In this series of cases, one bird died and eight were euthanatized. The interval between onset of symptoms as noted by the owner and death or euthanasia ranged from 3 days to 2 months. The main clinical signs reported were lethargy, loss of weight, diarrhea, abdomi-

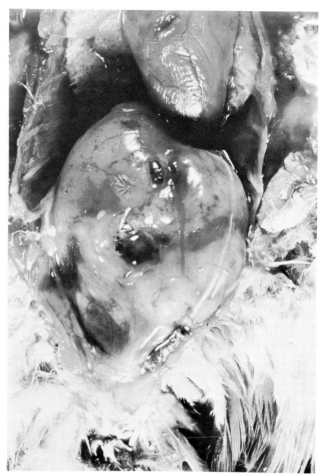

Fig. 27-32. *Embryonal nephroma in the kidney of a budgerigar.*

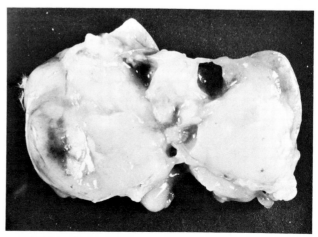

Fig. 27-33. *Cut section through the embryonal nephroma pictured in Figure 27-32.*

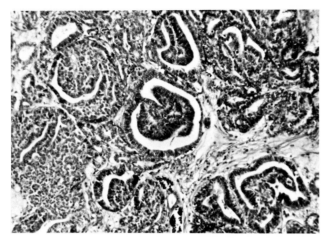

Fig. 27-34. *Embryonal nephroma of the kidney. Irregular epithelial tubules are surrounded by immature connective tissue.* ×100.

nal distention, dyspnea, and weakness. One bird had paralysis of the right leg.

On gross examination this tumor (Figs. 27-32, 27-33) cannot be differentiated from adenocarcinoma of the kidney, described above; histological features are also similar. There is, however, greater variation within individual embryonal nephromas than in adenocarcinomas. Lobules of epithelial cells are arranged in solid masses, tubular structures of variable size, or irregular strands and fronds. Acini or tubules that contain a small clump of epithelial cells and mimic poorly formed glomeruli also occur (Fig. 27-34).

A greater amount of immature connective tissue is associated with embryonal nephromas than with adenocarcinomas. Some resemble immature smooth muscle, and some are composed of widely spaced stellate cells, resembling embryonic mesenchyme. Embryonal nephromas also appear to have a richer vascular supply than adenocarcinomas of similar size, and are more likely to have large areas of necrosis. In biologic behavior the two tumors are apparently similar.

Beach[5] recorded 1 embryonal nephroma in a collection of 42 kidney tumors in budgerigars. Blackmore[7] listed the majority of his 44 kidney tumors as embryonal nephromas.

Testis

SEMINOMA

Seminoma of the testis occurred in two budgerigars, 5 and 6 years old. Symptoms and signs were related to the effects of a gradually enlarging abdominal mass.

Decreasing activity and appetite, increasing dyspnea, and loose droppings were the main symptoms and signs noted. Physical examination revealed a soft, bulging abdomen and a moderate loss of condition.

Necropsy in each bird revealed a testicular mass that was firm and smooth, and varied in color from cream-white to cream-pink. One tumor was globular and measured 2 cm. in diameter; the other was ovoid and measured 2.5 × 2 × 1 cm. The cut surface was smooth and glistening, and pale in color.

These tumors occupied the entire testis, but were encapsulated. They were composed of round cells of variable size with round hyperchromatic nuclei surrounded by a small amount of uniformly staining polychromatophilic cytoplasm. Cytoplasmic borders were easily distinguished except where the cells were closely grouped together. Narrow connective tissue trabeculae extended in an irregular pattern throughout the tumors, but seminiferous tubules could not be distinguished. There were frequent mitotic figures in the neoplastic cells.

Rewell[18] described the occurrence of a seminoma in a collared turtle dove (*Streptopelia risoria*). The bird was 4 years old and had a vague history of indisposition and emaciation for several months before death. Necropsy revealed a smooth-surfaced ovoid tumor, about 4 × 2 cm., which occupied the site of the left testis. Sectioning disclosed a soft, uniformly spongy, hemorrhagic tissue. Lombard and Witte[15] listed the occurrence of a seminoma in a Jardine babbler (*Turdoides bi-color*). Arnall[1] recorded the occurrence of 5 seminomas among 54 tumors in budgerigars. He mentioned that the main and sometimes only symptom was respiratory embarrassment. The largest tumor seen measured 2.5 × 2 × 1 cm. Metastases to the liver were found in one case. Frost[10] listed 6 seminomas among 199 tumors in budgerigars. Beach[5] recorded the occurrence of nine seminomas in pet budgerigars ranging in age from 4 to 7 years. Five of the nine birds showed atrophy of the other testis, and three showed change of cere color from blue to brown. Grossly the seminomas could not be distinguished from Sertoli cell tumors. The majority ranged from 2 to 3 cm. in maximal measurement, but in one case the neoplastic testis was shrunken to 0.3–0.5 cm., the other testis being atrophic and of similar size. The 9 seminomas were from a group of 210 tumors observed in budgerigars. Blackmore[7] listed the occurrence of a seminoma which metastasized in an amazon green parrot. He further wrote of 39 testicular tumors from a group of 168 tumors in budgerigars, but did not place the tumors into definite classifications, in the belief that many of the tumors cannot yet be put into a specific category. Ten of the testicular tumors had metastasized, mainly to the liver. He found that these tumors occurred most commonly in birds over 5 years of age and were, therefore, seen more commonly in pet birds.

INTERSTITIAL CELL TUMOR

An interstitial cell tumor of the testis occurred in a 9-year-old budgerigar, found dead in its cage one morning. The owner had trimmed the beak the day before and had noted nothing abnormal at that time. The bird was in good flesh, but it was noted that the cere was peeling off, the exfoliating portion being brown and the fresh surface blue. The abdomen was bulging moderately.

Several abnormalities were found at necropsy. One testis had an irregular surface, was firm and cream-white, and measured 2.5 × 1.5 × 1 cm. The other testis measured only 0.5 × 0.5 × 0.25 cm. The liver was very firm, creamy beige, and slightly enlarged, and contained a round green cyst measuring 1.5 cm. in diameter.

Histological examination revealed well-encapsulated bilateral interstitial cell tumors, with multiple foci of necrosis and hemorrhage. No normal testicular tissue was recognized. The neoplastic cells were round to polyhedral, with small round hyperchromatic nuclei and finely vacuolated eosinophilic cytoplasm. Thin fibrous trabeculae and blood vessels divided the mass into irregular groups of cells.

The liver showed moderately severe fibrosis, thrombosis of a large intrahepatic vein, and osseous tissue in the walls of dilated veins. The over-all impression of the pathologic process in the liver was lymphoma. The heart showed atherosclerosis of the coronary arteries.

A tumor of this type might be removed surgically under optimal conditions.

Beach[5] listed the occurrence of two interstitial cell tumors in budgerigars. One bird was 6 years old. In both birds the tumor was cystic, and the remaining testis atrophic. These tumors were from a group of 210 observed in budgerigars.

SERTOLI CELL TUMOR

Sertoli cell tumor of the testis occurred in five budgerigars ranging from 4 to 7 years of age. Clinical symptoms and signs were related to the effects of a gradually enlarging abdominal mass. Increasing lethargy, cessation of speech, diminishing appetite, and labored respirations were the most prominent symptoms. In addition, some birds had loose droppings, pasting of the vent, and difficulty in passing the droppings. Generally the birds were in good flesh and had a marked abdominal bulge. A brown cere appeared on one bird.

In gross appearance (Fig. 27-35) the tumors were

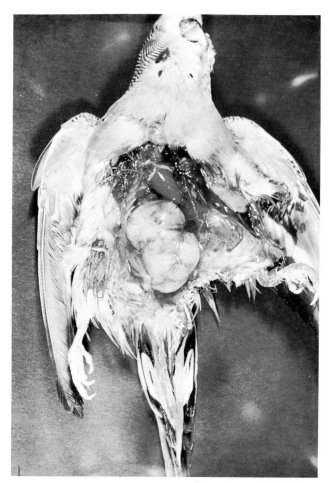

Fig. 27-35. *A very large Sertoli cell tumor in a budgerigar.*

spherical to ovoid, lobulated, and well encapsulated, and they ranged from 0.2 to 3 cm. in maximal measurement. They were firm and smooth-surfaced, and varied from cream to orange in color. One tumor was cystic. The solid cut surface was firm, glistening, and homogeneous, and was white, yellow, or grey in color. In three birds only one testis was involved and the other was atrophic.

Histologically each tumor was well encapsulated and occupied the entire testis. They were composed of multiple small nests of cells separated by a moderate amount of fibrous connective tissue (Fig. 27-36), probably derived from the walls of the seminiferous tubules. The neoplastic Sertoli cells had uniform round to oval nuclei and lacy or vacuolated cytoplasm with indistinct borders. Unlike in the counterpart in mammals, there was little tendency for the cells in these tumors to be elongated and to lie parallel within nests. The appearance was the same throughout the tumors, and they were relatively avascular.

Arnall[1] listed 1 Sertoli cell tumor among 54 tumors in budgerigars; Frost[10] reported 9 Sertoli cell tumors

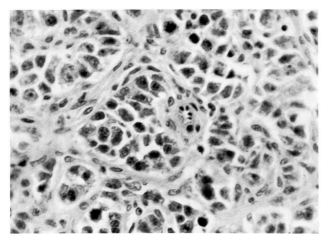

Fig. 27-36. *Sertoli cell tumor of testis. Small nests of Sertoli cells are separated by fibrous connective tissue. ×450.*

among 199 tumors in the species. Arnall[4] recorded 8 testicular tumors occurring in budgerigars, among 166 tumors in cage birds, but did not specify the exact number of Sertoli cell tumors. Beach[5] wrote of 24 Sertoli cell tumors among 210 tumors in budgerigars. Affected birds were evenly distributed between the ages of 3 and 7 years. The cere was brown in seven cases, and showed partial change in seven more. In two cases both testes were involved. The remaining testis was atrophic in 15 cases, in 6 of which it could not be found. In two other cases the remaining testis was cystic. Blackmore[7] listed 39 of 168 tumors in budgerigars as testicular but did not classify them, believing that many of the testicular tumors are hard to identify and that a great deal of work needs to be done before a reliable classification can be made.

Under optimal conditions this type of tumor might be removed surgically.

LEIOMYOSARCOMA

A leiqmyosarcoma of the testis occurred in a 10-year-old budgerigar. Clinical signs were those associated with a gradually enlarging mass in the abdominal cavity. Increasing dyspnea, decreasing vitality, difficulty in expelling droppings, and gradual loss of condition occurred.

Necropsy revealed an irregularly lobulated, smooth-surfaced mass in the testicular region. It was moderately firm and cream-white in color, with blood vessels scattered over the surface, and measured 4 × 2.5 × 1.5 cm. The cut surface was smooth, glistening, homogeneous, and cream-white. Its gross appearance did not differ from that of a Sertoli cell tumor.

The origin of this tumor could not be determined with certainty, but it was attached to and blended with the capsule of the testis. Histological features were essentially the same as those described for leiomyosarcoma of the spleen.

Under optimal conditions this type of tumor might be removed surgically.

HEMANGIOMA OF TESTICULAR CAPSULE

Hemangioma of the testicular capsule occurred in a 4-year-old budgerigar. Clinical signs and symptoms had consisted of intermittent passing of blood in the droppings for several weeks, and increasing depression and dyspnea. Physical examination revealed a bird in good flesh, with a soft bulging abdomen. The bird died.

Necropsy revealed a soft, ovoid, pink, pulpy mass, measuring 2.1 × 1.5 × 1.3 cm., attached to a testis. The liver was yellow-tan in color, with rounded edges.

The mass attached to the testis had characteristic histological features of hemangioma as described under hemangioma of the subcutis. Microscopical examination of the liver showed areas of necrosis, and it was believed that liver disease was the cause of death.

Under optimal conditions this type of tumor might be removed surgically.

Oviduct

LEIOMYOSARCOMA

Leiomyosarcoma of the oviduct occurred in a 4-year-old and an 8-year-old budgerigar. Clinical symptoms varied. The younger bird had never laid eggs; the other had been egg-bound at 2 years of age. The younger bird had not been eating well for 4 days before examination, and was euthanatized. The other bird was found dead; the owner had not noted any symptoms relating to the abdominal tumor. Each bird had a bulging abdomen.

In gross appearance the tumors were as follows: In the 8-year-old—a firm, white, U-shaped mass, one arm 3 cm. long and 1.5 cm. in diameter, and the other arm 1.5 cm. long and 1 cm. in diameter. The cut surface was red-brown and contained a roughly circular area 1 cm. in diameter that was mottled yellow in color. In the 4-year-old—an irregularly globular, firm white mass measuring 2.7 × 2 × 1.5 cm. was very loosely attached to the hilus of the liver.

Each tumor had originated from smooth muscle of the oviduct. They had similar microscopical features, as described under leiomyosarcoma of the spleen. The larger tumor from the 8-year-old female was more vascular than the other and contained a central focus of necrosis that was noted grossly as a yellow area.

Hasholt[13] described the surgical technique for the removal of a diseased oviduct.

Ovary

GRANULOSA CELL TUMOR

Granulosa cell tumor of the ovary occurred in five budgerigars ranging in age from 4 to 9 years. Clinical signs of illness associated with the presence of this tumor were related to pressure exerted on the thoracic and abdominal organs. When presented for examination, all five birds showed marked abdominal distention, and consequently had some degree of dyspnea and were less active than normal. Pressure on the bowel caused soft droppings in some birds, tenesmus, and pasting of the vent. All birds were euthanatized.

In gross appearance, the tumors varied somewhat. Three were composed of combined solid and cystic structures (Fig. 27-37), and two were completely solid. Of those with cysts, two had cystic portions larger than the amount of solid tissue, and one was a mixture of solid tissue and cysts. In one the cysts contained clear fluid; in the other two they contained dark fluid. The solid tissue was firm and white-yellow in color. On cut surface the stroma was white-yellow or yellow. Size varied from 1 to 5 cm. in maximal measurement, with the largest tumor being totally solid. They were botryoid, irregularly lobulated, or ovoid (Fig. 27-38).

Histological features of the different tumors varied somewhat. With but one exception the tumors consisted either of solid masses of cells with little or no connective tissue stroma, or small nests of cells separated by thin bands of connective tissue. Individual cells com-

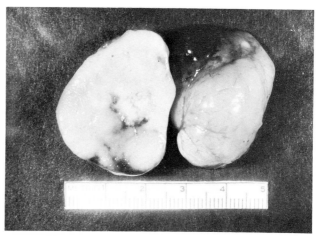

Fig. 27-38. *Cut section of the granulosa cell tumor pictured in Figure 27-37.*

posing the tumors were similar; nuclei were round or oval, and vesicular. Cytoplasm was foamy or vacuolated, and had indistinct borders. Those tumors in which the cells were divided into nests resembled Sertoli cell tumors of the testis. Necrosis and hemorrhage were common in each type.

In one tumor, the cells were arranged in small follicles or rosettes (Fig. 27-39). The nuclei were oval to elongate, and the cytoplasm was basophilic without vacuoles.

Under optimal conditions such tumors might be removed surgically.

Frost[10] listed 3 granulosa cell tumors among 199 tumors in budgerigars. Beach[5] wrote of 8 granulosa cell tumors among 210 tumors in this species. Seven of these occurred in birds from 2 to 9 years old, and one was in a bird under 12 months of age. Three of these hens had shown permanent or temporary change of the cere

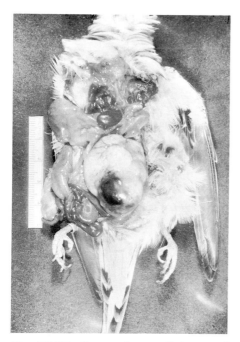

Fig. 27-37. *A granulosa cell tumor of the ovary in a budgerigar.*

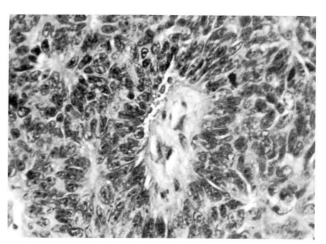

Fig. 27-39. *Granulosa cell tumor of the ovary. Neoplastic cells are forming small rosettes.* ×450.

to the blue color characteristic of the male. Five of these were pet birds, and three were breeders' birds. One bird had laid an egg only three weeks before being euthanatized. The tumors measured 1.5–2.5 cm. in maximal dimension, and were associated with watery cysts sometimes as large as 2.5 cm. in diameter. Blackmore[7] recorded 28 ovarian tumors among a group of 168 tumors in budgerigars, but did not classify the ovarian tumors into definite subdivisions. Twenty-two occurred in pet birds and 6 in breeders' birds. The ages ranged from 2 to over 10 years.

ADENOCARCINOMA

Adenocarcinoma of the ovary occurred in three budgerigars and one cockatiel (*Nymphicus hollandicus*). The cockatiel and one budgerigar were 3 years old, and the two other budgerigars were 5 years old.

All the budgerigars had shown signs of illness for 1 or 2 months. Abdominal distention, dyspnea, and difficulty in passing droppings were common to all. One bird had bilateral paresis for 2 months and had become totally paralyzed shortly before examination. The abdomen of one bird, formerly distended, had regressed in size but had subsequently been enlarging for 2 months. All birds were euthanatized.

The cockatiel had been sick intermittently over a period of 7 months, with extended periods of apparent good health between episodes of illness. The first illness began with a cessation of droppings for 3 days and the bird's acting as though it were straining to lay an egg. A few days later, severe dyspnea and diarrhea developed, and the bird became very depressed. On about the tenth day of illness, it passed a plug of pink-white mucoid material approximately 1.5 cm. in diameter and immediately began to return to a normal state. The bird was seen 5 months later, with a history of being incoordinated at times. The bird had laid an egg the day before, and was brought to the hospital for an injection of depot testosterone to suppress egg laying. Two months later the bird was presented with a history of having suddenly become very ill. It died on the examination table.

In gross appearance, the adenocarcinoma could not be distinguished from a granulosa cell tumor. Two of the tumors were composed of firm tissue, and two were partially cystic. They varied in size from approximately 2 cm. in maximal diameter in the budgerigar, to a trilobed mass each lobe of which measured 4 × 1.4 × 1 cm., in the cockatiel (Fig. 27-40). The shape of the tumor was usually irregular, because of the combination of cysts and solid tissue. The cysts contained clear yellow fluid and the stroma was firm and white, pink-white, or yellow-white. In the paralyzed budgerigar the

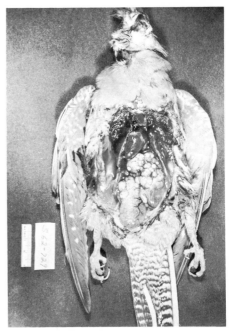

Fig. 27-40. *Adenocarcinoma of the ovary in a cockatiel.*

growth had invaded the kidney region and caused pressure on the sciatic nerve. One tumor metastasized to the liver.

The tumors also appeared similar microscopically. They were composed of uniformly sized cuboidal cells on delicate basement membranes. The cells were arranged in short fronds or strands and small tubules, with little or no connective tissue. Nuclei were of similar size, round and vesicular, with a prominent nucleolus. They were positioned near the basement membranes; light eosinophilic cytoplasm surrounded the nuclei and extended away from the basement membranes. Cysts visible grossly were lined with similar cells and appeared to be tubules or acini distended with proteinaceous fluid. Metastatic lesions had a similar appearance.

Ratcliffe[17] reported adenocarcinoma of the ovary in a budgerigar exhibited 52 months and in a sulfur-crested cockatoo (*Kakatoe galerita*) exhibited 66 months. These were from a collection of 42 tumors in psittacine birds. Lombard and Witte[15] recorded 1 carcinoma of the ovary in a canary among 27 tumors in passerines. Frost[10] listed 1 ovarian carcinoma among 199 tumors in budgerigars. Arnall[4] reported 7 ovarian tumors in budgerigars from a collection of 166 tumors in cage birds, but didn't classify the growths further. Beach[5] listed 1 adenocarcinoma of the ovary among 210 tumors in budgerigars. Blackmore[7] recorded the occurrence of 28 ovarian tumors among 168 tumors in budgerigars, but didn't subdivide them into specific categories.

ENDOCRINE SYSTEM

Thyroid Glands

ADENOCARCINOMA

Adenocarcinoma of the thyroid gland occurred in one female and three male budgerigars. The ages were 3, 4, and 11 years. The diverse clinical pictures presented by the two birds manifesting symptoms relating to presence of the tumor are as follows:

(1) The 4-year-old male evidenced decreasing activity and appetite for 1 month prior to examination. Dyspnea of increasing severity had developed, and when the bird was presented for examination the wings were completely extended and seemed to be assisting in respiration. The bird was very thin, trembled, and would fall from the perch. Euthanasia was performed.

(2) In the 11-year-old male, a globular, firm, yellow subcutaneous mass had been noted for 4 months in the mid-cervical region. Since the bird seemed to be in good physical condition, the mass was excised. Surgery was successful, and the bird was discharged on the second postoperative day.

Upon gross examination, the tumors varied somewhat in appearance. The 4-year-old male had bilaterally symmetrical, globular, dark-brown masses in the locations of the thyroid glands. They were smooth-surfaced with yellow specklings, and measured 1.5 cm. in diameter. The tumor in the 11-year-old male measured 1 cm. in diameter; its cut surface was glistening, acellular, pale yellow, and bulging.

The tumors in the two other birds were unilateral, moderately firm, smooth-surfaced, and homogeneously pink in color. One was ovoid and measured $0.7 \times 0.5 \times 0.2$ cm.; the other took the form of an equilateral triangle measuring 1 cm. on each side, and 1 cm. thick, with the base of the triangle resting on the heart-base. The cut surface of each mass reflected the appearance of its external surface.

The tumors were circumscribed, but poorly encapsulated. They consisted of small and irregularly shaped follicles and solid nests of follicular cells separated by thin, vascular connective tissue septa. In some portions of the tumor, single rows of epithelial cells formed long, irregular fronds. The cells were cuboidal with medium-sized, centrally located basophilic nuclei. Cytoplasm appeared granular when stained with hematoxylin and eosin. The tumors were well vascularized and contained occasional foci of hemorrhage. There was no colloid (Fig. 27-41).

Cancer of the thyroid is rare in birds. Feldman and Olson[8] did not list this tumor in their extensive review on neoplasms of the chicken. Murray[16] recorded a case

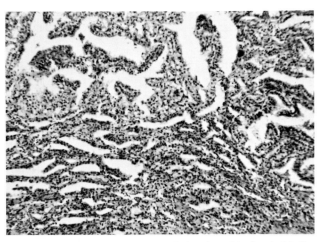

Fig. 27-41. *Adenocarcinoma of the thyroid gland. Malignant epithelium is forming irregular follicles and fronds. Colloid is absent.* ×100.

of thyroid cancer in a scarlet macaw (*Ara macao*). In the malignant tumor of the thyroid in a male budgerigar described by Fox[9] the mass on the right measured $1.0 \times 0.6 \times 0.4$ cm., and that on the left measured $0.5 \times 0.3 \times 0.2$ cm. The tumors were well circumscribed, yellow-grey, and moderately firm. Lombard and Witte[15] listed 1 thyroid carcinoma among 42 tumors in psittacine birds. Arnall[4] recorded 18 thyroid tumors among 166 tumors in budgerigars, but did not classify them further. Beach[5] found 1 thyroid carcinoma in a 2-year-old male budgerigar among 210 tumors in the species.

Pituitary Tumors

Pituitary tumors occurred in four budgerigars—three males and one female, ranging in age from 1 to 4 years.

One bird had polydipsia and very watery droppings for 6 months and was thought to be blind for 1 month prior to euthanasia. Another bird was apparently normal until the day of examination, when it was found on the floor of the cage, unable to perch. Placed on a finger the bird was able to perch, but when placed in a standing position on a flat surface, it pitched forward on its head and sternum. Appetite and droppings were normal. The bird died approximately 8 hours after examination.

Postmortem examinations revealed no gross abnormalities in the brain. The liver of the bird with loose droppings was enlarged, moderately firm, and pink-white. The kidneys in this bird were light brown.

In each case, when the brain was sectioned and examined microscopically, a poorly circumscribed tumor encroaching on the hypothalamus from the area of the pituitary was discovered. The lesions were similar, being

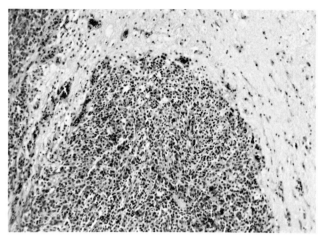

Fig. 27-42. *Section of brain in case of tumor of the pituitary. Neoplastic tissue is invading the hypothalamus.* × *100.*

highly cellular and moderately vascular. They obliterated the pituitary glands and replaced portions of the hypothalamus (Fig. 27-42).

The neoplastic cells had round nuclei that varied considerably in size. Some were small and basophilic; others were medium sized and moderately vesicular. All the cells had granular, slightly eosinophilic cyto-plasm with distinct borders. They were arranged in solid masses separated by thin connective tissue trabeculae. It was not possible to determine the portion of the pituitary from which the tumors had originated.

The liver described grossly was seen on microscopical examination to be rich in glycogen, and the kidneys of this same bird contained protein casts in some convoluted tubules.

Schlumberger[20] reported on 50 cases of spontaneous chromophobe pituitary tumors in budgerigars. Incidence was approximately equal in the two sexes. Forty per cent of Schlumberger's group showed diffuse enlargement of the pituitary; 56 per cent of the tumors were locally invasive, and 40 per cent had metastasized. Clinical signs and symptoms included unilateral or bilateral exophthalmos, blindness, somnolence, polyuria, polydipsia, convulsions, and obesity. The average age of the affected birds was 2½ years. Schlumberger[21] and Hubben *et al.*[14] succeeded in transplanting the pituitary tumor subcutaneously in budgerigars, and Schlumberger also transplanted it intracerebrally.

Unlike Schlumberger, other workers have not found a high incidence of pituitary tumors in budgerigars. Blackmore[7] listed 1 pituitary tumor among 168 tumors in budgerigars, and Beach[5] recorded 8 such tumors among 210 neoplasms in the species.

References

1. ARNALL, L.: Experiences with cage-birds. Vet. Rec. *70:*120–128, 1958.

2. ARNALL, L.: Some common surgical entities of the budgerigar. Vet. Rec. *72:*888–890, 1960.

3. ARNALL, L.: Anaesthesia and surgery in cage and aviary birds. Vet. Rec. *73:*139–142, 173–178, 188–192, 237–241, 1961.

4. ARNALL, L.: Further experiences with cagebirds. Vet. Rec. *73:*1146–1154, 1961.

5. BEACH, J. E.: Diseases of budgerigars and other cage birds. A survey of *post-mortem* findings. Vet. Rec. *74:*10–15, 63–68, 134–140, 1962.

6. BEACH, J. E.: Some of the major problems of budgerigar pathology. J. small anim. Pract. *6:*15–20, 1965.

7. BLACKMORE, D. K.: The pathology and incidence of neoplasia in cage birds. J. small anim. Pract. *6:*217–223, 1965.

8. FELDMAN, W. H., and OLSON, C.: Neoplastic Diseases of the Chicken. In *Diseases of Poultry,* 5th ed., H. E. Biester and L. H. Schwarte, eds. Ames. Iowa State University Press, 1965. Pp. 863–924.

9. FOX, H.: *Disease in Captive Wild Mammals and Birds.* Philadelphia, J. B. Lippincott, 1923. Pp. 284–286; 473, 480–482.

10. FROST, C.: Experiences with pet budgerigars. Vet. Rec. *73:*621–626, 1961.

11. GANDAL, C. P., and SAUNDERS, L. Z.: The surgery of subcutaneous tumors in parakeets (*Melopsittacus undulatus*). J.A.V.M.A. *134:*212–218, 1959.

12. GRAY, H.: The diseases of cage and aviary birds, with some reference to those of furred and feathered game. Vet. Rec. *16:*417–425, 1936.

13. HASHOLT, J.: Diseases of the female reproductive organs of pet birds. J. small anim. Pract. *7:*313–320, 1966.

14. HUBBEN, K., SHIRER, J. F., and ENOLD, G. L.: Transmissible pituitary chromophobe adenoma in the parakeet. Avian Dis. *8:*203–208, 1964.

15. LOMBARD, L. S., and WITTE, E. J.: Frequency and types of tumors in mammals and birds of the Philadelphia Zoological Garden. Cancer Res. *19:*127–141, 1959.

16. MURRAY, J. A.: The zoological distribution of cancer. Sci. Repts. Imp. Cancer Res. Fund *3:*41–60, 1908.

17. RATCLIFFE, H. L.: Incidence and nature of tumors in

captive wild mammals and birds. Am. J. Cancer *17:*116–135, 1933.

18. REWELL, R. E.: Seminoma of the testis in a collared turtle dove (*Streptopelia risoria*). J. Path. Bact. *60:*155, 1948.

19. SANGER, V. L., and LAGACE, A.: Avian xanthomatosis. Etiology and pathogenesis. Avian Dis. *10:*103–111, 1966.

20. SCHLUMBERGER, H. G.: Neoplasia in the parakeet. I.

Spontaneous chromophobe pituitary tumors. Cancer Res. *14:*237–245, 1954.

21. SCHLUMBERGER, H. G.: Neoplasia in the parakeet. II. Transplantation of the pituitary tumor. Cancer Res. *16:*149–153, 1956.

22. SCHLUMBERGER, H. G.: Tumors characteristic for certain animal species. A review. Cancer Res. *17:*823–832, 1957.

23. STONE, R. M.: Personal communication, 1965.

NOTE: The cost of the photomicrographs appearing in this Chapter was borne in part by the R. T. French Company, Rochester, New York.

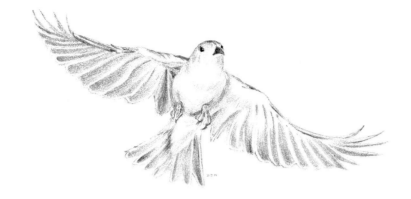

28

Metabolic and Miscellaneous Conditions

Obesity, Abdominal Rupture, Senility, and Shock
Lawrence Minsky

Gout
Jens Hasholt

OBESITY

Obesity is one of the more common problems encountered in pet birds, especially in budgerigars. Obesity is relative, and evaluation of the condition must be based on the particular bird in question. Experience in handling many birds of normal weight will provide a background for diagnosing the condition. Although physiological disturbances undoubtedly account for some instances of the problem, I am not aware of any critical work to support this hypothesis.

Dieting has proved valuable in many instances to reduce the weight to within normal range. Experimenting with the amount of ration given to the bird, starting with one-half to three-fourths of a level tablespoonful of a regular budgerigar seed mix per day as the sole source of feed, should lead to establishment of the proper amount for a particular bird.

It is my opinion that many birds are encouraged to become obese by the large number of food containers and the excessive variety of food stuffs constantly offered them. Imagine a housewife trying to keep her weight down with an open box of candy or cookies on every table and shelf in the house to tempt her as she goes about her daily chores.

Fat pads which develop over the breast, abdomen, and other areas may reach pathological proportions (Fig. 28-1). In some instances such fat masses have been successfully removed surgically from breast areas. This procedure was resorted to particularly when it was thought the masses were becoming neoplastic in character, as evidenced by alteration in their consistency. Nodular areas within a fat mass should be regarded with suspicion.

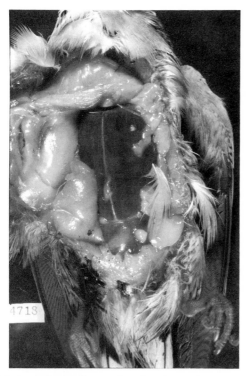

Fig. 28-1. *A budgerigar, showing large fat pads which have covered breast and abdomen.*

ABDOMINAL RUPTURE

Abdominal rupture, other than that caused by injury which would be treated with routine surgical procedures, generally has been seen in conjunction with a peculiar brownish discoloration of the skin and the fat in the abdominal wall, a xanthomatous reaction.

The muscular tissue of the abdominal wall is sometimes weakened, probably by degenerative changes, to the extent that the viscera protrude through to the subcutaneous layer. Surgical removal of the portion of the abdominal wall that is affected, sometimes including an area of skin if there has been considerable ballooning, has usually proved only temporarily successful. Sometimes the area of abdominal wall which is diseased is so extensive as to preclude surgical repair.

SENILITY

Senility in birds is very difficult to evaluate, because a variety of signs may be seen when a bird is presented for examination. Frequently the advanced age of the bird may suggest senility, but the question arises whether the symptoms or lesions noted should be attributed to senility since the same signs are also seen in younger birds. Such conditions as arthritis, gout, alopecia, and unexplained emaciation, which one might expect to see in old birds, are often seen in young birds as well.

In my practice, I seldom see budgerigars more than 10 or 11 years old. Canaries may live slightly longer, perhaps as long as 12 or 14 years.

SHOCK

One subject that has been bandied about a great deal and may deserve some comment here is the matter of shock occurring in birds during examination. It is not unusual to see in print or hear in discussion the assertion that birds generally and canaries particularly are prone to go into shock and die when handled. This has not proved to be the case in my experience in many years of handling pet birds. The relatively few deaths that occurred during examination were in very sick birds, especially those in which dyspnea was an outstanding sign. It is suggested that undue pressure on the thorax, resulting in suffocation, may be the cause of death in these cases, rather than shock.

GOUT

Gout is a metabolic disorder of obscure etiology. It is characterized by uric acid and urates being deposited in various parts of the organism instead of being excreted by way of the kidneys.

The deposits always occur extracellularly; they are never seen in the blood or lymph vessels, or in the spaces of the central nervous system. They are localized in joint cavities and tendon sheaths, as well as in spaces of different sizes in connective tissue adjacent to joints and tendons. They also occur on fairly large fasciae. Further, such deposits may be found on the surfaces of serous membranes, most often the epicardium and pericardium, and on the surface of the liver. In the parenchymatous organs—liver and kidneys—deposits may be seen in the interstitial connective tissue and under the capsular lining. However, in the kidneys, in most cases the deposits are to be sought in the excretory ducts.

The deposits consist of needle-shaped or amorphous crystals. In the joint cavities and connective tissue spaces the deposits (tophi) constitute a more or less viscid or thick mass; on the serous membranes the deposits occur as dry plastery patches.

Synovial gout and visceral gout are differentiated according to site. Synovial gout is usually regarded as the chronic form, and visceral gout as the acute. The two forms may occur separately or in combination. Finally, the term renal gout is sometimes used in the literature for cases with deposits in the kidneys alone.

INCIDENCE

The disease is definitely best known in fowl, its presence being demonstrated in 1 or 2 per cent of all such birds necropsied. Most of these birds show visceral gout or mixed forms, whereas pure synovial gout is comparatively rare.

Among the cage birds, the psittacine birds—budgerigars, parakeets, and parrots—are the most frequently affected. All writers, with the single exception of Gray,[4] state that the disease is rare in passerine birds, although it may occasionally be seen in canaries and Gouldian finches (*Poephila gouldiae*). Svensson[13] claimed to have found a relationship between season and incidence in fowl, but no such relationship has been noted in cage birds. In the British literature visceral gout is stated to be the most frequent form. This disagrees with observations made at the Veterinary Hospital, Copenhagen, where the ratio of the synovial to the visceral form has been found to be 50 to 1. It may be mentioned further that during the 6-month period before this Chapter was written no more than 10 cases had been seen in this Hospital. These 10 patients were all budgerigars with synovial gout. In this connection, it is remarkable that renal changes were noticed in only one case. (Within the same period urate deposits in the kidneys were incidental findings at necropsy in three birds, the question being raised whether the deposits might have appeared after death.)

A single writer, Kemna,[8] stated that hummingbirds are particularly liable to develop the disease, a statement which I have been unable to confirm. Kemna also mentioned that the disease is well known among birds of prey and ratites, whereas it is very rare among web-footed birds, waders, and pigeons.

ETIOLOGY

Gout, as stated earlier, is characterized by deposition in the body of uric acid and urates. Uric acid is a product resulting primarily from metabolism of the purines (adenine, guanine, and xanthine), but, in addition, some is produced from ammonia, the amino acid metabolite.

The synthesis of uric acid takes place not, as previously supposed, in the liver alone, but also in the kidneys. The processes are not well understood. It is known, however, that hypoxanthine is produced in the liver of fowl and pigeons, and that this compound is oxidized into uric acid by means of xanthine oxidase—in the liver in fowl and in the kidneys in pigeons. In pigeons, only the kidneys contain xanthine oxidase. It is not known whether this is in any way responsible for the rare occurrence of gout in pigeons.

In birds, uric acid is the most important waste product of protein metabolism, and it is excreted through the kidneys. The uric acid synthesized in the liver can, however, reach the kidneys only by way of the blood, which consequently must contain a certain amount of uric acid. The portion synthesized in the kidneys may possibly be excreted directly. However, it may also be possible that more uric acid is produced than even a normal kidney can excrete, and that the excess amount passes into the blood, either directly or by fluid absorption. Its direct passage is probably the more likely, considering the solubility characteristics of uric acid.

Regarding the question of concentrations of uric acid in various organs, the information available for fowl is sketchy and unsatisfactory, and no information whatever is available for cage birds. According to Levine et al.,[9] 10 per cent of the urates in chicken's blood are in solution, 18 per cent are protein-bound, and about 70 per cent are present as an ultrafiltrable or colloidal fraction. It is not known whether this ratio is stable, or whether only a single fraction is influenced by physiological and/or pathological changes of the uric-acid concentration.

The figures given for the concentration of uric acid in the blood, or, rather, the blood plasma,[10,11,12] differ somewhat, ranging from 1.2 to 8 mg. per 100 ml. (average 4.5 mg./100 ml.). The variations are due partly to differences between species and partly to influences of physiological factors, such as the reproductive state, the state of health, and the amount and kind of feed.

The concentration of uric acid in the blood is known to be pathologically raised in human patients with gout. Further, a rise may be associated with such diseases as leukemia and pneumonia, in which an extensive disintegration of cells leads to intensification of biosynthesis of purine. Finally, such an increase is not infrequently observed in arteriosclerosis, a disease that is known to occur in parrots.

A similar morbid rise of the plasma level of uric acid has been shown to take place in birds, too. Values of 18.9 mg./100 ml. have been recorded[7] in poultry suffering from avian monocytosis; Shaw[11] recorded 12 mg./100 ml. in web-footed birds exposed to poisoning. Finally, Folin et al.[2] and Levine et al.,[9] in experiments on ducks and fowl, respectively, obtained values of 224 and 304 mg. per 100 ml., respectively, by completely arresting uric acid excretion by ligating the ureters. Folin et al.[2] also showed that the concentration of uric acid differs in various organs (Table 28-1). All of the ducks in which the ureters had been ligated died of uremia after 12 to 24 hours, but, unfortunately, nothing was stated regarding possible deposition of urates.

The observation that complete obstruction of the excretion of uric acid results in a maximal—lethal—rise of the concentration of this metabolic waste product in

Table 28-1. Concentration of Uric Acid Observed[2] **in Various Tissues from Normal Ducks and Ducks with Ureters Ligated**

Condition	Tissue			
	Blood	Muscles	Kidneys	Liver
Normal	6.7	1.8	70.5	22.2
Ureters ligated	224.0	30.2	354.0	101.0

blood and organs is in keeping with the previously prevailing theory that gout is due to nephritis with an associated, greater or lesser impairment of function of the kidney and a consequent accumulation of uric acid in the blood.

Accordingly, the reflections concerning etiology of the condition have been concentrated particularly on the factors that might interfere with renal function. Exposure to cold and dampness, excessive protein consumption, vitamin A deficiency, intoxications, and certain infectious diseases have been mentioned as factors deserving particular attention. Bird *et al.*[1] found the offspring of poorly nourished parents to be particularly liable to the deposition of urates. They also claimed to have noticed a definitely preventive action of vitamin B_{12} in such cases. The problem, however, is not so simple as that. It is known from necropsy evidence that renal diseases may occur without associated gout, and that the opposite is also true. In other words, the renal disease may just as well be a consequence of gout as the cause of it.

I agree that the increased deposition of uric acid in the organism is largely responsible for the development of gout—whether the increase is due to impaired renal function or to surplus production of uric acid. However, conclusions cannot be drawn from the plasma level alone, because deposits are not found in either blood or lymph, not even in cases with the most extreme rises in uric acid in the plasma.

If, however, one looks at the sites at which deposits are found, it is seen that, except for the parenchymatous organs—liver and kidneys, they are all fluid-filled spaces where the fluid present is to be regarded as a dialysate of blood plasma to which has been added some substances, for example, albumin and globulin. Alterations of the solubility, electrolyte balance, and osmotic pressure of synovial fluid, for instance, in relation to the blood plasma cannot alone be responsible for the deposition. If they were, an equal deposition should be expected in all joints and tendon sheaths, and such has not been observed.

The disease often starts in one or a few joints. I have never seen the hip joint or shoulder joint affected. Variations of the environmental temperature—especially excessive cooling—to which a certain provocative importance has been attached, may, perhaps, merit consideration in the case of poultry. This is not true in the case of cage birds, which are generally kept in an environment with a fairly constant high temperature.

Whether the cell barrier—synovial capsule, tendon sheath, serous membrane, or connective tissue—may in any way influence the deposition of urates, or whether it plays a part in their passage, is an open question. The mild inflammatory reaction usually found in these tissues is in all likelihood a consequence of a purely mechanical irritation by the uric acid crystals.

A toxic effect, as occasionally suggested, is very unlikely, the toxicity of uric acid being so low that the substance can be introduced into the allantois, for instance, without damage to the fetus.

There is reason just to mention that the cerebrospinal fluid is not a dialysate of blood plasma but is a product secreted by the choroid plexus.

The results of reflecting on the foregoing facts are not encouraging. Exact knowledge of gout does not extend beyond demonstration of the deposited urates. It cannot even be said whether the deposits are harmful or whether they may constitute a defense measure taken by the organism, an attempt to stem a menacing rise of the level of uric acid in the plasma.

SIGNS AND SYMPTOMS

There are no diagnostic signs or symptoms typical of visceral gout. Failing appetite, changing moods, varying consistency of droppings, emaciation, and faintness are signs that are common to many diseases. The bird grows increasingly listless and feeble; it may suddenly be found dead on the floor of the cage, or it may waste away. If, however, the disease is combined with deposition of urates in joints and tendon sheaths, the diagnosis is no problem.

Birds suffering from articular gout are alert in the early stages of the disease and eat normally, seeming only to be somewhat restless. They change places frequently, and keep shifting from one leg to the other. The restlessness is particularly conspicuous just before the bird goes to roost. At a fairly early stage of illness the bird begins to have difficulty perching, becoming unsteady and swaying forward and backward on the perch. It prefers the thickest perches, or even the floor of the cage. This difficulty results from the bird's inability to grasp the perch properly, the foot remaining extended, with toes outstretched. The toes, and especially the tarsus, are rigid, swollen, warm, and tender. Within a short

Metabolic and Miscellaneous Conditions

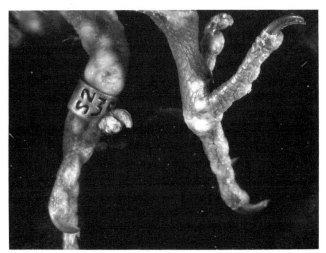

Fig. 28-2. *The feet of a budgerigar, showing multiple tophi. Note the tight-fitting metal band.*

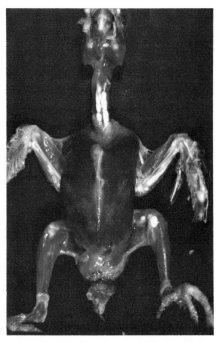

Fig. 28-3. *A budgerigar with the skin removed, showing urate deposits in the feet, knees, wrists, elbows, and ventral cervical region. Urate deposits were also present along the dorsum of the spine.*

time small rounded, light spots will be seen adjacent to one or more joints (Fig. 28-2). They increase rapidly in size, and project as hemispherical or padlike intumescences, each with a whitish yellow center surrounded by a faintly reddish hyperemic zone. In advanced cases, these bodies (tophi) become particularly prominent, partly because they become filled to the breaking point and partly because the surrounding swelling subsides, giving the rest of the foot an almost shriveled appearance.

In some instances the bird is no longer able to fly, and one wing—more rarely both—begins to droop. This is due to corresponding changes in the carpus and elbow. The tophi seem to have a special predilection for the peripheral articulations, the earliest signs nearly always occurring there. Next, the tarsus and heel become involved, rarely the knee, and never the hip joint. Concurrently, swelling is seen in adjoining tendon sheaths and tissues. In the wings, the phalanges and carpus, as well as the tendon sheaths of the forearm, are mainly involved, rarely the elbow joint, and never the shoulder joint. Deposits are found occasionally in cervical articulations and muscles (Fig. 28-3).

Gradually, as the disease progresses, the bird suffers increasing pain. It is evident that moving causes such distress that this more than anything else makes the owner decide to have the bird euthanatized. It is worth noting, however, that some birds remain remarkably unaffected by the disease, considering the size and extent of the deposits.

In the initial stages a mistaken diagnosis of plantar abscesses, infectious arthritis, or sprains may be made, owing to the tenderness of the legs; as soon as the white tophi become visible, however, the diagnosis should cause no difficulty. Demonstration of uric acid in a node

by the murexide test* is conclusive proof of the nature of the deposit.

PROGNOSIS

The chances of recovery from gout, whatever its site, are very small. The disease may run an extremely protracted course, extending over months, and it is often difficult to say with certainty whether a treatment instituted has any effect, because only the general condition can be influenced, not the deposition of urates that has already taken place.

THERAPY

Notwithstanding the poor prognosis, treatment should nearly always be attempted, at least for pet birds. The treatment to be considered is partly dietary, partly systemic drug therapy, and partly local treatment.

The sick bird should be kept at a fairly constant temperature and drafts must be avoided. The perches must be smooth, flat, broad, and of soft wood, and be placed at a low level because of the difficulty the bird

---

*A minute amount of material from an incised tophus is placed on a white porcelain surface with a drop of nitric acid and most carefully evaporated to dryness over a small free flame. When cool, the spot is touched with a drop of ammonia. Appearance of a reddish purple color is indicative of the presence of uric acid.

has in climbing. The food and water containers should also be placed within easy reach. The protein content of the food is to be lowered as much as possible. Concentrates, especially those of animal origin, are taboo. Low-protein seed mixtures should be provided, along with a rich supply of vegetables and fruit, supplemented by vitamin A. Vitamin B supplementation, on the other hand, is unlikely to have any effect in such cases—at least any curative effect.

For general treatment a great variety of drugs have been tried, most often sodium bicarbonate (0.5–2%) or lithium carbonate (1%). However, no unquestionable response to these has been noticed, at least not in budgerigars. The anti-gout drugs, colchicine and salicylic acid, so well known in human medicine, have been tried but were abandoned long ago, as doing more harm than good. Atophan (2-phenylquinoline-4-carboxylic acid), or cinchophen (N.F.), is recommended for budgerigars, 120 mg. once a day, and for fowl, 250 mg. twice daily.[3] In humans this drug has a palliative effect in acute cases, but not in chronic cases. This is probably due to the fact that the drug brings about an increased excretion of uric acid with a consequent fall of the level in the plasma, but it does not mobilize existing uric acid deposits. In birds suffering from articular gout presumably no more than arrest of the development can be expected at best, that is, that further deposits of uric acid in joints and tendon sheaths can be prevented. At the same time, however, the effect of the drug on the liver must be guarded against (compare the concept of cinchophen-provoked hepatitis in humans).

Corticosteroids are contraindicated because of the renal involvement.

Antibiotics, of which many different kinds have been tried, have had no effect. The indication for their use is, in fact, probably debatable.

Aspirin (acetylsalicylic acid) is given solely for its analgesic effect, since it has no curative properties. Dosage is 0.3 gm. (5 gr.) dissolved in 240 ml. (8 oz.) of water, given as drinking water or by means of a dropper.

For local treatment painting with undiluted tincture of iodine daily for 14 days has been recommended. Here, however, the question may be asked: Which is the more painful to the bird, the treatment or the illness?

Splitting and excochleation, followed by cauterization with a 1% solution of silver nitrate, may also be tried. However, it must be remembered that the wounds heal poorly, and that the deposition of urates will continue elsewhere.

No effective treatment for gout has yet been found. It is for the veterinarian to decide how long palliative treatment should be continued in the individual case.

NECROPSY FINDINGS

Visceral gout is evidenced by white to faintly grey plastery patches on the surface of the liver and on the pericardium. Such patches may also be found in several parts of the peritoneum, but deposits are never seen in the air sacs. Although the patches are found on the surfaces of the serous membranes only, they become adherent with surprising rapidity.

The kidneys are enlarged, swollen, and light in color. A distinct tubular marking is generally noticed, because the tubules are excessively filled with urates. Owing to the deposits, the ureters may sometimes appear as thick grey-white cords. In birds found at necropsy to have a scant deposit of urates in the kidneys alone, the possibility cannot be excluded that the material was deposited after death.

In joints and tendon sheaths the cavities are seen to be filled with thick whitish masses consisting of needle-shaped or amorphous urate crystals and desquamated epithelial cells undergoing fatty degeneration. The synovial membrane is swollen and red owing to hyperemia and scattered superficial inflammatory infiltrations. The great majority of lining cells are desquamated, and the surface is covered with a small amount of fibrin in which are embedded lumps of urate deposits. The cartilage is usually unchanged. The crystals always lie on the surfaces of the cartilage and synovial membrane, never in them. In advanced cases the synovial capsule and tendon sheath show fibrous thickening. Outside the synovial cavities the deposits may become quite large. The tophi are surrounded by mildly swollen, inflamed connective tissue. Spontaneous disruption may occur, both of the bodies in the synovial cavities and of the tophi. The resulting wounds show very little tendency to heal.

References

1. BIRD, H. R., RUBIN, M., WHITSON, D., and HAYNES, S. K.: Effectiveness of dietary supplements in increasing hatchability of eggs and viability of progeny of hens fed a diet containing a high level of soybean oil meal. Poultry Sci. *25*:285, 1946.

2. FOLIN, O., BERGLUND, H., and DERICK, C.: The uric acid problem. An experimental study on animals and man, including gouty subjects. J. Biol. Chem. *60*:361, 1924.

3. FRITZSCHE, K., and GERRIETS, E.: Geflügelkrankheiten. Berlin/Hamburg, Verlag Paul Parey, 1959.

4. GRAY, H.: The diseases of cage and aviary birds, with

some reference to those of furred and feathered game. Vet. Rec. *16:*343, 1936.

5. HASHOLT, J.: Fuglesygdomme. Aa. Poulsen: Prydfjerkæ, Skibby bogtrykkeri, 1959.

6. HASHOLT, J.: Current diseases of cage birds. J. small anim. Pract. *2:*97, 1961.

7. JUNGHERR, E., and POMEROY, B. S.: Avian Monocytosis (So-Called Pullet Disease), Infectious Nephrosis and Blue-comb Disease of Turkeys. In *Diseases of Poultry,* ed. 5, H. E. Biester and L. H. Schwarte, eds. Ames, Iowa State University Press, 1965. Pp. 844–862.

8. KEMNA, A.: Krankheiten der Stubenvögel. Minden, Philler Verlag. 1959.

9. LEVINE, R., WOLFSON, W. Q., and LENEL, R.: Concentration and transport of true urate in the plasma of the azotemic chicken. Am. J. Physiol. *151:*186, 1947.

10. NEWTON, L. G., and SIMMONS, G. C.: Avian nephritis and uraemia. Austral. Vet. J. *39:*135, 1963.

11. SHAW, P. A.: Duck disease studies. I. Blood analyses in diseased birds. Proc. Soc. Exper. Biol. Med. *27:*6, 1929; II. Feeding of single and mixed salts. *ibid.* *27:*120, 1929.

12. STURKIE, P. D.: The effects of age and reproductive state on plasma uric acid levels in chickens. Poultry Sci. *40:*1650, 1961.

13. SVENSSON, S.: Gikt hos höns. Skandinavisk Veterinär-Tidsskrift *27:*381, 1937.

Suggested Reading

APPLEBY, E. C.: Some observations on the dieases of finches and parrot-like birds kept in aviaries. Proc. B.S.A.V.A. Congress I. 19, 1958.

ARNALL, L.: Conditions of the beak and claw in the budgerigar. J. small anim. Pract. *6:*135, 1965.

BACHRACH, A.: Gout. In *Current Veterinary Therapy.* 1966–1967, R. W. Kirk, ed. Philadelphia, W. B. Saunders Company, 1966, Pp. 539–540.

BEACH, J. E.: Diseases of budgerigars and other cage birds. A survey of *post-mortem* findings. Vet. Rec. *74:*10, 63, 134, 1962.

BLOUNT, W. P.: *Diseases of Poultry.* London, Bailliere, Tindall & Cox, 1949.

COFFIN, D. L.: *Angell Memorial Parakeet and Parrot Book.* Winthrop-Stearns Inc., U.S.A., 1953.

COFFIN, D. L.: Diseases of Parrots. In *Parrots and Parrot-like Birds,* by Duke of Bedford, Fond du Lac, Wis., All-Pets Books, Inc., 1954.

FROST, C.: Experiences with pet budgerigars. Vet. Rec. *73:*621, 1961.

GEYER, S.: Klinische Erfahrungen bei Krankheiten der Stubenvögel. Tierärztl. Umsch. *14:*234, 1959.

GRATZL, E.: Gicht (Uricosis). In *Lexikon der prakt. Therapie und Prophylaxe für Tierärzte.* Wien, Urban-Schwarzenberger, 1948. Vol. 1, p. 357.

GRAY, E.: *Diseases of Poultry.* London, Crosby Lockwood and Son, Ltd., 1955.

GROTH, W.: Pathologisch-anatomische und histologische Be-
funde bei einigen Hühnerkrankheiten. Veteriñr-Medizinische Nachrichten *4:*205, 1961.

GRZIMEK, B.: *Krankes Geflügel,* 6th ed. Stuttgart/Berlin, Fritz Pfenningstorff, 1950.

HILBRICH, P.: *Krankheiten des Geflügels.* Schwenningen am Neckar, Verlag Hermann Kuhn, 1963.

KEYMER, I. F.: The diagnosis and treatment of common psittacine diseases. Mod. vet. pract. *39*(21):22, December 15, 1958.

KEYMER, I. F.: The diagnosis and treatment of some diseases of seed-eating passerine birds. Mod. vet. pract. *40*(7):30, April 1, 1959.

LESBOUYRIES, G.: *Pathologie des oiseaux de basse-cour.* Paris, Vigot Freres, 1965.

LINDT, S.: Beitrag zur Pathologie und Klinik der Stubenvögel (Volièrehaltung). Kleintier-Praxis *9:*4, 1964.

THE MERCK VETERINARY MANUAL: Merck and Co., Inc., U.S.A., 1955, p. 1157.

PLAZIKOWSKI, U.: *Boken om Burfåglar.* London/Stockholm/New York, S. E. Bergs Forlag, 1959.

REINHARDT, R.: *Lehrbuch der Geflügelkrankheiten.* Hannover, M.-H. Schaper, 1950.

TALBOTT, J. H., and TERPLAN, K. L.: The Kidney in Gout. In *Diseases of the Kidney,* M. B. Strauss and L. G. Welt, eds. Boston, Little, Brown and Company, 1963. Pp. 633–651.

WAILLY, P. de: L'amateur des oiseaux de cage et de volière. Paris, J.-B. Bailliere et fils, 1964.

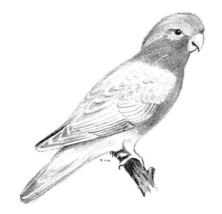

29

Poisoning and Other Casualties

Poisoning
Irving E. Altman

Wild Bird Casualties
Katharine Tottenham

Oil Pollution
Katharine Tottenham

POISONING

Very little information is available on poisoning of birds. Poisoning is usually accidental, being seen more often in birds that are permitted to fly free in the house, or in rooms and barns used as aviaries.

Losses in birds may be attributed to autointoxication or to poisoning by drugs, other chemicals, and foods. In isolated small birds, the diagnosis of poisoning is usually made too late to help the individual bird. In large flocks of birds, such diagnosis may permit preventive measures to be taken to avoid further trouble.

Self-poisoning, or autointoxication, is due to absorption of waste products of decomposition in the intestinal tract after injudicious feeding. Symptoms are loss of appetite, thirst, depression, weakness, and prostration.

Mouse and rat poisons are often the cause of poisoning in pet birds. Plain canary seed saturated with strychnine is commonly used for poisoning mice. Birds flying about a house in which this is used will find it and eat it. Strychnine is readily absorbed from the digestive tract and has a cumulative action. Clinical signs are tetanic spasms, paralysis, and respiratory failure, leading to death. Preventive measures are the only remedy.

Arsenic is also commonly used in mouse and rat baits. When such material is carelessly distributed around the home a bird may locate and eat it. Clinical signs and symptoms of arsenical poisoning are ruffled feathers, drooping of the wings, depressed appetite, regurgitation, and ataxia.

In homes where a good deal of smoking is done and butts are allowed to accumulate, birds may ingest tobacco and develop nicotine poisoning. If toxic quantities of tobacco are consumed, great depression is followed by prostration, and death occurs in a short time.

Carbon monoxide poisoning has been the cause of large losses. In one instance several thousand canaries were being transported by truck from ship to warehouse. On arrival at their destination, the birds in the center line of crates were all found dead. A leak from the exhaust had permitted carbon monoxide to enter the truck, and the center line of crates had received the greatest concentration of the gas. Some of the birds recovered when they were placed in fresh air. Necropsy showed very little pathologic change because of the suddenness of death. The lungs and blood of some of the birds whose death occurred later seemed to be cherry red in color.

In another case, a kindly owner put the cage of her pet bird on top of the gas range with only the pilot light on to keep the bird warm on cold winter nights. Apparently, enough gas escaped to cause the bird's death. After the loss of several birds and some investigation, the owner was advised not to put the cage on the gas range, and the losses ceased. Necropsy in these cases showed no macroscopic changes.

Arnall[1] reported the deaths of two budgerigars and one parrot occurring very soon after intramuscular injection of streptomycin. Many practitioners have had similar experiences after injection of procaine penicillin, the procaine being considered the cause of death.

According to Gray,[2] paints containing lead, arsenic, or zinc, because of their toxicity, should not be applied to cage or aviaries.

Alcoholic intoxication is not uncommon, especially in budgerigars. They very readily learn to sit on the rim of a beverage glass, and imbibe freely of the contents. Intoxication occurs frequently at parties where the pet bird is encouraged in the practice. Clinical symptoms are depression, the tendency to sit quietly with closed eyes, regurgitation, and loose droppings. Unconsciousness may result in severe cases. As with humans, time is the healer.

Some house plants may contain toxic principles, and care should be exercised when a bird is allowed freedom in their vicinity. The philodendron is a good example of such a toxic plant commonly found in the home.

Many other substances (*e.g.,* hydrocarbons, drugs, and other chemicals) may cause poisoning, but cases of poisoning caused by such agents are comparatively rare, and losses are insignificant.

WILD BIRD CASUALTIES

It must be realized that a wild bird that is damaged or weak enough to allow itself to be picked up by a human hand is likely to be very near death. This means that the mortality expectation is high, but prompt and speedy treatment followed by absolute quiet may save a number of such casualties.

Speed is necessary for much the same reason that in pre-anesthesia days doctors amputated a limb in a matter of seconds in order to diminish the effects of pain and shock. A wild bird can stand just so much handling, and no more.

Common sites of injury are the limbs; wings and legs are liable to fracture when a flying bird is hit by an automobile or strikes an overhead wire. Fractures near the shoulder joint are very difficult to cure, and in these cases it is often best to destroy the bird, unless it is of a species that will not be too handicapped by permanent pinioning and can live in a zoo enclosure. Obvious examples include wildfowl, pheasants, and other game birds, and waders (Fig. 29-1).

Contrary to the policy following other accidents, after an amputation a bird should be placed in the largest possible enclosure or aviary with an easily visible supply of water and appetizing food. If the bird is of a species

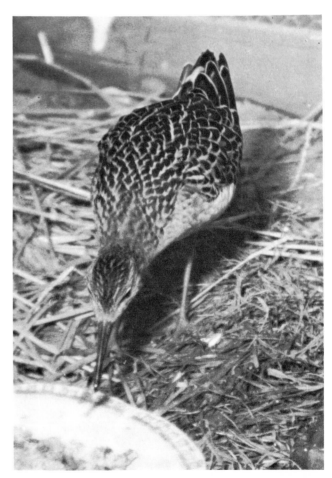

Fig. 29-1. *An adult ruff (Philomachus pugnax), a few days after amputation of complete wing, which had been fractured in two places.*

that will take it, live food is best. This partial freedom allows the bird to hide away while it orients itself to a flightless existence, and gives it the opportunity to feed and restore weight lost as a result of the accident or perhaps of a period of starvation that followed, if there was a lapse of time between the accident and discovery of the victim.

Not all wing fractures, however, are hopeless, and if the break is at a point where a splint can be used effectively healing may be suprisingly rapid. The main difficulty is one of weight; clearly, plaster bandages or wooden splints are unsuitable, as they would result in immobilization of the bird.

Birds other than passerine species will not be unduly crippled if a stiffened leg joint is unavoidable. Amputation, on the other hand, is not humanely justifiable for these biped animals.

Subluxation of the carpal joint is a frequent consequence of trauma that is sometimes mistaken for fracture of the wing. If the wing strikes against a hard object the primary feathers jolt the "wrist" and cause a sprain, which is then continually aggravated by the weight of the quills. When this happens the wing flails helplessly when the bird attempts to fly, and when the bird is at rest the flight feathers drag on the ground, giving the impression that the wing is broken.

Cure of this condition is very simple, as once the weight is removed recovery from the sprain is rapid. To achieve this the flight feathers are clipped off short with sharp scissors, avoiding the blood quills where they appear pink toward the root. No other treatment is necessary, and the major problem is keeping the bird fit and properly housed until the next molt, when the flight feathers will be renewed and it can fly once again.

The manner of housing convalescent wild birds depends on the species and the extent of the injuries. In general, passerine birds are best kept in a box cage of the type used for breeding budgerigars, or a large perching bird may be housed in a rabbit hutch. This cage design gives the bird a sense of security, and it is likely to accept captivity under these conditions until it is fit for release or transfer to an aviary.

Ground and water birds do not take kindly to cages and thrive better in an outdoor enclosure or a partitioned corner of an out-building. Shade and quiet are of great therapeutic value to injured or ailing birds, and if the condition is serious the bird will benefit from heat as well, which may be provided by using a hospital cage as described for nestling birds (see Chapter 8).

Food is of major importance because of the high rate of metabolism of birds. Most small birds show symptoms of starvation after only a few hours without food. If identity of the species is in doubt, then the provision of both seeds and live food is the best course.

The care of injured wild birds is enormously interesting but it is seldom a short-term undertaking, for unless the bird is truly fit to find its own living in the wild within a week or so after its capture it cannot be released until the late summer. This is because its territory will be lost and it will have no place to call its own until the breeding season ends, when both young and adult birds are on the move in the countryside and the presence of a stranger in their midst will not matter.

OIL POLLUTION

Most casualties among sea birds result from the effects of oil pollution, and there is more to their treatment than merely washing off the oil and returning the birds to the sea. Cleaning of the plumage, consideration of the weakness of the bird's heart, and provision of a balanced diet are, in that order, the major problems, and unless the bird can be cared for over a period of six months or even longer, it is generally kinder to destroy it at once. Almost inevitably, severe oiling and subsequent cleaning operations will destroy the delicate structure of the plumage, and the bird is unfit to return to its wild life until a molt has been completed (Fig. 29-2).

In a sea bird the down and the quills growing among it are interspersed with pockets of air, providing a pneumatic jacket with the dual purpose of retaining the body heat and providing buoyancy. The visible plumage spreads over this "under clothing," each feather preened and lacquered with preen oil to form a smooth but elastic surface which actively repels water.

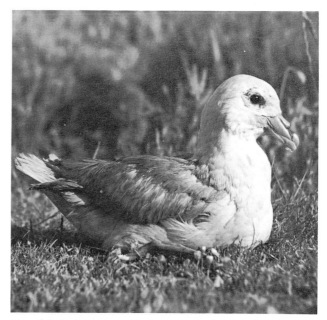

Fig. 29-2. *A fulmar* (Fulmarus glacialis), *showing the lacklustre plumage following severe fuel oil pollution cleaning.*

The cloying touch of fuel oil spoils this waterproof, buoyant insulation, allowing cold water to penetrate to the sensitive skin and releasing the air pockets that lace the plumules (down feathers). The result is disaster for the victim. A swan entirely divested of feathers can still float on water, but most other waterfowl and all sea birds depend on their plumage and perhaps the secretion of the preen gland for their buoyancy. If these mechanisms break down they are doomed to die, either by drowning or from exposure.

If a bird succeeds in coming ashore and survives the threat of respiratory tract infection due to chilling, it is still faced with further hazards. The most immediate one is heart failure, usually resulting from an aneurysm, evidently caused by the literally heart-bursting effort of struggling out of the sea on to dry land. It is not surprising then that a high proportion of the birds found washed up on the beach are already dead. Indeed, one is astonished that any of them manage to survive the ordeal of exposure to oil-polluted waters.

With a newly-arrived oiled bird the cleaning of the plumage should be delayed until it is warm, dry, and well fed. Wrapping in warm flannel or cotton wool will achieve the first, and as the bird generates heat within this cocoon, the feathers will steam and dry themselves.

Food for most sea birds means fish, of which sprats are the most popular. When these are out of season, small strips of herring or cod, cut lengthwise with the skin adhering to one side, prove satisfactory. To initiate the feeding response it is usually necessary to pry open the beak between forefinger and thumb, and to insert the fish as far as the back of the bird's tongue. Once food has been tasted and swallowed, most birds will take the next meal voluntarily. A vitamin–mineral mix may be added to the food.

Murres, razorbilled auks, puffins, petrels, shearwaters, gannets, and other diving birds seldom *learn* to feed from a dish and must be hand fed; gulls and ducks will not tame so easily but soon feed themselves, and for this reason are on the whole easier to manage.

The provision of water is often a serious problem because many oil victims show a horror of it for some time. However, a daily intake is essential for their well-being, and the kidneys will degenerate, causing death, if the bird refuses to drink. In stubborn cases the only answer is to feed with flaky white fish that has been soaked for several hours in a bowl of water and has absorbed enough for the bird's need. Salt water is unnecessary.

After 12 hours or so an oiled bird must be cleaned, and here one meets the major problem connected with the plumage. The tarry oil will have damaged the fine mesh of interlocking barbules that join the vanes of the polluted feathers, and it is all too easy to make matters worse in an attempt to clean the plumage with warm water and suds. Admittedly the bird will be clean after this treatment, but all the feathers will be damaged beyond repair; in a severe case this may not be of consequence, as the plumage must be molted out anyway, but when pollution is only minor it is a far from satisfactory method.*

Recently (1968) an oil solubilizer* has been used to remove oil from plumage with very good results.

The alternative is use of some form of "dry shampoo," a substance that is neutral and certainly not alkaline, and has a high absorption capacity. Fuller's earth is best for this purpose, as it can be dusted over the polluted feathers, left to act for a while, and then rinsed out with lukewarm water. Several applications may be necessary to clear badly polluted feathers.

Surgical spirit (isopropyl alcohol) may be used on the flight and tail feathers, but not on the plumage of the body, and all traces must be washed off before the bird has a chance to preen.

Fuel oil is actively poisonous to sea birds; respiratory tract infection, starvation, and heart failure are also causes of death, and these hazards are often increased by efforts to clean the plumage too soon. Birds that have swallowed fuel oil while attempting to preen may die from poisoning or as a result of blockage in the respiratory or digestive tract.

Once a sea bird has recovered from its first weakness it can be housed in an aviary or other enclosure where it can paddle in shallow water and enjoy sunshine and fresh air. On no account should such a bird be released into the sea until it has completely recovered; otherwise it will either drown or starve.

* An oil solubilizer (Polycomplex A-11, Ocean-Wide Marine Supply Co., Inc., P.O. Box 827, Huntington, N.Y. 11743) has recently (1968) been used to remove oil from plumage, with very good results.

References

1. ARNALL, L.: Experiences with cage-birds. Vet Rec. *70:*120–128, 1958.

2. GRAY, H.: The diseases of cage and aviary birds, with some reference to those of furred and feathered game. Vet. Rec. *16:*378–386, 1936.

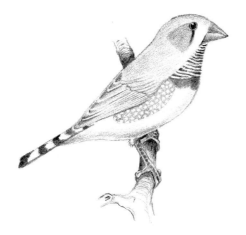

30

Bird-Borne Diseases in Man

Carlton M. Herman

In the development of knowledge of disease through research in recent times, particularly the knowledge of those diseases in which we have come to recognize microscopic organisms as the causative agents, we have become increasingly aware of a great number of such agents that have a wide host range. When man or his domesticated animals have shared as hosts of disease agents which also occur in wild animals, these diseases are classified as zoonoses. Research on such diseases forms an important segment of public health investigations. Control of such diseases in man requires not only an understanding of their transmissibility but also a knowledge of their occurrence and significance in the lower forms of animals, either as they affect the survival of these lower forms or as these lower forms may serve as sources of infection in man.

The list of diseases classified as zoonoses[12] is continually increasing, as more knowledge is gained on the biology and range of hosts of agents that are involved in human disease. Over 150 diseases of man are now classified as zoonoses, although in only a small number (less than one fourth of these) are birds involved.

VIRUS AND VIRUS-LIKE INFECTIONS

ORNITHOSIS

Perhaps the most significant bedsonial infection of birds transmissible to man is ornithosis (psittacosis). In this case birds serve as the primary reservoir of infection for man. A full discussion of this disease is presented in Chapter 24 of this book.

ENCEPHALITIDES

A group of arboviruses that cause diseases classified as encephalitides[9,10,12,13,15,16] occur in a wide range of vertebrate hosts, including birds. These diseases include mosquito-borne western, eastern, and Venezuelan equine encephalomyelitis, St. Louis, California, Japanese B, and Murray Valley encephalitis, and tick-borne Russian spring-summer encephalitis. These viral diseases are presumably transmitted from animals to man rather than from man to man. Man is usually considered an accidental host and, as such, plays no part in the essential biological cycle. These viruses, particularly those with "equine" in their designation, cause severe clinical disease in horses, as they often do in man. But here, too, the horse is considered an accidental host. Other animals are considered to be the source, there being no evidence of transmission from horse to horse.

Birds, even though they usually present no signs of disease when infected, are considered by many public health–oriented investigators as an essential link in the transmission cycle. Most diagnoses of infection in birds are based on the demonstration of antibodies in blood samples. Viremia, when disclosed, is usually of a low intensity and of short duration, often lasting less than a day. On occasion viremia of longer duration has been reported. Eastern equine encephalomyelitis virus has been shown to cause clinical manifestations and death in pheasants. Death in house sparrows (*Passer domesticus*) and ducks has been attributed to it. However, in view of the usual low-grade viremia in birds, my hypothesis is that birds, too, are usually accidental hosts, obtaining their infections from vertebrate sources other than birds. This is further supported by evidence that snakes manifest a substantial viremia for extended periods. Although it is suggested that the low-grade viremia usual in infected birds is generally insufficient to cause infection of potential mosquito vectors, just as the viremia in horse and man is insufficient to cause such infection, some investigators have demonstrated that infection may be transmitted by bird mites. Even though the infection is short-lived in the mites, the possibility exists that they may provide a mechanism for a bird-to-bird cycle.

An important facet of the encephalitides problem in birds, particularly among birds in captivity, is evidence that eastern equine encephalomyelitis virus can be transmitted from pheasant to pheasant by pecking.[9] It has been demonstrated by studies on captive flocks in New Jersey that, once infection is established in a flock, it can spread rapidly by this mechanical means.

Because of the usual short-lived low-grade viremia recognized in bird hosts, it is unlikely that migrating birds provide a mechanism for spread of the viral encephalitides. It is postulated that introduction of the disease into an aviary by new birds that are carriers is unlikely and that infection, should it occur, is more likely the result of mosquito transmission of an agent endemic in the area where the aviary is located. When feasible, screening of the quarters would greatly reduce this potential danger. Several times Venezuelan equine encephalomyelitis virus has caused infection in laboratory personnel working with the agent, and eastern equine encephalomyelitis virus has occurred among pheasant handlers as well as among persons investigating an outbreak of the disease. Although the greatest risk to handlers of infected birds is through the bite of infected mosquitoes, the possibility that the disease may be transmitted to man mechanically, as it is from pheasant to pheasant, should not be overlooked.

ROCKY MOUNTAIN SPOTTED FEVER

Recently antibodies of Rocky Mountain spotted fever have been reported from birds and bird ticks. Although as yet we cannot interpret the significance of this finding or say whether birds play a role in the natural biological cycle of this rickettsial disease, it is possible that birds and bird ticks spread this disease to other hosts and man. Ticks and other ectoparasites should be removed from newly acquired birds before they are placed in an aviary.

NEWCASTLE DISEASE

Newcastle disease is a viral infection frequently recognized in poultry.[12] Many avian species are susceptible, particularly pheasants. An Asiatic strain of the virus is most virulent, and exotic oriental pheasants are often carriers of the infection. Cases have been known to occur in handlers of infected birds, as well as in laboratory personnel working with the infectious agent.

In birds, pneumonic and neurologic symptoms dominate the clinical picture. In man, the most common symptom is an acute granular conjunctivitis. However, the infection is not always confined to the eyes, and a systemic syndrome of fever, chills, headache, and general malaise may be accompanied by mild leukopenia and relative lymphocytosis. Nasal and lacrimal secretions and saliva have been proved to be infectious. Recovery is usually complete in one or two weeks, without sequelae.

OTHER VIRAL DISEASES

Birds have been implicated as passive transmitters of at least two other viral diseases of domestic livestock. Circumstantial evidence has been presented on several occasions in Europe suggesting that migrating birds can carry the virus of foot-and-mouth disease of cattle, primarily by contamination of their feet with material containing the infective agent.[14]

The same mechanism has been suggested in implicating birds in the spread of transmissible gastroenteritis in pigs in midwestern United States. Evidence that birds may carry these viruses internally for extended periods is rather inconclusive. It is unlikely that birds in aviaries could become involved in the natural cycles of occurrence of either of these infections if good sanitation practices have been followed, even if free-living birds have access to the aviary.

BACTERIAL AND FUNGAL INFECTIONS

BACTERIAL DISEASES

Bacterial organisms classified as *Salmonella* constitute man's greatest health hazard evolving from birds. A variety of strains have been reported from birds, and some of them are the cause of extensive losses, the most important being *S. pullorum* in poultry (see Chapter 24). Many of these bacteria cause food poisoning in man. Infected eggs and meat products of poultry and other birds provide one of the chief sources of food poisoning in man. With the exception of poultry and other species of birds raised specifically for human food or food products, most birds in captive collections are of little concern in this regard, since they rarely end up on the dinner plates of man. However, the possibility of transfer to handlers exists if they do not avoid contamination of their own food with the feces of their charges.

Another common cause of food poisoning in man is the consumption of toxin from *Clostridium botulinum*. Several types of this organism are recognized. Type C, a common cause of extensive losses among wild waterfowl and other birds, occurs in poultry and other captive species. Type E is considered primarily of fish origin in cases of human infection, but birds are also susceptible.

The health hazard of *Salmonella* and botulism in aviaries is not that of man's becoming infected, but is rather the possibility of infection of the bird collection by feeding infective fish, meat, or egg products. A human carrier of *Salmonella* who serves as a food handler for birds can be just as great a hazard to the bird collection as a potential spreader of infection as the classical "typhoid Mary" was to the human population.

Several other bacterial diseases of man have been reported from birds,[12] or experimental exposure has shown birds to be susceptible. These include brucellosis, hemorrhagic septicemia, listerellosis, pseudotuberculosis, endemic relapsing fever, swine erysipelas, and tularemia, but in none of these are birds the primary source of infection. Avian tuberculosis,[6] frequently observed in both captive birds, such as poultry, and wild birds, has only rarely been authenticated as the cause of human infection. Suspected human cases should be fully and carefully studied to confirm and document existence of the avian type of tubercle bacilli of bird origin. The human type of tuberculosis has been reported from birds, particularly psittacines.

MYCOSES

One of the most widespread diseases of birds is the fungal disease aspergillosis. This disease is common in poultry, waterfowl, gulls, predatory birds, and penguins, and the list of hosts includes several species of passerine birds.[1] Although moldy food is often suggested as the source of infection, aspergillosis is a respiratory ailment contracted by inhalation. Although birds are not a source of infection to man, the same sources of contamination that produce the disease in birds might well cause infection in man. The *Aspergillus* organisms are ubiquitous. Most mycologists consider aspergillosis as a secondary infection in man,[8] since most cases are recognized only in conjunction with or following other lung or systemic ailments.

Much attention has been focused in recent years on the role of birds in certain other fungal infections of man, particularly histoplasmosis. The fungus which is the etiologic agent of this disease[3,4,5] grows well in bird droppings, and concentrations of bird feces at roosting sites have been implicated in outbreaks of the disease, particularly in children. However, the likelihood of this occurring in aviaries or among caged birds is rather slight.

PARASITIC DISEASES

The animal parasites of birds are not considered of much importance as a menace to the health of man. *Toxoplasma gondii,* the causative agent of toxoplasmosis in man and other mammals, has been reported from pigeons and chickens, but there is no epizootiological evidence that they are involved in a natural cycle to man. A parasite with some morphological similarities occurs widely in bird hosts and was thought to be a *Toxoplasma* but has more recently been shown to be an entirely different genus, *Lankesterella,* which has not been reported from man. *Sarcocystis,* a sporozoan parasite occasionally reported from man, is very common as a parasite of waterfowl and other birds. Some investigators have claimed that birds are a source of the human infection, but the morphology of the parasite described from man is sufficiently different from that of the forms observed in birds to rule out this possibility. When one considers the frequency of occurrence of this parasite in waterfowl, certainly many more cases would be reported in man if this were a source of human infection.

Schistosome blood flukes occur frequently in birds. One stage of the life cycle of these worms occurs in snails, from which they escape as free-swimming forms. They infect the vertebrate host by penetrating the skin, and are most prevalent in water birds. Man also can become infected.[2] The worms often infect swimmers in infested waters. Although they penetrate the skin of man, they are unable to complete their life cycle in man and they die in the skin. In some people they set up a severe itching, variously called "swimmer's itch," "clam-digger's itch," or another term appropriate to the situation. In some areas where water birds are kept in semi-natural conditions, a snail population could exist to provide a potential source for human infection.

Occasionally other parasites of birds have been reported from man. When found, they can be identified readily by competent taxonomists and usually are of interest mainly because of their rarity.

Bird mites, on occasion, will infest man and cause a severe dermatitis.[11] Lice of the order Mallophaga are often abundant on some species of birds and frequently crawl onto bird handlers. They do not establish themselves on the human hosts, for the food necessary for their existence does not occur on man. However, there have been cases where man develops a phobia with itching and other concurrent symptoms, with inflammation brought on by the scratching by the subject rather than biting by the arthropod.

With some species of birds, particularly swallows, large colonies of Cimicidae develop in the nesting material. These "bedbugs" often leave the nest after the young birds have fledged and migrate to adjacent quarters to feed on man.

ALLERGIES

Perhaps the least understood of public health hazards of birds is their relationship to allergic reactions in man. Many people have been shown to have severe allergic reactions with asthmatic attacks caused by contact with feathers. Usually removal of the contact alleviates the condition. Pigeon and budgerigar breeders or fanciers may develop a pulmonary disease which resembles farmer's lung[7] and which affects the peripheral gas-exchanging tissues. The disease is caused by inhalation of the antigens in the avian excreta.

When an allergic reaction is suspected in bird handlers, care should be taken to rule out mite dermatitis and histoplasmosis.

METHODS OF DIAGNOSIS

Methods of diagnosis have deliberately been left out of the brief discussion of the conditions mentioned in this Chapter. Some have been covered elsewhere in the book, and practitioners are urged to consult standard textbooks of diagnosis where full coverage is more appropriate. The practitioner should always strive to guide the bird keeper toward good housekeeping procedures, particularly sanitation, as the best preventive measure in avoiding transfer of disease from his charges to himself.

References

1. CHUTE, H. L., O'MEARA, D. C., and BARDEN, E. S.: *A Bibliography of Avian Mycosis.* Misc. Publ. 655, Maine Agric. Expt. Sta., 1962. 120 pp.

2. CORT, W. W.: Studies on schistosome dermatitis. XI. Status of knowledge after more than twenty years. Am. J. Hyg. *52:*251–307, 1950.

3. D'ALESSIO, D. J., HEEREN, R. H., HENDRICKS, S. L., OGILVIE, P., and FURCOLOW, M. L.: A starling roost as the source of urban epidemic histoplasmosis in an area of low incidence. Am. Rev. Resp. Dis. *92:*725–731, 1965.

4. DODGE, H. J., AJELLO, L., and ENGELKE, O. K.: The association of a bird-roosting site with infection of school children by *Histoplasma capsulatum.* Am. J. Publ. Health *55:*1203–1211, 1965.

5. EMMONS, C. W.: Histoplasmosis. Animal reservoirs and other sources in nature of the pathogenic fungus, *Histoplasma.* Am. J. Publ. Health *40:*436–440, 1950.

6. FELDMAN, W. H.: *Avian Tuberculosis Infections.* Baltimore, Williams & Wilkins Co., 1938. 483 pp.

7. HARGREAVE, F. E., PEPYS, J., LONGBOTTOM, J. L., and WRAITH, D. G.: Bird breeder's (fancier's) lung. Lancet *1:*445–449, 1966.

8. HEFFERNAN, A. G. A., and ASPER, S. P., Jr.: Insidious fungal disease. A clinicopathological study of sec-

ondary aspergillosis. Bull. Johns Hopkins Hosp. *118:*10–26, 1966.

9. HERMAN, C. M.: The role of birds in the epizootiology of eastern encephalitis. Auk *79:*99–103, 1962.

10. HERMAN, C. M.: Birds and Our Health. In *Birds in Our Lives,* Washington, D.C., U.S. Government Printing Office, 1966. Pp. 284–291.

11. HERMS, W. B., and JAMES, M. T.: *Medical Entomology.* New York, Macmillan, 1961. 616 pp.

12. HULL, T. G., ed.: *Diseases Transmitted from Animals to Man,* 4th ed. Springfield, Ill., Charles C Thomas, 1955. 717 pp.

13. LOCKE, L. N., SCANLON, J. E., BYRNE, R. J., and KNIS-LEY, J. O., Jr.: Occurrence of eastern encephalitis virus in house sparrows. Wilson Bull. *74:*263–266, 1962.

14. McDIARMID, A.: *Diseases of Free-Living Wild Animals.* FAO Agricultural Studies No. 57. Rome, Food and Agriculture Organization of the United Nations, 1962. 119 pp.

15. REEVES, W. C.: The encephalitis problem in the United States. Am. J. Publ. Health *41:*678–686, 1951.

16. STAMM, D. D.: Relationships of birds and arboviruses. Auk *83:*84–97, 1966.

17. SCHWABE, C. W.: *Veterinary Medicine and Human Health.* Baltimore, Williams & Wilkins Co., 1964. 516 pp.

Index

Folio numbers in *italics* refer to illustrations; f following a folio number refers to a footnote, and t following folio number refers to a table.